Electron Spin
Double Resonance Spectroscopy

Electron Spin Double Resonance Spectroscopy

LARRY KEVAN

DEPARTMENT OF CHEMISTRY
WAYNE STATE UNIVERSITY
DETROIT, MICHIGAN

LOWELL D. KISPERT

DEPARTMENT OF CHEMISTRY
THE UNIVERSITY OF ALABAMA
TUSCALOOSA, ALABAMA

A WILEY-INTERSCIENCE PUBLICATION

JOHN WILEY & SONS

New York • London • Sydney • Toronto

Copyright © 1976 by John Wiley & Sons, Inc.

All rights reserved. Published simultaneously in Canada.

No part of this book may be reproduced by any means, nor transmitted, nor translated into a machine language without the written permission of the publisher.

Library of Congress Cataloging in Publication Data:
Kevan, Larry.
    Electron spin double resonance spectroscopy.

    "A Wiley-Interscience publication."
    Includes bibliographical references and index.
    1. Electron paramagnetic resonance spectroscopy.
I. Kispert, Lowell D., 1940–   joint author.
II. Title.

QD96.E4K48   543'.085   75-44418
ISBN 0-471-47340-5

Printed in the United States of America

10 9 8 7 6 5 4 3 2 1

Preface

During the past few years the electron magnetic double resonance techniques of electron nuclear double resonance (ENDOR) and electron-electron double resonance (ELDOR) have been increasingly used in structural determination of free radicals and in studying the interaction of radicals with their environment. The motivation has been not only to improve spectral resolution over ordinary ESR but also to develop a broader array of techniques sensitive to molecular and radical motion and to weak interactions of radicals with their matrix or solvent. One expanding frontier in magnetic resonance is to obtain more incisive information about radicals in disordered solid or viscous systems as often found in biological macromolecules. ENDOR and ELDOR show considerable promise in this area.

As these techniques are now relatively well understood by magnetic resonance experts, it seemed appropriate to write a book that could introduce the nonresonance expert to these important electron double resonance techniques. In this book we use a minimal amount of formal mathematical and quantum mechanical treatment of the subject. We include many figures in Chapter 1 to demonstrate the concepts that are essential to the understanding of ENDOR and ELDOR. In Chapter 2 we review the experimental techniques involved and discuss the operation of commercial spectrometers in terms of fundamental principles. Chapters 3 and 4 present numerous examples in liquid and solid phase ENDOR, amplifying the concepts discussed in Chapter 1. The interpretation of *matrix* ENDOR in disordered solids is discussed in some detail. A comprehensive set of tables summarize the ENDOR literature through 1974. Chapters 5 and 6 contain a similar discussion pertaining to liquid and solid phase ELDOR, with a review of the ELDOR literature through 1974. Chapter 7 is devoted to biochemical applications of ENDOR and ELDOR. The description of the approach to be taken in determining the structural parameters of biological radicals should prove useful for future biological applications, especially in disordered systems. In addition, stress is placed on the environmental and motional information about the active or paramagnetic site in biological systems that can be obtained.

We thank a number of our colleagues: Mike Bowman, Kichoon Chang, Stan Clough, Jim Hyde, Ichiro Miyagawa, D. P. Lin, Harold Moore, Carolyn Mottley, P. A. Narayana, and Shula Schlick for their helpful criticism of various chapters of the manuscript. Bob Sneed was especially helpful in obtaining figures of the ENDOR and ELDOR spectrometers. We also are grateful to Agnes Wirtz for her careful job in preparing the figures and to Maureen Murphy, Sue London, and the secretarial staff at the University of Alabama for typing the manuscript.

LARRY KEVAN
LOWELL D. KISPERT

Detroit, Michigan
Tuscaloosa, Alabama
March 1976

Contents

1. ESR and Double Resonance — 1
2. Experimental Methods — 58
3. Liquid Phase ENDOR — 95
4. ENDOR in Solids — 165
5. Liquid Phase ELDOR — 254
6. Single Crystal and Powder ELDOR — 303
7. Biochemical Applications — 388

Index — 415

Electron Spin
Double Resonance Spectroscopy

1. ESR and Double Resonance

1.1 Introduction
1.2 Magnetic Relaxation
1.3 Types of Double Resonance
1.4 ENDOR
    1.4.1 Energy Levels
    1.4.2 ENDOR Mechanisms
        1.4.2.1 ΔT_{1e} Mechanism—Transient ENDOR
        1.4.2.2 ΔT_{1e} Mechanism—Steady State ENDOR
        1.4.2.3 Packet-Shifting Mechanism
        1.4.2.4 Distant ENDOR or Depolarization Mechanism
        1.4.2.5 Lineshift Mechanism
    1.4.3 Enhancement of rf Field at Nucleus
    1.4.4 Sign of ENDOR Response
        1.4.4.1 Absorption Signals
        1.4.4.2 Dispersion Signals
    1.4.5 ENDOR Resolution
        1.4.5.1 Resolution in Liquids
        1.4.5.2 Resolution in Solids
1.5 ELDOR
    1.5.1 Energy Levels
    1.5.2 ELDOR Mechanisms
        1.5.2.1 Transient ELDOR
        1.5.2.2 Steady State ELDOR
    1.5.3 Spin Packet Model of Linewidths
    1.5.4 Modulation Frequency Dependence
    1.5.5 ELDOR Resolution
        1.5.5.1 Resolution in Liquids
        1.5.5.2 Resolution in Solids
References

2 ESR AND DOUBLE RESONANCE

1.1 INTRODUCTION

Electron spin resonance (ESR) is a powerful tool for the study of free radicals and triplet states in chemistry. ESR is particularly useful because of its high specificity for detection, identification, and monitoring of reactive paramagnetic intermediates in chemical and biochemical reactions. This phenomenon is simply magnetic resonance spectroscopy between unpaired electron energy levels. The interaction of an unpaired electron with magnetic nuclei introduces hyperfine interaction that greatly increases the number of magnetic energy levels between which transitions may occur. A fundamental limitation of ESR, as with any spectroscopic technique, is its resolution. Electron magnetic double resonance methods are becoming of increasing importance because they can increase the effective resolution of ESR spectra. Modern instrumentation is making electron magnetic double resonance methods increasingly available to a variety of chemists and biochemists for application to their particular problems. In addition, since double resonance depends on relaxation between magnetic energy levels, these methods are proving useful for studying magnetic relaxation mechanisms and magnetic energy transfer. Because of double resonance techniques, we may expect that magnetic relaxation will become an increasingly important parameter in characterizing and studying free radicals.

In this book we examine electron magnetic double resonance techniques. These techniques will be described in a simple theoretical fashion with emphasis on how to obtain and analyze actual double resonance spectra. Applications to radicals in solution and in disordered solids are stressed as well as applications to radicals in single crystals.

1.2 MAGNETIC RELAXATION

First, let us consider the ESR phenomenon itself. An unpaired electron is characterized by a spin vector $\mathbf{S}$, which gives the value of the spin angular momentum vector $\hbar\mathbf{S}$. The magnetic moment of the electron is proportional to $\hbar\mathbf{S}$ and is given by

$$\boldsymbol{\mu}_e = -\gamma\hbar\mathbf{S} = -g\beta\mathbf{S} \tag{1.1}$$

where γ is a constant called the magnetogyric ratio of the electron and equals 1.76×10^7 rad sec^{-1} G^{-1}, g is a dimensionless constant called the electron g factor, which equals 2.0023 for a free electron and is about 2.0 for most organic free radicals, and $\beta = |e|\hbar/2mc = 0.927 \times 10^{-20}$ erg G^{-1} and is termed the *electronic Bohr magneton*. The g and γ are simply proportionality constants in different units between the spin angular momentum and the magnetic moment of an electron.

A magnetic moment implies interation with a magnetic field **H**; the interaction energy is represented by

$$E = -\boldsymbol{\mu}_e \cdot \mathbf{H} = g\beta \mathbf{S} \cdot \mathbf{H} \tag{1.2}$$

If we define the magnetic field direction to be the z direction and recall that m_s is the symbol for the z component of the spin vector, we have

$$E = g\beta H m_s \tag{1.3}$$

For electrons $\mathbf{S} = \frac{1}{2}$ and m_s has the two values $\pm\frac{1}{2}$. The two energy states are shown in Fig. 1-1; the lower state has spin down ($m_s = -\frac{1}{2}$) and the

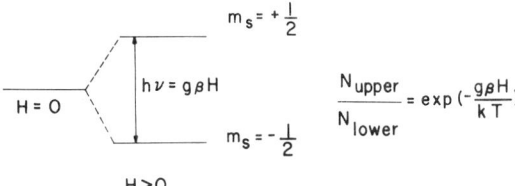

Figure 1-1. Simple ESR energy level diagram where H is the magnetic field. The ratio of the number of spins in the upper and lower levels is given by the Boltzmann factor.

spin is antiparallel to the applied magnetic field. For a fixed magnetic field, transitions between the two energy states can be induced by an oscillating magnetic field perpendicular to H of frequency $\nu = g\beta H/h$. Such transitions constitute magnetic resonance.

The energy between the magnetic energy levels at 3000 G, $g\beta H$, is only 10^{-3} of kT at 300 K. At thermal equilibrium the Boltzmann factor, $\exp(-g\beta H/kT)$, gives the population ratio of the two levels so the levels are almost, but significantly not, equally populated. The application of microwave energy in the proper orientation (microwave magnetic field perpendicular to the static magnetic field) causes transitions between the magnetic levels. The microwave field stimulates transitions in both directions with a rate that depends on the microwave power and on the number of spins in each level. Transitions from the lower to upper levels absorb energy whereas upper to lower level transitions emit energy. Since the population is slightly greater in the lower level, there will be a net absorption of microwave energy; this provides the observed ESR signal. Under steady application of the microwave field with no other interactions the populations in the magnetic energy levels would soon become equal; there would then be no net absorption of microwave energy and no ESR signal.

4   ESR AND DOUBLE RESONANCE

However the spin system is subject to other interactions, the very interactions that bring about thermal equilibrium, which can collectively be called spin-lattice interactions. They comprise radiationless interactions between the spin system and the thermal motion of the "lattice" or surroundings. The rate of such transitions between two electron spin energy levels is symbolized by W_e. The inverse of the total rate of spin-lattice-induced transitions is described by a characteristic time called the spin-lattice relaxation time and is denoted by the symbol T_{1e}.

At sufficiently low microwave powers the spin-lattice relaxation processes are fast enough to maintain a thermal equilibrium population between the magnetic energy levels. As the microwave power is increased, the net upward rate of microwave-induced spin transitions from the lower to upper states is increased and eventually competes with the spin-lattice-induced net downward rate. The spin populations in the two magnetic states become more equal and the ESR signal intensity decreases; this is known as power saturation.

In addition to spin-lattice relaxation in which energy is transferred from the spin system to the lattice, there exist spin-spin relaxation mechanisms in which energy is redistributed within the spin system. One may think of this redistribution as a modulation of the spin energy levels. In both fluid and solid phases the net local magnetic fields are rapidly varying because of different types of molecular motion, and a given electron spin energy level at $m_s g \beta H$ is therefore modulated. At high spin concentrations direct spin-spin exchange and dipolar interaction can also occur. The characteristic time for spin-spin relaxation within a single spin system is symbolized by T_{2e}.

In double resonance we will also be concerned with nuclear spin systems. The same principles apply. The rate of spin-lattice-induced transitions between two nuclear spin energy levels is symbolized by W_n and the analogous relaxation times are denoted by T_{1n} and T_{2n}.

In a single spin system, either electron or nuclear, the spin-lattice, T_1, and spin-spin, T_2, relaxation times can be given a precise classical and quantum mechanical description. A collection of spins has a magnetic moment vector **M** that can be resolved into three components, M_x, M_y, and M_z. Before a magnetic field is applied the number of spins in the two magnetic energy states for $S = \frac{1}{2}$ is equal; after the field is applied some of the spins begin flipping to achieve a thermal equilibrium distribution between the two states. For an applied magnetic field in the z direction the spin flips cause M_z to change toward a steady value M_o, which is proportional to the measured static magnetic susceptibility. M_z approaches M_o with a time constant T_1 such that $M_z = (1/e)M_o = 63\% M_o$ in time T_1. To observe resonance the microwave magnetic field H_1 is applied perpendicular to the external field H_z. If the intensity of H_1 is increased greatly with a pulse of microwaves, the spin system saturates. This means the populations in the upper and lower spin states are equalized, $M_z = 0$, and the resonance absorption disappears. After the pulse the recovery of M_z toward M_o with a time constant T_1 can be observed by the growth of the resonance line. T_1 is also called the longitudinal relaxation time because it refers to relaxation along the magnetic field axis.

The M_x and M_y components of **M** are zero in the absence of H_1. Application of H_1 in the xy plane rotates M_z and produces finite M_x or M_y components. When H_1 is removed, the M_x or M_y components decay by 63% in time T_2. T_2 is also called the transverse relaxation time because it refers to relaxation of magnetization components transverse to the external magnetic field.

1.3 TYPES OF DOUBLE RESONANCE

To understand what electron nuclear double resonance (ENDOR) and electron-electron double resonance (ELDOR) transitions are, let us consider the energy levels of a system containing one unpaired electron ($\mathbf{S} = \frac{1}{2}$) and one nuclear spin ($\mathbf{I} = \frac{1}{2}$) such as a hydrogen atom. Since the electron spin and nuclear spin can each be oriented up or down with respect to the external magnetic field, there are four possible energy levels, as shown in Fig. 1-2. The two electron spin eigenfunctions are denoted by α_e and β_e, whereas the two nuclear spin wavefunctions are denoted by α_n and β_n. An important selection rule in electron spin resonance is that the electron spin flips but the nuclear spin does not flip in an ESR transition to first

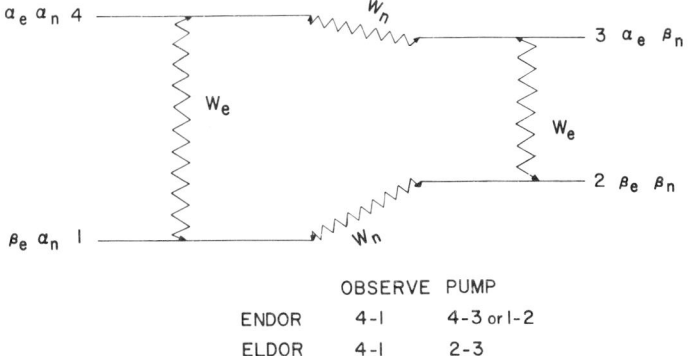

Figure 1-2. Energy level diagram for $\mathbf{S} = \frac{1}{2}$, $\mathbf{I} = \frac{1}{2}$ system showing the observed and pumped transitions that correspond to ENDOR and ELDOR. W_e and W_n refer to the electronic and nuclear relaxation rates.

6 ESR AND DOUBLE RESONANCE

order. Thus in Fig. 1-2 an ESR transition will occur between energy levels 1 and 4 and a second ESR transition will occur between energy levels 2 and 3. Let us focus attention on the observation of the ESR transition between energy levels 1 and 4. The intensity of this transition will depend on the population difference between these two energy levels. If one then applies a nuclear frequency to the system, which corresponds to either the energy difference between levels 4 and 3 or the energy difference between levels 2 and 1, one will induce nuclear spin flips that will change the populations in energy levels 4 or 1, respectively. This will in turn change the intensity of the observed ESR signal, and this change in intensity is called an ENDOR response. Note that there is a common energy level between the observed ESR transition and the pumped nuclear magnetic resonance (NMR) transition.

In ELDOR one uses two different microwave frequencies rather than one microwave frequency and one radiofrequency as in ENDOR. Essentially in ELDOR one ESR transition is observed while another ESR transition is pumped with the second microwave frequency. For example, in Fig. 1-2 the 4–1 transition may be observed and the 2–3 transition may be pumped. If the pumping of the 2–3 transition causes a change in the spin population in levels 1 or 4, then the observed ESR signal intensity will change. This constitutes an ELDOR response. Note that there are no common energy levels between the observed transition and the pumped transition in ELDOR. The population changes that do occur are carried by spontaneous nuclear spin-flips.

In both ENDOR and ELDOR a change in the intensity of an ESR signal is observed as a second frequency is applied to the system. It is easily seen that this will allow new hyperfine information to be obtained by using double resonance as well as allowing detailed study of the various magnetic relaxation processes themselves.

1.4 ENDOR

1.4.1 Energy Levels

In order to show what magnetic parameters are measured by ENDOR let us first consider the energy levels for a $S=\frac{1}{2}$, $I=\frac{1}{2}$ system as given by the following spin Hamiltonian where g_n is a dimensionless nuclear

$$H = g\beta \mathbf{H} \cdot \mathbf{S} - g_n \beta_n \mathbf{H} \cdot \mathbf{I} + hA\mathbf{S} \cdot \mathbf{I} \qquad (1.4)$$

g factor, β_n is the nuclear magneton that equals 5.05×10^{-24} erg G^{-1}, and A is an isotropic hyperfine coupling in hertz. Note that g_n and A may be positive or negative. Here we have assumed that g and A are isotropic scalars as would be the case for a radical in solution. We shall consider the anisotropic case in Chapter 4 on ENDOR of radicals in solids. The first term is the electronic Zeeman interaction and is typically much larger than the nuclear Zeeman and hyperfine interactions for magnetic fields greater than 3000 G. We can then use the strong field approximation in which **H** is taken as the z direction and m_s and m_I are valid quantum numbers. This approximation ignores second order hyperfine terms of order $h^2A^2/g\beta H$. The energy levels in hertz are then given by

$$\frac{E}{h}(m_s, m_I) = \frac{g\beta H m_s}{h} - \frac{g_n\beta_n H m_I}{h} + Am_sm_I = \nu_e m_s - \nu_n m_I + Am_sm_I \quad (1.5a)$$

where

$$\nu_n = \frac{g_n\beta_n H}{h}$$

Figures 1-3 and 1-4 show the energy levels for $A < 0$ and the two cases $\nu_n > |A|/2$ and $\nu_n < |A|/2$, respectively. We must use the absolute value of

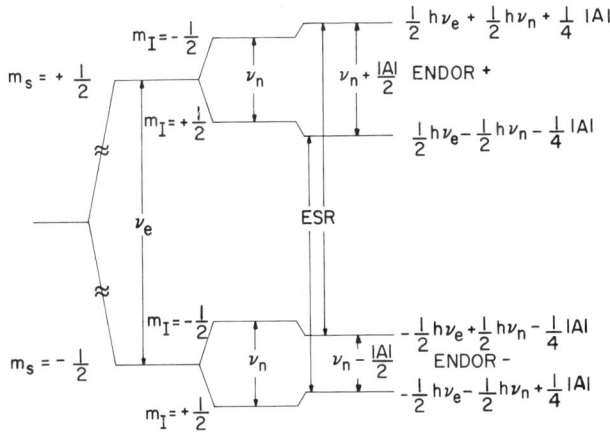

Figure 1-3. Energy levels (Hz) for $S = \frac{1}{2}$ and $I = \frac{1}{2}$ system: $\nu_n = (g_n\beta_nH)/h > |A|/2$ and $A < 0$, $g_n > 0$.

the coupling constant since the frequency is taken to be positive. $A < 0$ is typical for aromatic organic radicals. Note that the ordering of the energy levels depends on the sign of A and on the relative magnitudes of ν_n and $|A|/2$. In later figures (see Fig. 1-6) we will often use $A > 0$, and the energy level order will change accordingly. For reference, values of ν_n at 9.5 and 35 GHz are given in Table 1-1 for common nuclei. In both Figs.

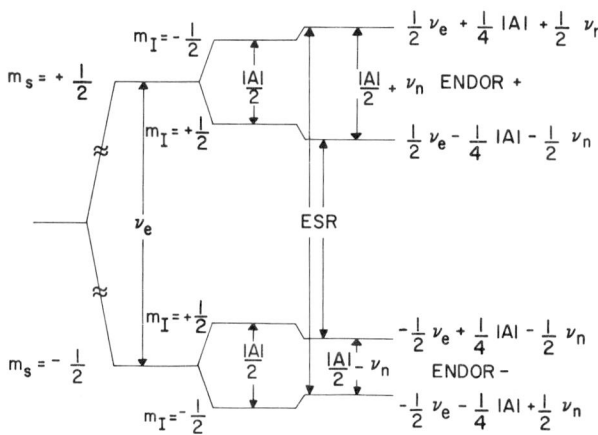

Figure 1-4. Energy levels (Hz) for $S=\frac{1}{2}$ and $I=\frac{1}{2}$ system: $|A|/2 > \nu_n = (g_n\beta_n H)/h$ and $A<0$, $g_n>0$.

1-3 and 1-4 the ESR transitions are governed by the selection rules $\Delta m_s = \pm 1$, $\Delta m_I = 0$, and are identical.

$$\Delta E(\text{ESR}) = \nu_e \pm \frac{|A|}{2} \qquad (1.5b)$$

It is for this reason that the nuclear Zeeman interaction is usually left out of the spin Hamiltonian for radicals in solution; it subtracts out for all allowed ESR transitions. However, the ENDOR transitions given by $\Delta m_I = \pm 1$ depend on the nuclear Zeeman interaction. ENDOR spectra are shown in Fig. 1-5. For $\nu_n > |A|/2$ (Fig. 1-3), as is common for proton ENDOR, the two ENDOR transitions are given by $\nu_n \pm |A|/2$. Two ENDOR lines are observed separated by $|A|$ and centered at ν_n. Note that the same two ENDOR transitions are observed when *either* ESR line is monitored and in both cases the ENDOR lines are split by exactly $|A|$. However, since ν_n depends on H, there will be a shift in the center of the spectrum as different ESR lines are monitored by sweeping the magnetic field. For $\nu_n < |A|/2$ (Fig. 1-4) the two ENDOR transitions are given by $|A|/2 \pm \nu_n$. Two lines are observed separated by $2\nu_n$ and centered at $|A|/2$. The same two ENDOR transitions are observed when either ESR line is monitored, but their separation differs slightly since ν_n depends on H. If $|A|/2 = \nu_n$, then only one ENDOR line will be observed at $\nu_n + |A|/2$. In general, the ENDOR frequencies in solution are given by eq. 1.6:

$$\nu_\pm = \left| \nu_n \pm \frac{A}{2} \right| \qquad (1.6)$$

Table 1-1. Nuclear Frequencies for Common Nuclei at 9.5 GHz (3390 G) and 35 GHz (12,488 G) ESR Frequencies

Nucleus	ν_n at 9.5 GHz (3390 G)	ν_n at 35 GHz (12,488 G)
^{1}H	14.4 MHz	53.2 MHz
^{2}H	2.22	8.16
^{7}Li	5.61	20.7
^{11}B	4.63	17.1
^{13}C	3.63	13.4
^{14}N	1.04	3.83
^{15}N	1.46	5.39
^{19}F	13.6	50.0
^{23}Na	3.82	14.1
^{27}Al	3.76	13.9
^{29}Si	2.87	10.6
^{31}P	5.84	21.5
^{35}Cl	1.41	5.21
^{37}Cl	1.18	4.34
^{39}K	0.67	2.48
^{41}K	0.37	1.36
^{51}V	3.97	14.0
^{55}Mn	3.58	13.2
^{57}Fe	0.47	1.72
^{59}Co	3.42	12.6
^{63}Cu	3.83	14.1
^{65}Cu	4.10	15.1
^{79}Br	3.62	13.3
^{91}Br	3.90	14.4
^{85}Rb	1.39	5.13
^{87}Rb	4.72	17.4
^{127}I	2.89	10.6
^{133}Cs	1.89	6.97

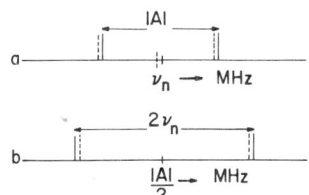

Figure 1-5. ENDOR spectra for (a) $\nu_n > |A|/2$ and (b) $\nu_n < |A|/2$. In both cases the solid lines give the spectrum observed when the high field ESR line is monitored and the dashed lines give the spectrum observed when the low field ESR line is monitored. The absolute value of the hyperfine constant must be used because the nuclear frequency is always taken as positive.

10 ESR AND DOUBLE RESONANCE

From Fig. 1-5 is seen that both $|A|$ and ν_n can be determined from the ENDOR spectrum. Since $\nu_n = |g_n|\beta_n H/h$ we see that $|g_n|$ is determined. The hyperfine interaction $|A|$ can sometimes be determined from the ESR spectrum in solution; however, we will see in Section 1.4.3 that ENDOR offers much improved resolution and accuracy for obtaining $|A|$. The nuclear g factor can only be determined from the ENDOR spectrum, and since g_n is known for all ordinary nuclei, one can unambiguously identify the nucleus that gives rise to the hyperfine interaction. This is particularly important in solids where unknown paramagnetic impurities are more likely to be present. Note that only the absolute values of $|A|$ and $|g_n|$ are determined directly by experiment. In special cases the signs of these quantities can be determined; examples are given in Chapters 3 and 4. Also, in solids anisotropic hyperfine couplings and quadrupole couplings (for $I \geq 1$) can be determined from ENDOR measurements.

1.4.2 ENDOR Mechanisms

1.4.2.1 ΔT_{1e} Mechanism—Transient ENDOR

To consider an ENDOR response from an elementary mechanistic point of view we first treat the various relaxation pathways and consequent energy level populations for the simple $\mathbf{S} = \frac{1}{2}$, $\mathbf{I} = \frac{1}{2}$ four level spin system shown in Fig. 1-6. We initially consider the four levels to be in thermal

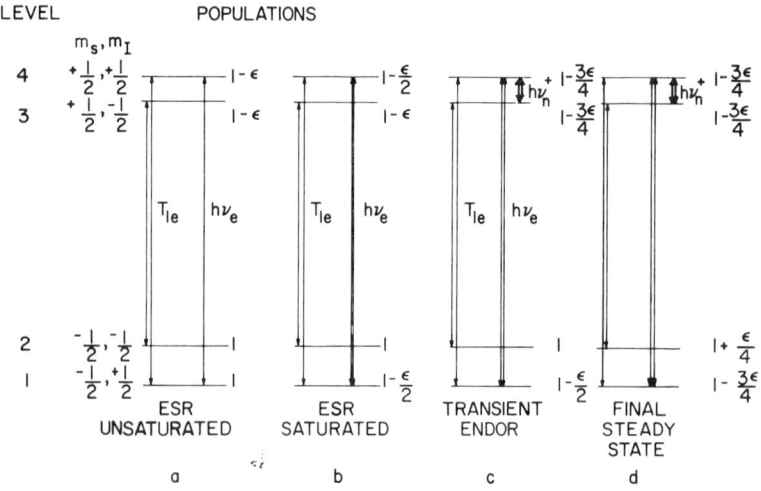

Figure 1-6. Population diagram for transient ENDOR with $\mathbf{S} = \frac{1}{2}$, $\mathbf{I} = \frac{1}{2}$, $A > 0$, $g_n > 0$, $|A|/2 > \nu_n$ (note difference from energy level order in Fig. 1-4 where A was negative) where T_{1e} is finite and all other relaxation times are so long as to be effectively infinite.

equilibrium with each other. This implies the existence of spin-lattice relaxation processes. In this example we consider T_{1e} to be finite and all other relaxation processes to be long enough to be considered effectively infinite. At temperatures above a few Kelvins the electronic Boltzmann factor can be expanded as in eq. 1.7.

$$\frac{N_4}{N_1} = \exp\left(-\frac{g\beta H}{kT}\right) = 1 - \frac{g\beta H}{kT} \qquad (1.7)$$

The population difference between the nuclear levels 3 and 4 and between 1 and 2 can be neglected since these differences are of the order of $g_n\beta_n H/kT$, which is about 10^{-3} of the population difference between the electronic energy levels. If we let $\varepsilon = g\beta H/kT$, we have the initial energy level populations as shown in Fig. 1-6a. If we induce ESR transitions between levels 1 and 4 with sufficiently low microwave power to avoid saturation, these thermal equilibrium populations will be maintained by the electronic spin-lattice relaxation interactions. However if we increase the microwave power so the induced absorption rate competes with the electronic spin relaxation rate, we will saturate the ESR transition and equalize the relative populations of the two energy levels involved as shown in Fig. 1-6b. Under the condition of complete saturation no ESR response would be observed. Of course in reality complete saturation is seldom achieved, but at least a much smaller ESR signal is observed under saturation conditions. Finally in Fig. 1-6c we apply a nuclear radiofrequency (rf) between levels 3 and 4. Since we have assumed the nuclear spin-lattice relaxation rate to be effectively zero, the rf field will saturate this transition and equalize the populations as shown. The net result is to produce an inequality in the populations of the two energy levels corresponding to the ESR transition, namely, levels 1 and 4. Thus the application of the nuclear radiofrequency partially desaturates the ESR signal and increases the ESR response. This increase in the ESR signal constitutes an ENDOR response. For the example shown a maximum response of 25% of the unsaturated ESR signal is expected. Note that if a nuclear frequency is applied between levels 1 and 2, the ESR signal is also desaturated and a second ENDOR signal appears. The partial desaturation of the ESR signal by the rf field can be regarded as a decrease in the effective T_{1e}. This decrease is characteristic of the most general ENDOR mechanism.

In the example shown in Fig. 1-6 one would only obtain a transient ENDOR response. This is because in the presence of a saturating microwave field and a saturating rf field the three energy levels involved would all eventually become equally populated at a population ε less than level 2 and again there would be no ESR signal as in Fig. 1-6d. This transient ENDOR signal decays with the electronic spin-lattice relaxation time.

ENDOR was first observed by Feher in 1956.[1] He studied the phosphorus-doped silicon system in which the odd valence electron on phosphorus renders the system paramagnetic. At 1.25 K $T_{1e} \sim 40$ min and the other relaxation times (T_{1n} and T_x, which are discussed later) are longer than 10 hours.[2] Thus this system approximately satisfies the assumptions made for the ENDOR mechanism illustrated in Fig. 1-6. Figure 1-7 shows some experimental results on this system adapted from

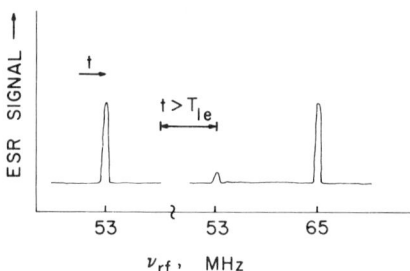

Figure 1-7. Experimental ENDOR results from ^{31}P in P-doped Si at $H_o \sim$ 3200 G. With reference to Fig. 1-6, the $h\nu_n^+$ transition occurs at 53 MHz and decays in time $t > T_{1e}$. The $h\nu_n^-$ transition occurs at 65 MHz. Adapted from G. Feher, *Phys. Rev.*, **114**, 1245 (1959) and from E. C. McIrvine et al., *Phys. Rev.*, **136**, A 467 (1964).

Feher[3] and from McIrvine, Lambe, and Laurance.[4] The $h\nu_n^+$ signal at 53 MHz is shown to be transient because it is much decreased after $t > T_{1e}$. However, if the rf field sweep is continued, the $h\nu_n^-$ transition at 65 MHz is observed. Note that this is expected from Fig. 1-6. When the populations in levels 1 and 2 of Fig. 1-6d are equalized by saturation, the population of level 1 $(1 - \varepsilon/4)$ becomes greater than the population of level 4 $(1 - 3\varepsilon/4)$ and ENDOR is observed.

The ENDOR transitions in Fig. 1-7 correspond to interaction of the unpaired electron with ^{31}P nuclei. This is known since either $\nu_n^+ + \nu_n^- = 2\nu_n$ or $|\nu_n^+ - \nu_n^-| = 2\nu_n$, depending on the relative magnitude of ν_n and $|A|/2$. The sum of the ENDOR frequencies gives $|g_n| \sim 24$ from $h\nu_n = |g_n|\beta H$, which is larger than g_n for any known nucleus. The difference of the ENDOR frequencies gives $|g_n| \sim 2.4$, which identifies ^{31}P. In this solid sample it turns out that the hyperfine coupling to ^{31}P is purely isotropic so $\nu_n^+ + \nu_n^- = |A| \sim 118$ MHz. These values of $|A|$ and $|g_n|$ are approximate because with this magnitude of $|A|$ we are on the borderline of validity for the strong field approximation on which eqs. 1.5 and 1.6 are based. If the exact solution to the spin Hamiltonian[5] is used, the values obtained from Feher's results are $|g_n| = 2.265 \pm 0.004$[1] and $|A| = 117.53 \pm 0.02$ MHz.[3] These values show the high accuracy obtainable from ENDOR experiments.

1.4.2.2 ΔT_{1e} Mechanism—Steady State ENDOR

Transient ENDOR can only be observed if the response time of the ESR spectrometer is less than T_{1e}. With typical spectrometers it takes several seconds to sweep through the ENDOR line so a T_{1e} much longer than this is required to observe transient ENDOR. The P-doped silicon system has atypically long relaxation times and then only at very low temperatures, which allows observation of transient ENDOR. But by 4.2 K, T_{1e} in this system has shortened to ~ 10 sec. For most chemically interesting systems at 77 K and above and for radicals in solution electron relaxation times are typically 10^{-2} to 10^{-6} sec. Thus to observe ENDOR in such systems a steady state mechanism is required. We may still consider the mechanism discussed for transient ENDOR in which T_{1e} is effectively shortened by the application of the rf field. But to achieve a steady state effect we must consider a relaxation pathway that parallels the T_{1e} pathway. Then the effective T_{1e} will be decreased just as the resistance of a circuit is decreased when another resistance of similar magnitude is added in parallel.

Figure 1-8 shows our four level spin system in which the relaxation times T_{1e}, T_{1n}, and T_{x1} are all considered. T_{x1} refers to a cross-relaxation process in which both electron and nuclear spin flips occur simultaneously with $\Delta(m_s + m_I) = 0$. There is another cross-relaxation process T_{x2}, which corresponds to $\Delta(m_s + m_I) = \pm 2$, but it is unimportant for purely isotropic hyperfine interaction so we ignore it for the moment. In Fig. 1-8a it can

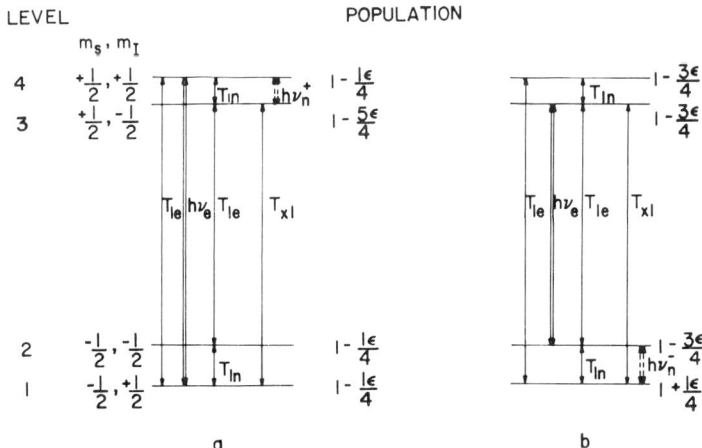

Figure 1-8. Population diagram for steady state ENDOR with $S=\frac{1}{2}$, $I=\frac{1}{2}$, $A>0$, $g_n>0$, $|A|/2 > \nu_n$. The populations shown are for the case where $T_{1e} \sim T_{x1} \ll T_{1n}$ and one ESR transition is saturated. In (a) only $h\nu_n^+$ and in (b) only $h\nu_n^-$ will lead to ENDOR signals.

be seen that for saturation of the 1–4 electronic transition there are two possible relaxation paths in addition to T_{1e}. We will use (m_s, m_I) to denote the states involved in these pathways. One path involves T_{1n} from $(\frac{1}{2}, \frac{1}{2})$ to $(\frac{1}{2}, -\frac{1}{2})$, T_{1e} from $(\frac{1}{2}, -\frac{1}{2})$ to $(-\frac{1}{2}, -\frac{1}{2})$, and T_{1n} from $(-\frac{1}{2}, -\frac{1}{2})$ to $(-\frac{1}{2}, \frac{1}{2})$. The other path involves T_{1n} from $(\frac{1}{2}, \frac{1}{2})$ to $(\frac{1}{2}, -\frac{1}{2})$ and T_{x1} from $(\frac{1}{2}, -\frac{1}{2})$ to $(-\frac{1}{2}, \frac{1}{2})$. Either or both of these paths can produce a steady state ENDOR response.

For paramagnetic centers in solids one typically finds the statement that generally $T_{1e} < T_{x1} \ll T_{1n}$,[6] and consequently relaxation pathways involving T_{1n} are ignored. However for radicals in solution $T_{1e} \sim T_{1n} < T_{x1}$ is often found for proton ENDOR and it seems probable that this may also apply for radicals in solids that are not strongly coupled to the vibrational modes of the matrix in contrast to the strong coupling of transition metal ions in substitutional sites in crystals. Let us first consider the case $T_{1e} \sim T_{1n} \ll T_{x1}$. Then in the presence of a saturating microwave field, the total relaxation rate will be proportional to the sum of the reciprocals of the two resistances or relaxation times, which is given as $T_{1e}^{-1} + (T_{1n} + T_{1e} + T_{1n})^{-1}$ or $1^{-1} + 3^{-1} = 1.33$ where $T_{1e} = T_{1n} = 1$. In the presence of an additional saturating rf field applied at either $h\nu_n^+$ or $h\nu_n^-$ one of the nuclear relaxation pathways is short-circuited and the total relaxation rate will be proportional to $1^{-1} + 2^{-1} = 1.5$. Thus the steady state effect is one of enhancement of the ESR signal by a factor of $1.5/1.33 = 1.12$. If $T_{1n} > T_{1e}$ the enhancement will be less. Note that in this particular case both $h\nu_n^+$ and $h\nu_n^-$ transitions are predicted to occur with equal intensity because both transitions short-circuit the same nuclear relaxation path to the same degree. In Fig. 1-9 is a proton ENDOR spectrum of benzophenone anion

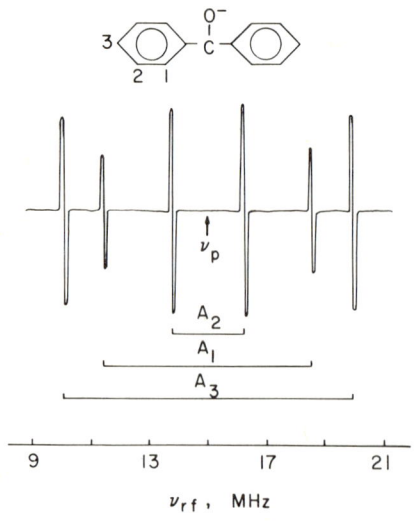

Figure 1-9. Proton ENDOR spectrum of benzophenone anion in liquid dimethoxyethane at 210 K. Each type of proton gives a pair of lines centered around the free proton frequency ν_p and separated by the hyperfine constant A. In this example the intensities of the two ENDOR lines corresponding to a given type of proton are equal; however, these ideal intensity patterns are not typical of ENDOR spectra of organic radicals. Adapted from K. Mobius and K. P. Dinse, *Chimia*, **26**, 461 (1972).

radicals in liquid dimethoxyethane at 210 K. There are three different types of equivalent protons in this radical (ortho, meta, and para) and each type is expected to give two ENDOR lines corresponding to the $h\nu_n^+$ and $h\nu_n^-$ transitions. It can be seen that six lines, consisting of three pairs of equal intensity symmetrically disposed around ν_n, are in agreement with the T_{1e}, T_{1n} relaxation pathway.

Now let us consider the case of predominance of the other alternate relaxation pathway in Fig. 1-8, which involves T_{1n} and T_{x1}. If $T_{1n} \gg T_{x1} \sim T_{1e}$, only the T_{1e} relaxation path is effective for the electronic transition in the absence of a saturating rf field. In the presence of a saturating microwave field applied to the 1–4 transition the steady state populations are as shown in Fig. 1-8a; both the T_{1e} and T_{x1} processes maintain the thermal equilibrium population difference between the levels they connect, except for the transition that is saturated. Then application of $h\nu_n^+$ short-circuits the T_{n1}, T_{x1} relaxation path and produces an ENDOR signal. The total relaxation rate is increased from $1^{-1} + \sim 100^{-1} = 1$ before $h\nu_n^+$ is applied to $1^{-1} + 1^{-1} = 2$ after $h\nu_n^+$ is applied where $T_{1e} = T_{x1} = 1$. This implies that the $h\nu_n^+$ pumping rate is not only greater than the T_{1n}^{-1} relaxation rate but also greater than the T_{x1}^{-1} relaxation rate. Thus a maximum steady state enhancement factor of 2 is predicted. Note that only one ENDOR line is predicted. Application of the rf at $h\nu_n^-$ gives no effect since the populations of levels 1 and 2 are already equal. However, if the ESR transition 2–3 is saturated, as shown in Fig. 1-8b, the same relaxation processes lead to the steady state spin population shown there, and application of only $h\nu_n^-$ leads to an ENDOR response.

An example of the predominance of the T_{x1} relaxation path is shown in Fig. 1-10 for ENDOR spectra of ^{32}P-doped silicon.[8] Although both ENDOR transitions are observed, one transition is much more intense than the other, in qualitative agreement with the picture in Fig. 1-8. Feher cleverly used this intensity inequality to determine the sign of

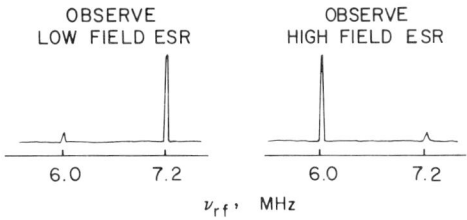

Figure 1-10. Schematic ENDOR spectra of ^{32}P-doped silicon at $H_o \simeq 3190$ G at 1.2 K. The intensity difference of the ENDOR lines for the different ESR transitions is used to deduce that the magnetic moment of ^{32}P is negative; see the population diagram in Fig. 1-11. Actually ^{32}P has $\mathbf{I} = 1$ instead of $\frac{1}{2}$ but the argument in Fig. 1-11 remains valid. Adapted from G. Feher et al., *Phys. Rev.*, **107**, 1462 (1957).

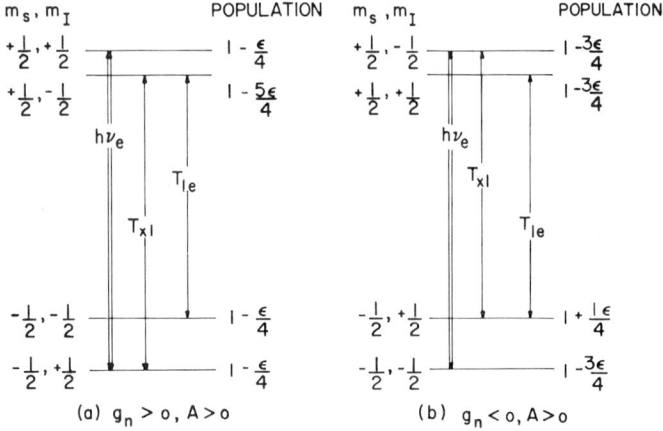

Figure 1-11. Population diagrams for steady state ENDOR with $S=\frac{1}{2}$, $I=\frac{1}{2}$, $|A|/2 > \nu_n$ and positive (a) and negative (b) nuclear magnetic moments. When the low field ESR transition is saturated, only the higher energy ENDOR transition is observed in the example in Fig. 1-10, which indicates that (b) is correct.

$g(^{32}P)$. As shown in Fig. 1-11 the lower energy ENDOR transition is expected to be more intense for $g_n > 0$ and the higher energy ENDOR transition is expected to be more intense for $g_n < 0$. This prediction requires that the sign of A be known as it is for an unpaired electron in an orbital on a given atom such as phosphorus. The experimental results in Fig. 1-10 demonstrate that g_n of ^{32}P is negative.

The intensity inequality of higher energy and lower energy ENDOR transitions is unfortunately common in both solid phase and liquid phase spectra. This means that the relative intensity of a given ENDOR transition cannot be used indiscriminately as a reliable indication of the number of nuclei contributing to a given transition. The dominance of T_{x1} relaxation is only one of several mechanisms that lead to intensity inequalities. Other mechanisms are discussed in Chapters 3 and 4.

Let us now return to Fig. 1-8 and consider the case where $T_{1e} \sim T_{1n} \sim T_{x1} = 1$. Then we have three relaxation pathways in parallel. The effective relaxation rate goes from $1 + 3^{-1} + 2^{-1} = 1.83$ in the absence of a saturating nuclear frequency to $1 + 2^{-1} + 1^{-1} = 2.5$ in the presence of a saturating nuclear frequency $h\nu_n^+$. Thus a maximum enhancement factor of $2.5/1.83 = 1.36$ is predicted for $h\nu_n^+$ ENDOR. In a similar way an enhancement factor of $2.0/1.83 = 1.09$ is predicted for $h\nu_n^-$ ENDOR. As long as the T_{x1} pathway makes a significant contribution to the total electronic relaxation rate, an intensity inequality for the two ENDOR transitions is predicted.

Up to now we have neglected the T_{x2} relaxation process $\Delta(m_s + m_I) =$

±2 since it is often not important. However when the hyperfine interaction is anisotropic the T_{x2} process is generally at least partially allowed and under certain conditions it is also allowed for isotropic hyperfine interaction.[6] Figure 1-12 shows the relaxation pathways for the $\mathbf{S}=\tfrac{1}{2}$, $\mathbf{I}=\tfrac{1}{2}$ system when T_{x2} is included. We first note that if $T_{x2}=T_{x1}$ both $h\nu_n^+$ and

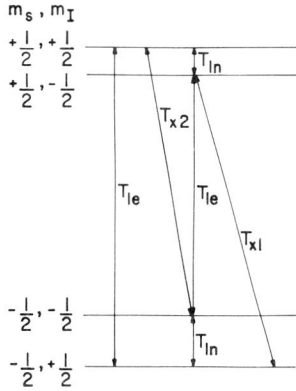

Figure 1-12. Relaxation pathways for steady state ENDOR in a $\mathbf{S}=\tfrac{1}{2}$, $\mathbf{I}=\tfrac{1}{2}$, $A>0$, $g_n>0$, $|A|/2>\nu_n$ system with anisotropic hyperfine interaction.

$h\nu_n^-$ ENDOR transitions are expected to occur with equal intensity regardless of the relative importance of the T_x and T_{1n} relaxation pathways. This system is now too complex to write down steady state level populations from simple considerations. However for the case $T_{1e}=T_{1n}=T_{x1}=T_{x2}$ we can predict a maximum ENDOR enhancement factor of $3.0/2.33=1.29$ for the four parallel relaxation pathways.

Let us briefly consider what determines the probability of the T_{x2} process. At very low temperatures, typically below 5 K, electronic relaxation often occurs by a "direct" process involving the absorption and emission of phonons at the microwave frequency. Then the electronic relaxation rates and the ESR transition probabilities depend on similar physical factors. The ESR transitions corresponding to the T_{x1} and T_{x2} processes are usually termed *forbidden* ESR transitions because a nuclear spin-flip must occur as well as an electron spin-flip. These forbidden ESR transitions become partially allowed because of anisotropic hyperfine terms in the spin Hamiltonian.[9] Consequently the cross-relaxation probabilities are given by[6]

$$T_{x1}^{-1} \sim T_{1e}^{-1}\left(\frac{A_x+A_y}{4h\nu_e}\right)^2 \qquad T_{x2}^{-1} \sim T_{1e}^{-1}\left(\frac{A_x-A_y}{4h\nu_e}\right)^2 \qquad (1.8)$$

where A_x and A_y refer to principal values of the hyperfine interaction. If the hyperfine interaction is isotropic ($A_x=A_y$), then T_{x2}^{-1} goes to zero, although T_{x1}^{-1} is still finite. An example is provided by P-doped silicon at

18 ESR AND DOUBLE RESONANCE

1.2 K, shown in Fig. 1-10, where the ENDOR spectrum reflects that the T_{x2}^{-1} rate is much less than the T_{x1}^{-1} rate.

For solid systems at higher temperatures (>50 K) and for liquids, the electron spin relaxation process is usually "indirect" and involves two phonon or Raman scattering events. This process can arise from vibrational modulation of hyperfine interactions, which in turn gives rise to finite T_{x2}^{-1} rates even for only isotropic hyperfine interaction.

Up to this point we have only considered relaxation processes within a single spin system that affect the ENDOR response. Spin exchange between different spin systems may also affect it. In general, spin exchange decreases the ENDOR response. Thus one cannot increase the radical concentration to improve the ENDOR signal intensity beyond the concentration where spin exchange becomes important. Figure 1-13

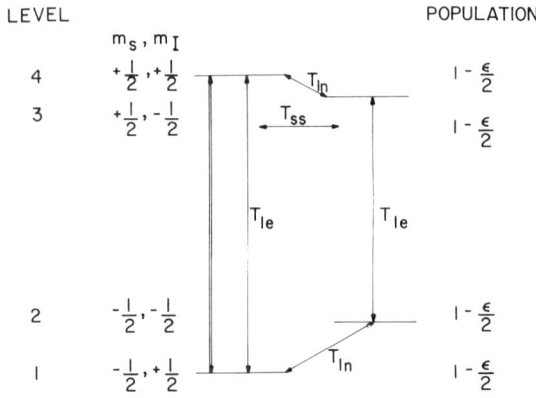

Figure 1-13. Population diagram for steady state ENDOR with $S = \frac{1}{2}$, $I = \frac{1}{2}$, $A > 0$, $g_n > 0$, $|A|/2 > \nu_n$. The populations shown are for the case where $T_{ss} \ll T_{1e}$. Thus all level populations are equalized and no ENDOR response is possible. In general, spin exchange processes (T_{ss}) decrease ENDOR enhancements.

shows a population diagram for the extreme case where the spin exchange time T_{ss} is much shorter than T_{1e}. The T_{ss} process corresponds to an α spin flipping to a β spin and a β spin flipping to an α spin. This effectively acts like nuclear relaxation in both α and β electron spin states. In this case the saturated ESR transition transfers its saturation to the initially unsaturated levels of other spin systems. Since $T_{ss} \ll T_{1e}$, the T_{1e} processes become saturated and no ENDOR is possible. If the spin exchange process is not controlling ($T_{ss} \ll T_{1e}$) but only significant ($T_{ss} \sim T_{1e}$), partial transfer of saturation occurs and the ENDOR enhancement in the absence of spin exchange is decreased.

The experimental effect of spin exchange was first shown by studies on

P-doped silicon at 4.2 K under visible illumination.[4] The light produces free electron carriers that produce rapid spin exchange between the paramagnetic phosphorus centers. For typical light intensities $T_{ss} \sim 1$ sec compared to $T_{1e} \sim 10$ sec.[2] For a sample in which ENDOR is observed in the dark, the ENDOR signal disappears within a few seconds after the light has been turned on. The effect of spin exchange has also been observed, although not so dramatically, in concentration dependent studies of free radicals in solution. Hyde found that the ENDOR enhancement of tetracene cation in concentrated sulfuric acid at 273 K decreased by a factor of 2.5 when the tetracene concentration was increased from 10^{-3} to 10^{-2} M.[10]

In discussing spin exchange effects on ENDOR it is pertinent to distinguish between Heisenberg exchange and chemical exchange. Heisenberg exchange is spin-spin exchange between pairs of free radicals. The illuminated P-doped silicon system is an example of this type of exchange. Chemical exchange is spin-spin exchange between a free radical and a diamagnetic molecule such as between tetracene cation and tetracene. Freed has quantitatively treated the ENDOR response expected from such exchange mechanisms.[11] He shows that Heisenberg exchange diminishes ENDOR enhancements as indicated by the qualitative arguments based on Fig. 1-13. He also shows that chemical exchange, in which the diamagnetic species are polarized by the radicals under ESR saturation, has effects identical with Heisenberg exchange. If the diamagnetic species are not polarized, chemical exchange can lead to ENDOR enhancements, but generally polarization is expected.

Finally we consider an example of spin exchange in the presence of a finite cross-relaxation (T_{x1}) process. The population diagram is illustrated in Fig. 1-14. The saturation of the 1–4 ESR transition is transferred to the 2–3 ESR transition by the spin exchange process. Since $T_{ss} \ll T_{1e}$, the T_{1e} process cannot maintain thermal equilibrium between the levels it connects. However the T_{x1} process does not compete with T_{ss} and can maintain thermal equilibrium populations between the two levels it connects. Thus the steady state level populations are as given in the figure. When the low energy $h\nu_n^+$ transition is saturated by applied radiofrequency, ENDOR enhancement is observed as shown in Fig. 1-14a'. But when the high energy $h\nu_n^-$ transition is saturated, the ENDOR signal is negative and corresponds to microwave emission as shown in Fig. 1-14b'. This situation has been observed experimentally in illuminated P-doped silicon at 4.2 K (see Fig. 1-15). Under these conditions $T_{x1} \sim 10$ min, and although no ENDOR response is seen after illumination for several minutes as described earlier, the ENDOR responses in Fig. 1-15 are seen after ~ 10 min.

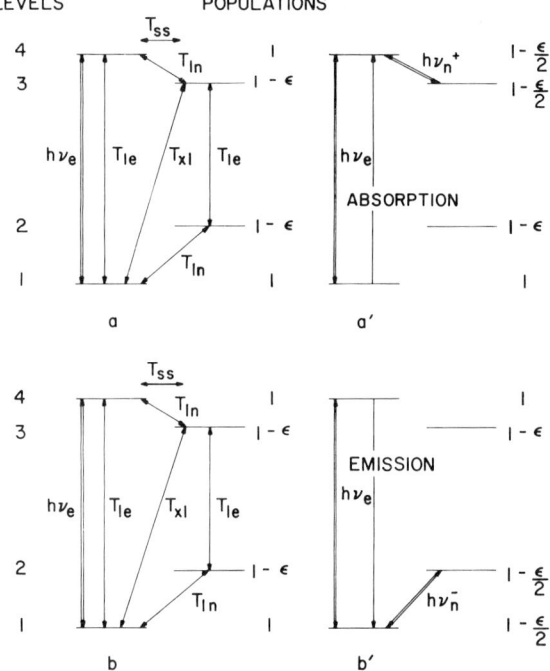

Figure 1-14. Population diagram for steady state ENDOR with $S=\frac{1}{2}$, $I=\frac{1}{2}$, $A>0$, $g_n>0$, $|A|/2>\nu_n$. The populations shown in (a) and (b) are for the case where $T_{ss} \ll T_{1e} \lesssim T_{x1} \ll T_{1n}$. When saturating nuclear energy $h\nu_n^+$ is applied, the populations change to those in (a') and an ENDOR enhancement occurs; but when saturating nuclear energy $h\nu_n^-$ is applied, the populations change to those in (b') and a negative ENDOR signal (microwave emission) occurs.

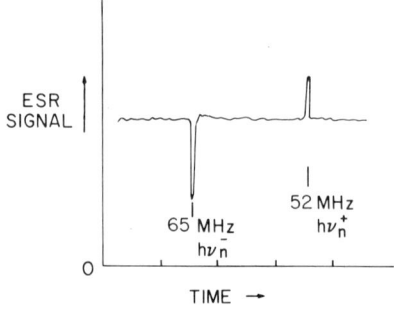

Figure 1-15. Example of the ENDOR response corresponding to the population diagram of Fig. 1-14 observed in illuminated P-doped silicon at 4.2 K. Adapted from E. C. McIrvine et al., *Phys. Rev.*, **136**, A467 (1964).

Table 1-2. Summary of Maximum ENDOR Enhancements for Different Relaxation Conditions

Relaxation Conditions[a]	$h\nu_n^+/h\nu_n^-$ [b]	Maximum ENDOR Enhancements (%)[c]	Figure
$T_{1e} = T_{1n} \ll T_{x1}$	1	12	1-8
$10T_{1e} = T_{1n} \ll T_{x1}$	1	4	
$T_{1e} < T_{1n} \ll T_{x1}$	1	<12	
$T_{1e} = T_{x1} \gg T_{1n}$	∞	100	1-8
$10T_{1e} = T_{x1} \ll T_{1n}$	∞	10	
$T_{1e} < T_{x1} \ll T_{1n}$	∞	<100	
$T_{1e} = T_{1n} = T_{x1}$	4	36	1-8
$T_{1e} = T_{1n} = T_{x1} = T_{x2}$	1	29	1-12
$T_{ss} \ll T_{1e} \ll T_{x1} < T_{1n}$	–	0	1-13
$T_{ss} \ll T_{1e} < T_{x1} \ll T_{1n}$	−1	>0	1-14

[a] T_{x2} is considered infinite where not mentioned. Symbols are defined in text.
[b] For saturation of the 1–4 transition $(-\tfrac{1}{2}, +\tfrac{1}{2} \rightarrow +\tfrac{1}{2}, +\tfrac{1}{2})$ where $h\nu_n^+$ and $h\nu_n^-$ are defined as in Fig. 1-8.
[c] Percent of ESR signal.

The results of this section are summarized in Table 1-2. The maximum ENDOR enhancements as a percent of the ESR signal depend on the relaxation time conditions, as do the relative intensities of the $h\nu_n^+$ and $h\nu_n^-$ ENDOR transitions. Typically enhancements of 1 to 10% are observed for steady state ENDOR.

1.4.2.3 Packet-Shifting Mechanism

The packet-shifting ENDOR mechanism is a special case of the ΔT_{1e} mechanism that is applicable to inhomogeneously broadened lines. It was first discussed by Feher as an explanation of his original ENDOR experiments.[3,12] An inhomogeneously broadened ESR line is the overall envelope of homogeneous spin packet substructure, as shown in Fig. 1-16a. Each spin packet corresponds to those spins that "see" the same net local magnetic field and can be described as a homogeneously broadened line. In solids the differing spin orientations of magnetic nuclei surrounding an unpaired electron produce differing net local fields and hence correspond to differing spin packets that resonate at different

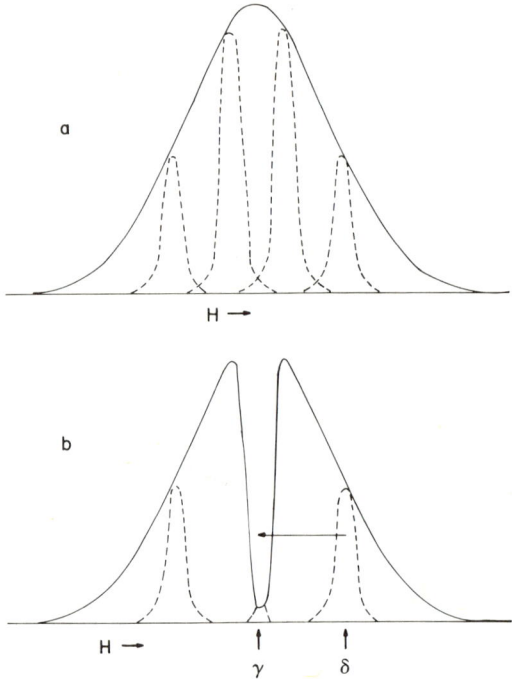

Figure 1-16. (a) Inhomogeneously broadened ESR line showing the homogeneously broadened spin packet substructure. (b) Schematic of packet-shifting mechanism for ENDOR. Spin packet γ is saturated, but application of a nuclear frequency shifts spin packets δ to γ to partially desaturate γ and produce an ENDOR response.

frequencies. Now let us suppose that one region of an inhomogeneous line containing one or a few spin packets is saturated as shown in Fig. 1-16b. If there is little spin diffusion between spin packets, the rest of the line will remain unsaturated and one can treat each spin packet as belonging to a separate energy level. To do ENDOR we apply a nuclear frequency that can flip a nucleus to change the nuclear spin orientation around unpaired electrons originally in spin packet δ to a new nuclear spin orientation found in spin packet γ. This has the effect of shifting spin packet δ to γ, as shown in Fig. 1-16b, and partially desaturating the center portion of the line to give an ENDOR response.

Of course the nuclear frequency can also flip a nucleus around unpaired electrons originally in spin packet γ. If this is followed by T_{x1} or $T_{1e} + T_{1n}$ processes to return those electrons to spin packet γ, this is the same ΔT_{1e} mechanism discussed in the preceding subsection.

Thus when ENDOR is done on inhomogeneously broadened ESR lines, either packet shifting may occur or the electrons in the saturated spin packet or packets may have their effective T_{1e} changed. Different electrons are involved in these two mechanisms. However it is not normally possible to distinguish experimentally between these mechanisms. The ΔT_{1e} mechanism can apply to either homogeneously or inhomogeneously broadened ESR lines, but the packet-shifting mechanism applies only to inhomogeneously broadened lines. In effect, the packet-shifting mechanism can be considered as a special case of the ΔT_{1e} mechanism that utilizes a different set of unpaired electrons to change the effective T_{1e} of the set of electrons constituting the saturated portion of the ESR line.

1.4.2.4 Distant ENDOR or Depolarization Mechanism

A distinctly different ENDOR mechanism was found by Lambe and co-workers in experiments with ruby (Al_2O_3; 0.05% Cr^3).[13,14] The fundamental characteristic of this mechanism is that the ENDOR response decays, after removal of the rf power, with a time constant of order T_{1n} instead of T_{1e}. This implies that host nuclei having no direct interaction with the electron spin are involved in the ENDOR response and led Lambe et al. to propose a depolarization mechanism.[14]

In simple terms this mechanism can be described as shown in Fig. 1-17. Saturation of the electron spin system leads to nuclear spin polarization of

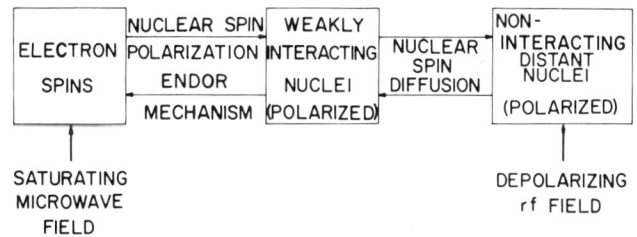

Figure 1-17. Schematic of distant or depolarization ENDOR mechanism.

surrounding nuclei that have only weak isotropic and/or anisotropic hyperfine interactions with the electrons. (Discussion of the mechanism by which this polarization occurs is deferred for the moment.) The nuclear polarization can then be transferred to noninteracting "distant" nuclei by nuclear spin diffusion in a time of order T_{1n} or somewhat shorter. One now does essentially an NMR experiment on the bulk nuclei in the sample in that these nuclei only absorb their unperturbed NMR frequencies. However they are coupled on the electron spins by virtue of their polarization. If a saturating rf field is applied, the bulk (distant) nuclei absorb their NMR frequencies and depolarize. This depolarization

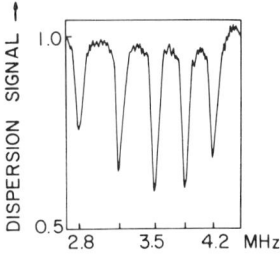

Figure 1-18. Distant ENDOR spectrum in ruby; the effect on the dispersion ESR signal as the radiofrequency is scanned through the region corresponding to the ^{27}Al nuclear frequencies. The measurements were made near 3300 G at 4.2 K without magnetic field modulation. Data taken from J. Lambe et al., *Phys. Rev.*, **122**, 1161 (1961).

is carried back to the electron spin system by the reverse path to cause a change in the electron spin level populations and hence an ENDOR response. The time scale will be of order T_{1n} or nuclear spin diffusion times.

The classic distant ENDOR spectrum in ruby is shown in Fig. 1-18. The bulk ^{27}Al nuclei have a spin of $\frac{5}{2}$ and hence, because of quadrupole interaction, give rise to $2I = 5$ NMR transitions, which are in this case detected by ENDOR. The positions of the lines are unshifted from their NMR positions in pure Al_2O_3 with no paramagnetic impurities. Distant ENDOR can realistically be called ESR detection of NMR with about 10^3 times more sensitivity and resolution than straight NMR detection.

The remaining question revolves about the mechanism by which the nuclear polarization is set up. Two different mechanisms for this have been demonstrated. The first involves saturation of so-called forbidden transitions in which both an electron spin and a nuclear spin are flipped. That this process leads to net nuclear polarization is shown in Fig. 1-19. The level populations are determined by thermal equilibrium from T_{1e} processes, which are assumed to be faster than the unsaturated T_x processes. The nuclear polarization is defined as $\langle I_z \rangle / I$, where $\langle I_z \rangle$ is the sum of the I_z's times their level population divided by the total number of levels. The allowedness of such transitions depends on the ratio of the dipolar field from the unpaired electron at the nucleus to the externally applied field. When this ratio is ~ 0.5 to 0.1, the nuclear spin-flip transitions are most allowed. Because these are the nuclei that interact relatively weakly with the electron spin, if they are polarized there is little energy barrier to nuclear spin diffusion to more distant nuclei. Nuclei strongly coupled to a paramagnetic center are not at the same resonance frequency as distant nuclei, so there is an energy barrier for spin diffusion between such nuclei and the uncoupled bulk nuclei.

A consequence of nuclear polarization via forbidden nuclear spin-flip transitions is that the maximum ENDOR signal arises from the wings, rather than from the center, of the ESR line where the spin-flip transitions occur. This can be clearly seen if the direct absorption signal, rather

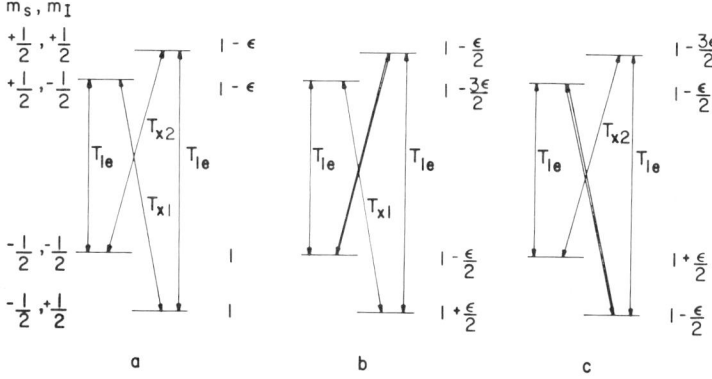

Figure 1-19. Population diagram showing nuclear polarization after saturation of a forbidden transition in which both electron and nuclear spins flip. (a) Thermal equilibrium populations. (b) Populations after saturation of a T_{x2} transition. The nuclear polarization is given by $\langle I_z \rangle / I$ and is $+\varepsilon/2$. (c) Populations after saturation of a T_{x1} transition. The nuclear polarization is $-\varepsilon/2$. Note that the T_{1e} processes maintain thermal equilibrium while the slower unsaturated T_x processes do not.

than its first derivative, is detected;[14] it is a characteristic feature of this ENDOR mechanism. Analysis of the population dynamics of this mechanism via the Bloch equations shows that upon application of rf power, the absorption ESR signal shows a small increase and the dispersion ESR signal shows a large decrease.[14] Thus detection of the dispersion signal affords much better sensitivity for this ENDOR mechanism.

The second mechanism of nuclear polarization leading to distant ENDOR involves saturation of the allowed ESR transitions in which only an electron spin flips. This leads to nuclear polarization if there is strong dipolar coupling within the electron spin system, which is in turn coupled to the nuclear Zeeman system.[15] The theoretical treatment is somewhat complex and will not be given here, but the theory appears to agree well with experimental results on copper Tutton salts of formula $(Zn, Cu)X_2SO_4 \cdot 6H_2O$ where $X = K$, Rb, or Cs. The ENDOR effect is predicted to be an enhancement of the absorption ESR signal, as is observed. The time response is again of the order of T_{1n}. This mechanism may be distinguished from the previous one in that it predicts an ENDOR enhancement when sitting on the center of the ESR absorption line as well as a significant ENDOR effect at microwave powers sufficient to saturate the allowed transitions but not the forbidden ones.

It should be emphasized that distant ENDOR mechanisms can occur simultaneously with ΔT_{1e} ENDOR mechanisms. In particular, both mechanisms are observed in dilute ruby with 0.01% Cr^{+3} in Al_2O_3.[14]

However in more concentrated ruby (0.1% Cr^{+3}) the distant ENDOR mechanism decidedly dominates. This concentration effect probably reflects a longer T_{1n} in dilute ruby. If T_{1n} is too long, nuclear spin diffusion is slow and distant ENDOR becomes difficult to detect. Likewise it appears that low rf power is sufficient to see distant ENDOR because T_{1n} is long, whereas higher rf power is needed for ΔT_{1e} ENDOR because the relevant T_{1n} in this mechanism is shortened by interaction with a close electron spin.

The observation of ENDOR signals at the free nuclear frequency is not a good criterion for distant ENDOR. Signals at the free nuclear frequency often occur in disordered solids. These have been termed *matrix* ENDOR lines and appear to be due to a ΔT_{1e} mechanism under the conditions of observation, namely, high rf power and high frequency detection.[16] The best criterion for distinction between distant and matrix ENDOR signals seems to be the response time of the ENDOR signal. Distant ENDOR decays on a T_{1n} scale and matrix ENDOR decays on a T_{1e} scale. This suggests that distant ENDOR can be selectively discriminated against by using suitably high frequency detection. However if T_{1n} and T_{1e} become comparable at a given temperature and electron spin concentration, the time criterion between the two mechanisms becomes blurred.

1.4.2.5 Line-Shift Mechanism

In principle an ENDOR signal can also arise if application of rf power causes the ESR line to shift in frequency because this will change the ESR intensity at a fixed field observation point. In this case it is not always necessary to saturate the ESR line. This mechanism applies when the unpaired electron spin has contact interaction with the nuclei in contrast to distant ENDOR, which mainly involves dipolar interactions. Then when the nuclei are polarized by saturating the ESR line, they produce a new effective field for the unpaired electron that slightly shifts the ESR line. An example of this shift for conduction electrons in colloidal Li particles is given in Fig. 1-20 by Feher and Isaacson.[17] If one observes the ESR at position A in this figure while sweeping with a depolarizing rf field, an ENDOR signal is observed when the Li resonant frequency is reached and depolarizes the nuclei to change the effective field. Then the ESR line shifts back to its unsaturated position (see Fig. 1-21).

The field shift from this mechanism is given by

$$H_n = \left(\frac{8\pi}{3}\right) |\Psi(0)|^2 \gamma_n \hbar \left[I(I+1) \frac{\hbar \gamma_n H}{3kT} \right] \frac{\gamma_e}{\gamma_n} Z \qquad (1.9)$$

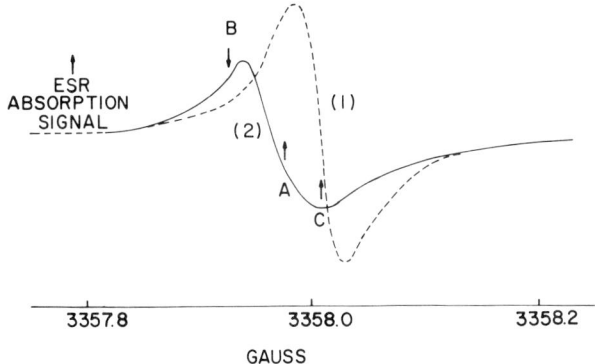

Figure 1-20. ESR signal from conduction electrons in colloidal Li particles in a LiF crystal at room temperature at (1) unsaturating (~0.1 mW) and (2) saturating (~2.0 mW) microwave powers. The field shift is due to the nuclear polarization of the lithium nuclei caused by saturating the ESR line. Point A shows the optimum field position for carrying out an ENDOR experiment (see Fig. 1-21). Points B and C indicate field positions where negative ENDOR signals may be observed. Adapted from G. Feher and R. A. Isaacson, *J. Magn. Resonance*, **7**, 111 (1972).

where $\Psi(0)$ is the electron wavefunction at the nucleus, Z is the electron spin saturation parameter equal to $\gamma_e^2 H_1^2 T_{1e} T_{2e}$, and the other symbols have been defined. For ^{7}Li at $T = 300$ K, $H = 3300$ G, and $Z = 1$, H_n is about 0.1 G. The field shift is less for ^{6}Li because it has a smaller magnetic moment and spin than ^{7}Li. Also ^{6}Li is only 7.4% abundant, but a weak ^{6}Li ENDOR signal can still be seen, as is shown in Fig. 1-21.

In the colloidal Li example the mobile conduction electron has a contact interaction with a large number of Li nuclei and a very narrow

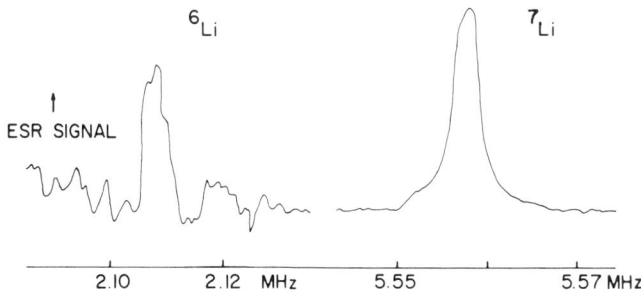

Figure 1-21. Room temperature ENDOR spectra from ^{6}Li (7.4% abundance) and ^{7}Li (92.6%) in colloidal lithium particles in a LiF crystal. The ESR absorption signal was detected. The gain used for the ^{6}Li spectrum is ~40 times higher than for the ^{7}Li spectrum. The magnetic field was set to that denoted by point A in Fig. 1-20. Adapted from G. Feher and R. A. Isaacson, *J. Magn. Resonance*, **7**, 111 (1972).

28 ESR AND DOUBLE RESONANCE

linewidth. Because the field shifts (H_n) are so small, the lineshift ENDOR mechanism can only be applied to very narrow lines. An aromatic organic radical in solution may be a candidate for this ENDOR mechanism, but only if the hyperfine structure is well resolved.

Feher and Isaacson[17] also show that ENDOR can be observed from an unsaturated ESR line by the lineshift mechanism. It is only required to produce the nuclear polarization by some means other than saturating the ESR line. This can be done by thermal equilibrium spin polarization of nuclei at a very low temperature of order 1 to 2 K.

1.4.3 Enhancement of rf Field at the Nucleus

All the preceding ENDOR mechanisms require a saturated nuclear transition, so a basic requirement for successful ENDOR is sufficient rf power. Nuclear saturation is defined by

$$\gamma_n^2 H_2^2 T_{1n} T_{2n} \geq 1 \tag{1.10}$$

where H_2 is the amplitude of the rf magnetic field in the rotating frame. Thus for small γ_n a large H_2 is required for nuclear saturation. Since H_2 is generally limited by experimental factors to ~ 10 G, it would appear that ENDOR on nuclei with small γ_n would be precluded in many cases. Fortunately, because the effective rf field at the nucleus is enhanced via the hyperfine field in most cases, this limitation on ENDOR is not so severe. In fact, the enhancement is greatest for those nuclei with small γ_n.

The rf enhancement effect is most clearly explained in terms of the classical picture in Fig. 1-22 by Abragam and Bleaney.[6] The isotropic hyperfine interaction for a system of electron spins and nuclear spins creates an "electronic" magnetic field at the nucleus due to the electronic

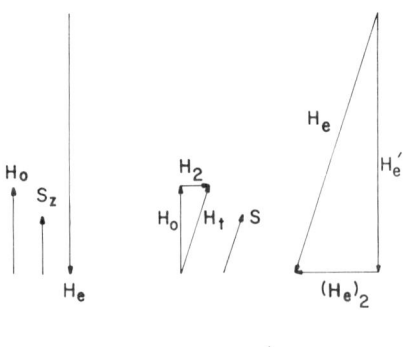

Figure 1-22. Classical explanation of rf enhancement effect. (a) Directions of external field H_o, S_z component of electron spin and electronic field (hyperfine field) at a nucleus, H_e, in the absence of an rf field. (b) Application of rf field H_2 produces resultant field H_t about which S and H_e precess to produce the additional rf field $(H_e)_2$ at the nucleus. For typical experimental conditions $H_o \gg H_2$ so $H_o \approx H_t$ and $H_e' \approx H_e$.

magnetic moment. The size of this electronic magnetic field H_e is given by equating the hyperfine interaction energy term to the form of a nuclear Zeeman interaction energy as in eq. 1.11 where the isotropic coupling A is in reciprocal seconds.

$$hAS_zI_z = -g_n\beta_nH_eI_z \qquad (1.11)$$

Then H_e in $G = hAm_s/-g_n\beta_n = 2\pi Am_s/-\gamma_n$. The H_e field is directed opposite to the applied external field H_o direction if A/γ_n is positive, as shown in Fig. 1-22a. Application of an rf field H_2 in the x direction gives a total field H_t that precesses at the nuclear frequency of H_2. The electron spin and resultant H_e will align along H_t, since the electron frequency is much greater than the nuclear frequency. In other words, the electronic motion can follow the field changing at nuclear frequencies. H_e will then have a component in the x direction $(H_e)_2$ that oscillates at the frequency of H_2 and adds to the total H_2 field seen by the nucleus. From Fig. 1-22b it is seen that $(H_e)_2 = H_2(H'_e/H_o) \simeq H_2(H_e/H_o)$, since $H'_e \simeq H_e$ for typical values of H_o and H_2, and that $(H_e)_2$ is oppositely directed to H_2 for A/γ positive. For $(H_e)_2 \gg H_2$ the rf enhancement factor is (H_e/H_o). The total effective H_2 can be conveniently written as

$$H_2^{\text{eff}} = H_2 + (H_e)_2 = H_2\left|\left(1 - \frac{m_sA'\gamma_e}{H_o\gamma_n}\right)\right| \qquad (1.12)$$

where $A = A'\gamma_e$ and A' is now measured in gauss. Note the absolute value sign.

The rf enhancement factor is significant only for nuclei having an isotropic hyperfine constant of ≥ 10 G. Also note that there is no enhancement if $m_s = 0$. This will be important for some triplet states and transition metal ion complexes. Let us take some typical examples of spin $\frac{1}{2}$ radicals. For protons with $A' = -5$ G, $H_2^{\text{eff}} = H_2|(1+0.5)|$; for ^{13}C with $A' = 10$ G, $H_2^{\text{eff}} = H_2|(1-4)|$; and for ^{14}N with $A' = 15$ G, $H_2^{\text{eff}} = H_2|(1-21)|$. These hyperfine constants are typical of organic radicals. ^{14}N shows a relatively large enhancement factor for hyperfine couplings typical of nitroxide radicals.

1.4.4 Sign of ENDOR Response

1.4.4.1 Absorption Signals

In the ΔT_{1e} and depolarization ENDOR mechanisms discussed earlier the ENDOR response was always an enhancement of an absorption ESR signal. Let us call this a positive ENDOR response. However if one examines the ENDOR spectra in the literature, it is found that both positive and negative ENDOR responses are observed. The simple theoretical predictions of positive ENDOR do not include the effect of magnetic field modulation or rapidly pulsed rf power. These modulations clearly affect the passage times of the microwave and nuclear magnetic fields through different portions of the absorption line and may give rise to negative ENDOR effects. No anomalous sign ENDOR responses seem to have been observed with cw rf fields in the absence of magnetic field modulation. Of course magnetic field modulation is generally required because of signal-to-noise considerations.

To illustrate the apparent sign contradictions, consider several examples of ENDOR due to depolarization mechanisms. ENDOR of Al nuclei in ruby shows a positive absorption signal in the absence of field modulation[14] and a negative absorption signal in the presence of 5 kHz field modulation.[13] ENDOR in copper Tutton salts shows a positive absorption signal in the absence of field modulation.[15] However ENDOR of protons in x-irradiated malonic acid gives a negative absorption signal in the presence of 100 kHz field modulation.[18]

In addition to modulation effects, it also appears that negative ENDOR absorption signals can arise from the application of intense rf fields of the order of 10 G or more. Atherton et al. have observed a change from positive to negative ENDOR responses for protons in Coppinger's radical as the rf power is increased.[19] In this case the rf power was pulsed at 6 kHz and the magnetic field was modulated at 40 Hz. Similar results have been reported by Miyagawa et al. from radicals in x-irradiated organic crystals[20] (see Fig. 1-23). In the second case a cw rf field was used together with 15 kHz field modulation. An interesting feature of these negative ENDOR results is that the negative ENDOR signal at high rf

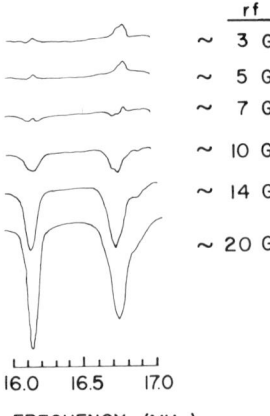

Figure 1-23. Rf field dependence of proton ENDOR signals from an x-irradiated crystal of N-acetylglycine for the applied magnetic field perpendicular to the *bc* plane. As the rf field is increased the ENDOR signals change from positive to negative. The absolute rf field magnitude is only approximate. From I. Miyagawa et al., *J. Magn. Resonance*, **10**, 156 (1973).

power seems to be several times more intense than the maximum positive ENDOR signal observed at lower rf power. Thus some signal-to-noise improvement seems possible.

Negative ENDOR absorption signals due to high rf power can be qualitatively understood in terms of a rf coherence effect.[21] A strong rf field mixes and shifts the energy levels and makes forbidden transitions allowed. This results in a splitting of the ESR line. The line splitting can produce a negative ENDOR response since the peak maximum of the unsplit ESR line will decrease toward the baseline as the line splits. For the experimental cases of negative ENDOR mentioned earlier it is not clear whether the rf fields were strong enough to cause ESR line splittings. So this explanation must be regarded as tentative, especially since the theory does not include the effects of pulsed rf or magnetic field modulation. Nevertheless the empirical features of negative ENDOR at high rf power are of interest.

Finally one should note that the lineshift ENDOR mechanism can produce negative ENDOR. Consider Fig. 1-20. If the ESR line is observed at points B or C, negative ENDOR will be observed upon depolarization of the nuclei. In this case the negative and positive ENDOR mechanisms are the same and are predicted independently of field modulation or high rf power.

The overall conclusions of this section are that the sign of the ENDOR absorption response does not always agree with simple theory and that the sign may depend on the nature of the experimental apparatus.

1.4.4.2 Dispersion Signals

ENDOR dispersion signals have not been discussed much, but the original work by Feher used dispersion detection. Both ΔT_{1e} and depolarization ENDOR mechanisms predict a decrease in the ESR dispersion signal[14] for the ENDOR response (i.e., negative). This was confirmed in experiments carried out on ruby in the absence of field modulation.[14] In the presence of 100 Hz field modulation, the silicon ENDOR dispersion signal in P-doped silicon at 1.25 K[3] and the potassium and chlorine ENDOR dispersion signals from F centers in KCl at 1.25 K[22] do show a decrease (i.e., negative) as expected. However, in P-doped silicon at 1.25 K with 100 Hz field modulation, the phosphorus ENDOR dispersion signal shows an increase (i.e., positive).[3]

The difference is apparently due to the different electronic and nuclear relaxation times of the different species coupled with field modulation effects. Thus dispersion ENDOR signals can also show apparently anomalous signs.

1.4.5 ENDOR Resolution

1.4.5.1 Resolution in Liquids

ENDOR offers an increase in effective spectral resolution in liquids compared to ESR, principally because of the lower spectral density in ENDOR spectra. Typical linewidths of 100 kHz are observed in both liquid phase ENDOR and ESR. So there is little difference in the absolute spectral resolution of the two methods. However the effective resolution depends on the spectral density or number of lines per unit spectral width.

The average spectral density of an ESR spectrum is given by eq. 1.13.[23]

$$\text{ESR spectral density} = \frac{\prod_{k=1}^{K}(2N_k I_k + 1)}{\sum_{k=1}^{K} 2 A_k N_k I_k} \qquad (1.13)$$

The numerator corresponds to the number of ESR hyperfine lines, assuming no degeneracy, from a radical with K groups of equivalent nuclei with nuclear spin I_k and number N_k in each group. The denominator is the total width of the ESR spectrum in megahertz, where A_k is the hyperfine constant in megahertz of the kth group of equivalent nuclei. Note that forbidden transitions and m_I dependent and second order contributions to the ENDOR linewidth have been ignored. The product in the numerator of eq. 1.13 increases the spectral density rapidly with each additional group of inequivalent nuclei; an additional inequivalent proton will double the spectral density.

In ENDOR, as seen from eq. 1.6, only two ENDOR lines arise from each group of equivalent nuclei, and the spectral width equals the largest hyperfine constant A_{max}. Then the average spectral density is given by eq. 1.14.

$$\text{ENDOR spectral density} = \frac{2K}{A_{max}} \qquad (1.14)$$

It is seen that the spectral density increases by a factor of $(K+1)/K$ as K increases assuming that A_{max} does not change. So the ESR spectral density increases much faster with K than does the ENDOR spectral density.

The ENDOR spectral density is smaller than the ESR spectral density, and the ratio of these is a measure of the improved effective resolution obtainable by ENDOR. Results for several liquid phase radicals are summarized in Table 1-3, and Fig. 1-24 compares ESR and ENDOR spectra for the triphenylmethyl radical.

Table 1-3. Effective Spectral Resolution Enhancement for Radicals in Liquids Obtainable by ENDOR

Radical	Protons	Groups of Equivalent Protons	ESR Lines	Effective Resolution Enhancement[a]
Tetracene cation	12	3	125	4.5
Triphenylmethyl	15	3	196	4.7
Coppinger's radical	41	3	370	26
Triphenylphenoxyl	17	7	4050	36

From J. S. Hyde, in *Magnetic Resonance in Biological Systems*, A. Ehrenberg, B. G. Malmström, and T. Vänngard, eds., Pergamon, London, 1967.
[a] ESR spectral density divided by ENDOR spectral density.

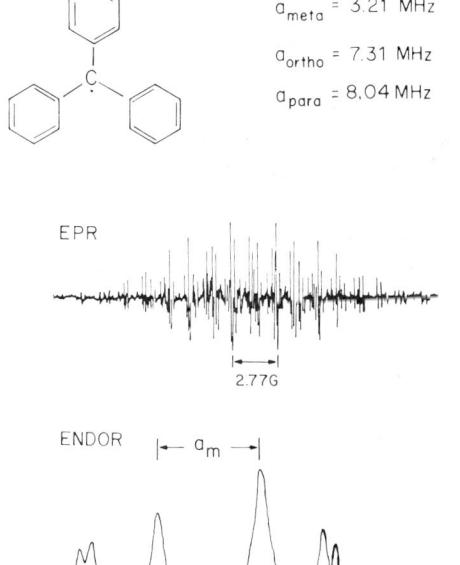

TRIPHENYLMETHYL RADICAL

$a_{meta} = 3.21$ MHz
$a_{ortho} = 7.31$ MHz
$a_{para} = 8.04$ MHz

Figure 1-24. ESR and ENDOR spectra of triphenylmethyl radical showing the decrease in spectral density in the ENDOR spectrum. The effective resolution enhancement from ENDOR compared to ESR is 4.7 (see text).

1.4.5.2 Resolution in Solids

In solids the ESR lines of most radicals are broadened by unresolved hyperfine interaction with surrounding magnetic nuclei. This produces an inhomogeneously broadened line (recall Fig. 1-16) whose linewidth is generally of the order of a few gauss or more. With reference to the preceding subsection, the ESR hyperfine lines are so dense in inhomogeneously broadened lines that they overlap to produce one broad line. Here ENDOR provides a dramatic increase in actual resolution and essentially detects the homogeneous spin packet substructure of an inhomogeneous ESR line. The increase in resolution is approximately given by the ratio of electron magnetic moment to nuclear magnetic moment, or about 1000.

The classic example of ENDOR resolution of unresolved hyperfine substructure in an inhomogeneously broadened ESR line is the case of trapped electrons in alkali halide crystals (F centers).[22] The trapped electron in a chloride ion vacancy in crystalline KCl has a single ESR line with a full width at half height linewidth of 55 G, or 154 MHz.

Figure 1-25 shows part of the ENDOR spectrum of this system from which the hyperfine interaction to the nearest neighbor chlorines can be determined. The ENDOR linewidth (full width at half height) is about 50 kHz, so the resolution has been enhanced by a factor of 3000. For radicals in organic crystals the ESR linewidth is typically 28 MHz (10 G) and the ENDOR linewidth is typically 100 kHz for a resolution enhancement of 280.

ENDOR resolution is decreased somewhat if the interacting nucleus has a quadrupole moment, as does chlorine. Then the number of

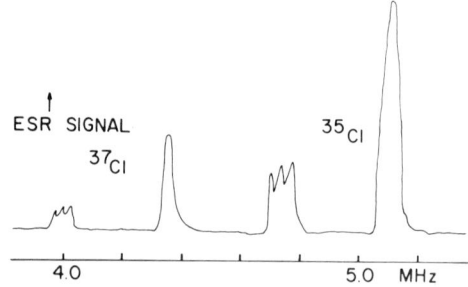

Figure 1-25. ENDOR spectrum of a trapped electron (F center) in a single crystal of KCl interacting with the nearest chlorines at 1.2 to 77 K. The magnetic field is oriented parallel to the 100 direction. Two ENDOR transitions are observed for each chlorine isotope with some quadrupole fine structure appearing on the lower energy transition. The ENDOR linewidth is ~50 kHz compared to an ESR linewidth of 55 G or 154 MHz. Thus the resolution enhancement of ENDOR is 3000 in this example.

ENDOR lines increases, as shown in Fig. 1-25, and the ENDOR spectral density increases. However, to first order, quadrupole interactions do not affect the ESR spectrum, so the ESR spectral density in unchanged.

Another factor affecting resolution is the presence of forbidden ESR transitions in which both electron spins and nuclear spins flip simultaneously. These transitions occur commonly in solids when the nuclear Zeeman interaction is of comparable magnitude to the electron-nuclear dipolar interaction. Although the presence of forbidden ESR transitions increases the ESR spectral density, the number of ENDOR lines, and hence the ENDOR spectral density, is unchanged. Thus the resolution enhancement of ENDOR is even more favorable when the ESR spectrum is complicated by forbidden transitions.

The preceding comments about resolution apply generally to radicals in single crystals and also to radicals in polycrystalline or glassy disordered matrices if the hyperfine interaction is purely isotropic. However the existence of anisotropic or dipolar interactions will generally broaden the ENDOR lines in disordered matrices, sometimes to the point where they are not detectable. Specific examples are discussed in Chapter 4.

Finally Abragam and Bleaney[6] have discussed the broadening effect of cross relaxation both between two electron spins and between two nuclear spins on ENDOR linewidths in solids. Since cross relaxation between two nuclear spins appears to increase the ENDOR linewidth by only about twofold in actual examples, it does not appear to be of great importance. Broadening due to cross relaxation between two radicals depends on the local concentration of radicals and can be minimized by optimizing the radical concentration.

1.5 ELDOR

1.5.1 Energy Levels

In order to show what magnetic parameters are measured by ELDOR, let us again consider the energy levels for a radical in solution where $S = \frac{1}{2}$, $I = \frac{1}{2}$. The anisotropic case is considered in Chapter 6 on ELDOR of radicals in solids. As in Section 1.4.1, the magnetic fields are assumed to be greater than 3000 G, in which case the electronic Zeeman term is usually larger than the nuclear Zeeman and hyperfine interactions. Thus the energy levels are given by eq. 1.5a, as discussed in Section 1.4.1, where second order hyperfine terms of the order of $A^2/g\beta H$ have been neglected. Figure 1-26 shows the energy levels for $A/2 > \nu_n$, a typical situation for most ELDOR studies recently reported. Even though the

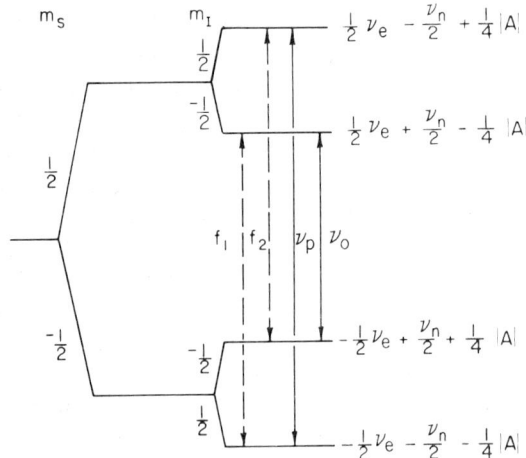

Figure 1-26. The energy level diagram (in Hz) at constant magnetic field for $S=\frac{1}{2}$, $I=\frac{1}{2}$ where $A>0$, $g_n>0$ and $A/2>\nu_n$. In an ELDOR experiment the allowed ESR transition ν_o is observed while the allowed ESR transition ν_p is pumped. Forbidden lines occur whenever $\Delta m_I = \pm 1$ and are given by frequencies f_1 and f_2.

ordering of the energy levels depends on the sign of A and on the relative magnitude of ν_n and $|A|/2$ as in Figs. 1-3 and 1-4, it is not necessary to consider the cases $A>\nu_n$ and $A<\nu_n$ separately as we did for ENDOR. Rather it is necessary to determine the pumped (ν_p) and the observed (ν_o) ESR transition frequencies, since ELDOR lines occur only at frequencies equal to the difference between these ESR transition frequencies. For example, in Fig. 1-26 $\nu_o = \nu_e - \frac{1}{2}|A|$ and $\nu_p = \nu_e + \frac{1}{2}|A|$, so an ELDOR transition will occur at $\nu_p - \nu_o = |A|$. A plot of the resulting ELDOR spectrum as a function of $(\nu_p - \nu_o)$ is given in Fig. 1-27a. Because both transitions are allowed ($\Delta m_s = \pm 1$, $\Delta m_I = 0$), we refer to the spectral line as an allowed-allowed ELDOR transition, the name of the ELDOR

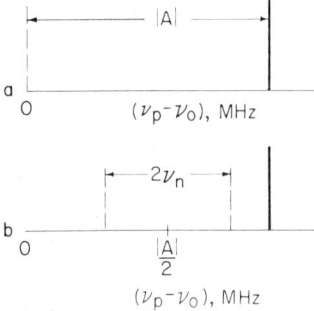

Figure 1-27. The observed ELDOR spectrum for the four energy level diagram given in Fig. 1-26 when (a) only allowed-allowed transitions occur, and (b) when allowed-allowed (solid line) and forbidden-allowed transitions (dashed lines) occur.

transition being constructed from the name of the pumped ESR transition followed by the name of the observed transition. Note also that the allowed-allowed transition does not depend on the nuclear Zeeman frequency ν_n but only on $|A|$. In the case of a radical with several nuclei interacting with an electron, second order corrections of the order $A^2/g\beta H$ must be taken into account. This is discussed in more detail in Chapter 6.

Other transitions are also possible when forbidden ($\Delta m_s = \pm 1$, $\Delta m_I = \pm 1$) ESR lines are pumped. For example, in Fig. 1-26 if frequency $f_2 (f_2 = \nu_e - \nu_n)$ is pumped and frequency $\nu_o (\nu_e - \frac{1}{2}|A|)$ is observed, a forbidden-allowed ELDOR transition is predicted at $\frac{1}{2}|A| - \nu_n$. On the other hand, if frequency $f_1 (f_1 = \nu_e + \nu_n)$ is pumped and frequency ν_o is observed, a forbidden-allowed ELDOR transition is predicted at $\frac{1}{2}|A| + \nu_n$. With significant transition probability for all possible forbidden-allowed ELDOR transitions, the ELDOR spectrum in Fig. 1-27b will result.

Further ELDOR experiments are also possible if forbidden ($\Delta m_s = \pm 1$, $\Delta m_I = \pm 1$) ESR signals are experimentally observed, as can quite often be the case in solids. In this event the forbidden ESR transition f_2 can be observed when the transition f_1 is pumped or the role of the pumped and observed transitions can be interchanged. In both situations a line is predicted to occur at $2\nu_n$. Note that in contrast to ENDOR, only when forbidden lines are pumped do the positions of the observed ELDOR lines depend on the magnitude of the magnetic field. Of course, whether these forbidden lines are experimentally observed depends on the transition probability of the forbidden pumped ESR transition and the amount of pump microwave power applied (see Section 1.5.2). In fact, the transition probability for forbidden ESR lines of radicals in solution is extremely small and the intensity of forbidden-allowed or forbidden-forbidden ELDOR lines is normally much weaker than that of the allowed-allowed ELDOR lines. So in liquids a pattern such as those given in Fig. 1-27a or b will result with intense lines at $|A|$ in addition to some weak forbidden lines. In the case of more than one equivalent interacting nucleus, intense allowed-allowed lines at $|A|$ and multiples of $|A|$ are observed.

In solids forbidden-allowed lines at $\frac{1}{2}|A| + \nu_n$ and $\frac{1}{2}|A| - \nu_n$ are typically much stronger and under certain conditions may make up the entire spectrum. In this case all the ELDOR line positions are field dependent, not just the weak ELDOR lines.

For the example given in Fig. 1-27, the pump frequency was chosen to be larger than the observing frequency. Experimentally the pumping frequency can also be smaller than the observing frequency, in which case

38   ESR AND DOUBLE RESONANCE

the ELDOR spectrum is plotted against $v_o - v_p$. The ELDOR spectra obtained will appear exactly like those given in Fig. 1-27.

1.5.2 ELDOR Mechanisms

1.5.2.1 Transient ELDOR

To consider an ELDOR response from an elementary point of view we will treat the various relaxation pathways and resultant population distribution assuming somewhat the same conditions as were used in Fig. 1-6 for ENDOR spectroscopy. That is, the four energy levels will be assumed to be in thermal equilibrium with T_{1e} and T_{1n} finite and all other relaxation processes will be assumed long enough to be considered effectively infinite. If we induce ESR transitions between levels 2 and 3 of Fig. 1-28a with microwave power sufficiently low to avoid saturation, the thermal equilibrium populations will be maintained by T_{1e} processes and will be equal to those given in Fig. 1-28a, where $\varepsilon \sim 10^{-3} = \beta H/kT$. Again the population differences between levels 4 and 3 and between 1 and 2 can be neglected because they are of the order of $g_n\beta_n H/kT$ ($\sim 10^{-6}$). In Fig. 1-28b we apply a second intense microwave frequency between

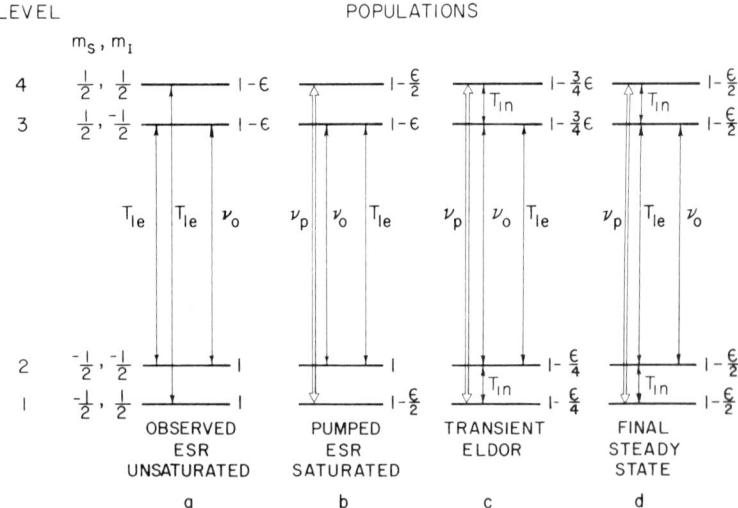

Figure 1-28. Population diagram for transient ELDOR with $S = \frac{1}{2}$, $I = \frac{1}{2}$, $A > 0$, $g_n > 0$, $|A|/2 > v_n$ (note similarity to Fig. 1-26) where T_{1e} and T_{1n} are finite and all other relaxation times are effectively infinite. In (c) the transient effect on populations when T_{1n} is short is shown, and when $T_{1n} \ll T_{1e}$ the final steady state in (d) is obtained.

levels 4 and 1. If sufficiently high microwave power is applied, levels 4 and 1 become saturated and equal to $1-\varepsilon/2$. In reality, the ability to saturate these levels completely will depend on the electron spin-lattice relaxation time. A portion of the spin population of level 4 will next be transferred to level 3 (or equivalently spin population in level 2 will be transferred to level 1) if the nuclear spin-lattice time (T_{1n}) is competitive with the electron spin-lattice relaxation time (T_{1e}). This results in a decrease in the population difference between levels 3 and 4 and 2 and 1 as given in Fig. 1-28c, causing a decrease to be observed in the ESR intensity of the transition 3–2. The difference in the observing ESR intensity before and after the pumping frequency has been applied is called ELDOR. Qualitatively it can be seen that the more nearly levels 1 and 4 are saturated, the greater the number of spins that can be transferred to level 3. Thus it follows that the ELDOR intensity increases with increasing pump power. The partial saturation of levels 2 and 3 can be looked at as an *increase* in the effective T_{1e}, and not as a decrease in the effective T_{1e}, as was the case for most ENDOR mechanisms discussed in Section 1.4.2. In Fig. 1-28 the magnitude of the pumping frequency is chosen to be larger than the observing frequency. Notice that this ELDOR mechanism will also permit an ELDOR response to be observed when the magnitude of the observing frequency is larger than that of the pumping frequency and the labels of the pumping and observing transitions are interchanged.

For the example given in Fig. 1-28, one would only obtain a transient ELDOR response, as all energy levels would eventually become equally populated (Fig. 1-28d) in the presence of a saturating pumping frequency and strong nuclear spin-lattice relaxation rates $(T_{1n} \ll T_{1e})$. Thus the observed ESR signal eventually decreases to zero intensity and a 100% reduction of the unsaturated ESR signal is observed.

1.5.2.2 Steady State ELDOR

Just as in the ENDOR studies, the response of a commercial ELDOR spectrometer is several seconds; so transient ELDOR cannot be obtained since T_{1e} is on the order of 10^{-2} sec or shorter for radicals in solution or for radicals in solids above 77 K. Thus the ELDOR spectra obtained with a commercial spectrometer result from steady state relaxation mechanisms. In the discussion of steady state ENDOR mechanisms, the steady state rate equations for the populations reduce to equations identical to those of an electrical circuit. In both ENDOR and ELDOR a change in the ESR intensity is analogous to a change in voltage between the observed energy levels. In the ENDOR case the rf power saturation of levels 3 and

4 in addition to the microwave power saturation of levels 2 and 3 effectively means that the voltage drop across 2 and 3 is the same as that across 2 and 4. This in turn implies that the change in voltage can be calculated simply as the voltage drop across two resistors placed in parallel. Thus a calculation of the change in resistance as done in Section 1.4.2.2 is adequate for predicting ENDOR enhancements.

The situation for ELDOR is not quite as straightforward. The four level energy diagram given in Fig. 1-29a depicts the relaxation times T_{1e}, T_{1n}, T_{x1}, and T_{x2} as defined in Section 1.4.2.2. An equivalent electrical circuit[24] is given in Fig. 1-29b with resistors T_{1e}, T_{1n}, T_{x1}, and T_{x2} and batteries V used to simulate the differences in the steady state population. Saturating levels 1–4 places a short circuit at 1–4 in Fig. 1-29b and results in Fig. 1-29c. The values of R_1, and R_2 for the equivalent circuits defined in Fig. 1-29d, are given by

$$\frac{1}{R_1} = \frac{1}{T_{n1}} + \frac{1}{T_{x1}} \quad \text{and} \quad \frac{1}{R_2} = \frac{1}{T_{n2}} + \frac{1}{T_{x2}} \qquad (1.15)$$

since resistors T_{1n} and T_{x1} as well as T_{1n} and T_{x2} are connected in parallel.

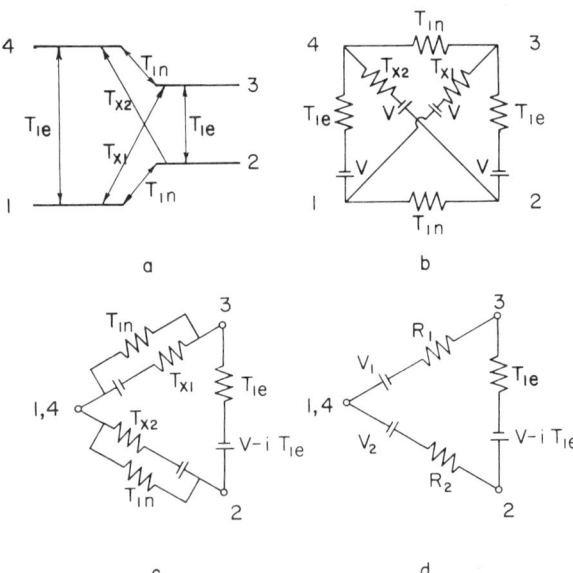

Figure 1-29. Electrical circuit analog for a steady state ELDOR: (a) four level energy diagram with relaxation times T_{1e}, T_{1n}, T_{x1}, and T_{x2}, (b) equivalent electrical circuit with resistors T_{1e}, T_{1n}, T_{x1}, and T_{x2} and batteries V, (c) equivalent electrical circuit when pathway 1 to 4 is short-circuited, (d) equivalent parallel circuit diagram for (c) in terms of resistors R_1 and R_2, voltages V_1 and V_2 where $1/R_1 = 1/T_{1n} + 1/T_{x1}$ and $1/R_2 = 1/T_{2n} + 1/T_{x2}$ and current i.

The voltages V_1 and V_2 can be calculated by application of Thevenin's theorem (a result of Kirchhoff's rules for electrical circuits). For instance, to calculate V_1 the circuit in Fig. 1-29c is first disconnected at points 1, 4, and 3, leaving only the upper portion of the circuit remaining. V_1 can then be calculated as the voltage drop across resistor T_{1n} for the partial circuit that includes T_{1n}, T_{x1}, and a battery V and is equal to

$$V_1 = \frac{VT_{1n}}{T_{x1} + T_{1n}}. \tag{1.16}$$

Further application of Thevenin's theorem to the partial circuit between point (1, 4) and 2 yields the value of V_2.

$$V_2 = \frac{VT_{1n}}{T_{x2} + T_{1n}}. \tag{1.17}$$

The short circuit changes the voltage across levels 2–3 from V to $V - iT_{1e}$ where iT_{1e} is the voltage drop across T_{1e} and i is the current, which is equal to

$$i = \frac{V - V_1 - V_2}{R_1 + R_2 + T_{1e}}. \tag{1.18}$$

The voltages V_1 and V_2 have opposite polarity to V and thus are negative in eq. 1.18. In this case the ELDOR reduction factor R (this is not a resistance) is defined as $V - (V - iT_{1e})/V = R$. Substituting V_1, V_2, R_1, and R_2 from eqs. 1.15, 1.16, and 1.17 into eq. 1.18 followed by substituting i into the definition of R gives

$$R = \frac{iT_{1e}}{V} = \frac{(1/T_{1n})^2 - (1/T_{x1}T_{x2})}{\left(\dfrac{1}{T_{1e}}\right)\left(\dfrac{2}{T_{1n}} + \dfrac{1}{T_{x1}} + \dfrac{1}{T_{x2}}\right) + \left(\dfrac{1}{T_{1n}} + \dfrac{1}{T_{x1}}\right)\left(\dfrac{1}{T_{1n}} + \dfrac{1}{T_{x2}}\right)} \tag{1.19}$$

upon rearranging.

This same result has been rigorously derived by Freed and co-workers[25,26] by solving for the reduction factor using a time dependent spin Hamiltonian. They found that the reduction factor is equal to the ratio of the double cofactor[7] $C_{oo',pp'}$ of the transition probability matrix W for the observed (o–o') and pumped (p–p') transitions to the double cofactor $C_{pp',pp'}$ of the transition probability matrix for the pumped transition. So we have

$$R = \frac{C_{oo',pp'}}{C_{pp',pp'}} \tag{1.20}$$

where $C_{oo',pp'}$ is the $o'p'$th cofactor of C_{op}, which is the opth cofactor of W. A cofactor C_{op} is equal to $(-1)^{o+p}$ times the matrix obtained by deleting the oth row and pth column of W. As an example of the calculation of R, the relaxation probability matrix for the four level diagram in Fig. 1-29a can be constructed[26] as eq. 1.21

$$W = \begin{array}{c} \\ \textcircled{1} \\ \textcircled{2} \\ \textcircled{3} \\ \textcircled{4} \end{array} \begin{bmatrix} \textcircled{1} & \textcircled{2} & \textcircled{3} & \textcircled{4} \\ W_n + W_e + W_{x1} & -W_n & -W_{x1} & -W_e \\ -W_n & W_n + W_e + W_{x2} & -W_e & -W_{x2} \\ -W_{x1} & -W_e & W_n + W_e + W_{x1} & -W_n \\ -W_e & -W_{x2} & -W_n & W_n + W_e + W_{x2} \end{bmatrix}$$

(1.21)

where W_n and W_e are the lattice-induced nuclear spin-flip and electron spin-flip transition probabilities, respectively, and W_{x1} and W_{x2} are the combined electron and nuclear spin transition probabilities. These transition probabilities are related to the relaxation times by the following relations:

$$W_n = \frac{1}{T_{1n}} \quad W_e = \frac{1}{T_{1e}} \quad W_{x1} = \frac{1}{T_{x1}} \quad W_{x2} = \frac{1}{T_{x2}} \quad (1.22)$$

Thus a short relaxation time T becomes a large probability W. The diagonal matrix elements are the negative sum of all the relaxation probabilities contained in the same row. The off-diagonal elements are simply the transition probabilities between the two states. For instance, W_{12} is just $-W_n$, which is the probability of a nuclear spin-flip proceeding from level 1 to level 2. The ordering of the elements of the matrix in eq. 1-21 is in the order of the energy levels 1, 2, 3, 4. The reduction factor from eq. 1.20 when observing transition 2–3 while pumping levels 1–4 equals

$$R = \frac{C_{23,14}}{C_{14,14}}. \quad (1.23)$$

To evaluate R the value of the double cofactor $C_{23,14}$ must be determined. To do this the cofactor C_{21} is first determined by striking out the second row and first column of eq. 1.21 to give eq. 1.24.

$$C_{21} = (-1)^3 \begin{bmatrix} \textcircled{2} & \textcircled{3} & \textcircled{4} \\ -W_n & -W_{x1} & -W_e \\ -W_e & W_n + W_e + W_{x1} & -W_n \\ -W_{x2} & -W_n & W_n + W_e + W_{x2} \end{bmatrix} \begin{array}{c} \textcircled{1} \\ \textcircled{3} \\ \textcircled{4} \end{array} \quad (1.24)$$

Next the C_{34} cofactor of matrix 1.24 is determined by striking out the row labeled 3 and the column labeled 4 to give

$$C_{34} = (-)(-1)^7 \begin{vmatrix} -W_n & -W_{x1} \\ -W_{x2} & -W_n \end{vmatrix} \begin{matrix} ① \\ ④ \end{matrix} = W_n W_n - W_{x1} W_{x2} = C_{23,14} \quad (1.25)$$

(columns labeled ② and ③)

Further application of this method yields the value of $C_{14,14}$ from which R can be evaluated by eq. 1.23.

$$R = \frac{W_n W_n - W_{x1} W_{x2}}{W_e(W_n + W_n + W_{x1} + W_{x2}) + (W_n + W_{x1})(W_n + W_{x2})} \quad (1.26)$$

Setting $W_n = 1/T_{1n}$, $W_e = 1/T_{1e}$, etc., shows that eq. 1.26 is equivalent to eq. 1.19 obtained by the electrical circuit analog. Because both the circuit analog and the matrix methods involve a fair amount of algebra, only the final reduction factor expressions will be given for the examples that follow.

A typical condition for the relaxation pathway of radicals in solution is $T_{1e} \sim T_{1n} \ll T_{x1}$ or T_{x2} or in the notation of Freed,[7] W_{x1} and $W_{x2} \approx 0$, with significant W_e and W_n processes. To derive the steady state populations in the presence of a saturating microwave pumping frequency the following conditions are noted for the four level diagram given in Fig. 1-28. The population of level 1(3) equals that of level 2(4) ($P_1 = P_2$ as well as $P_3 = P_4$) by thermal equilibrium (negligible differences occur from W_n processes); and the population of level 4 equals that of level 1 ($P_1 = P_4$) as a result of the saturating microwave pumping field. Solving for the populations and using the fact that $P_1 + P_2 + P_3 + P_4 = 4 - 2\varepsilon$ results in a population of $1 - \varepsilon/2$ for each level, as shown in Fig. 1-28*d*. Thus the observing transition ν_o intensity decreases to zero, or a 100% reduction is observed. Evaluating the reduction factor using eq. 1-26 gives $R = W_n(2W_e + W_n)^{-1} = T_{1n}^{-1}(2/T_{1e} + 1/T_{1n})^{-1}$. It is noted here that $R = 100\%$ only when $W_n \to \infty$, which is to say $T_{1n} \ll T_{1e}$. This is a quite unrealistic condition for radicals in solution. If $T_{1n} = T_{1e}$, then $R = \frac{1}{3}$, a 33% reduction. In addition, as the relaxation time T_{1n} increases, the reduction factor decreases until T_{1e} becomes much shorter than T_{1n}, in which case $R = 0\%$ and only T_{1e} processes predominate. Significant T_{1n} processes have been found by Freed and his co-workers[25] for nitroxide radicals in solution where electron-nuclear dipolar (END) relaxation dominates. This mechanism requires the electrons to relax back to the lower level of the pumped transition via a nuclear flip followed by an electron flip followed by a nuclear flip process.

Other dominant relaxation paths are also possible. For instance, when the relaxation probabilities are dominated by isotropic hyperfine modulation, then $T_{1n} \sim T_{x2} \gg T_{x1} \sim T_{1e}$ is possible, as previously discussed in

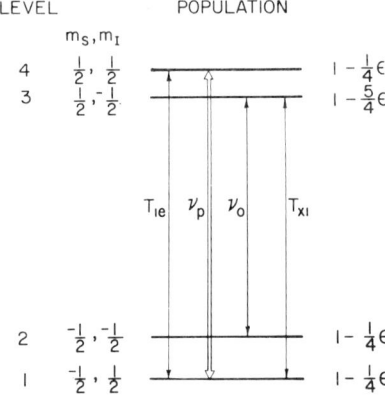

Figure 1-30. Population diagram for steady state ELDOR with $S=\frac{1}{2}$, $I=\frac{1}{2}$, $A>0$, $g_n>0$, and $|A|/2>\nu_n$. The populations shown are for the case where $T_{1e} \approx T_{x1} \ll T_{1n}$, T_{x2}, ν_p is the allowed ESR transition that is pumped and ν_o is the allowed ESR transition that is observed. A reduction factor of 0% is predicted.

Section 1.4.2.2 and shown in Fig. 1-30. Solving for the steady state population difference of level 2 and 3 from the requirements that $P_1 = P_4$ (saturation), $P_3 = P_1 - \varepsilon$ (thermal equilibrium), and $P_1 = P_2$ (thermal equilibrium) results in a difference of ε. This is the same difference as that found for the unsaturated four level case in the absence of a saturating microwave frequency; thus no change occurs in the observed ESR line and therefore $R = 0\%$. Evaluating R from eq. 1.26 gives the same result since $W_n = W_{x2} = 0$. A reduction factor equal to zero also occurs when $W_n^2 = W_{x1} W_{x2}$.

Significant T_{x1} and T_{x2} processes can occur when the relaxation is dominated by the modulation of the hyperfine anisotropy. The steady state population of the four level system when $T_{x1} \sim T_{x2} \sim T_{1e} < T_{1n}$ occurs is given in Fig. 1-31 for the condition $P_1 = P_4$ (saturation), $P_4 = P_2 - \varepsilon$, and $P_3 = P_1 - \varepsilon$ (thermal equilibrium). The population difference equals 2ε or an increase of ε over that for the unsaturated, four level case in the absence of pumping microwave power. Therefore an enhancement of the ESR line is observed. From eq. 1.26 with $W_n = 0$, the reduction factor is $R = -W_{x1} W_{x2} [W_e(W_{x1} + W_{x2}) + W_{x1} W_{x2}]^{-1}$. If $W_{x1} = W_{x2} = W_e = 1$, then $R = -\frac{1}{3}$, or a 33% enhancement of the ESR line. As W_n^2 increases, the magnitude of the enhancement will decrease until the product W_n^2 exceeds the product $W_{x1} W_{x2}$. At this point a reduced ELDOR line will be observed. This type of behavior is observed for the $(CH_3)_2\dot{C}COOH$ radical[27] where the variation in the rotational correlation time of the methyl groups with temperature alters the magnitude of W_{x2} and thus the sign of R.

Allowed-allowed ELDOR transitions do not give the only possible lines. If forbidden lines are pumped and allowed lines are observed,

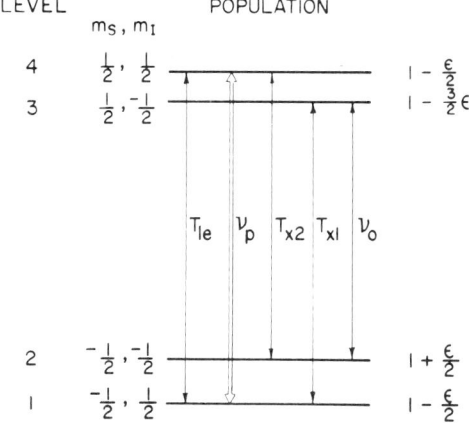

Figure 1-31. Population diagram for steady state ELDOR with $S=\frac{1}{2}$, $I=\frac{1}{2}$, $A>0$, $g_n>0$, and $|A|/2>\nu_n$. The populations shown are for the case where $T_{x1} \simeq T_{x2} \simeq T_{1e}$ and T_{1n} is infinite. An enhancement of the observed, allowed ESR intensity is predicted when the allowed ESR transition ν_p is pumped.

significant ELDOR intensity can be observed, providing that the transition probability of the forbidden line is not less than 10^{-4} of the main lines. The steady state population that occurs when strong T_{x1} or T_{1n} processes exist for a four level system is given in Figs. 1-32a and 1-32b, respectively, where the forbidden transition 2–4 is pumped and the allowed transition 2–3 is observed. A complete saturation of the observed transition is predicted in both cases. Calculation of $R = C_{23,24}/C_{24,24}$ by

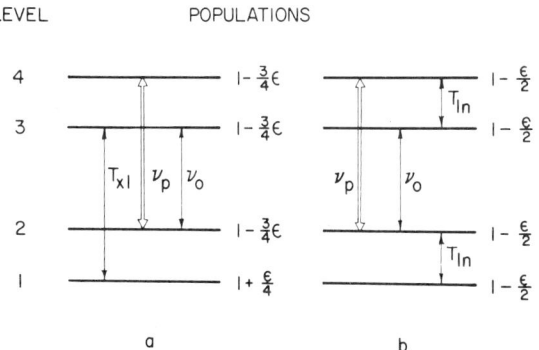

Figure 1-32. Population diagram for the steady state ELDOR with $S=\frac{1}{2}$, $I=\frac{1}{2}$, $A>0$, $g_n>0$, and $|A|/2>\nu_n$. The populations shown are for the cases where (a) $T_{x1}<T_{1e}$ and (b) $T_{1n}<T_{1e}$ and all other relaxation times are infinite. The observed ESR transition (ν_o) is allowed and the pumped ESR transition (ν_p) is forbidden. Large reductions are predicted in both cases.

the procedure given in eqs. 1.23 to 1.26 gives $R = (W_n + W_{x1}) \times [W_n + W_e + 2W_{x1}]^{-1}$. This implies that $R = 100\%$ when $W_n \gg W_e$ or W_{x1}, or in other words, when strong W_n processes exist. More typically, $W_n \sim W_{x1} \sim W_e$ so that for $W_n = W_{x1} = W_e = 1$, $R = 50\%$. In the event $W_{x1} = 0$ and $W_n = W_e = 1$, R also equals 50%. As either W_n or W_{x1} decreases, R decreases until $R = 0$, where only W_e processes dominate. Note also from the previous discussion that when allowed lines are pumped $R = 0$ for $W_n^2 = W_{x1}W_{x2}$, yet nonzero forbidden-allowed lines are observed under these conditions. This effect has been observed for the ELDOR lines from the $\dot{C}H(COOH)_2$ radical in irradiated malonic acid.[28] A similar case occurs if the forbidden transition 1–3 is pumped and the allowed transition 2–3 is observed. In this case $R = (W_n + W_{x2})[W_n + W_e + 2W_{x2}]^{-1}$ so that R depends on the magnitude of W_n or W_{x2} relative to W_e. Note that in both forbidden-allowed situations the R values can only be positive; thus only reductions are observed.

When ELDOR studies are carried out for radicals in single crystals, it is possible to observe forbidden ESR transitions; thus it is important to calculate the reduction factor and its dependence on the relaxation factors. As an example, if the forbidden 1–3 transition is observed and the forbidden 2–4 transition is pumped, $R = (W_n - W_e) \times [W_n + W_e + 2W_{x1}]^{-1}$. In this case a reduced ELDOR line will appear if $W_n > W_e$, whereas an enhanced line will occur if $W_e > W_n$. Since $W_e > W_n$ is a usual case in most situations, enhanced forbidden-forbidden lines are predicted. This has been demonstrated experimentally by Iwasaki and his co-workers[29] for a radical in irradiated single crystals of potassium hydrogen maleate. In fact in the limit of large W_e or when $W_{x1} = W_n = 0$, a 100% enhancement occurs. This, of course, assumes that the forbidden ESR lines can be observed in the ESR spectrum. Note also that in this example, predominant W_e processes give rise to enhanced lines, whereas ELDOR lines are absent whenever W_e processes predominate in the allowed-allowed or forbidden-allowed experimental situations described earlier.

In still another experiment, if the 1–3 forbidden ESR transition is observed and the 2–3 allowed transition is pumped, the calculated reduction factor in this case equals $(W_n + W_e)(W_n + 2W_e + W_{x2})^{-1}$. Again a reduction is predicted for all values of W_n, W_{x2}, and W_e. Particularly interesting is the fact that $R = 50\%$ for both $W_{x2} = W_n$ and $W_n = W_{x2} = 0$. Here again is a situation where ELDOR lines appear when only W_e processes predominate. Similarly, if the forbidden 2–4 transition is observed and the 2–3 allowed transition is pumped, $R = [(W_n + W_e)(W_n + W_{x1})][(W_n + 2W_e + W_{x2})(W_n + W_{x2})]^{-1}$; and again only a reduced line is observed. If W_e processes predominate, $R = 0\%$.

These reduction factor equations for an $S = \frac{1}{2}$ and $I = \frac{1}{2}$ four energy level system are summarized in Table 1-4 as a function of the observed and pumped transitions and different relaxation conditions.

So far we have only considered relaxation processes with a single spin system that affect the ELDOR signal intensity. As in ENDOR, spin exchange (such as Heisenberg exchange, chemical exchange, and spectral diffusion) between different spin systems alters the ELDOR intensity. Whereas spin exchange decreases ENDOR signals, it increases the ELDOR response. This can be seen by referring to Fig. 1-13 where the allowed 2–3 transition (of one radical) is observed and the 1–4 transition (of another radical) is pumped. The T_{ss} processes will transfer the saturation from the 1–4 levels to the 2–3 levels, causing a decrease in the observed ESR intensity. This means an increase in the ELDOR spectral intensity. In fact, calculation of R in the presence of significant T_{1n} and T_{ss} processes[25] shows that $R = C/(2+C)$ where $C = T_{1e}/T_{1n} + T_{1e}/2T_{ss}$. As $T_{ss} \to 0$, $C \to \infty$ and $R = 100\%$. It is to be noted that the T_{ss} process tends to equalize the population difference between all pairs of hyperfine levels and therefore can be regarded as a source of pseudonuclear spin-flips. Whereas certain intramolecular cross-relaxation processes can give rise to enhanced ELDOR spectra, the T_{ss} processes always result in reduced ELDOR spectra.

Although the four level energy diagram is extremely instructive for many ELDOR applications, multiple energy level schemes must be briefly discussed in order to introduce certain additional relaxation pathways that have been found to be important in some applications.

For the case of two nonequivalent protons,[30] eight energy levels must be considered corresponding to the two orientations of the electron and the four orientations of two nonequivalent protons (see Fig. 1-33). The rate of the induced nuclear spin transition W_n, the induced electron spin transition W_e, or the cross-relaxation pathway W_x in which one electron and one nuclear spin are simultaneously flipped can still be predominant; however, additional induced transitions as given in Fig. 1-33 are possible. For instance, a W'_n relaxation pathway where both nuclear spins and the electron spin are flipped can be an important relaxation pathway. In fact, it has been shown[30] that a cross-relaxation path W'''_x that is slightly different from W_x or W''_x is a particularly important relaxation pathway when two nonequivalent protons become symmetrically equivalent with increasing temperature. This causes the central four energy levels corresponding to the nuclear spin configuration $\alpha_n^1 \beta_n^2$ to become equivalent to the nuclear spin configuration $\beta_n^1 \alpha_n^2$. As these levels become degenerate a significant increase in the W'''_x processes indicated in Fig. 1-33 by the dashed lines is observed. This causes a strong variation in the intensity of

Table 1-4. ELDOR Reduction Factor Equations as a Function of the Type of Observed and Pumped Transitions and the Relaxation Conditions for a $S = \frac{1}{2}$ and $I = \frac{1}{2}$ Four Energy Level System

Relaxation Condition	Transition Pumped	Transition Observed	Reduction Factor R
$W_{x1} = W_{x2} = 0; W_n \neq W_e \neq 0^a$	1–4 (allowed)	2–3 (allowed)	$W_n/(2W_e + W_n)$
$W_n = W_{x2} = 0; W_{x1} \neq W_e \neq 0^b$	1–4 (allowed)	2–3 (allowed)	0
or			
$W_{n1}W_{n2} = W_{x1}W_{x2}$			
$W_n = 0; W_{x1} \neq W_{x2} \neq W_e^c$	1–4 (allowed)	2–3 (allowed)	$-W_{x1}W_{x2}/[(W_e(W_{x1} + W_{x2}) + W_{x1}W_{x2})]$
$W_n \simeq W_{x1} \simeq W_e^d$	2–4 (forbidden)	2–3 (allowed)	$W_n + W_{x1}/(W_n + W_e + 2W_{x1})$
$W_n \simeq W_{x1} \simeq W_e^d$	1–3 (forbidden)	2–3 (allowed)	$(W_n + W_{x2})/(W_n + W_e + 2W_{x2})$
$W_n \neq W_e \neq W_{x1} \neq W_{x2}^d$	2–4 (forbidden)	1–3 (forbidden)	$(W_n - W_e)/(W_n + W_e + 2W_{x1})$
$W_n \neq W_e \neq W_{x2} \neq W_{x1}^d$	2–3 (allowed)	1–3 (forbidden)	$(W_n + W_e)/(W_n + 2W_e + W_{x2})$
$W_n \neq W_e \neq W_{x2} \neq W_{x1}$	2–3 (allowed)	2–4 (forbidden)	$\dfrac{(W_n + W_e)(W_n + W_{x1})}{(W_n + 2W_e + W_{x2})(W_n + W_{x2})}$
$W_n \neq W_{ss} \neq 0$	1–4 (allowed)	2–3 (allowed)	$(W_n/W_e) + W_{ss}/2W_e$

[a] See Fig. 1-28.
[b] See Fig. 1-30.
[c] See Fig. 1-31.
[d] See Fig. 1-32.

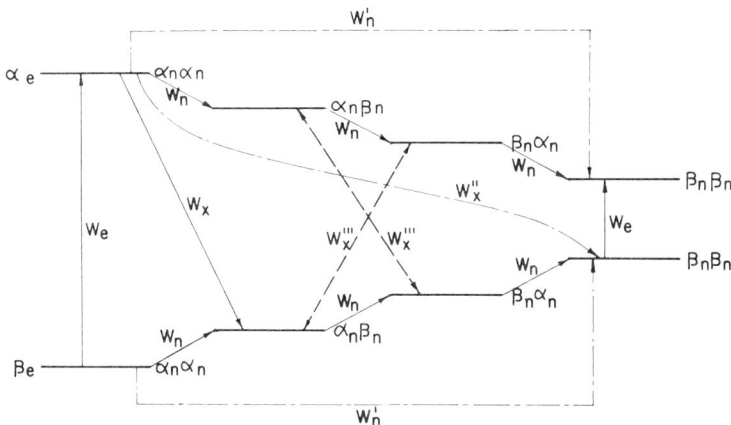

Figure 1-33. The eight level energy diagram for $S=\frac{1}{2}$, $I_1=\frac{1}{2}$, $I_2=\frac{1}{2}$, $A>0$, $g_n>0$, and $|A|/2>\nu_n$ showing the cross-relaxation pathways W_x, W_x'', and W_x''' that occur when there are two nonequivalent protons.

the observed ELDOR lines with temperature. In this instance the observed ELDOR spectrum reflects the "shorting out" of certain cross-relaxation times with respect to the electron spin-lattice relaxation time. Further discussions of these processes will be given in Chapter 6.

1.5.3 Spin Packet Model of ELDOR Linewidths

In Section 1.4.2.3, the packet-shifting and the ΔT_{1e} mechanisms were defined, and it was shown that the presence of either of these mechanisms in the absence of spin diffusion resulted in an ENDOR response for an inhomogeneous ESR line. An ELDOR response can also be observed from an inhomogeneous line by somewhat the same mechanisms if the definition of the spin packet width is redefined. The limiting spin packet width for the ENDOR response in solids depends on the neighboring nuclear-nuclear dipolar interaction, whereas the spin packet width associated with the ELDOR response depends on the neighboring electron-nuclear dipolar interaction. Thus the ELDOR linewidth can be 1000 times broader than the ENDOR linewidth (the ratio of the nuclear to electron moments), so lower resolution is observed. Despite this, the spin packet width, and the degree, if any, of spin diffusion between spin packets can be estimated by simulating the ELDOR line.

As an example let us consider the field swept ELDOR line given in Fig. 1-34 obtained from the one line ESR spectrum of the trapped electron in 10 M NaOH aqueous glass[31] at 77 K. A field swept ELDOR line is

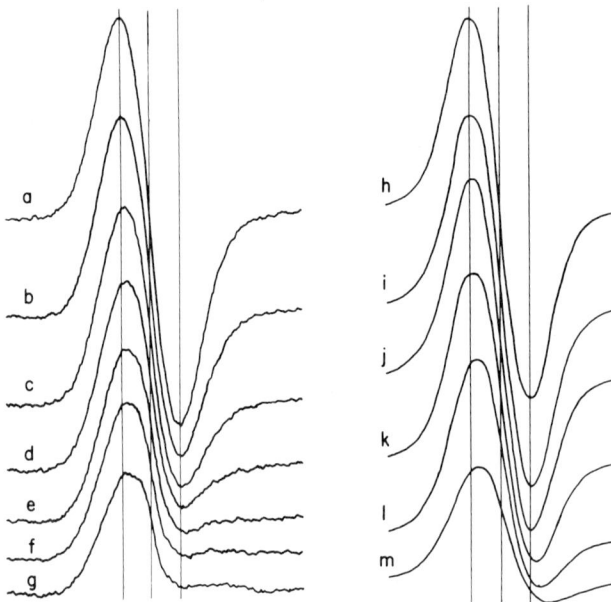

Figure 1-34. Field swept ELDOR spectra of trapped electrons in γ-irradiated 10 M NaOH glass at 115 K with $\nu_p - \nu_o = 20$ MHz. Observed spectra are shown on the left at various pumping powers: (a) −39 dB, (b) −25 dB, (c) −20 dB, (d) −15 dB, (e) −10 dB, (f) −5 dB, and (g) 0 dB. Simulated spectra are shown on the right for the saturation parameter S equal to (h) 0, (i) 0.1, (j) 0.3, (k) 1.0, (l) 3.0, and (m) 10.0 with the inhomogeneity parameter $a = 0.37$. From H. Yoshida, D. F. Feng, and L. Kevan, *J. Chem. Phys.*, **58**, 3411 (1973).

recorded as a function of varying the magnetic field while maintaining constant pump and observing frequencies at a fixed frequency separation. In the limit of zero pump power, the field swept ELDOR line is identical to the ESR line. To simulate the ELDOR response as a function of pump power and $\Delta\nu$, the difference in the pumping (ν_p) and observing (ν_o) microwave frequencies, the spin packet shape function is taken as Lorentzian with a half width at half height $\Delta\omega_L T_{2e}^{-1}$ and a Gaussian distribution of spin packets. The halfwidth at half height of the Gaussian line is taken as $\Delta\omega_G$ and the centers of the spin packets (ω') form a Gaussian distribution about ω_o, the center of the observed line. Since the spin packets are assumed not to interact, the pumping and the observing frequencies must be applied to the same spin packet to have any effect. After explicit forms of the lineshape functions are substituted into the equation for the imaginary part of the magnetic susceptibility χ'' at the observing frequency, χ'' can be calculated as a function of an inhomogeneity parameter a where $a = \Delta\omega_L/\Delta\omega_G$ and a saturation parameter S where $S = \gamma^2 H_{1p}^2 T_{1e} T_{2e}$, and H_{1p} is the microwave magnetic field of the pumping frequency. The observed ELDOR lineshape depends on whether the field modulation cycle time is more or less than T_{1e}.[31] For the example in Fig. 1.33 T_{1e} is longer than the field modulation time, and the derivative of χ'' with respect to the observing frequency $\omega_o(d\chi''/d\omega_o)$ must be calculated. The theoretical field swept ELDOR spectra given in Fig. 1-34h to m were obtained by using the parameters S and a that gave the best fit to the experimental spectra. The value of parameter a gives the spin packet width. Other parameters needed for the calculation of χ'', such as ω_p (the pump frequency), ω_o, and $\Delta\omega_G$, are experimentally known. It is to be noted that as the pump power increases, the high field peak decreases more rapidly than the low field peak and then both peaks shift slightly toward higher fields. The typical field swept ELDOR spectral lineshape observed as a function of $(\nu_p - \nu_o)$ is given in Fig. 1-35. As

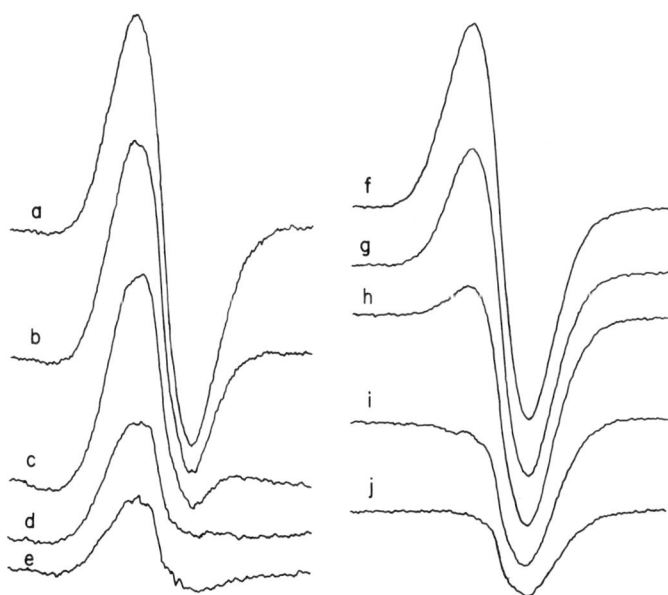

Figure 1-35. Field swept ELDOR spectra of trapped electrons in γ-irradiated 10 M NaOH glass at 77 K and measured at 115 K with $\nu_p - \nu_o$ equal to (a) 90, (b) 60, (c) 40, (d) 20, and (e) 10 MHz, and $\nu_p - \nu_o$ equal to (f) −90, (g) −50, (h) −40, (i) −20, and (j) −10 MHz at a pump power of 0 dB. From H. Yoshida, D. F. Feng, and L. Kevan, *J. Chem. Phys.*, **58**, 3411 (1973).

$(\nu_p - \nu_o)$ is decreased from 90 MHz, the high field part of the derivative spectrum decreases, then disappears; and then the low field part of the spectrum decreases. This process is interchanged when the pump frequency is less than the observing frequency and is in agreement with theory.

From the values of S and a, the values of T_{1e} and T_{2e} can be determined as a function of pump power; methods for determining T_{1e} and T_{2e} are given in ref. 31. If a unique set of values for T_{1e} and T_{2e} is calculated that is not dependent on pump power, then it is concluded that the noninteracting spin packet model is a correct model for the description of the inhomogeneous ESR line. However, for the example of trapped electrons in 10 M NaOH glass, a nonunique set of T_{1e} and T_{2e} values is obtained. This arises because spin diffusion actually occurs between spin packets so that desaturation of the observed spin packet occurs. This causes the experimental spectra to saturate more slowly with power than the simulated spectra, which assume no spin diffusion. As the pump power increases, the spin diffusion rate increases, which results in an apparent decrease in T_{1e}. Another way of saying this is that spin diffusion provides an additional relaxation path that is equivalent to

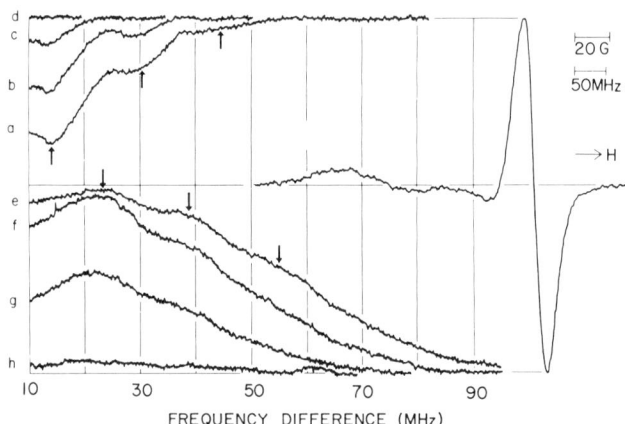

Figure 1-36. Frequency swept ELDOR spectra of trapped electrons in 10 M NaOH glass recorded at 115 K as a function of the frequency difference $\nu_p - \nu_o$ with $\nu_p > \nu_o$. The spectra were recorded at a pumping power level of (a) 0 dB, (b) −10 dB, (c) −20 dB, and (d) −39 dB when observing at the low field peak of the derivative ESR spectrum and at a pump power level of (e) 0 dB, (f) −10 dB, (g) −20 dB, and (h) −39 dB while observing at the high field peak of the ESR spectrum given at the right-hand side of the figure. Structure in the ELDOR spectrum is depicted by the arrows. From H. Yoshida, D. F. Feng, and L. Kevan, *J. Chem. Phys.*, **58**, 3411 (1973).

spin-lattice relaxation. Analysis of this effect shows that the apparent T_{2e} is approximately independent of pumping power.

Using a spin packet model in the presence of spin diffusion, the calculated frequency swept ELDOR spectra (obtained by maintaining the magnetic field and observing frequency ν_o constant while sweeping the pumping frequency ν_p and recording the spectra as a function of $\nu_p - \nu_o$) of an inhomogeneous line is shown to be a smoothly decreasing curve as the frequency difference $\nu_p - \nu_o$ increases. This is what is generally observed for the inhomogeneous line of the trapped electron in 10 M NaOH glass (Fig. 1-36) and for the inhomogeneous ESR line of the F-center studied by Moran[32] in x-irradiated KCl at 300 K. The frequency swept ELDOR lineshape will be discussed in further detail in Chapter 5. In both cases definite structure is observed. This structure can be attributed to hyperfine couplings or to second order transitions involving simultaneous spin-flips of e_t^- and neighboring nuclei. It is important to note that a frequency swept ELDOR line may give rise to structure that could not have been anticipated from the ESR spectrum. Such structure can be deduced by field swept spectra only if an exhaustive set of field swept ELDOR spectra are recorded with different pumping and observing frequency differences.

1.5.4 Modulation Frequency Dependence

In Section 1.5.5.2 the magnitude of the reduction (denoted by a positive R factor) or an enhancement (denoted by a negative R factor) of an ESR line for a four level system was shown to depend only on the relative magnitudes of the relaxation probabilities W_n, W_{x1}, and W_{x2} in relation to W_e. Experimentally the magnitude and the sign of the reduction factor have also been found to depend on the modulation frequency used in the experiment. The failure of the theory in Section 1.5.2.2 to predict this dependence is due to the fact that the R factors are calculated assuming the absence of any applied magnetic field modulation. ELDOR spectra can be obtained without using such modulation; however, magnetic field modulation is normally needed for sensitivity reasons. Qualitatively the modulation dependence arises in the following way.

If the modulation cycle time is slow compared to T_{1e}, the spin packets can relax in a manner dependent on W_e, W_n, W_{x1}, and W_{x2}. For instance, if $T_{1e} = 10^{-6}$ sec and the modulation frequency equals 100 Hz, the angular frequency $\omega_m = 2\pi \times 10^2$ sec and the cycle time is 1.6×10^{-3} sec, which is slow with respect to T_{1e}. However, when the modulation cycle time is comparable to or faster than T_{1e}, then there is insufficient time for the individual spin packets to relax via W_n, W_{x1}, or W_{x2} processes during each magnetic field modulation cycle. For instance, if $T_{1e} = 10^{-6}$ sec and the modulation frequency equals 100 kHz, the cycle time equals 1.6×10^{-6} sec, which is comparable to T_{1e}. Thus before the spin packets can relax, they are brought through resonance again, giving rise to a pseudorelaxation time dependent on modulation frequency. Since the reduction factors depend on the transition probabilities, which are inversely proportional to relaxation times, the reduction factors depend on the modulation frequency used and are especially sensitive to modulation cycle times of the same magnitude as T_{1e}.

Signals are also observed in various ESR experiments when the detectors are set 90° out of phase with the field modulation.[33,34] On the surface this appears difficult to understand, for we commonly say that no signal should be observed. In order to observe in-phase signals ($\theta = 0°$) but no out-of-phase signals ($\theta = 90°$) the magnetization M must follow the effective field H_{eff} (the resultant field due to the externally applied field, the microwave field, and the applied modulation field) during resonance. The condition that governs this is referred to as *adiabatic rapid passage*. Qualitatively this condition requires that H_{eff} must be swept through resonance fast enough with respect to T_{1e} that the magnetization does not relax back to a direction parallel to the applied magnetic field H_o during passage of H_{eff}. On the other hand, H_{eff} must not be swept through resonance so rapidly that the magnetization cannot maintain the initial relative angle between the magnetization and H_{eff}. When this angle does change, out-of-phase signals can be observed. Three effects can cause such a change in angle, namely, tumbling rates, high modulation frequencies, and large modulation amplitudes.

For example, in solution rotational diffusion processes cause individual spins of a radical to pass through resonance at varying rates because of the g and hyperfine splitting anisotropy. This can result[33,34] in a change in the phase relationship between M and H_{eff}. Similar effects can be observed when high modulation frequencies (comparable to T_{1e}) are employed. Of course the modulation amplitude can also influence this phase relationship as small changes in H_{eff} occur with modulation amplitude.

Because of the phase relationship between M and H_{eff}, the deduction of a relaxation time or other related parameters from the magnitude of the reduction factors must include the modulation phase amplitude and frequency. Such a calculation is not only difficult but may give rise to nonunique relaxation parameters.[34d] An examination of the magnitude of this effect will be given in Section 5.2.5 for radicals in solution and viscous media and in Section 6.2.9 for radicals in single crystals. Since T_{1e} is typically equal to 10^{-6} sec or longer for many organic radicals in solution, the R factors are usually dependent on modulation frequency when 100 kHz magnetic field modulation is used. However, in this book we quote the uncorrected reduction factors as given in the literature.

1.5.5 ELDOR Resolution

1.5.5.1 Resolution in Liquids

In Section 1.5.1 it was shown that if the observing frequency is set on a high field line of a well resolved ESR spectrum of an organic free radical and the pumping frequency is swept to higher frequencies, then each ESR line on the low field side of the spectrum is associated with an ELDOR line. In such an example the number of ELDOR lines equals the number of ESR lines. In general, the relative ELDOR line intensities are different from the ESR line intensities. For instance, combination lines often appear as a result of a change of more than one nuclear quantum number of a particular spin configuration in order to convert a molecule contributing to a pumped transition into a molecule contributing to an observed transition. These lines are generally weaker in intensity than transitions involving a single nuclear relaxation process. Thus it is not the number of lines as in ENDOR but rather the relative intensities of the ELDOR lines that determine the effective resolution.

It has also been found[35] that the intensity of the combination lines varies with temperature to a greater degree than the primary transitions, a feature that can be used to distinguish the two types of lines. It is also useful to obtain ELDOR spectra from different portions of the ESR spectrum, because different combination lines and thus different intensities do appear for these lines. By noting the different intensities, the primary line can be identified. The nitrogen hyperfine splittings for DPPH have been determined[35] by this latter technique.

The ELDOR linewidth also depends on the ESR spin packet width. If an inhomogeneously broadened ESR line such as obtained for DPPH is studied,[35] a significant increase in resolution can be obtained. However, because the experimental ELDOR linewidths have been found to be wider than the calculated spin packet width, it is difficult to predict the increase in resolution obtainable.

Field modulation can also decrease the resolution. The ELDOR lineshape of a well resolved ESR spectrum where the pump is swept is calculated to be a saturated Lorentzian[25] in the absence of field modulation. When field modulation is used,[35] the lineshape changes from $1/(1+\Delta\omega_p^2 T_{2e}^2 + d_p^2 T_{2e}\Omega_p)$ to $1/(1+\Delta\omega_p^2 T_{2e}^2 + d_p^2 T_{2e}\Omega_p)^2$ where T_{2e} is the transverse relaxation time, d_p is the transition moment for the electron spins and equal to $\frac{1}{2}\gamma_e H_1$, Ω_p is the saturation factor, subscript p prefers to pumping modes, and $\Delta\omega_p$ is the frequency deviation from the center of the pumped ESR lines.

It appears that ELDOR techniques are preferable to ENDOR when measuring large hyperfine splittings. This is because the nuclear relaxation is generally fast, which makes it difficult to saturate the nuclear transition as required for ENDOR. The short T_{1n} for such systems favors observation of ELDOR. Small hyperfine splittings are usually associated with longer T_{1n}, which make it difficult to observe ELDOR. Thus ELDOR spectra exhibit optimum resolution for a radical with one or two large splittings along with a number of smaller splittings such as for DPPH.[35] We discuss the analysis of DPPH in more detail in Chapter 4.

1.5.5.2 Resolution in Solids

The ESR spectral linewidth of organic radicals in crystals where resolvable hyperfine structure is not observed is approximately 8 to 12 MHz.[27] Typically the ELDOR linewidth is 3 to 5 MHz, which may be a decrease in the spectral linewidth by a factor of 2 to 3. In other cases in which fine structure is observed, such as for the $NH_2D^+\dot{C}DCOO^-$ radical in irradiated glycine,[36] where the inhomogeneous linewidth is 50 MHz, the ELDOR linewidth is still approximately 5 MHz. A particularly impressive increase in resolution occurs for chlorinated radicals,[37] where quadrupole relaxation enhances W_n-type processes so that only two intense ELDOR lines occur, whereas little intensity occurs from the forbidden ESR lines that give rise to a large number of lines in the ESR spectrum. In short, solid phase ELDOR spectra obtained from an inhomogeneous ESR line containing a large number of small splittings along with a few large splittings show the greatest effective resolution enhancement.

REFERENCES

1. G. Feher, *Phys. Rev.*, **103**, 834 (1956).
2. G. Feher and E. A. Gere, *Phys. Rev.*, **114**, 1245 (1959).
3. G. Feher, *Phys. Rev.*, **114**, 1219 (1959).
4. E. C. McIrvine, J. Lambe, and N. Laurance, *Phys. Rev.*, **136**, A467 (1964).
5. G. Breit and I. I. Rabi, *Phys. Rev.*, **38**, 2072 (1931).
6. A. Abragam and B. Bleaney, *EPR of Transition Ions*, Oxford University Press, London, 1970, Chapter 4.
7. J. H. Freed, *J. Chem. Phys.*, **43**, 2312 (1965).
8. G. Feher, C. S. Fuller, and E. A. Gere, *Phys. Rev.*, **107**, 1462 (1957).
9. G. R. Trammell, H. Zeldes, and R. Livingston, *Phys. Rev.*, **110**, 630 (1958).

10. J. S. Hyde, *J. Chem. Phys.*, **43**, 1806 (1965).
11. J. H. Freed, *J. Phys. Chem.*, **71**, 38 (1967).
12. G. Feher, *Physica*, **24**, 580 (1958).
13. R. W. Terhune, J. Lambe, G. Makhov, and L. G. Cross, *Phys. Rev. Lett.*, **4**, 234 (1960).
14. J. Lambe, N. Laurance, E. C. McIrvine, and R. W. Terhune, *Phys. Rev.*, **122**, 1161 (1961).
15. W. Th. Wenckebach, L. A. H. Schreurs, H. Hoogstraate, T. J. B. Swanenburg, and N. J. Poulis, *Physica*, **52**, 455 (1971).
16. J. S. Hyde, G. H. Rist, and L. E. G. Eriksson, *J. Phys. Chem.*, **72**, 4269 (1968).
17. G. Feher and R. A. Isaacson, *J. Mag. Res.*, **7**, 111 (1972).
18. R. C. McCalley and A. L. Kwiram, *Phys. Rev. Lett.*, **24**, 1279 (1970).
19. N. M. Atherton, A. J. Blackhurst, and I. P. Cook, *Chem. Phys. Lett.*, **8**, 187 (1971).
20. I. Miyagawa, R. B. Davidson, H. A. Helms, and B. A. Wilkinson, *J. Mag. Res.*, **10**, 156 (1973).
21. J. H. Freed, D. S. Leniart, and J. S. Hyde, *J. Chem. Phys.*, **47**, 2762, (1967).
22. G. Feher, *Phys. Rev.*, **105**, 1122 (1957).
23. J. S. Hyde, in *Magnetic Resonance in Biological Systems*, A. Ehrenberg, B. G. Malmström, and T. Vänngard, eds., Pergamon, London, 1967, p. 63.
24. S. Clough, personal communication.
25. J. S. Hyde, J. C. W. Chien, and J. H. Freed, *J. Chem. Phys.*, **48**, 4211 (1968).
26. J. H. Freed, *Electron Spin Relaxation in Liquids*, L. T. Muus and P. W. Atkins, eds., Plenum, New York, 1972, pp. 503–530.
27. L. D. Kispert, K. Chang, and C. M. Bogan, *J. Chem. Phys.*, **58**, 2164 (1973).
28. G. H. Rist and J. H. Freed, personal communication.
29. M. Iwasaki, K. Toriyama, and K. Nunome, *J. Chem. Phys.*, **61**, 106 (1974).
30. L. D. Kispert, K. Chang, and C. M. Bogan, *J. Phys. Chem.*, **77**, 629 (1973).
31. H. Yoshida, D. F. Feng, and L. Kevan, *J. Chem. Phys.*, **58**, 3411 (1973).
32. P. R. Moran, *Phys. Rev.*, **135**, A247 (1964).
33. J. S. Hyde and L. Dalton, *Chem. Phys. Lett.*, **16**, 568 (1972).
34. J. S. Hyde and D. D. Thomas, *Ann. N. Y. Acad. Sci.*, **222**, 680 (1974); (b) L. A. Dalton, J. L. Monge, L. R. Dalton, and A. L. Kwiram, *Chem. Phys.*, **6**, 166 (1974); (c) P. W. Percival, J. S. Hyde, L. A. Dalton, and L. R. Dalton, *J. Chem. Phys.*, **62**, 4332 (1975); (d) A. Abragam, *The Principles of Nuclear Magnetism*, Clarendon, Oxford, 1961, p. 85.
35. J. S. Hyde, R. C. Sneed, Jr., and G. H. Rist, *J. Chem. Phys.*, **51**, 1404 (1969).
36. L. D. Kispert, K. Chang, and P. S. Wang, *J. Mag. Res.*, **14**, 339 (1974).
37. L. D. Kispert, K. Chang, and C. M. Bogan, *Chem. Phys. Lett.*, **17**, 592 (1972).

2. Experimental Methods

2.1 Introduction—ESR Instrumentation
    2.1.1 The Resonant Cavity—ESR
    2.1.2 Cavity Sensitivity
    2.1.3 Microwave Source
    2.1.4 Modulation
2.2 Introduction—ENDOR Instrumentation
    2.2.1 Types of ENDOR Spectrometers
    2.2.2 Varian ENDOR Cavity
        2.2.2.1 ENDOR Cavity—External View
        2.2.2.2 ENDOR Cavity—Internal View
        2.2.2.3 ENDOR Cavity—Microwave Modes
2.3 Critical Operating Parameters—ENDOR
    2.3.1 Sensitivity and Magnetic Field Homogeneity and Stability
    2.3.2 Sample Size
    2.3.3 Introduction of rf Power into Cavity
    2.3.4 Rf Power Level—Cw Versus Pulsed Schemes
    2.3.5 Mode of Detection and Modulation Scheme
2.4 Introduction—ELDOR Instrumentation
    2.4.1 Varian ELDOR Cavity
        2.4.1.1 ELDOR Cavity—External View
        2.4.1.2 ELDOR Cavity—Internal View
        2.4.1.3 ELDOR Cavity—Microwave Modes
    2.4.2 ELDOR Spectral Presentation
    2.4.3 Traveling Wave Helix
2.5 Critical Operating Parameters—ELDOR
    2.5.1 Isolation of Microwave Modes
    2.5.2 Temperature Control
    2.5.3 Magnetic Field Stability

2.6 Limitations—ENDOR
    2.6.1 Frequency Range of Commercial ENDOR Instruments
    2.6.2 Sensitivity
    2.6.3 Saturable Transitions
2.7 Limitations—ELDOR
    2.7.1 Frequency Range
    2.7.2 Radical Concentration
    2.7.3 Temperature Range
    References

2.1 INTRODUCTION—ESR INSTRUMENTATION

There are many excellent books that explain the experimental details of an ESR spectrometer. The beginner will find the books by Wertz and Bolton[1] and by Atherton[1] to be excellent descriptions of the fundamentals of ESR spectroscopy; more technical details can be found in books by Poole,[2] Wilmshurst,[3] and Alger.[4] Before typical ENDOR and ELDOR experimental setups are described, a brief review is given of the terms and the basic phenomena essential to the understanding of the operations of ESR, ENDOR, and ELDOR spectrometers.

Both ENDOR and ELDOR spectrometers include a standard ESR spectrometer plus additional apparatus to produce the second frequency used. The most frequently used ESR spectrometer operates at a microwave frequency of 9.5 GHz (3.1 cm wavelength), which requires a magnetic field of approximately 3200 G for ESR signals to be observed from most organic radicals. The heart of the ESR, ELDOR, and ENDOR spectrometers is the resonant cavity, which contains the sample and directs and controls the microwave beam to and from the sample. The absorption of microwaves by the sample is monitored, amplified, and recorded by the detection and modulation systems. To provide a resonant condition requires a stable, linearly variable, and homogeneous magnetic field of arbitrary magnitude.

2.1.1 The Resonant Cavity—ESR

To understand the behavior of an ESR cavity at microwave frequencies, analogy can be made to the behavior of nearly any closed vessel or resonant cavity at acoustic frequencies. As a specific example consider the operations of a trombone. Different musical notes can be obtained from a trombone, depending on the position of the slide. A given musical note will be produced when the fundamental wavelength of the sound is a multiple of the dimension of the slide (resonant cavity). Intermediate positions will produce dischordant sounds resulting from destructive interference at wavelengths that are not multiples of the resonant cavity dimension. In a somewhat similar manner the fundamental resonant frequency in an ESR cavity is determined by the cavity dimensions. For cavity dimensions of $1.7 \times 0.9 \times 0.45$ in., the fundamental frequency occurs at a microwave frequency of 9.5 GHz. Any absorption of this fundamental resonance by a sample will disturb the resonance frequency, which can in turn be detected by the proper circuitry.

A given microwave frequency consists of a magnetic field component that lies perpendicular to an electric field component. The magnetic field (H_1) component of the microwaves is used to detect free radicals by monitoring the changes in the net magnetic dipole of the free radicals. In order to accomplish this, only a few of the many wave patterns (modes) that can be produced in a cavity resonator are used. The particular mode used depends on the shape and size of the cavity, which permits the placement of the sample at the maximum H_1 field and maintains H_1 perpendicular to the static field. For the often used rectangular-parallelepiped cavity, this is normally the TE_{102} mode, where TE stands for transverse electric and the subscripts designate the number of half-wavelengths along the A, B, and C directions, respectively (see Fig. 2-1).

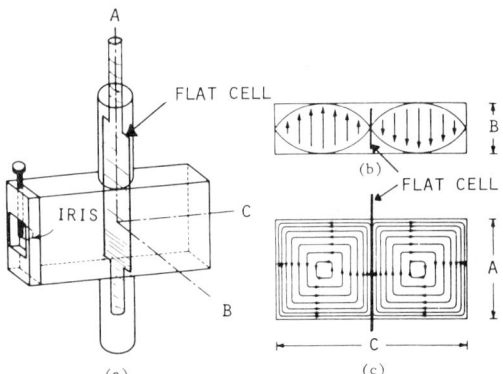

Figure 2-1. A rectangular parallelepiped TE_{102} microwave cavity. (*a*) A flat cell sample holder is positioned parallel to the B direction in the center of the cavity by the cylindrical extensions above and below the cavity. The microwave energy is coupled into the cavity through the iris hole. (*b*) The electric field contours in the BC plane. The flat cell is positioned so as to be in the nodal plane of the electric field. (*c*) Magnetic field flux in the AC plane. The flat cell is positioned in the plane of the maximum microwave magnetic field. The A direction is approximately one half-wavelength and C is exactly two half-wavelengths. Adapted from J. E. Wertz and J. R. Bolton, *Electron Spin Resonance*, McGraw-Hill, New York, 1972.

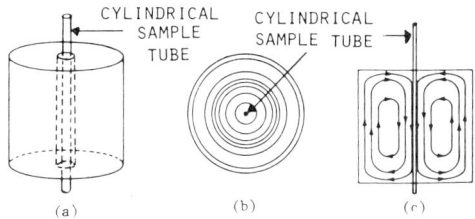

Figure 2-2. A cylindrical TE$_{011}$ microwave cavity. (a) The capillary sample tube is placed at the center of cylindrical cavity. (b) Electric field contours. The sample is placed along a line where $E = 0$. (c) Magnetic field contours. The sample is situated where the magnetic field is a maximum. Adapted from J. E. Wertz and J. R. Bolton, *Electron Spin Resonance*, McGraw-Hill, New York, 1972.

For a TE$_{102}$ mode the microwave magnetic field is found to be a maximum in a plane that bisects the center of the cavity. In this plane the electric field is a minimum (effectively zero). Another often used cavity is the cylindrical cavity. In this case a TE$_{011}$ mode is used where the maximum microwave magnetic field is found in a cylindrical area (a line) at the center of the cavity and H_1 is typically higher by a factor of $\sqrt{3}$ than in the TE$_{102}$ rectangular cavity (see Fig. 2-2).

In some cases the ESR cavity is replaced by a microwave helix. A microwave helix is a broad-band device that consists of a helical coil approximately 3 mm in diameter made of gold wire which can support a microwave frequency over a wide range of frequencies. The H_1 field varies periodically along the helix with a maximum in the center of the helical coil.

2.1.2 Cavity Sensitivity

The ability of the cavity to respond to an absorption of energy, which is proportional to H_1^2, is represented by the symbol Q. The larger the Q, the more sensitive is the cavity to small changes in energy absorption. However, at a certain value of Q, an increase in Q also means an increase in noise. Since the optimum signal-to-noise ratio obtainable is normally required for a successful performance of an ESR experiment, a cavity with an optimum Q is used. The rectangular and cylindrical cavities used today usually possess unloaded Q's (without sample or variable temperature dewar) of 7000 and 20,000, respectively. On the other hand, the Q of the microwave helix is less than that of the rectangular and cylindrical cavity and is typically no larger than 1200.

The cavity sensitivity is also dependent on the number of hyperfine lines associated with a given radical. As the number of hyperfine lines increases, the signal height of any individual line decreases, and thus the ability to detect a free radical decreases. This occurs because the single ESR line produced by an electron is split into additional lines for each interaction with a nuclear spin. For example, when the electron interacts with a proton or with a fluorine or carbon-13 nucleus, the electron ESR line is split into two lines. The importance of this can be demonstrated by the following example.

The theoretical minimum concentration of radicals detectable by a spectrometer operating at 9.5 GHz is approximately 10^{-9} M for a sample that requires 100 mW of microwave power to produce a one line ESR spectrum with a linewidth of 1 G.[1] However, many ESR investigations are carried out at lower microwave powers such as 1 mW to avoid serious saturation and thus serious distortion of the ESR line. Since the ESR signal intensity increases with the square root of the microwave power, the best that one can hope to detect at 1 mW is 10^{-8} M. Even this assumes that only one line will be observed in the ESR spectrum. Since most spectra of interesting radicals do contain hyperfine lines, the minimum detectable number of radicals is increased by D_i/D_k, where D_k is the degeneracy of the most intense line and D_i is the sum of the degeneracies of all the lines in the spectrum. Calculations for systems of chemical interest show that approximately 10^{-7} M is a practical limit of radicals detectable.

The cavity sensitivity is also related to the type of cavity used to study a given sample. If the sample has been dissolved in a very polar solvent, such as water or sulfuric acid, only very small sample tubes (1 mm i.d. capillary tubes for cylindrical cavities, as in Fig. 2-2, and flat cells for rectangular cavities, as in Fig. 2-1) can be used. This is to ensure that when the sample is placed in the cavity, the solution will be located where the microwave H_1 field is at or near a maximum and the microwave electric field is at or near zero. This prevents a severe loss of ESR signal intensity due to the absorption of microwaves by the electric field interacting with the large dielectric constant of the polar solvent; this is generally referred to as a high dielectric loss. It turns out that for polar materials a rectangular cavity gives the best signal-to-noise ratio primarily because the flat cell (0.05 cm^3) contains five times the volume of an optimum-sized capillary tube (0.01 cm^3). On the other hand, if a sample is limited in size, which occurs for many biological materials, or if the samples have very small or no dielectric loss (nonpolar materials such as paramagnetic defects in irradiated organic crystals, triplet states in glasses and crystals, or dilute radicals in nonpolar solvents such as ethylbenzene or toluene), a signal-to-noise ratio larger by 1.5 to 2.25 will be obtained from a cylindrical cavity because of the higher cavity Q while maintaining the same sample size.

When a microwave helix is used, the sample size for nonpolar materials is limited by the dimensions of the helix, which is typically 3 mm o.d. and 40 mm in length. However, for polar samples the dielectric loss limits the size to approximately 1 mm o.d. and 40 mm in length. Because of the greater filling factor, the sensitivity is similar to that of a rectangular or cylindrical cavity despite the lower Q.

Sensitivity can be increased by going to higher frequency such as 30 to 40 GHz because sensitivity is proportional to the frequency squared. However, the cavity dimensions at 35 GHz are only a few millimeters and the sample volume in a flat cell decreases to 0.02 cm^3. So the effective sensitivity is little increased unless samples are size limited. The dielectric loss also increases with frequency, which makes it difficult to study aqueous samples at higher frequencies. However, work at 35 GHz can be profitable for single crystals and samples with low dielectric loss.

2.1.3 Microwave Source

The microwave radiation needed for an ESR transition to occur at 3200 G is produced by a vacuum tube called a klystron. This vacuum tube can be tuned only over a very small frequency range, and thus most ESR spectrometers operate at a constant klystron frequency. The microwave energy from the klystron is coupled to the cavity by a small hole in the cavity body referred to as an iris (see Fig. 2-1). The iris prevents the reflection of microwaves from imperfections in the construction of the cavity, or from the different sizes and shapes of the waveguides. If this is not done, standing waves result from these reflections and appear at the detector, effectively decreasing the sensitivity of the instrument. With a properly adjusted iris, microwave power changes at the detector arise only from the absorption of microwave energy by the sample. When a microwave helix is used, the impedance of the helix must be matched to the transmission line by using microwave shielding and a reflector plate at one end of the helix.

To vary the level of microwave power incident upon the sample, an attenuator is placed between the output of the klystron and the sample. The attenuator contains an absorptive element that blocks a portion of the power from the klystron from reaching the sample and causing an ESR transition.

2.1.4 Modulation

Unless the sample contains a high concentration of radicals, the signal to the detector normally is so weak that noise components over a wide range

64 EXPERIMENTAL METHODS

of frequencies compete with or mask the ESR signal. Therefore a small alternating magnetic field at a known frequency (referred to as modulation) is superimposed on the static field by a field modulation unit. In this way the magnetic field passes periodically through the resonant field of the radical, resulting in a superposition of this modulation frequency on the ESR absorption signal. The combination of signals along with a large number of noise components is fed to a phase sensitive detector. This detector will amplify only those signals that contain the superimposed modulation frequency and phase and will reject other signals occurring out of phase and frequency. Thus only the ESR signal is amplified. An input absorption signal, modulated by the magnetic field, to this type of detector always appears as a first derivative of the absorption signal at the output.

2.2 INTRODUCTION—ENDOR INSTRUMENTATION

A simplified block diagram of an ENDOR spectrometer is shown in Fig. 2-3 with that portion that belongs to a basic ESR spectrometer outlined by the narrowly ruled lines. The ESR spectrometer consists of a klystron, which supplies the microwave frequency; field modulation coils, which support the modulation frequency and produce a modulation magnetic field in a direction parallel to the external field direction; the microwave and phase sensitive detectors; the cavity; a temperature and magnetic field controller; the magnet that supplies the magnetic field; and a recorder for displaying the ESR spectrum as a function of the magnetic field.

The ENDOR spectrometer is comprised of those components schematically outlined by heavy lines. This includes the rf oscillator and the rf power amplifier. The rf power must be of sufficient magnitude (as high as 200 W average) to saturate NMR transitions within the sample under investigation. The rf coils are placed inside the ESR cavity in such a manner that the rf magnetic field is perpendicular to the applied external static magnetic field. When the ESR cavity is replaced by a microwave helix, the rf coils are placed outside the helix.

The frequency output of the rf oscillator also serves as the drive for the X axis (frequency axis) of the recorder. The ENDOR signal output from the phase sensitive detectors is applied to the Y axis of the recorder.

Before an ENDOR spectrum can be observed, an ESR spectrum is obtained by sweeping the magnetic field, using magnetic field modulation whose amplitude is less than the ENDOR linewidth in kilohertz divided

INTRODUCTION—ENDOR INSTRUMENTATION

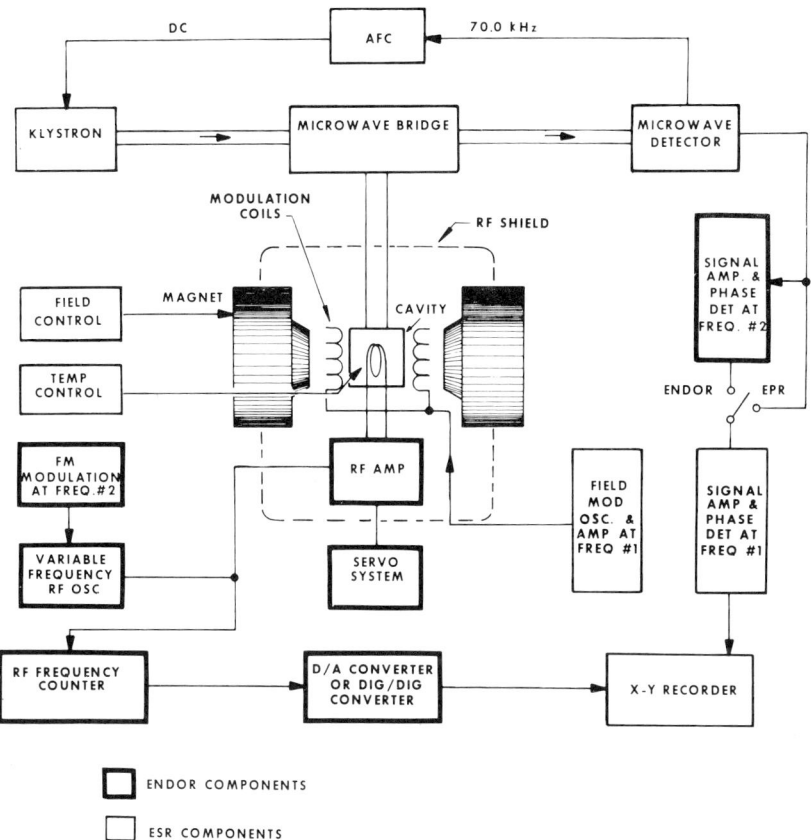

Figure 2-3. Block diagram of an ENDOR spectrometer. The heavily ruled lines outline the components added to a standard ESR spectrometer. In particular a variable frequency oscillator and amplifier, a second modulation and phase detector in addition to a rf counter are required. Reproduced by courtesy of the Varian Instrument Division.

by the gyromagnetic ratio of a proton (4.2 kHz G^{-1}) and using a microwave power that produces partial saturation. Next the applied magnetic field is positioned on an ESR line of interest, and the radio frequency is swept over the expected range for NMR transitions. Any change in the ESR line caused by a change in the populations of the energy levels, when an NMR transition occurs, results in a change in the output of the phase sensitive detector that serves as the Y axis drive for the recorder. In addition, the X axis of the recorder is driven by the output of the rf oscillator so that a spectrum of radiofrequency versus difference in ESR signal amplitude (ENDOR signal) is recorded.

2.2.1 Types of ENDOR Spectrometers

ENDOR spectrometers fall into two classes, low power and high power. Two types of low power ENDOR spectrometers have been described.[5-19] One type is used to carry out ENDOR investigations on solid samples with extremely long relaxation times (~1 to 10 sec or longer), where only field modulation and continuous rf power of approximately 0.1 W are used. A second type that is used to investigate samples, usually solids, having intermediate relaxation times (10^{-4} to 1 sec) employs somewhat higher rf power (~1 W) along with some combination of magnetic field or nuclear rf amplitude modulation. At these low rf power levels the rf range can extend from 1 to 400 MHz. High power ENDOR (10 to 500 W) is used for studying liquids as well as solids having short ($<10^{-4}$ sec) relaxation times. Various modulation schemes are used. However, as in the case of low power ENDOR, the modulation frequencies must be lower than the relaxation probabilities so that the spin system can follow the modulations. There are two types of high power ENDOR spectrometers: continuous wave (cw)[20-25] and pulsed.[26] The cw high power ENDOR spectrometers employ wideband (1 to 220 MHz) power amplifiers (10 to 500 W) that enable experiments to be carried out with the radiofrequency being continuously swept and detected from 1 to 200 MHz. The pulsed high power ENDOR simultaneously pulses the rf field and the detectors on and off as the frequency is swept. Normally 1000 W of radiofrequency are pulsed over a frequency range of from 5 to 50 MHz. Commercial ENDOR spectrometers are currently available from Varian Instrument Division, JEOL, and Bruker.

The commercial JEOL[25] ENDOR spectrometer (Model ES-EDX1) consists of a cylindrical ESR cavity with the rf coils placed inside in addition to a broad-band amplifier (3 to 50 MHz) that provides 10 to 200 W rf power and is therefore classed as a cw high power ENDOR spectrometer. The JEOL ENDOR unit also uses a frequency of 6.5 kHz to frequency-modulate the radiofrequency, in addition to an 80 Hz magnetic field modulation. A portion of the ESR signal detected by the microwave detector is amplitude-modulated at 80 Hz, whereas that portion of the ESR signal occurring as a result of the presence of a radiofrequency (ENDOR) is amplitude-modulated at both 6.5 kHz and 80 Hz. Passage of this signal through a phase sensitive detector at 6.5 kHz amplifies all 6.5 kHz modulation components of the ESR signal. However, this amplified ESR signal will still contain the 80 Hz component. Phase sensitive detection of this signal at 80 Hz will amplify only the ENDOR portion of the ESR signal. By using this combination of modulation frequencies, an increase in sensitivity can be obtained[26] over that when only a single modulation frequency is used.

The commercial Bruker ER 420 ENDOR spectrometer[20] employs a microwave helix instead of a microwave cavity. The microwave helix has a diameter of 3 mm and is embedded in a Teflon mounting to provide mechanical stability. An rf coil, having a diameter of 12 mm, constructed from two coils connected in parallel, each consisting of 13 turns of silver-plated copper wire, is wrapped around the microwave helix. This arrangement allows for rf fields up to 18 G in the rotating frame to be reached using a 20-W rf amplifier. Because of the size of the microwave helix, the sample size is limited to less than 3 mm o.d. diameter tubes. By using interchangeable rf coils, an rf sweep range from 1 to 80 MHz can be obtained; however, typically a sweep range of from 8 to 38 MHz is possible with one coil. A 20-W amplifier is used with amplification possible from 250 kHz to 80 MHz. The ENDOR signals are obtained by frequency-modulating the radiofrequency at 9.3 kHz followed by phase sensitive detection. It is also possible to detect ENDOR signals by field modulation at this frequency followed by phase sensitive detection.

On the other hand, the rf power is pulsed in the commercial Varian E-700 ENDOR spectrometer attached to the Varian E-line ESR spectrometers.[26,27] A block diagram of the Varian ENDOR spectrometer is given in Fig. 2-4. The 1000 W of rf power are frequency-modulated at 6 kHz. In order to reduce the sample and cavity heating arising from the intense rf fields, the rf fields are pulsed with a duty cycle that can vary from 10 to 50% so that the average power dissipated to the cavity varies from 100 to 500 W. By turning the detector on during the time that the radiofrequency is pulsed on, the ESR signals are amplified only during the rf pulses, thus preventing the amplification of noise during the off time. The magnetic field is also modulated at 35 Hz and the signal is phase sensitive detected at 35 Hz.

If the observed ESR linewidths are smaller than about 3 G, then the magnetic field and the klystron frequency must be held very constant so that the resonant condition does not change and detection always occurs at the peak of the ESR line. In normal ESR an automatic frequency control (AFC) stabilizes the microwave frequency and a Hall Probe feedback loop separately controls the magnetic field stability. Increased stability for ENDOR is provided by a field frequency lock system that stabilizes the field and frequency together rather than separately. The field frequency lock unit locks the magnetic field to the ESR signal of a sample of DPPH located in a microwave helix situated in the magnet gap. The same microwaves are used to excite the DPPH sample as are used in producing the ESR signal under study. Any drift in the microwave source results in an appropriate corrective change in the magnetic field; similarly, any drift in the field can be corrected by an applied voltage to the magnet power supply. The radiofrequency can be swept from 6 to

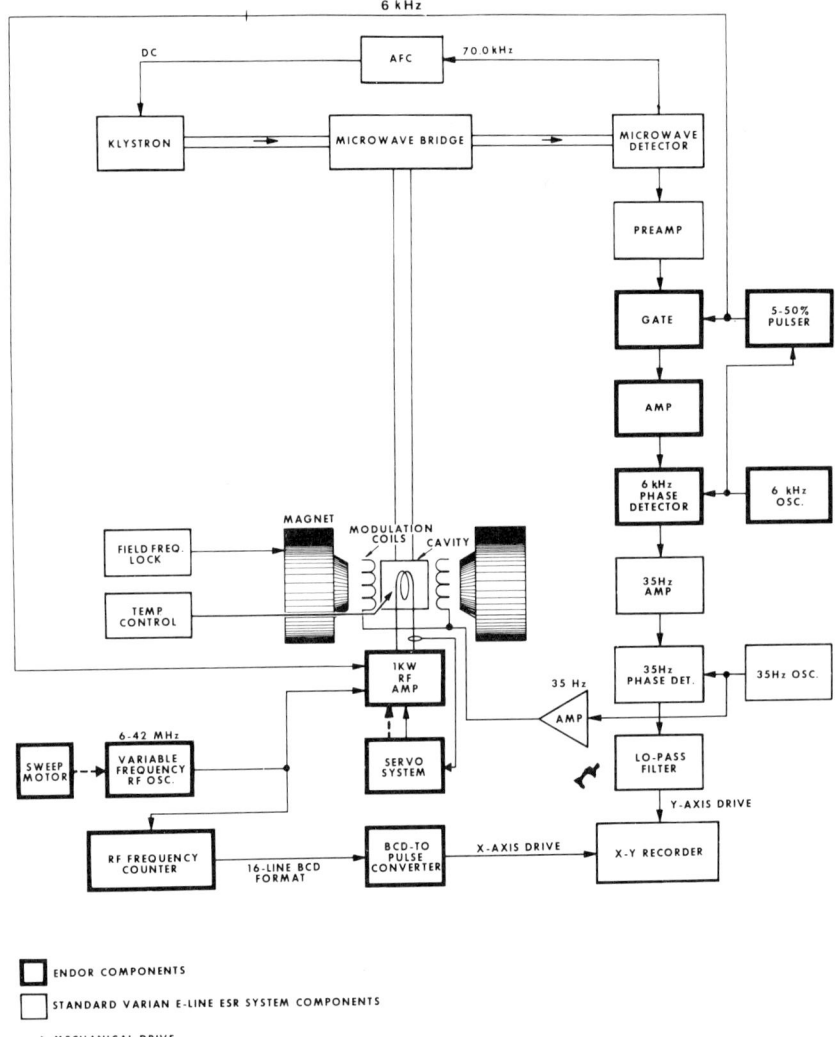

Figure 2-4. Block diagram of the Varian E-700 ENDOR spectrometer. The blocks containing the heavily ruled lines contain those components that are added to a standard Varian E-line ESR spectrometer. Reproduced by courtesy of the Varian Instrument Division.

42 MHz at 1 kW of rf power. Low power ENDOR can be carried out at liquid helium temperatures if special liquid helium dewars are constructed. At these power levels the upper frequency of the rf oscillator can be increased to 90 MHz. Since many commercial Varian ENDOR spectrometers are currently being used, a more detailed description is given in the next section.

2.2.2 Varian ENDOR Cavity

2.2.2.1 ENDOR Cavity—External View

An exterior view of the Varian ENDOR cavity is shown in Fig. 2-5. This is basically a Varian E-235 large sample access cylindrical cavity that has

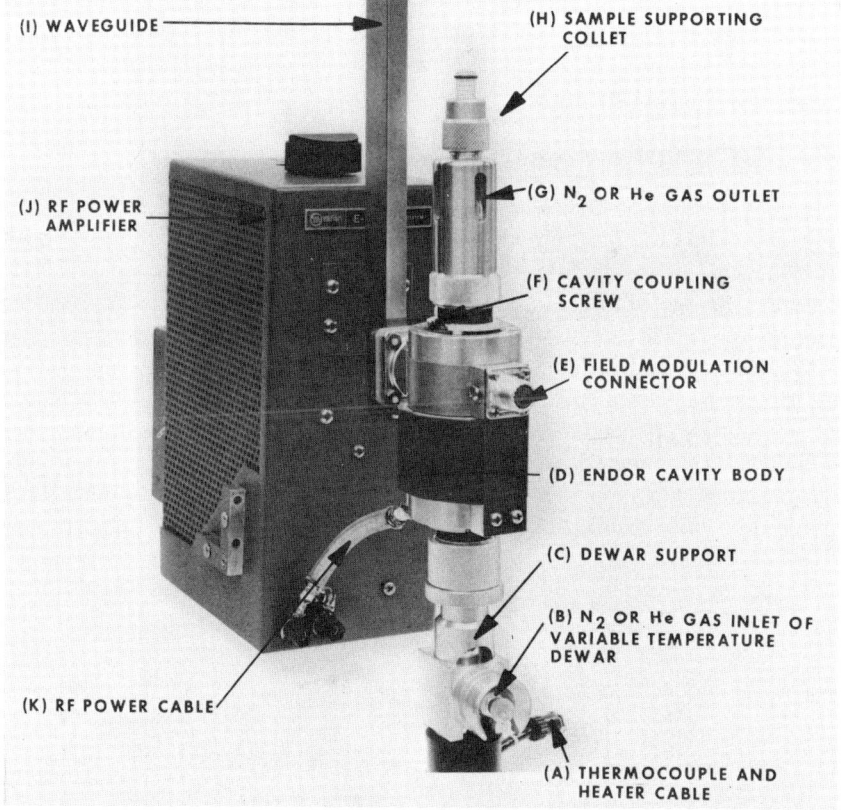

Figure 2-5. The exterior view of the Varian ENDOR cavity attached to the rf power amplifier. Reproduced by courtesy of the Varian Instrument Division.

70   EXPERIMENTAL METHODS

a special built-in rf coil. The variable temperature housing (C) shown in Fig. 2-5 is attached to the bottom of the cavity housing (D) by a screw-on flange. A variable temperature quartz dewar insert is held in place inside the cavity by this housing. Cold nitrogen or helium gas is blown into the dewar at position B and subsequently forced past the sample, which is suspended inside the dewar and exits at G. Variable temperature is obtained by applying a current to a heater coil located beneath the ESR sample inside the dewar that warms the cold nitrogen or helium gas to the required temperature. The temperature can also be adjusted by varying the cold gas flow rate. The cable that connects the heater and thermocouple to a variable temperature controller is located at A. The ESR sample is held firmly in the center of the cavity by the supporting collets at H. Current input to drive the modulation coils embedded in epoxy at position D is through a twinex connector located at E. The rf power is transmitted by the coaxial cable located at K to the cavity from the rf power amplifier (J) situated behind the cavity. The microwave frequency is transmitted by the waveguide at I from the klystron and is coupled to the cavity by the iris at F.

2.2.2.2 ENDOR Cavity—Internal View

Figure 2-6 shows a cutaway view of the ENDOR cavity housing (D) in Fig. 2-5. The modulation coils are located at (Q) and are exterior to both the sample and cavity. An approximate 15-G field is achieved at 35 Hz whereas 8 G is obtainable at 6 kHz. The cavity walls are composed of wound silver wire embedded in epoxy. The rf coils are formed by four $\frac{1}{16}$-in. silver-plated brass rods (M) passing through the cavity, parallel to its axis and electrically insulated from the cavity. The rods are connected at (L) and (N) in such a way as to form one turn of a loop as indicated in I below or connected to form a two turn loop as in II. The variable temperature dewar located at the center of the sample access ports O is made up of two concentric quartz tubes of approximately 17 mm o.d. and

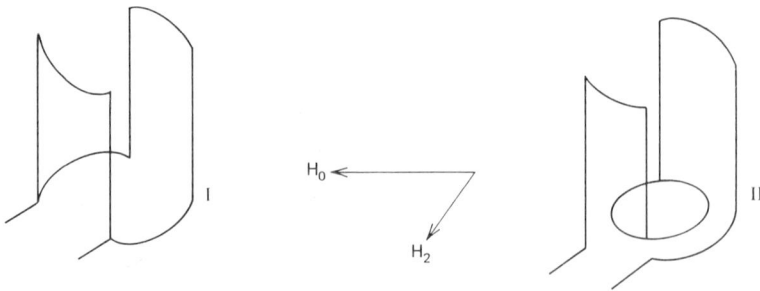

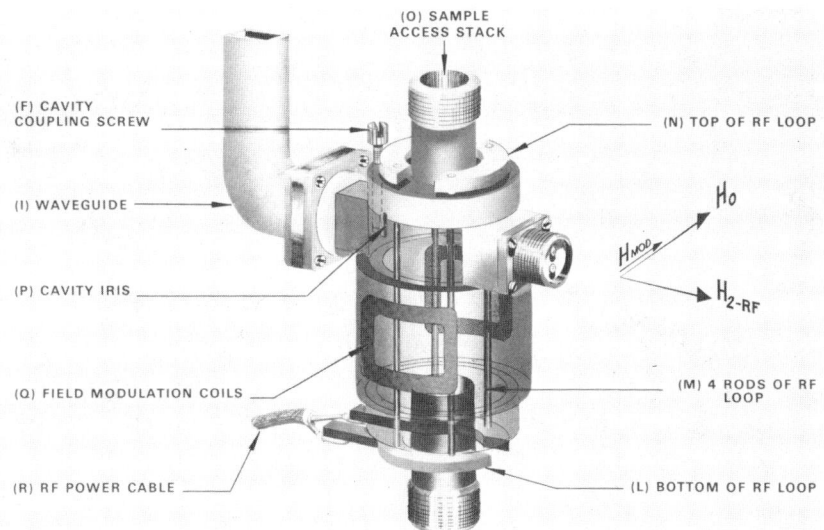

Figure 2-6. Cutaway view of the Varian ENDOR cavity showing the location of the field modulation coils and the rods of the rf loop. Reproduced by courtesy of the Varian Instrument Division.

11 mm i.d. Thus variable temperature ENDOR studies can be carried out on samples up to 11 mm o.d. (outside diameter). The cavity is normally adjusted in length and the iris (P) is properly spaced so that the TE_{102} mode resonates at 9.4 GHz and the cavity plus dewar can be properly coupled to the microwaves entering at P. If other dewars are used, small metal sleeves may have to be added or removed to the sample access stack to accommodate this change properly. However, normal 11-mm o.d. and 16-mm o.d. liquid nitrogen dewars can easily be used in this cavity.

2.2.2.3 ENDOR Cavity—Microwave Modes

A schematic diagram of the microwave modes used in the ENDOR cavity is given in Fig. 2-7. The microwave magnetic field maximum for a TE_{102} mode (T) is found at the center of the cavity (U) where the sample is located. The modulation coils (Q) for sweeping the magnetic field sinusoidally at a rate of 35 Hz through resonance are placed perpendicular to the microwave magnetic field (H_1). The output of the modulation coils drives the X axis of an oscilloscope for ESR display of the ESR resonance. The modulation amplitude is usually set to a level that gives the largest ESR signal. Even if the ESR spectrum is overmodulated, ENDOR lines are not broadened as long as magnetic field modulation amplitude H_m (G) × 4.2 < ENDOR linewidth (kHz).

72 EXPERIMENTAL METHODS

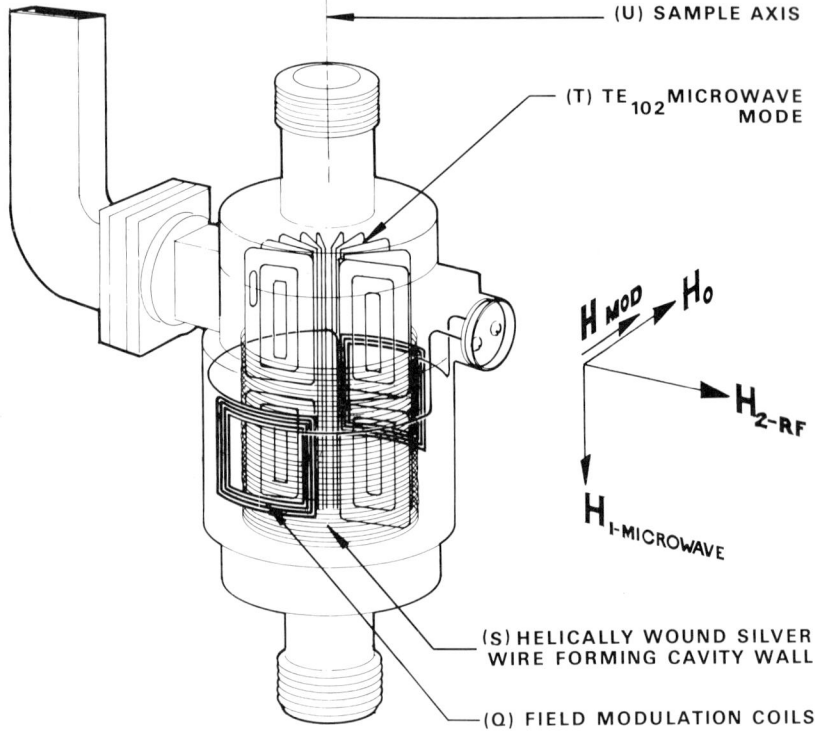

Figure 2-7. A schematic diagram of the microwave modes in the Varian ENDOR cavity. Reproduced by courtesy of the Varian Instrument Division.

2.3 CRITICAL OPERATING PARAMETERS—ENDOR

2.3.1 Sensitivity and Magnetic Field Homogeneity and Stability

Since the ENDOR signal-to-noise ratio is always some fraction of the ESR signal-to-noise ratio (for liquids, typically 1% of the ESR height), it is necessary to have a well tuned ENDOR spectrometer. This requires that the ESR spectrometer be in perfect working order and ideally be capable of producing a signal-to-noise ratio of at least 100:1 or better from a standard Varian weak pitch sample. The Varian weak pitch (0.00033% pitch in KCl) sample contains 1×10^{13} spins cm^{-1} providing the ESR signal is recorded with a 1.7-G linewidth. Most good commercial instruments can achieve such a signal-to-noise ratio for 10^{13} spins (the effective length of a rectangular cavity is 1 cm). The magnetic field homogeneity of most commercial magnets used in ESR experiments is

±10 milligauss (mG), which is quite adequate. A homogeneity of this magnitude is usually necessary in order to properly investigate organic free radicals in solution where frequently ESR linewidths of 60 mG or smaller are encountered. Deuterium ENDOR may require slightly better homogeneity.[28]

The most serious problem is one of magnetic field and microwave frequency stability. After setting the field to coincide with a selected position of the ESR line, the magnetic field and the microwave frequency should be invariant for the duration of the experiment. Since the experiments may take several hours, special attachments are added to the standard ESR spectrometers to provide adequate magnetic field and microwave oscillator stability required for ENDOR investigations. Normally, microwave oscillators, even with automatic frequency controls (AFC), will drift because of changes in the temperature of the ESR cavity and to a lesser degree other small changes in the circuitry. Small drifts in magnetic field can also occur because of temperature changes in the immediate surroundings.

There are two methods that can be used to correct this situation. First, the field and frequency can be prevented from drifting by using a field frequency lock system, which has been described in Section 2.2.1. An alternative method appears to work adequately whenever the cavity can be immersed in a refrigerant. Cook[19] describes an ENDOR spectrometer operating at 35 GHz where the cavity is immersed in a refrigerant and helium gas is admitted to the cavity to provide thermal contact between the sample supported by the rf coil and the refrigerant. In this case the cavity can be kept at constant temperature, and thus the microwave frequency remains reasonably constant for the duration of each ENDOR experiment. However, the magnetic field stability still remains a problem. ESR experiments at 35 GHz require ESR fields around 12.5 kG. Assuming 0.5 G for linewidth requires a magnetic field stability of 1 part in 10^5 or better over the duration of each ENDOR experiment. This type of stability can be obtained by locking the field to the nuclear magnetic resonance signal of deuterium (obtained by an NMR gaussmeter). Any change in the deuterium NMR signal is amplified and applied to a pair of coils on the magnet that compensate for any changes in the main magnetic field. The system reported by Cook[19] has a stability of 1 part in 10^6 per 30 min.

2.3.2 Sample Size

Sample shape and size are not really critical parameters. However, it is usually advantageous to have as large a sample size as possible to take advantage of the cavity-filling factor. The ESR signal intensity depends on the total number of spins in the active part of the cavity and not on the concentration per unit volume. Therefore signal intensity can be gained if the largest sample tube is used, which in the case of the Varian ENDOR cavity is an 11-mm o.d. tube when a variable temperature dewar is used or up to 16 mm when no variable temperatures are used (room temperature). However if the sample is at all polar, the microwave electric field will be absorbed by the electric dipole of the sample, and this may prevent detection of the magnetic dipoles by the microwave magnetic field. Physically this phenomenon is observed to be a loss of cavity Q. However, excellent solvents with low dielectric constants, such as ethyl benzene and toluene, do exist and are highly recommended for carrying out ENDOR investigations in solution. When a polar sample (i.e., ice) is frozen to a sufficiently low temperature (i.e., <100 K) the dielectric constant drops to nonpolar values and ENDOR can easily be done. Polycrystalline or glassy samples generally have broad ESR lines and thus both ESR and ENDOR sensitivity is decreased. With a large sample access cavity it is possible to carry out successful ENDOR experiments on frozen glasses[29-30a,30b] or powder samples.[31-32] Most crystals can also be used. Thus the sample size or shape does not limit one from observing ESR and/or ENDOR spectra. However a severe problem can arise in collecting ENDOR data from a crystal. In order to determine accurately the principal hyperfine splittings, ENDOR data must be collected from three orthogonal crystal planes. In many cases[33] the crystal needs to be aligned to 2 minutes of an arc, so very precise alignment is required.

2.3.3 Introduction of rf Power into Cavity

The method by which rf power is introduced into the cavity depends largely on the type of ENDOR experiment. For instance, ENDOR experiments on samples (transition metal complexes or semiconductors) that are carried out at 4 K normally require rf power levels on the order of 0.1 W or less because the paramagnetic relaxation times are long. As the temperature is raised above 4 K, relaxation times shorten and larger rf powers are required. Near room temperature rf powers of 10 to 20 G are typically needed to observe free radicals in solution.[20-25] When rf powers of 0.1 W or less are used, the rf coil can be wrapped around the sample and the entire sample and rf coil immersed in the liquid helium refrigerant or in cooled gas without any difficulties from rf power dissipation. At high rf power levels (1 to 20 G), it would be impossible to carry out an ENDOR experiment using this rf coil configuration as the liquid helium would boil away as the rf power is dissipated.

However this problem can be eliminated by placing the rf coil on the inside of the cavity walls, outside of a dewar insert extending through the cavity. This removes the load on the cryogenic system and a successful experiment can be carried out. The large rf coil also allows a large access area in the cavity, permitting the investigation of large amounts of liquid, frozen glasses[29] or large single crystals.

On the other hand, I. Miyagawa and his co-workers[24] have shown that very intense rf fields can be used when the rf coil is wrapped around the sample (a crystal in their particular experiment) if the sample is cooled with chilled nitrogen gas. The experimental setup is similar to the Varian variable temperature arrangement with the sample held in place by the rf coil.

2.3.4 Rf Power Level—Cw versus Pulsed Schemes

Successful experiments have been carried out using high power wideband amplifiers[21-24] in which no pulsed rf is used. Instead, 100 to 500 W of continuous rf power is used to irradiate the sample. Whether the 1 kW pulsed ENDOR delivering 100 W of radiofrequency will be better than a cw spectrometer delivering 100 W of continuous rf power turns out to be dependent[27] on how easily the nuclear signal can be saturated. If the nuclear signal is easily saturated, using continuous rf irradiation is better than a pulsed rf by a factor of $10^{1/2}$. On the other hand, if the nuclear signal saturates with difficulty, the pulsed rf will give signals that are $10^{1/2}$ times more intense than those with continuous rf.

2.3.5 Mode of Detection and Modulation Scheme

Although a complete set of data does not exist, the results of several experiments show that the ENDOR lineshape and intensity depend critically on the detection and modulation scheme used.[27] However before the optimum field, rf modulation, and detection schemes can be established, it will be necessary to predetermine the ENDOR mechanism for each given free radical sample. This is unfortunately still not possible. Thus several different schemes are used, with a great deal of discussion being carried out on the merits of each. For instance, superheterodyne spectrometers have been used because it has been claimed that they have better ultimate sensitivity, although they do not give good results when high microwave power is required to saturate the ESR line.[34]

Miyagawa and co-workers[24] use 16 kHz field modulation and phase-detect at 32 kHz to obtain ENDOR spectra of irradiated single crystals.

76 EXPERIMENTAL METHODS

On the other hand, Mobius and co-workers[23] carry out ENDOR measurements at an rf power of 1 kW in a cw mode using 300 Hz magnetic field modulation and a 20 kHz frequency modulation of the rf field to investigate radicals in solution. Allendoerfer[21b] operates an ENDOR spectrometer using magnetic field modulation at 20 kHz and cw operation at 500 W.

2.4 INTRODUCTION—ELDOR INSTRUMENTATION

The only known commercial ELDOR spectrometer currently being used is the Varian E-800 frequency swept ELDOR spectrometer. Several homemade ELDOR spectrometers have been reported[35-39] and differ largely in the design of the bimodal cavity used. Most have used a bimodal cylindrical cavity or a rectangular cavity, although Vieth and Hausser[39] and Benderskii et al.[37] have used a cylindrical observing cavity and a helix to support the pump frequency. The discussion of the experimental setup will therefore be limited to that of the Varian ELDOR spectrometer (bimodal cavity) and the helical arrangement of Vieth and Hausser.

A simplified block diagram of the Varian E-800 frequency swept ELDOR spectrometer is shown in Fig. 2-8. Those components that make up an ESR spectrometer are outlined by the narrow lines and are the same as those used for the ENDOR spectrometer. Those components outlined in heavy lines are the added components necessary for the construction of an ELDOR spectrometer. The additional klystron referred to as the pump klystron can be continually swept from a frequency approximately 350 MHz above to about 100 MHz below the frequency of the ESR klystron referred to as the *observing klystron*. The geometry of the TE_{102} rectangular ESR cavity has been changed so that it can simultaneously support the variable microwave frequency and the fixed microwave frequency modes in such a way that they are orthogonal to each other and are isolated from one another. An AFC-controlled servomotor has been added to the cavity, in order that the pumping cavity section can be kept at resonance over the entire range of the swept-pumping klystron frequency. The frequency difference between the pumping klystron frequency and the observing klystron frequency is displayed on a counter. The digital output of the counter is converted to an analog signal that drives the X axis of the ESR recorder. The Y axis of the recorder is connected in the usual way to the output of the phase sensitive detector. In order to assure that no pumping power can reach the observing detector crystal directly, a transmission cavity filter tuned to

INTRODUCTION—ELDOR INSTRUMENTATION

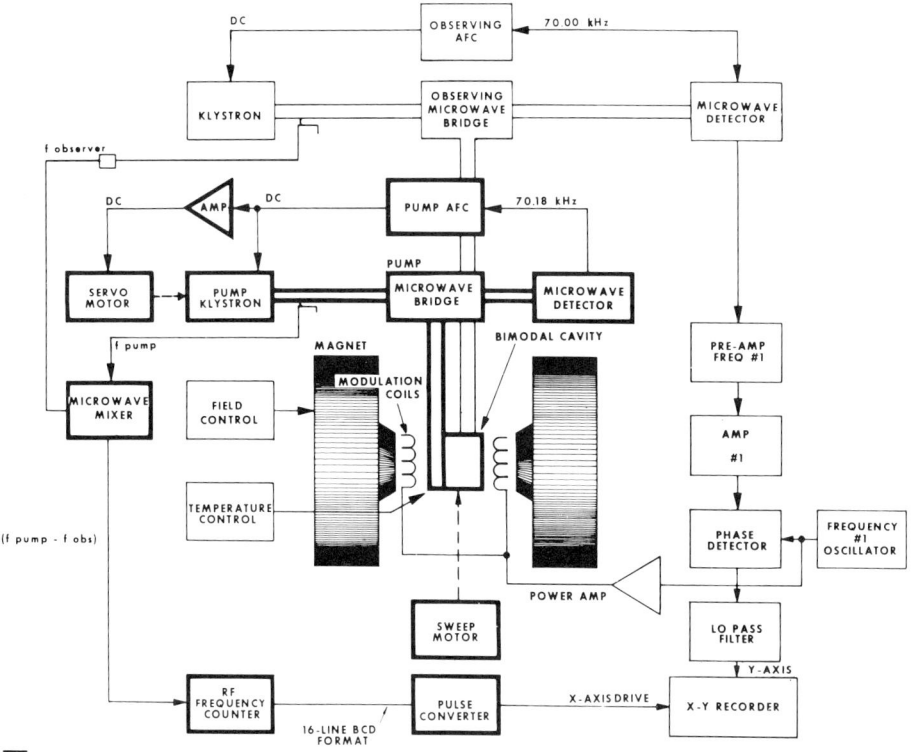

Figure 2-8. Block diagram of the Varian E-800 ELDOR spectrometer. The heavily ruled lines outline the components added to the standard ESR spectrometer. The modulation frequency can be either 100, 10, or 1 kHz or 270 or 35 Hz. Reproduced by courtesy of the Varian Instrument Division.

the observing frequency, which serves to eliminate the microwave path from the pumping klystron to the observing detector crystal, has also been added.

2.4.1 Varian ELDOR Cavity

2.4.1.1 ELDOR Cavity—External View

An external view of the rectangular bimodal Varian ELDOR cavity is given in Fig. 2-9. The straight section of rectangular pipe labeled *observing waveguide* (M) provides the electrical pathway for the transmission

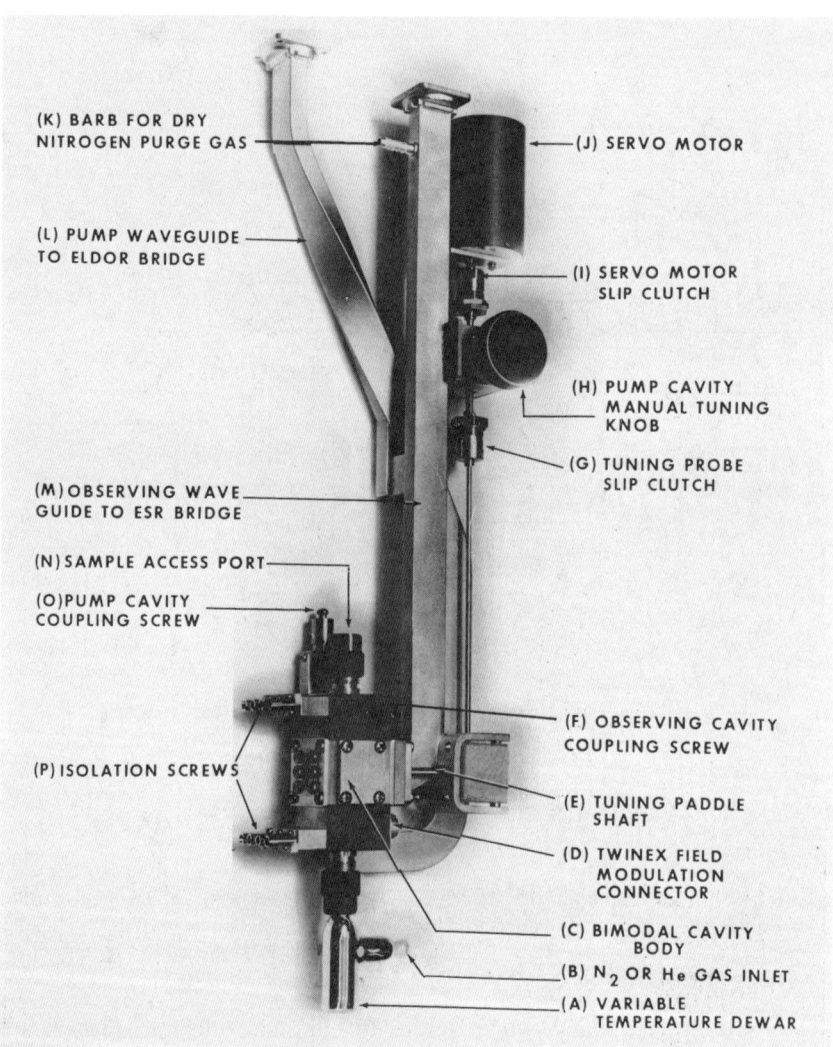

Figure 2-9. The external view of the Varian ELDOR cavity. Reproduced by courtesy of the Varian Instrument Division.

INTRODUCTION—ELDOR INSTRUMENTATION 79

of microwaves (held at a constant frequency) to the observing resonator portion of the bimodal ELDOR cavity (position X, Fig. 2-10). To a good approximation, the observing resonator of the ELDOR cavity is constructed similar to the Varian rectangular cavity and serves the same function. The other section of rectangular pipe, which resembles an inverted question mark L (labeled *pump waveguide*), provides the electrical pathway for the transmission of microwaves from the tunable klystron to the pumping resonator portion of the ELDOR cavity (position R, Fig. 2-10). This pump cavity is also rectangular and is oriented at 90° to the rectangular observing resonator so that the resulting structure of the two joined cavities forms a cross (see Fig. 2-10). The pump cavity resonant frequency is varied by simultaneously turning two tuning paddles, constructed in the shape of a T (see Fig. 2-10, position S) inside the pump

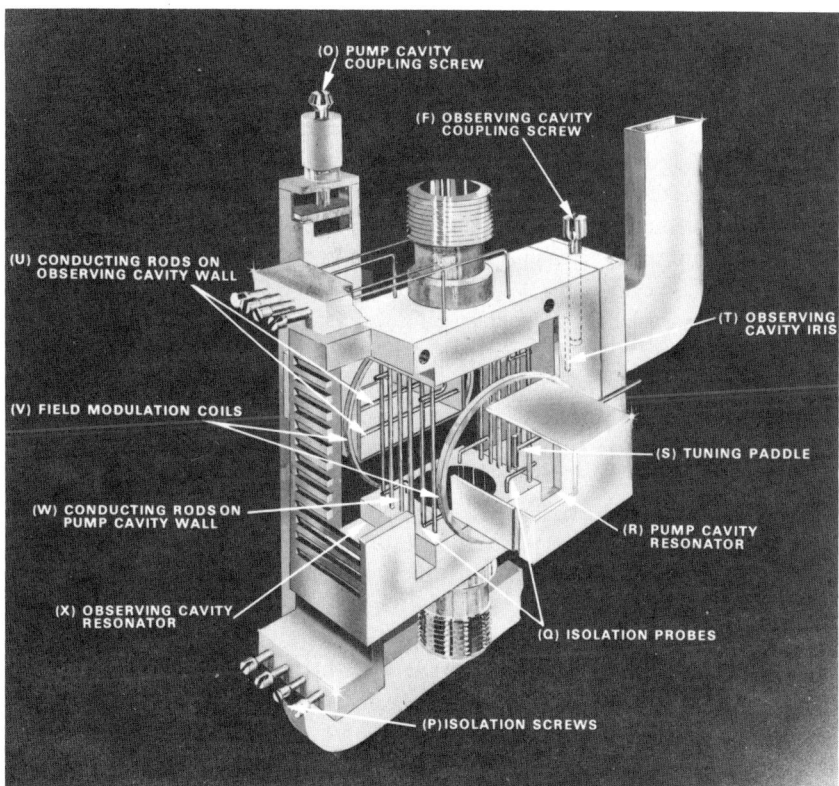

Figure 2-10. The internal view of the Varian ELDOR cavity, patent number 3,609,520 (Sept., 1971). Reproduced by courtesy of the Varian Instrument Division.

cavity. These two paddles are attached to the tuning paddle shaft E (Fig. 2-9) located on either side of the observing waveguide. The paddles can be turned automatically by the servomotor located at position (J) so that a continuous variation in the pump cavity resonant frequency can be achieved. The paddles are placed so that they do not perturb the resonant frequency or the coupling of the observing cavity upon rotation. The pump klystron frequency is changed by applying a correction voltage generated by an AFC circuit to a second servomotor located in the ELDOR bridge, which restores the pump microwave frequency to the new cavity resonant condition. Repeated application results in a continuously tunable pumping frequency. The pumping microwave frequency can also be varied manually by turning the manual tuning knob (H). A slip clutch (I) protects the servomotor during manual operation and another slip clutch at position (G) protects the servomotor when the gear train travels against the upper lower mechanical stop. Alternatively, the tuning paddle can be replaced by a set of rexolite rods, which are driven either into or out of the pumping cavity by the servomotor (J), resulting in a shift in the pump resonant frequency similar to the above.

The sample access area (N), 11 mm o.d. maximum and 5 mm o.d. with dewar, is located in a vertical cylinder at the center of the two cavities (center of the cross) where the microwave magnetic field H_1 is a maximum for both cavities. When the cavity is placed in the magnetic field both the pump and observing microwave magnetic fields are perpendicular to the magnetic field. Variable temperature quartz dewars (A) are needed to obtain ELDOR spectra as a function of temperature. However the more quartz that is inserted into the cavity, the smaller is the frequency difference range between the observing and pumping cavities. Therefore special thin wall ($\sim$0.5 mm) quartz variable temperature dewars are used in the ELDOR cavity in order to provide variable temperature capability while still maintaining an adequate ELDOR frequency range. The normal Varian ESR variable temperature or liquid nitrogen dewar can also be used at the expense of limiting the ELDOR frequency range. Normally this range would decrease and instead of being able to vary the pump from $\sim$350 MHz above to 100 MHz below the observing frequency, a frequency range from $\sim$200 MHz above to $\sim$75 MHz below the observing frequency is typical. Any slight nonorthogonality between the pumping and observing cavity modes is corrected by insertion of isolation screws (P), which appear on the front of the cavity. The quartz dewars, if not made of two closely concentric tubes, can also induce nonorthogonality between the pumping and observing cavity modes. In the case of randomly selected dewars some isolation problems can result.

2.4.1.2 ELDOR Cavity—Internal View

A cutaway view of the inside of the bimodal cavity body (C in Fig. 2-9) is shown in Fig. 2-10. The TE_{102} pumping microwave modes are coupled into the ELDOR cavity by the pumping cavity iris located below the pump cavity coupling screw, position (O); the observing TE_{102} microwave modes are coupled into the ELDOR cavity at position (T) by the observing cavity iris. The pump-coupling mechanism is a sliding short, a piece of metal that moves back and forth in the waveguide as the pump-coupling screw (O) is turned. It is located a fraction of a half wavelength beyond the pump cavity iris. Its purpose is to couple all the pump microwave energy into the pump cavity so as to prevent the microwave energy from reflecting toward the source. A small piece of conducting metal attached to a threaded Teflon rod serves as the observing frequency coupling screw.

As the two tuning paddles (S) are turned, the microwave resonant frequency of the pump cavity resonator (R) changes, causing a shift in the pumping klystron frequency via an AFC circuit. This results in a swept pump microwave frequency. In addition, as the pump frequency is swept, the pump cavity coupling changes, and thus the frequency sweep of the pump cavity must be halted at regular intervals in order to adjust the pumping cavity coupling screw. Recall that the tuning paddles (S) only perturb the resonant frequency of the pump resonator and not the frequency of the observing cavity resonator (X). In the area of the ELDOR cavity where the observing and pumping modes overlap, the walls of the observing cavity resonator are formed by horizontal conducting rods at position (U) whereas the walls of the pumping cavity resonator are bound by vertical rods at position (W). Even in a carefully built ELDOR cavity, the two microwave cavity modes are never quite orthogonal to each other, and the isolation screws (P) mentioned previously can be used to correct for any imperfections by introducing a compensating perturbation at (Q). It is possible to have a large asymmetric crystal sample holder that reduces the isolation; slight adjustments of the isolation paddles may compensate for this error. The field modulation coils (V) are wrapped around the outer portion of the pump cavity resonator.

2.4.1.3 ELDOR Cavity—Microwave Modes

The locations of the microwave TE_{102} modes are given in Fig. 2-11. The lines of microwave magnetic field of the observing cavity modes are the vertically placed modes at position (Y), whereas the horizontally positioned solid lines at (Z) are the pumping cavity modes. The reason for the

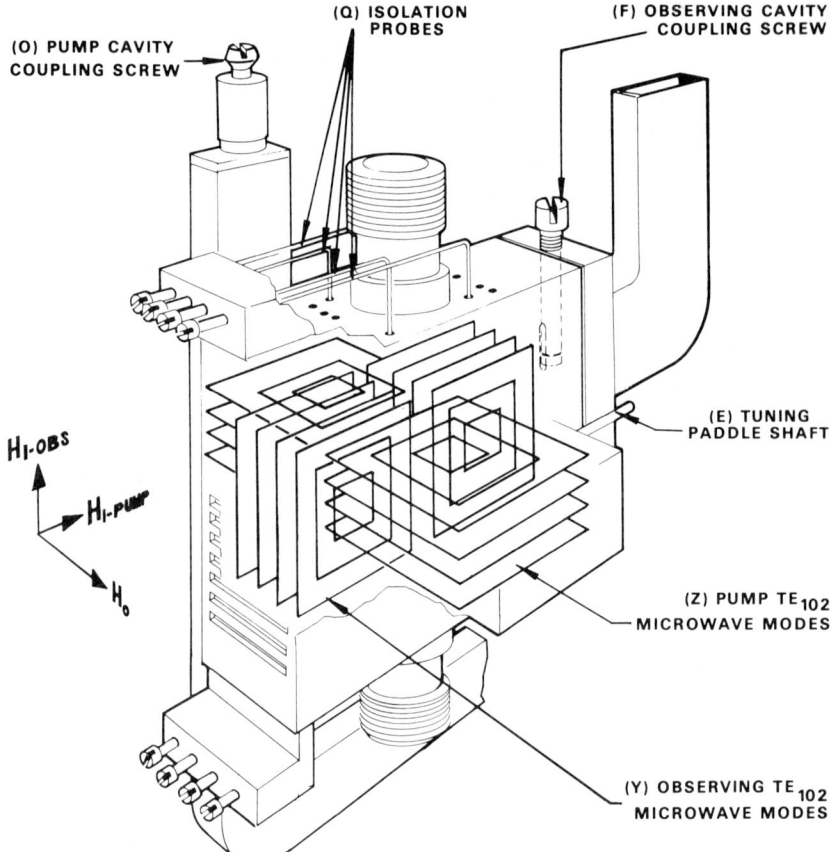

Figure 2-11. The microwave modes of the Varian ELDOR cavity. Reproduced by courtesy of the Varian Instrument Division.

conducting rods (U) and (W) in Fig. 2-10 is now clear, since the position of the rods permits a conductive pathway along which each mode can be supported. The microwave magnetic field maximum for the two modes occurs at the exact center of the cavity (i.e., at the center of the two intersecting planes). Because of the arrangement of the modes, a point sample like a single crystal serves as an ideal sample for investigation. However line samples are also commonly used.

2.4.2 ELDOR Spectral Presentation

Commercially there are two modes in which ELDOR spectra are recorded: frequency swept and field swept. In the frequency swept configuration the ESR magnetic field is positioned at the resonance field of one of the spectral peaks of the ESR spectrum while the observing microwave frequency is kept constant and the pumping microwave frequency is swept. If the observing magnetic field is positioned at a higher magnetic field than the field of other ESR lines to be probed, the pumping frequency (ν_p) is set to scan a frequency greater than the observing frequency (ν_o) (Fig. 1-36.) Alternatively the pumping frequency can be scanned below the observing frequency if the observed ESR line is located at a lower magnetic field than the ESR lines to be probed. The difference frequency between the observing and pumping klystron is displayed on a frequency counter having a range up to 500 MHz, permitting a selectable frequency resolution of either 0.01 or 0.1 MHz. These frequencies are connected to a digital output that advances the stepping motor of a special recorder or to a D-to-A converter that drives the X axis of an ordinary XY recorder. The Y axis of the recorder displays the change in the ESR amplitude as the pumping frequency is swept, resulting in a plot of spectral amplitude versus frequency difference.

On the other hand, a field swept ELDOR spectrum is recorded when the pumping microwave frequency is set to a predetermined frequency above or below the observing microwave frequency and the magnetic field is swept. The resulting spectrum appears similar to an ESR spectrum in that a plot of spectral amplitude versus magnetic field is observed; differences in line intensities occur, however (Fig. 1-34).

In both spectral presentations the observing klystron frequency is under automatic frequency control, which provides stability to approximately 1 part in 10^7. A continuous X-axis display is also assured by keeping the pumping frequency under automatic frequency control.

In order to assure better isolation of the pumping frequency mode from the observing microwave mode, a microwave filter is introduced. This filter is a transmission-type cavity that causes a 45-dB reduction in transmitted power from the pump klystron to the detector diode and a 3-dB reduction in power of the ESR signal coming from the observing cavity. This prevents the crystal detector from being damaged by excessive leakage of the pump klystron power.

The maximum isolation obtainable in a bimodal cavity between the pumping and observing cavities when both are operated at a fixed frequency can be as high as 60 to 80 dB. However inclusion of a variable pumping frequency generally reduces the isolation to around 40 dB.

Other spectral presentations that are not commercially available are also possible[36a] and are given in Table 2-1 along with those described earlier. The first two examples are the conditions for the observing and pumping frequencies as well as the magnetic field for the field swept and frequency swept ELDOR spectra, respectively, which were previously

Table 2-1. Different Types of Signal Display in Electron-Electron Double Resonance

Observing Frequency	Pumping Frequency	DC Magnetic Field	X-axis Variable	Comments
Fixed	Fixed	Swept	H_o	The technique of Ref. 36a, known as field swept ELDOR.
Fixed	Swept	Fixed	$\Delta\nu$	The technique of Ref. 36b, known as frequency swept ELDOR.
Swept	Fixed	Fixed	$\Delta\nu$	
Fixed	Swept	Swept	H_o	Magnetic field and frequency of pumping source locked to one hyperfine interval with ν_p/H constant.
Swept	Fixed	Swept	H_o	Magnetic field and frequency of observing source locked to one hyperfine interval with ν_o/H constant.
Fixed	Fixed	Fixed	Time	Transient experiment.

described. The fourth example listed, where the pumping frequency and the magnetic field are locked to a hyperfine interval and both are swept while the observing microwave frequency is set to a fixed value, holds some promise spectroscopically. In this mode it is theoretically possible to obtain values of T_{2e} and T_{1e} directly from the ELDOR line shapes, providing that the magnetic field modulation does not contribute to the lineshape. Experimentally this is a difficult situation to achieve. Currently such a mode of spectral display is possible with an ELDOR spectrometer built by Vieth and Hausser.[39] The third and fifth examples, where the observing frequency is swept, are less desirable modes of ELDOR detection, since the noise generated by the automatic tracking system can reach the observing microwave detector. Transient experiments are usually run according to the last example given.

2.4.3 Traveling Wave Helix

An ELDOR spectrometer recently constructed by Vieth and Hausser[39] and a similar arrangement employed by Benderskii et al.[37] use a microwave helix as the pumping microwave source. Because a microwave helix is a broad-banded device, it will support a wide range of frequencies without requiring a change in the physical dimensions as is necessary with cavities. The Vieth and Hausser[39] spectrometer can be swept over a frequency range of 1 GHz, although most sweeps are limited to 150 MHz. Thus ELDOR spectra potentially can be recorded when the difference between the observing and pumping is greater than 350 MHz (the present limit of the Varian ELDOR spectrometer). Because of some important applications at large frequency differences, this section is devoted to a brief description of the helical ELDOR spectrometer. Comments in other sections of this chapter generally refer to experiments carried out using the Varian commercial ELDOR spectrometer.

The microwave helix of Vieth and Hausser is constructed by gluing thin silver tape in a helical arrangement to the inner wall of a quartz tube. The quartz tube is inserted in the cylindrical cavity depicted in Fig. 2-12 such that the windings of the helix are perpendicular to the electrical field lines of the TE_{112} cavity mode. In this configuration the distortion of the observing microwave field is minimized. In order to achieve good isolation between the observing and pumping microwave modes (50 dB when

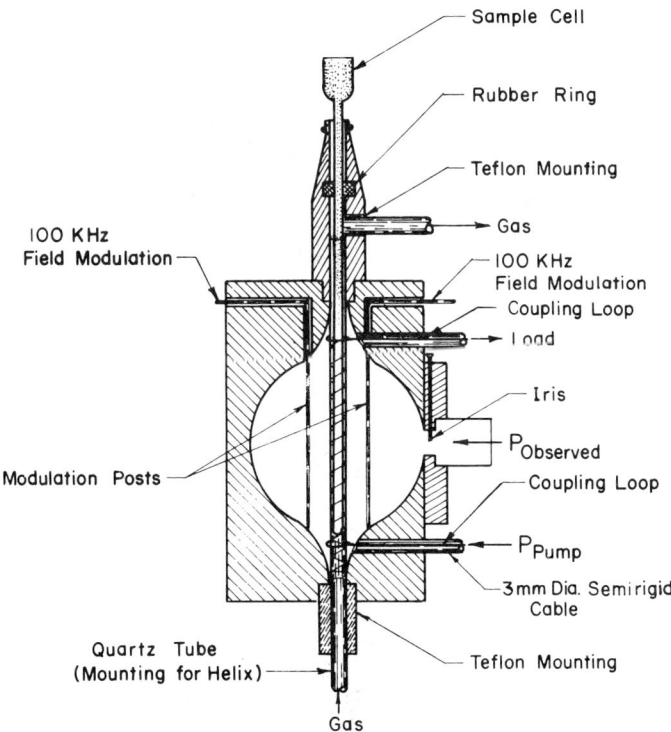

Figure 2-12. A cross-sectional view of the Vieth and Hausser ELDOR cavity using a microwave helix.

$\nu_p - \nu_o = \pm 10$ MHz) the axis of the helix and cavity must be orthogonal. In addition, the amount of microwave field from the helix that occurs outside the helical volume can be decreased by keeping the helical circumference small in comparison to the microwave wavelength. Of course this size is limited by the size of the sample. Furthermore the isolation is assured from sample to sample by using a band-pass filter in the observing part of the spectrometer.

Since the radial homogeneity of the helix field increases as the radius of the helix and the pitch angle of the windings decrease, an optimum diameter of 3.8 mm and a pitch of 3 mm occurs at 8.6 GHz ($\lambda = 35$ mm). Care must be paid to finding the optimum matching of the coupling device and the load so that microwave reflections are minimized, and thus good axial field homogeneity is required.

Because the helix has a low Q, a higher pump power is required to obtain the same amount of ESR saturation as obtained with a cavity. Thus the normal pump power is 5 W although pumping power as high as 220 W is possible with the Vieth and Hausser[39] ELDOR spectrometer.

In order to prevent the heating of the sample, the pump power is pulsed with a duty cycle of 4 to 50%. In this way the average power is less than 10 W. The observing klystron has a maximum output of 1.2 W. Variable temperature is achieved between 173 and 333 K by passing a stream of cooled gas though the quartz tube shown in Fig. 2-12.

The dimensions of the helix limit nonpolar samples to tubes 3.5 mm o.d. in diameter and 40 mm in length. For field swept ELDOR spectra, the sensitivity of this system is about $R \times 10^{12}$ spins G^{-1} of linewidth (R = ELDOR reduction factor). This figure is only approximate as it depends on the ease with which the ESR lines are saturated. An increase in sensitivity by nearly a factor of 10 can be achieved by signal averaging and digital filtering.

2.5 CRITICAL OPERATING PARAMETERS—ELDOR

2.5.1 Isolation of Microwave Modes

To produce a real ELDOR effect, the pumping microwave mode must be isolated from the observing microwave mode and vice versa. Cavities can now be constructed in which 60 dB of isolation can be obtained between the two microwave modes when the sample under investigation possesses cylindrical symmetry. A difficulty arises, however, when the sample geometry is not cylindrically symmetric. The anisotropic dielectric loss in the cavity due to the sample geometry causes a distortion of the orthogonality of the two microwave modes, thus decreasing the isolation.

To correct for this, isolation adjustment screws are used. Normally the investigation would be seriously hampered if these isolation screws had to be adjusted for each sample. However this adjustment need only be made once if cylindrically symmetric sample tubes of the same diameter are used. Normally, high purity quartz tubing devoid of paramagnetic impurities is necessary. Flat cells also can be used, as isolation adjustment can be performed once at the beginning of a series of samples. On the other hand, investigation of single crystals can prove to be troublesome, especially for those crystal mountings where cylindrical symmetry is lacking upon sample rotation. This occurs when the longest exterior face of the crystal is mounted perpendicular to the axis about which the crystal is rotated. Therefore if large crystals (4 mm in diameter) are necessary for the ELDOR investigation, a great deal of time may be spent adjusting the isolation. Small crystals (<2 mm) minimize this problem and are used whenever possible.

A crystal goniometer may be an additional isolation problem. In many cases the crystal must be mounted at a particular oblique angle to the crystal face. In order for this to be done the tip of the goniometer is machined to the required oblique angle. If the goniometer tip is constructed out of 4-mm o.d. glass rod, significant distortion of the microwave isolation can result. To eliminate this problem the tip can be constructed out of smaller diameter Pyrex rod (2-mm o.d.) or out of small diameter quartz or rexolite rod.

2.5.2 Temperature Control

Many ELDOR investigations have been reported where the ELDOR spectral intensity is a strong function of temperature. Temperature control is therefore important and it is necessary to report the temperature for each spectral measurement. Temperature control by flowing gas through a dewar gives control to ±1 to 2°C and appears to be adequate. A possibly more critical parameter is the cooling of the cavity exterior when investigations are being carried out at low temperature. In a variable temperature configuration the cooling gases exit from the stacks at the top of the cavity. The gases then spill over the cavity body, cooling the exterior. This causes klystron frequency drift, in addition to a possible change in the isolation between the microwave modes as a result of inhomogeneous cooling of the cavity exterior. To prevent difficulties from cavity cooling by the flow gas, the outside of the cavity must be insulated or the flow gas can be led some distance above the cavity with a plastic tube. It is also a good technique to blow dry nitrogen gas between the dewar and the cavity body to maintain constant temperature.

Samples investigated at the fixed temperature of a refrigerant do not have this problem.

2.5.3 Magnetic Field Stability

The magnetic field stability requirements for ELDOR investigations are not nearly as stringent as those needed for ENDOR investigations because ELDOR linewidths are generally comparable to the ESR linewidths. For example, in irradiated organic solids where typical ESR linewidths are 10 to 12 MHz, the ELDOR linewidths are found to be 5 to 6 MHz. So the field stability of 1 in 10^6 available from a well controlled Hall feedback loop system, as in many commercial magnets, is adequate. If investigations are carried out on ESR lines narrower than 3 MHz, such as in irradiated deuterated compounds or solution samples, additional stability may be required as with ENDOR.

2.6 LIMITATIONS—ENDOR

2.6.1 Frequency Range of Commercial ENDOR Instruments

The commercial Varian E-700 ENDOR spectrometer is limited to a frequency range of about 6 to 48 MHz at 1 kW of pulsed rf power. A similar frequency range is also available with the 200 W cw JEOL ES-EDX1 ENDOR spectrometer. The availability of this frequency range and rf power permits the ENDOR investigation of proton couplings (A_H) of organic free radicals in solution[5,26] in addition to the investigation of proton and nitrogen couplings in glasses[29,30,42] and powders.[31,32,40,43] The proton ENDOR spectrum appears as two lines, equally distributed about the free proton frequency ($\nu_H \cong 14$ MHz at 3300 G) for each nonequivalent proton (i.e., $\nu_{endor} = \nu_H \pm A_H/2$). As most of the proton hyperfine splittings of interest are smaller than 30 MHz, the ENDOR frequencies fall in the 6 to 48 MHz range. Nitrogen ENDOR lines will be observed over a similar frequency range, provided the hyperfine splitting (A_N) is approximately 60 MHz or less, as the nitrogen ENDOR frequencies occur at $|A_N \pm \nu_N \pm Q|$ where ν_N is the nitrogen Zeeman splitting ($\nu_N = 1.0$ MHz at 3300 G) and Q is the quadrupole splitting ($Q \cong 1$ MHz). The nitrogen and proton couplings of ligands attached to transition metals[30,31] can also be measured over the 6 to 48 MHz range, provided low temperatures are used (20 to 40 K). At lower power levels this frequency range has been adequate to measure fluorine couplings in rare earth materials[44,45] as well as sodium[46] and lithium[49] couplings in color centers and a portion of the proton or nitrogen ENDOR spectrum for irradiated organic crystals.[48] A large number of ENDOR studies in this frequency range have been carried out on the ring protons in ground state triplets[16,49] at 4.2 K as well.

On the other hand, some modification of the commercially available ENDOR frequency range would have to be done to study color centers where the ^{39}K (ref. 6) and ^{35}Cl (ref. 50) hyperfine splittings are a few megahertz and thus the ENDOR spectra occur below 6 MHz. An extension of the frequency range would be necessary to study fluorine interactions in color centers where a sweep range up to 75 MHz is required.[51] In fact, a rather large ENDOR frequency range of up to 400 MHz is required to determine accurately nuclear moments, hyperfine and quadrupole tensors and their signs as well as the effective spin for transition metal ions such as Nd^{+3} (ref. 52), Eu^{+2} (ref. 8), Yb^{+3} (ref. 53), Gd^{+3} (ref. 54), Tb^{+4} (ref. 55), Cu^{+3} (ref. 55), V^{+2}, Mn^{+2} (ref. 56), Ni^{+2} (ref. 57), Fe^{+3} (ref. 58), Cr^{+3} (ref. 59), and V^{+3} (ref. 60). However, usually low temperatures (1 to 4 K) as well as low rf power (0.1 W) are necessary for the observation of ENDOR spectra of transition metal ions. Spectrometers similar to that of Feher[6] can be used to scan over a 400 MHz rf range. The study of semiconductors[6] is carried out at 1 to 4 K in much the same way where the ENDOR results permit mapping of the donor wavefunction in a large volume around the paramagnetic center.

The reason for the limited rf range mentioned above is the difficulty of building a pulsed ENDOR spectrometer with high enough rf power to be able to saturate the NMR transitions of radicals in liquids. A continuous rf field of 100 to 1000 W of pulsed (10% duty cycle) rf power is usually required. The Varian spectrometer operates with 1000 W of pulsed radiofrequency, detecting ENDOR only during the "on" time. This level of rf power results in a great deal of rf interference and prevents large frequency scan ranges. Similar limitations occur with the 200 W cw ENDOR of JEOL. The original design philosophy of the Varian and JEOL instruments was to enable measurement of small hyperfine couplings from complex ESR spectra in solution, especially protons, as well as to gain resolution. Since the frequency range starts at 6 MHz, certain important experiments cannot be done, such as measuring deuterium ENDOR spectra, which have been shown by Kwiram[28] to be valuable. Other splittings by nuclei with both small nuclear Zeeman frequencies (<2 MHz) and small hyperfine splittings (<3 MHz) cannot be measured.

Several homemade ENDOR instruments do exist that operate over a frequency range from 1 to 100 MHz using cw techniques and operating at 200 W of rf power.[20,21,24] In addition, the Bruker ER 420 ENDOR spectrometer has the capability of sweeping from 1 to 80 MHz using interchangeable probeheads.

2.6.2 Sensitivity

Because the ENDOR intensity is usually about 1% of the ESR intensity, it is difficult to investigate radical concentrations below 10^{-4} M. The maximum sensitivity seems to be achieved by using a cavity with a large access hole (25-mm diameter) to permit large samples to be used. This is especially important if nonpolar solvents such as toluene or ethylbenzene can be used. With polar solvents capillary tubes must be used. There is usually considerable difficulty in getting as much sample in the cavity as would be ideal when using capillary tubes. Thus a more limited concentration range is found for liquid samples using polar solvents.

The large hole cavity does permit sizable samples of radicals in polycrystalline, powdered, or frozen glass media to be studied. ESR spectra from such media always appear somewhat weak because of the intensity loss due to the averaging of the ESR signals from the random orientation of microcrystallites. In addition, the ENDOR signal intensity from such media is inversely proportional to the proton or nitrogen anisotropy. Thus large splittings are difficult to observe. Radicals from conjugated or aromatic samples where the splittings are small should give substantial ENDOR signals.[29] Rather intense ENDOR signals are also observed from radicals in powdered media containing nearly isotropic splittings. Beside permitting very large powder samples to be investigated, the large access hole cavity also permits quite large single crystals to be studied and allows the use of a complex three circle goniometer.

2.6.3 Saturable Transitions

The ability to observe ENDOR signals, given that the ESR signal-to-noise ratio is greater than 100:1, depends on three conditions. First, the ESR transitions must be saturable at the microwave power levels available. If partial saturation occurs up to 10 mW, ENDOR signals generally are observed. Samples containing transition metals whose ESR transitions are difficult to saturate near room temperature are usually investigated at low temperatures (4 to 20 K) where saturation conditions are more favorable.

Second, the NMR transitions must be saturable with the available nuclear rf power. This can be difficult. For example, if the ratio W_e/W_n

equals 10 (where W_e = electron relaxation probability and W_n = nuclear relaxation probability) and $T_{1e} = 10^{-6}$ sec, an rf magnetic field of 4 G in the rotating frame is required to saturate the NMR transition.

Third, for the common T_{1e} ENDOR mechanism the nuclear relaxation time or the cross-relaxation time must be of similar magnitude as the electron relaxation time in order that a change in the ESR saturation can be observed when the nuclear resonance takes place. An optimum ratio of these relaxation times can often be obtained by varying the temperature. In fact, it has been found that the lowest temperature is not always the best.

2.7 LIMITATIONS—ELDOR

2.7.1 Frequency Range

The frequency range of the Varian E-800 ELDOR system is dependent on the thickness of the walls of the quartz dewars. The frequency range with 0.5-mm dewar walls extends from a pump frequency of about 350 MHz above the observing microwave frequency to a pump frequency of about 100 MHz below the observing microwave frequency. As the wall thickness of the variable temperature dewars increases, this range decreases. Typically a Varian liquid nitrogen dewar with 1-mm walls will reduce this range so that a frequency swept spectrum can only be obtained from ~200 MHz above the observing klystron frequency to ~75 MHz below the observer. Fortunately most radicals containing proton, nitrogen, chlorine, deuterium, and bromine nuclei have hyperfine splittings less than 340 MHz and thus can be studied over this frequency range. The hyperfine splittings for fluorine, phosphorus, and carbon-13 can exceed 340 MHz and thus can be studied only at crystal angles where the hyperfine splitting is less than 340 MHz or where the isotropic splittings in solution are small. In addition, the large dipolar anisotropy for these nuclei tends to give unfavorable relaxation times for ELDOR and makes detection difficult.[61]

2.7.2 Radical Concentration

As with many double resonance techniques, the radical concentration must be higher to observe ELDOR than to observe ESR. First, the unloaded Q of good rectangular cavities for ESR is decreased from about 7000 to about 4000 for the observing section of the Varian bimodal

ELDOR cavity. In addition, the microwave filter, which provides 45 dB of isolation between the pump microwave power and the observing detector crystal, has a minimum insertion loss of approximately 3 dB when tuned to the observing bridge frequency. These two factors mean that the observing ESR signal level will be decreased by a factor of 1.9. In addition, the ELDOR effect is typically 5 to 50% of the ESR signal height. Intense ELDOR signals (50% of the ESR height) occur when the radicals undergo favorable intramolecular motion.[62,63] The ELDOR signal height is then lowered 5 to 50 times below the ESR signal observed in a good ESR spectrometer. Of course, in an ELDOR experiment the ESR signal is first observed with the ELDOR cavity and bridge, and the ELDOR signal can be expected to be 5 to 50% of this ESR signal. The microwave filter can be removed if care is taken in operating the ELDOR spectrometer to prevent the pumping klystron frequency from becoming unlocked from the resonance mode of the pumping cavity. In this way a factor of $\sqrt{2}$ in the signal-to-noise ratio can be gained.

2.7.3 Temperature Range

To obtain optimum relaxation conditions it is critically important to have the temperature well regulated but variable over a wide range. Flow gas systems using liquid nitrogen ≥ 100 K (or liquid helium ≥ 10 K) are adequate.[45,64,65] The temperature range can be extended to 5 K by using a liquid helium transfer system (Helitran) available from Air Products, Inc. This system has the provision to vary the temperature between 5 and 300 K by use of an auxiliary heater that heats liquid helium just below the sample position in the ESR cavity. The quartz dewar supplied with the Helitran transfer system can be used with the Varian spectrometer. However it has a thicker wall than the Varian ELDOR dewars and so the frequency range decreases to 225 MHz above to 100 MHz below the observer frequency.

REFERENCES

Experimental Methods

1. J. E. Wertz and J. R. Bolton, *Electron Spin Resonance*, McGraw-Hill, New York, 1972; N. M. Atherton, *Electron Spin Resonance*, Halsted Press-Wiley, New York, 1973.
2. C. P. Poole, Jr., *Electron Spin Resonance: A Comprehensive Treatise on Experimental Techniques*, Wiley-Interscience, New York, 1967.

REFERENCES

3. T. H. Wilmshurst, *Electron Spin Resonance Spectrometers*, Hilger, London, 1967.
4. R. S. Alger, *Electron Paramagnetic Resonance Techniques and Applications*, Wiley-Interscience, New York, 1968.
5. A. L. Kwiram, *Ann. Rev. Phys. Chem.*, **22**, 133 (1971).
6. G. Feher, *Phys. Rev.*, **114**, 1219 (1959).
7. J. Lambe, N. Laurance, E. C. McIrvine, and R. W. Terhune, *Phys. Rev.*, **122**, 1161 (1961).
8. O. S. Leifson and C. D. Jeffries, *Phys. Rev.*, **122**, 1781 (1961); J. M. Baker and F. I. B. Williams, *Proc. Phys. Soc. A*, **267**, 283 (1962).
9. H. Seidel, *Z. Phys.*, **165**, 218 (1961).
10. W. C. Holton and H. Blum, *Phys. Rev.*, **125**, 89 (1962).
11. W. T. Doyle, *Phys. Rev.*, **131**, 555 (1963).
12. R. Gazzinelli and R. L. Mieher, *Phys. Rev.*, **175**, 395 (1968).
13. J. L. Hall and R. T. Schumacher, *Phys. Rev.*, **127**, 1892 (1962).
14. H. H. Woodbury and G. W. Ludwig, *Phys. Rev.*, **117**, 102 (1960).
15. G. D. Watkins and J. W. Corbett, *Phys. Rev. A*, **134**, 1359 (1964).
16. C. A. Hutchison, Jr., and G. A. Pearson, *J. Chem. Phys.*, **47**, 520 (1967).
17. P. Ehret and H. C. Wolf, *Z. Naturforsch.*, **23A**, 1740 (1968).
18. H. C. Box, H. G. Freund, and K. T. Lilga, *J. Chem. Phys.*, **46**, 2130 (1967).
19. R. J. Cook, *J. Sci. Instr.*, **43**, 548 (1966).
20. D. Schmalbein, A. Witte, R. Roder, and G. Laukien, *Rev. Sci. Instr.*, **43**, 1664 (1972).
21. (a) A. H. Maki, R. D. Allendoerfer, J. C. Danner, and R. T. Keys, *J. Amer. Chem. Soc.*, **90**, 4225 (1968); (b) R. D. Allendoerfer and D. J. Eustace, *J. Phys. Chem.*, **75**, 2765 (1971).
22. N. S. Dalal, D. E. Kennedy, and C. A. McDowell, *J. Chem. Phys.*, **59**, 3403 (1973).
23. K. P. Dinse, K. Möbius, and R. Biehl, *Z. Naturforsch.*, **28A**, 1069 (1973).
24. I. Miyagawa, R. B. Davidson, H. A. Helms, Jr., and B. A. Wilkinson, Jr., *J. Magn. Resonance*, **10**, 156 (1973).
25. T. Yamamoto, M. Kono, K. Sato, T. Miyamae, K. Mukai, and K. Ishizu, *JEOL News*, **10a**, 6 (1972).
26. J. S. Hyde, *J. Chem. Phys.*, **43**, 1806 (1965).
27. Varian Instrument Division Bulletin, *E-700 High Power ENDOR System*, 1971; J. S. Hyde, T. Astlind, L. E. G. Eriksson, and A. Ehrenberg, *Rev. Sci. Instr.*, **41**, 1598 (1970).
28. R. C. McCalley and A. L. Kwiram, *Phys. Rev. Lett.*, **24**, 1279 (1970).
29. J. S. Hyde, G. H. Rist, and L. E. G. Eriksson, *J. Phys. Chem.*, **72**, 4269 (1968).
30. (a) G. H. Rist, J. S. Hyde, and T. Vanngard, *Proc. Nat. Acad. Sci. U.S.*, **67**, 79 (1970); (b) J. Helbert, B. Bales, and L. Kevan, *J. Chem. Phys.*, **57**, 723 (1972).
31. G. H. Rist and J. S. Hyde, *J. Chem. Phys.*, **52**, 4633 (1970).
32. L. R. Dalton and A. L. Kwiram, *J. Chem. Phys.*, **57**, 1132 (1972).
33. J. M. Baker, J. R. Chadwick, G. Garton, J. P. Hurrell, *Proc. Roy. Soc. A*, **286**, 352 (1965).
34. E. R. Davies and J. P. Hurrell, *J. Phys. C*, **1**, 847 (1968).
35. P. P. Sorokin, G. J. Lasher, and I. L. Gelles, *Phys. Rev.*, **118**, 939 (1960); W. P. Unruh

and J. W. Culvahouse, *Phys. Rev.*, **129**, 2441 (1963); J. A. Giordmaine, L. E. Alsop, F. R. Nash, and C. H. Townes, *Phys. Rev.*, **109**, 302 (1958); P. R. Moran, *Phys. Rev.*, **135**, A297 (1964); S. Tanaka, A. Koma, and M. Kobayashi, *J. Phys. Soc. Japan*, **22**, 127 (1967).

36. (a) J. S. Hyde, J. C. W. Chien, and J. H. Freed, *J. Chem. Phys.*, **48**, 4211 (1968); (b) J. S. Hyde, L. D. Kispert, R. C. Sneed, and J. C. W. Chien, *J. Chem. Phys.*, **48**, 3824 (1968).
37. V. A. Benderskii, L. A. Blumenfild, P. A. Stunzas, and E. A. Sokolov, *Nature*, **220**, 365 (1968); E. A. Sokolov and V. A. Benderskii, *Pribar Tekh. Eksp.*, **2**, 232 (1969).
38. M. P. Eastman, G. V. Bruno, J. H. Freed, *J. Chem. Phys.*, **52**, 321 (1970).
39. H. M. Vieth, H. Brunner, and K. H. Hausser, *Z. Naturforsch.*, **26A**, 167 (1971); H. Vieth, personal communication.
40. G. H. Rist and J. S. Hyde, *J. Chem. Phys.*, **49**, 2449 (1968).
41. G. H. Rist and J. S. Hyde, *J. Chem. Phys.*, **50**, 4532 (1969).
42. J. S. Hyde, R. C. Sneed, Jr., and G. H. Rist, *J. Chem. Phys.*, **51**, 1404 (1969).
43. A. L. Kwiram, *J. Chem. Phys.*, **49**, 2860 (1968).
44. R. G. Bessent and W. Hayes, *Proc. Roy. Soc. A*, **285**, 430 (1965).
45. U. Ranon and J. S. Hyde, *Phys. Rev.*, **141**, 259 (1966).
46. H. Ohkura, K. Miyoshi, and Y. Mori, *J. Phys. Soc. Japan*, **27**, 790 (1969).
47. R. L. Mieher, *Phys. Rev. Lett.*, **8**, 362 (1962).
48. T. Cole, C. Heller, and J. Lambe, *J. Chem. Phys.*, **34**, 1447 (1961); M. A. Collins and D. H. Whiffen, *Mol. Phys.*, **10**, 317 (1966); J. W. Wells and H. C. Box, *J. Chem. Phys.*, **46**, 2935 (1967).
49. C. A. Hutchison, Jr., and G. A. Pearson, *J. Chem. Phys.*, **43**, 2545 (1965).
50. W. E. Blumberg and G. Feher, *Bull. Amer. Phys. Soc.*, **5**, 183 (1960).
51. W. C. Holton, H. Blum, and C. P. Slichter, *Phys. Rev. Lett.*, **5**, 197 (1960).
52. D. Halford, *Phys. Rev.*, **127**, 1940 (1962).
53. J. M. Baker, W. B. J. Blake, and G. M. Copland, *Phys. Lett. A*, **26**, 504 (1968).
54. J. P. Hurrell, *Brit. J. Appl. Phys.*, **16**, 755 (1965).
55. W. E. Blumberg, J. Eisinger, and S. Geschwind, *Phys. Rev.*, **130**, 900 (1963).
56. N. Lawrance and J. Lambe, *Phys. Rev.*, **132**, 1029 (1963).
57. P. R. Locher and S. Geschwind, *Phys. Rev. Lett.*, **11**, 333 (1963).
58. P. R. Locher and S. Geschwind, *Phys. Rev. A*, **139**, 991 (1965).
59. G. A. Woonton and G. L. Dyer, *Can. J. Phys.*, **45**, 2265 (1967).
60. R. H. Borcherts, L. L. Lohr, Jr., *J. Chem. Phys.*, **50**, 5262 (1969).
61. L. Kispert and K. Chang, *J. Magn. Resonance*, **10**, 162 (1973).
62. L. D. Kispert, K. Chang, and C. M. Bogan, *J. Chem. Phys.*, **58**, 2164 (1973).
63. L. D. Kispert, K. Chang, and C. M. Bogan, *J. Phys. Chem.*, **77**, 629 (1973).

3. Liquid Phase ENDOR

3.1 Introduction
3.2 Spectral Analysis of Proton ENDOR
    3.2.1 Chemical Analogy and ESR Simulation
    3.2.2 Relative Intensities
    3.2.3 Temperature Dependence of ENDOR Widths and Intensities
    3.2.4 Deuteration
    3.2.5 Coherence Effects
    3.2.6 Separation of Overlapping Spectra: ENDOR-Induced ESR
3.3 Rates of Intramolecular Motion
3.4 Applications to Electronic Structure
3.5 Nuclei Other than Protons
3.6 Liquid Crystal Solvents
    3.6.1 Sign of Isotopic Coupling Constants
    3.6.2 Quadrupole Coupling Constants
3.7 Theory of Liquid Phase ENDOR
    3.7.1 Freed's Theory
    3.7.2 Phenomenological Theory
        3.7.2.1 H_1 Dependence of ENDOR Response
        3.7.2.2 H_2 Dependence of ENDOR Response
        3.7.2.3 Dependence of ENDOR Response on Hyperfine Coupling
    3.7.3 Nuclear Relaxation Mechanisms
        3.7.3.1 Electron-Nuclear Dipolar Modulation
        3.7.3.2 Isotropic Hyperfine Modulation
        3.7.3.3 Experimental Criteria to Distinguish END and IH Mechanisms
    3.7.4 Rf Coherence Effects
    3.7.5 Dispersion Mode ENDOR
    References

3.1 INTRODUCTION

Although ENDOR was first carried out in the solid phase in 1959 it was not until 1964 that the first publication on liquid phase ENDOR appeared.[1] The lag was due basically to instrumentation and also partly to the lack of interest in the liquid phase on the part of physicists who first used ENDOR. As discussed in Chapter 2 a basic requirement for successful liquid phase ENDOR experiments is a high power rf field. This follows as a consequence of the much shorter relaxation times for radicals in liquids compared to radicals in solids. In the last 10 years liquid phase ENDOR has developed steadily and has been applied to an ever wider variety of chemical problems. Since good instrumentation is available commercially, the application of this technique will undoubtedly become more and more common. In this chapter we outline how to use liquid phase ENDOR to study the electronic structure of neutral and charged free radicals and to study conformations and rates of intramolecular motion in such radicals. The theoretical basis of liquid phase ENDOR is well developed but is treated in this chapter mostly from a phenomenological point of view. This seems more appropriate for practical application of ENDOR to solve chemical problems. We initially present the spectral analysis of proton ENDOR in relation to specific chemical examples and then briefly describe the theory of liquid phase ENDOR.

In the liquid phase proton ENDOR has been most commonly observed, but isolated studies have also demonstrated ENDOR from ^{14}N (ref. 2), ^{13}C (ref. 3), ^{31}P (ref. 4), ^{7}Li and ^{23}Na (ref. 5), ^{85}Rb, ^{87}Rb, and ^{133}Cs (ref. 6), and ^{19}F (ref. 7). As indicated in Chapter 1 it is easy to identify a particular nucleus that contributes to an ENDOR line because either the sum or difference of the two ENDOR frequencies associated with a given nucleus is directly related to the free nuclear frequency.

There are several different types of displays of ENDOR spectra in the literature and we summarize them briefly here for reference. Typically the absorption mode ESR spectrum is observed with some sort of magnetic field modulation so that a derivative presentation of the ESR spectrum results. The magnetic field is set on an ESR derivative peak and the rf field is swept to obtain an ENDOR spectrum. When the radiofrequency is pulsed (amplitude modulation) and low frequency magnetic field modulation is used, as in the commercial Varian ENDOR spectrometer, the ENDOR responses appear as absorption lines as shown in Fig. 3-1. When cw radiofrequency is used and modulated, typically at kilohertz frequencies, in addition to low frequency magnetic field modulation, as is found in the commerical JEOL spectrometer, the ENDOR responses appear as

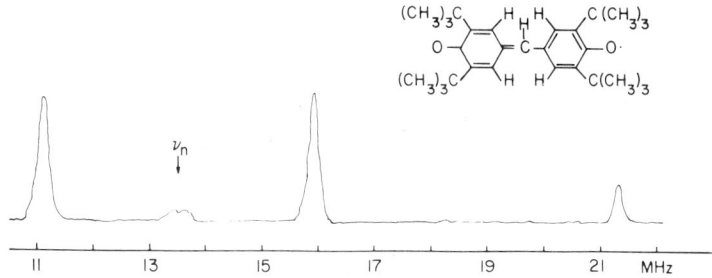

Figure 3-1. Absorption-type display of ENDOR spectrum for the proton on the central carbon (21.3 MHz), the ring protons (15.9 MHz), and the t-butyl protons (~ 13.5 MHz) for Coppinger's radical ($3 \times 10^{-4}\,M$ in n-pentane) at 188 K.

derivative lines as shown in Fig. 3-2. These two displays are the ones most commonly seen in the literature. Hyde[8] also introduced a differential pulse technique that can be used with a pulsed rf spectrometer. In this technique alternate pulses are at different frequencies with the difference depending on the setting of a variable capacitor. This is effectively amplitude and frequency modulation of the radiofrequency and the ENDOR display then appears as a derivative line.

Another type of display is ENDOR-induced ESR.[8] Here one basically detects the ESR spectrum due to the occurrence of ENDOR transitions. One sits on a particular ENDOR line at fixed radiofrequency and sweeps the magnetic field. The result is a derivative-type ESR spectrum that corresponds to the ENDOR line observed. Such ENDOR-induced ESR spectra can be obtained with either pulsed or cw radiofrequency. An

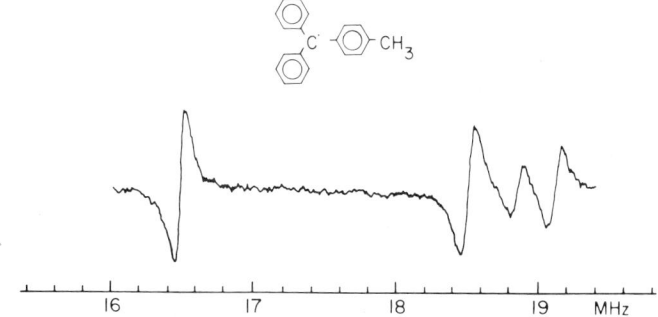

Figure 3-2. Derivative-type display of ENDOR spectrum for $\sim 10^{-3}\,M$ (p-tolyl)diphenylmethyl radical in toluene at 203 K. The free proton frequency occurs at 14.876 MHz and the ENDOR lines in order of increasing frequency are assigned to the meta protons, the ortho protons, the para protons, and the methyl protons in the tolyl ring, respectively. From R. D. Allendoerfer and A. H. Maki, *J. Amer. Chem. Soc.*, **91**, 1088 (1969).

98 LIQUID PHASE ENDOR

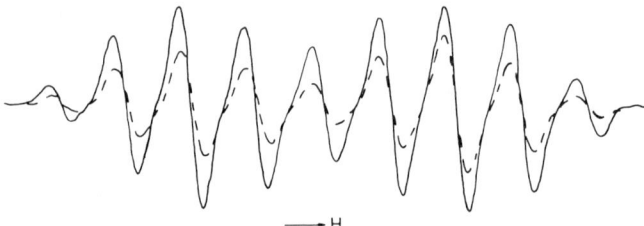

Figure 3-3. ENDOR-induced ESR display for Coppinger's radical. The solid and dashed lines correspond to scanning the magnetic field while sitting on the 15.9 and the 21.3 MHz ENDOR lines of Coppinger's radical, respectively (see Fig. 3-1). From J. S. Hyde, *J. Chem. Phys.*, **43**, 1806 (1965).

example of ENDOR-induced ESR is shown in Fig. 3-3. It will be shown later how ENDOR-induced ESR can be useful for separation of overlapping ESR spectra arising from two different radicals.

Both absorption and derivative presentation of ENDOR lines seem equally satisfactory in general. However since the derivative display suppresses broad ENDOR lines relative to narrow ones, the ability to look at both types of presentations may be useful in certain cases.

3.2 SPECTRAL ANALYSIS OF PROTON ENDOR

In aromatic radicals proton coupling constants are always less than 10 G so the proton ENDOR spectra consist of a pair of ENDOR lines for each set of equivalent protons centered around the free proton frequency (see Fig. 1-5). Only a first order perturbation treatment of the magnetic energy levels is necessary to interpret liquid phase proton ENDOR spectra. The ENDOR frequencies are then given by eq. 1.6, and a pair of ENDOR lines corresponding to one set of equivalent protons is exactly separated by the proton hyperfine constant and centered around the free proton frequency. With second order perturbation theory the average second order shift of the ENDOR lines is given by $A^2/4\nu_e$ where A is measured in frequency units. To second order the separation of the two ENDOR lines is still exactly the hyperfine frequency but both lines are shifted to slightly higher frequencies given by the second order term. For typical coupling constants this second order term is less than a few kilohertz. Since liquid phase ENDOR linewidths are typically 100 kHz or more, such small shifts cannot be detected experimentally. Thus first order treatment of the magnetic energy levels is perfectly satisfactory for liquid phase proton ENDOR. We will find that this is not true, however, for the liquid phase ENDOR of other nuclei.

With commercial ENDOR spectrometers one can typically sweep the radiofrequency from about 6 MHz to more than 30 MHz. If the ESR frequency is at 9.6 GHz, then the free proton frequency will be at 14.4 MHz. Thus for small coupling constants one can see both pairs of ENDOR lines on each side of the proton frequency, but for larger coupling constants only the high frequency ENDOR line will be observed. The ENDOR spectrum is typically simple and one can rapidly obtain a number of proton coupling constants from the ENDOR lines observed. However the assignment of these coupling constants to particular protons or particular sets of equivalent protons in the radical is not straightforward. The relative intensities of the ENDOR lines are sometimes useful but are not typically proportional to the number of equivalent protons corresponding to a particular ENDOR line. The major problem in the spectral analysis of proton ENDOR is to utilize a variety of approaches to assign accurately the ENDOR coupling constants to particular protons. The various methods of approach are summarized as follows.

3.2.1 Chemical Analogy and ESR Simulation

From previous ESR work and molecular orbital calculations a great deal is known about the coupling constants of protons in various types of aromatic radicals. Thus in assigning ENDOR spectra of unanalyzed radicals one can draw upon chemical analogy to a considerable degree. This is of less use, however, for the very small coupling constants that are usually the ones first revealed by ENDOR studies. The most common approach is to make a reasonable chemical assignment of a coupling constant to particular protons and then to simulate the ESR spectrum. The criterion of accurate assignment is the agreement of the simulated ESR spectrum with the experimental one. Although this is the most commonly used method, more definite assignments of ENDOR lines can be made by several of the approaches described in the following sections.

To give an example of this method, however, one may consider the ENDOR spectra of four triarylmethyl radicals in Fig. 3-4. At the time of this ENDOR study the triphenylmethyl radical had been assigned confidently by ESR but the other more complex radicals had not been assigned by ESR alone because of the extreme complexity of their hyperfine patterns. The triphenylmethyl radical at the top of the figure has three sets of equivalent protons, and three ENDOR lines above the free proton frequency (~14.9 MHz) are observed. In order of increasing coupling constant these may be assigned to the meta, ortho, and para protons, respectively.

100 LIQUID PHASE ENDOR

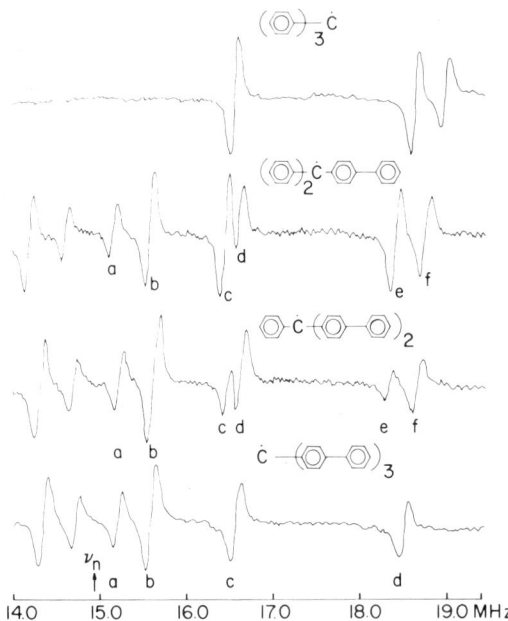

Figure 3-4. ENDOR spectra of the four triarylmethyl radicals indicated at ∼0.003 M in toluene at room temperature. The free proton frequency is ∼14.9 MHz. From A. H. Maki et al., *J. Amer. Chem. Soc.*, **90**, 4225 (1968).

For assignment of the ENDOR line to the other three compounds we summarize the reasoning of Maki et al.[9] Figure 3-5 shows the numbering of the carbon positions in triarylmethyl radicals. First consider the tris(p-biphenylyl)methyl radical whose ENDOR spectrum is at the bottom of Fig. 3-4. There are only four ENDOR lines observed above the free proton frequency, although from the geometry of the molecule there appear to be five sets of equivalent protons. Apparently two of these sets of protons must have about the same coupling constant to within the ENDOR linewidth of about 100 kHz. The inner ring is expected to be little affected by the phenyl substituent in the para position so the

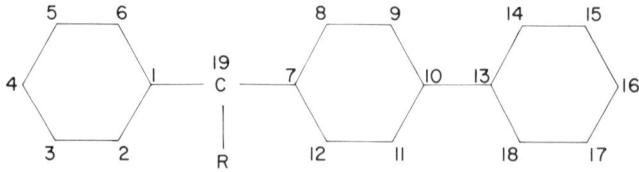

Figure 3-5. Numbering of the carbon positions in the triarylmethyl radicals shown in Fig. 3-4.

splitting constant of ENDOR line d is assigned to position 8 and ENDOR line c is assigned to position 9. The smallest splitting indicated by ENDOR line a is reasonably assigned to the meta protons in the outer ring, position 15. That leaves ENDOR line b to be assigned to the coupling constant of the protons at both positions 14 and 16.

The other two radicals whose ENDOR spectra are shown in the center of Fig. 3-4 both show six ENDOR lines and have eight possible nonequivalent coupling constants. Again some of the coupling constants of the nonequivalent protons are approximately equal. By analogy to the tris(p-biphenylyl)methyl radical, lines a and b can be assigned to positions 15 and to 14 and 16, respectively. Lines c and d must be assigned to the meta protons at positions 3 and 9. It is not obvious whether position 3 or position 9 has the larger coupling constant, so simulations of the ESR spectra were made for each choice for both compounds. In each case the best fit was obtained by assigning the larger coupling constant from ENDOR line d to position 9. This assignment is also in agreement with the approximate ENDOR intensities of lines c and d. For the (p-biphenylyl)diphenylmethyl radical the intensity ratio of line c to line d is approximately 2:1 as expected if line c is assigned to position 3. For the bis(p-biphenylyl)phenylmethyl radical the ratio of these two ENDOR lines is reversed as expected. Relative intensities of ENDOR lines can be useful if the two hyperfine constants are close together and the two types of protons to which they refer are similar (both ring protons, for example). The relative intensities of ENDOR lines will be discussed more quantitatively in the next subsection. The other two ENDOR lines e and f must be assigned to positions 2, 4, and 8. It is reasonably assumed that the coupling to position 4 will remain larger than the coupling to position 2 as in the triphenylmethyl radical so line f is assigned to position 4 and line e is assigned to position 2. The other coupling at position 8 must be the same as one of these and by comparison of simulated and experimental ESR spectra as well as of the relative intensities of lines e and f, it can be seen that ENDOR line f should also be assigned to position 8. This completes the assignment of this particular set of radicals. Although it seems relatively simple it should be recognized that the preceding assignments could not be made from the ESR spectra alone.

3.2.2 Relative Intensities

Here we consider the relative intensities of ENDOR lines from different sets of equivalent protons as observed above the free proton frequency. We will not consider the relative intensities of the high frequency and low

102   LIQUID PHASE ENDOR

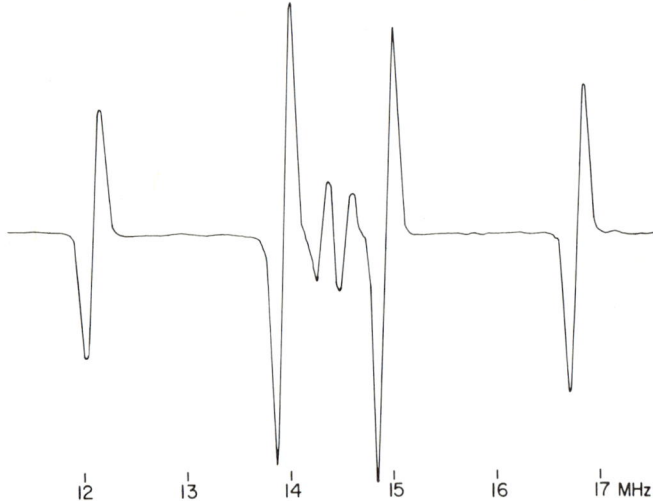

Figure 3-6. ENDOR spectrum of 10^{-3} M tri-t-butyl phenoxy radical in mineral oil at room temperature. From R. Allendoerfer and A. H. Maki, *J. Magn. Resonance*, **3**, 396 (1970).

frequency ENDOR lines from the same set of equivalent protons in this section. The relative intensities do not normally reflect the number of protons giving rise to a particular ENDOR transition. A dramatic example of this can be seen in Fig. 3-6 for the three types of protons in the tri-t-butylphenoxy radical. The assignment of the coupling constant to the different classes of protons is shown in Fig. 3-7 along with the observed relative intensities and the number of protons in each class. Most dramatically, the t-butyl protons in the ortho position seem to be far less intense than might be expected.

We can regard the most probable mechanism of the ENDOR response for protons in solution to be the ΔT_1 mechanism discussed in Chapter 1.

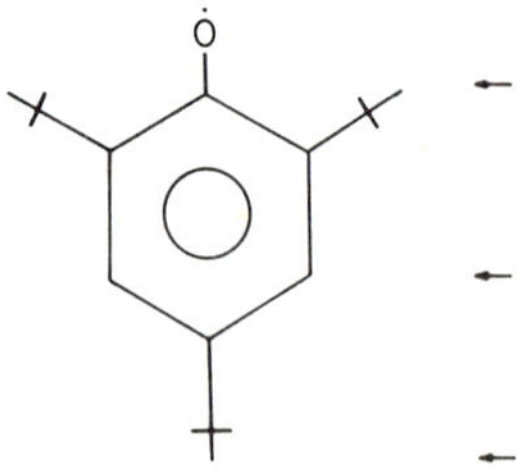

	COUPLING CONSTANTS	NO OF PROTONS	OBSERVED INTENSITIES	CORRECTED INTENSITIES
	0.072 G	18	0.7	21
	1.736 G	2	2.0	2
	0.365 G	9	3.3	9

Figure 3-7. Structure of the tri-t-butyl phenoxy radical with indicated coupling constants and intensities for the different proton classes. See text for additional explanation.

The expected maximum ENDOR enhancement will depend on the dominant relaxation pathway, as illustrated in Table 1-2. The dominant pathway depends on the details of the nuclear relaxation mechanism and may, in general, be expected to differ for different types of protons, such as aromatic ring protons versus t-butyl protons attached to an aromatic ring. In addition, Allendoerfer and Maki[10] have pointed out that ENDOR enhancements depend on the ability of the nuclear radiofrequency to reduce the population difference between the level of the saturated ESR line and the level of the unsaturated ESR lines that are connected by the radiofrequency. In the idealized diagrams in Chapter 1 we have always indicated saturation of only one ESR line in the multilevel system used to demonstrate the ENDOR effect. However if the ESR transitions connected by the radiofrequency are not well separated, several may be partially saturated, which would reduce the maximum ENDOR enhancement. An approximate treatment of this problem, which is discussed in more detail in Section 3.7 on ENDOR theory, results in

$$F_{obs} = F_{max} \frac{T_{2e}^2 \Delta\omega^2}{T_{2e}^2 \Delta\omega^2 + 2.5}. \tag{3.1}$$

Here F_{obs} is the observed ENDOR enhancement, F_{max} is the maximum ENDOR enhancement for the particular ENDOR line observed, and $\Delta\omega$ is the hyperfine splitting in angular frequency units (multiply experimental linear frequencies by 2π) for the class of protons being observed. To apply this equation one needs to know the electron spin-spin relaxation times. They may be obtainable from the well resolved ESR linewidth but if one has very small hyperfine couplings as from the t-butyl protons in the tri-t-butylphenoxy radical, then the ESR lines will be inhomogeneously broadened and will not reflect the value of T_{2e}. Nevertheless, usually a reasonable assumption for T_{2e} can be guessed; 2×10^{-7} sec seems typical for neutral radicals in solution near or somewhat below room temperature. It can also be seen from eq. 3.1 that the classes of protons with the smallest hyperfine coupling will need the largest correction to their observed intensities. This is qualitatively what is observed in the spectrum in Fig. 3-6. The application of eq. 3.1 to this spectrum has been carried out[10] and the results are shown as corrected intensities in Fig. 3-7. Now it can be seen that the corrected intensities approximately reflect the number of protons being observed in each ENDOR transition. This is found in spite of the fact that F_{max} may be expected to differ for each different class of protons. Nevertheless it has been found in a large number of aromatic radicals studied by ENDOR that F_{max} is rather similar for different classes of protons in aromatic radicals and that the

Table 3-1 Selected Results on Proton ENDOR Intensities: Application of Allendoerfer-Maki Intensity Correction

Radical Solvent, Temperature	Proton Types Observed Proton Intensities	Corrected Proton Intensities Ideal Proton Intensities	T_{2e} (sec) Coupling constants (MHz)
4-Formyl-2,6-di-t-butylphenoxy[a] mineral oil, room temperature	ring:formyl:t-butyl 2:0.37:0.35	2.1:1.0:19.5 2:1:18	1.7×10^{-7} 5.9:1.1:0.20
Tri-t-butylphenoxy[b] mineral oil, room temperature	ring:p-t-butyl:o-t-butyl 2:3.3:0.69	2.1:8.5:28 2:9:18	2×10^{-7} 4.9:1.0:0.20
(p-Tolyl)diphenylmethyl[c] toluene, 203 K	methyl:para:ortho:meta 3.0:2.0:4.7:4.7	3.1:2.0:4.8:5.4 3:2:6:6	2×10^{-7} 8.5:8.0:7.3:3.2
Bis(p-methoxyphenyl)nitroxide[d] toluene, 183 K	ortho:meta:methoxy 3.4:1.8:0.47	4.1:4.4:6.5 4:4:6	1×10^{-7} 5.5:2.1:0.70
2,5-Di-t-butyl-p-benzosemiquinone[e] ethanol, 253 K	ring:t-butyl 2:2:2	2:18 2:18	4.9×10^{-7} 6.13:0.19
3,6-Diethoxy-2,5-dimethyl-p-benzosemiquinone[e] ethanol, 253 K	methyl:methylene 6.0:1.3	6:4.1 6:4	9×10^{-7} 3.89:0.19
2,5-Dimethyl-p-benzosemiquinone[f] ethanol, 233 K ethanol, 273 K	methyl:ring 6:2 6:3	no correction indicated 6:2 6:2	$1-9 \times 10^{-7}$ 6.35:5.14 6.35:5.14

[a] R. D. Allendoerfer and D. J. Eustace. *J. Phys. Chem.*, **75**, 2765 (1971).
[b] R. D. Allendoerfer and A. H. Maki, *J. Magn. Resonance*, **3**, 396 (1970).
[c] R. D. Allendoerfer and A. H. Maki, *J. Amer. Chem. Soc.*, **91**, 1088 (1969).
[d] R. D. Allendoerfer and J. H. Engelmann, *Mol. Phys.*, **20**, 569 (1971).
[e] N. M. Atherton and A. J. Blackhurst, *J. Chem. Soc. Faraday II*, **68**, 470 (1972).
[f] N. M. Atherton and B. Day, *Mol. Phys.*, **27**, 145 (1974).

overlap correction of eq. 3.1 gives remarkably good results. As is discussed in the next subsection, the relative ENDOR intensities may also depend on temperature. This is reflected in eq. 3.1 by a temperature dependent T_{2e} and to a much smaller extent from a temperature dependence of the hyperfine coupling. Nevertheless for most ENDOR spectra of aromatic radicals that have been observed at temperatures corresponding to a near optimum signal, the overlap correction of eq. 3.1 has been very successfully used.[7,10-13] A summary of some of these results is shown in Table 3-1. It is remarkable that the overlap correction works so well for such widely varying types of protons.

On the basis of the overlap correction one can easily understand why relative intensities of two different protons with about the same hyperfine constant seem to be in about the correct ratio. Unless the coupling constant is extremely small, the correction factor for both such protons will be about the same, so their relative intensities, although reduced, should roughly reflect the relative number of protons contributing to the two ENDOR lines. This reasoning was used previously in the analysis of the ENDOR lines of the substituted triphenylmethyl radicals in Fig. 3-4.

Although eq. 3.1 seems to be very useful, one should still be aware that it is an approximation and that in certain cases different classes of protons contributing to two different ENDOR lines may have rather different values of F_{max}. Also in certain temperature ranges and particularly in very viscous solutions, where the dominant nuclear relaxation mechanisms may change, the correction of eq. 3.1 may be somewhat inaccurate.

A useful diagram based on eq. 3.1 is shown in Fig. 3-8. It can be seen

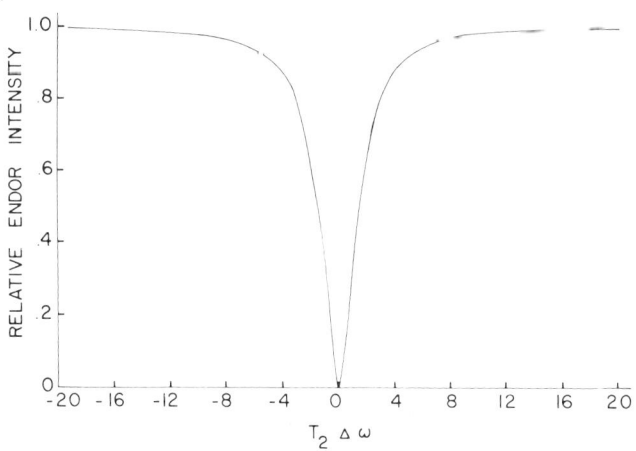

Figure 3-8. Relative ENDOR intensities as a function of $T_{2e}\Delta\omega$ as given by eq. 3.1. From R. D. Allendoerfer and D. J. Eustace, *J. Phys. Chem.*, **75**, 2765 (1971)

3.2.3 Temperature Dependence of ENDOR Widths and Intensities

ENDOR linewidths and intensities depend partly on the anisotropy of their hyperfine interactions. Since large anisotropies are averaged less efficiently than small anisotropies by molecular tumbling and internal rotation, the degree of averaging depends on temperature and leads to a temperature dependent linewidth and line intensity. Protons attached directly to aromatic rings have relatively large anisotropy amounting to about 50% of the isotropic coupling constant,[14] whereas the anisotropy of a rotating methyl group is only about 10% of the isotropic coupling constant.[15] Thus as the liquid viscosity increases at lower temperatures, ring protons broaden and diminish in intensity much more rapidly than do rotating methyl group protons. This is shown rather dramatically by the ENDOR spectrum of the tri-tolylmethyl radical in toluene in Fig. 3-9. In fact, methyl proton ENDOR can even be seen quite clearly in frozen

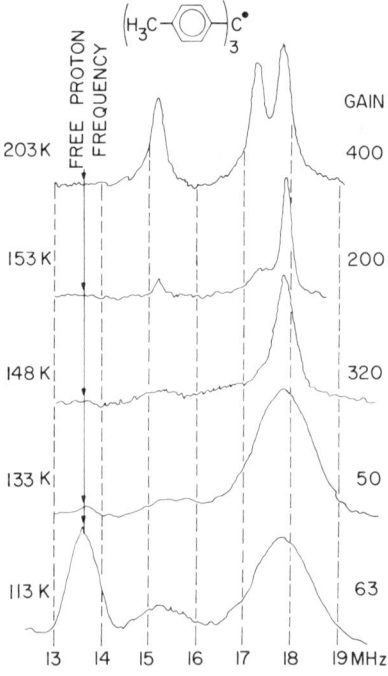

Figure 3-9. ENDOR spectra of tri-tolylmethyl radical in toluene as a function of temperature. As the temperature decreases the ring proton lines at 15.2 and 17.2 MHz broaden beyond detection whereas the methyl proton line at 17.9 MHz broadens but remains detectable. The appearance of the line at the free proton frequency is discussed in Chapter 4. From J. S. Hyde et al., *J. Phys. Chem.*, **72**, 4269 (1968).

glassy matrices, whereas ring proton ENDOR usually becomes unobservable in glassy matrices at low temperature.[16]

An example in which the effect of averaging the hyperfine anisotropy is directly used for the assignment of ENDOR lines occurs in the analysis of various para-methyl-substituted pentaphenylcyclopentadienyl radicals.[17] Figure 3-10 shows the structure of one of these radicals and its ENDOR

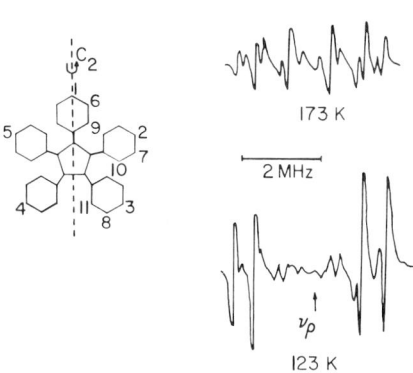

Figure 3-10. ENDOR spectra of 1,3,4-trimethylpentaphenylcyclopentadienyl radical in isopentane at two temperatures. The structure of the unsubstituted radical shows the positions of methyl substitution. The 1-methyl protons should give rise to one pair of ENDOR lines and the 3,4-methyl protons should give rise to another pair of ENDOR lines centered about the free proton frequency (denoted by ν_p). At the lower temperature the methyl proton ENDOR lines remain sharp thus enabling their assignment in the complex spectrum. From K. Möbius et al., *Mol. Phys.*, **20**, 289 (1971).

spectrum at two temperatures. The lines that remain sharp and intense as the temperature is lowered are assigned to methyl protons.

ENDOR intensities also depend on the ratio of viscosity to absolute temperature with a functional form that depends on the particular type of nuclear relaxation process that is important in the ENDOR mechanism. This type of intensity dependence has probably not yet been developed well enough to be of great aid in assigning ENDOR lines.

3.2.4 Deuteration

Deuteration of specific sites on a radical is a very useful way to assign ENDOR lines just as it is useful in assigning ESR spectra. In ESR spectra deuteration of a position with a relatively large hyperfine coupling only serves to complicate the spectrum by increasing the number of lines, since deuterium nuclei have $I = 1$, whereas proton nuclei have $I = \frac{1}{2}$. Of course if the deuteration occurs at a site with a small hyperfine coupling, the increased number of lines from deuteration is not resolved and only increases the linewidth of the ESR lines. In ENDOR spectra the deuteration of a particular proton position completely removes these proton ENDOR lines from the proton ENDOR spectrum. This occurs because the free deuteron frequency is 6.5 times lower than the free proton frequency, so that deuteron ENDOR lines contribute in a far different frequency range than do proton ENDOR lines. However the difficulty with specific deuteration in assigning ENDOR spectra is the same as for ESR spectra; namely, it may be difficult to obtain or to synthesize the specifically deuterated compounds one needs.

An excellent example of how deuteration can be used to assign a complicated ENDOR spectrum is Hyde's study of the triphenylphenoxy radical, which has seven sets of nonequivalent protons.[18] Figure 3-11

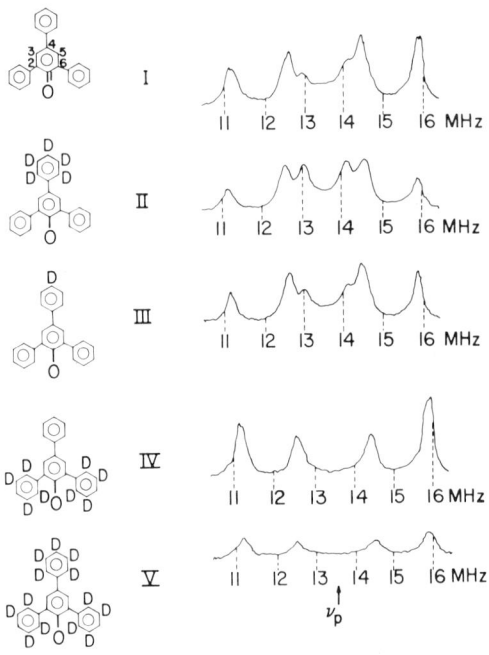

Figure 3-11. ENDOR spectra of variously deuterated triphenylphenoxy radicals, as shown at left, in benzene at 293 K. For analysis see text. From J. S. Hyde, *J. Phys. Chem.*, **71**, 68 (1967).

shows the ENDOR spectra of the various partially deuterated compounds studied. Even with deuteration this spectrum is not easy to analyze because several of the hyperfine couplings are very similar. The undeuterated compound I shows four sets of ENDOR lines corresponding to four hyperfine couplings with two of these almost overlapping to produce one broad line near 15.9 MHz. However the spectra together with the corrected intensity ratios based on eq. 3.1 can be unambiguously assigned. For example, the line near 15.9 MHz in compounds II and V is assigned to the 3,5 central ring protons with a coupling of 4.703 MHz. In compound III this line is shifted slightly to give a coupling of 4.589 MHz and is interpreted as arising from an overlap of two equally intense ENDOR lines that correspond to couplings of 4.703 MHz and 4.475 MHz, the latter being assigned to the ortho protons on the 4-phenyl ring. Because of the accuracy with which the ENDOR line positions can be measured, such reasoning regarding two unresolved ENDOR lines, as indicated earlier, can be applied with some confidence. A detailed discussion of the complete analysis is given in the original paper. The final set of coupling constants obtained was used to simulate the ESR spectrum and excellent agreement was obtained. The overall assignments are given in Table 3-2 and are compared with previous assignments based only on an ESR spectrum. The greater accuracy inherent in ENDOR is easily seen.

Table 3-2. Triphenylphenoxy Radical Hyperfine Constants Obtained by ENDOR and by ESR

Proton Position		ENDOR[a] MHz (G)	ESR[b] (G)
4-Phenyl	ortho	4.475 (1.60)	1.75
	meta	1.662 (0.59)	0.64
	para	4.84 (1.73)	1.75
2,6-Phenyls	ortho	2.03 (0.73)	0.7
	meta	1.070 (0.38)	0.37
	para	2.032 (0.725)	0.7
3,5 Ring protons		4.703 (1.68)	1.75

[a] J. S. Hyde, *J. Phys. Chem.*, **71**, 68 (1967).
[b] K. Dimroth et al., as quoted by Hyde, ibid.

It is also pertinent to remark that ENDOR can often tell whether or not the specifically deuterated compounds are deuterated in the position believed. For example, compound V in Fig. 3-11 was synthesized to contain protons only at the 3,5 central ring positions. In this case one would expect only one ENDOR line since these protons are equivalent. Since two are observed, one of the other positions in the molecule is clearly not completely deuterated. This turned out to be the para position on the 2,6-phenyl groups. Thus ENDOR may sometimes be useful in checking the purity of specifically deuterated compounds.

3.2.5 Coherence Effects

Because of the high rf fields used in liquid phase ENDOR, coherence effects that lead to splitting of certain ENDOR lines are observed.[10] Here we only give a qualitative description of coherence effects as they specifically pertain to the assignment of certain ENDOR lines. A more detailed discussion is given in Section 3.7. Three different types of coherence effects may be distinguished. Two types are electron-nuclear coherence effects in which the coupling of the microwave and rf fields causes ENDOR lines to split. This effect occurs for high microwave power or for very high rf power. Splitting dependent on microwave power is observed, but usually the available rf power is too small to cause splitting dependent on rf power to be observed. The third type of coherence effect is a nuclear-nuclear one in which the splitting of *certain* ENDOR lines is brought about by sufficiently strong rf fields that can cause double quantum transitions between the nuclear energy levels. This nuclear-nuclear coherence effect depends mainly on the rf field strength and hence can be distinguished from the microwave field dependent electron-nuclear coherence effect. The nuclear-nuclear coherence effect is of importance here because double quantum transitions can only be seen for spin systems that have a total nuclear spin greater than one-half. When dealing with proton ENDOR this means that the nuclear-nuclear coherence effects will only be seen for ENDOR lines that correspond to two or more equivalent protons in the radical. Thus coherence effects can unambiguously select out those ENDOR lines that correspond to more than one equivalent proton.

This was first demonstrated[19] for Coppinger's radical:

$$\text{(CH}_3)_3\text{C} \quad \text{H} \qquad \text{H} \quad \text{C(CH}_3)_3$$

[structure: ·O—(ring)—C=(ring)=O with (CH₃)₃C and H substituents]

$$\text{(CH}_3)_3\text{C} \quad \text{H} \quad \text{H} \quad \text{H} \quad \text{C(CH}_3)_3$$

This radical has three ENDOR lines corresponding to the single methide proton, the four ring protons, and the 36 *t*-butyl protons. Figure 3-12 shows the high frequency end of the ENDOR spectrum as a function of rf field. It can be seen that no splitting occurs for the ENDOR line corresponding to the single methylenyl proton whereas with maximum rf field a slight splitting is observed for the ring proton ENDOR line. It should be noted that this splitting is most prominently observed when the ENDOR line arises from monitoring the $m_I = 0$ ESR line of the ring protons. In the case of an ENDOR line from an odd number of equivalent protons the maximum splitting would be observed when monitoring the $m_I = \frac{1}{2}$ ESR line. This dependence on the m_I ESR line observed occurs because the net effect of the double quantum transitions

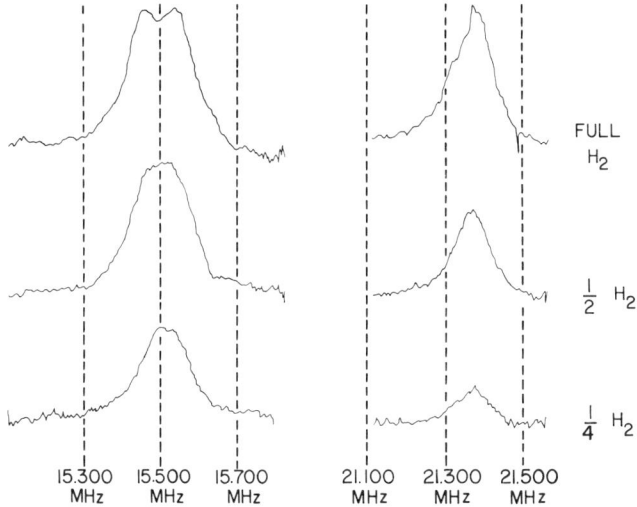

Figure 3-12. Effect of rf field (H_2) on two of the ENDOR lines from Coppinger's radical (3×10^{-4} M) in heptane at 188 K. The line at 15.51 MHz is from the four ring protons when the high field $m_I = 0$ ESR line is observed, and the 21.37 MHz line is from the methylenyl proton. The splitting of the 15.51 MHz line at full H_2 (~20 G) illustrates a nuclear-nuclear coherence effect. From J. H. Freed et al., *J. Chem. Phys.*, **47**, 2762 (1967).

to change the nuclear spin population depends on the m_I of the observed ESR level.

An interesting example of the application of this nuclear-nuclear coherence effect is provided by the ENDOR spectrum of 1-phenylnaphthalene anion.[20] Figure 3-13 shows the ENDOR spectra of 1-phenylnaphthalene anion at two different rf field strengths. A maximum of 12 hyperfine constants corresponding to 12 sets of nonequivalent protons is possible for this radical, but the ENDOR spectrum at the lower rf field strength in Fig. 3-13 only shows 10 ENDOR lines above the free proton frequency (the line from the largest splitting is not shown). Consequently one or two of these lines must correspond to more than one equivalent proton. It is seen that two of these lines do in fact broaden upon application of a high rf field, so these two lines must correspond to two equivalent protons each. Nuclear-nuclear coherence effects were also applied to the ENDOR spectrum of 2-phenylnaphthalene anion in which 11 of 12 possible ENDOR lines were observed above the free proton frequency. Again one of the lines split at high rf field strength, indicating that it corresponded to two equivalent protons. Of course, the overall assignment of the many lines in the ENDOR spectrum in Fig. 3-13 must be made on other grounds, such as those described earlier and discussed in the original work.[20]

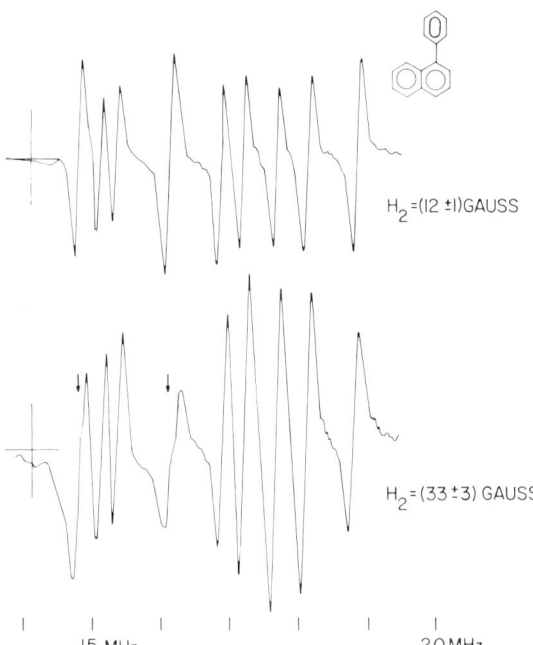

Figure 3-13. Effect of rf field (H_2) on the ENDOR spectra of 1-phenylnaphthalene anion in dimethoxyethane. The spectra above the free proton frequency (shown by the cross) are shown except for one line at 22.2 MHz corresponding to the largest splitting. The ENDOR lines showing broadening due to the nuclear-nuclear coherence effect are marked by arrows; these lines correspond to degenerate hyperfine couplings. From K. P. Dinse et al., *J. Magn. Resonance,* **6,** 444 (1972).

Although observation of the splitting of an ENDOR line because of a nuclear-nuclear coherence effect is positive proof that that ENDOR line corresponds to more than one equivalent proton, the opposite is not true. First of all the splitting depends critically on the amount of rf field strength available, and second the splitting appears to depend on the ENDOR linewidth. For example, in N-galvinoxyl radical in which the central carbon of the radical is replaced by N, the ENDOR lines are somewhat broader and no splitting of the ring proton ENDOR line is observed at the same rf power at which a splitting in galvinoxyl is observed.[19] Of course if higher rf field strengths are available, then one would expect to see a splitting of the ring proton ENDOR lines in N-galvinoxyl.

3.2.6 Separation of Overlapping Spectra: ENDOR-Induced ESR

Often ESR spectra are generated that do not belong to one radical species. The overlap of ESR spectra from two different radicals may make analysis prohibitively difficult. Although many lines of the two overlapping spectra may overlap, there will generally be at least some lines in the spectrum that correspond to only one radical species. In this case ENDOR can offer real advantages in simplifying and separating the overlapping spectra. The coupling constants of each radical can be obtained separately by ENDOR taken by sitting on a nonoverlapped ESR line corresponding to one of the radicals. An example of this is illustrated in a study of semiquinone radical anions produced by dissolving the quinone in alkaline ethanol.[21,22] If the quinone is 2,5-dimethyl-*p*-benzoquinone, then initially the ESR spectrum is the simple one shown in Fig. 3-14A, which corresponds to the expected semiquinone anion. However if one waits several hours at room temperature, the ESR spectrum

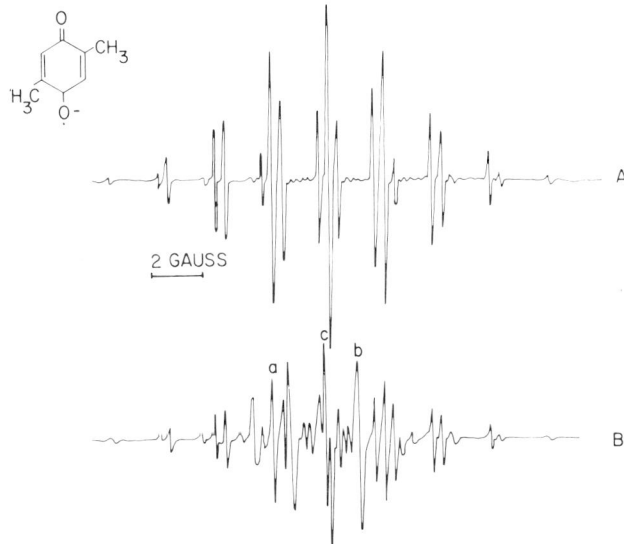

Figure 3-14. (*A*) ESR spectrum of the 2,5-dimethyl-*p*-benzosemiquinone radical anion in ethanol at room temperature. (*B*) ESR spectrum of the solution in *A* after partial reaction with ethanol solvent has occurred to create the secondary radical 3,6-diethoxy-2,5-dimethyl-*p*-benzosemiquinone. Lines marked *a*, *b*, and *c* were saturated to obtain the ENDOR spectra in Fig. 3-15. From N. M. Atherton et al., *J. Chem. Soc. Faraday II*, **68**, 470 (1972).

changes to that shown in Fig. 3-14*B*. The complexity of this spectrum suggests that a second radical is being produced and that at this stage there is a mixture of both radicals present. To separate the coupling constants corresponding to these two radicals one may obtain ENDOR spectra by sitting on the ESR lines marked *a*, *b*, and *c*. ENDOR spectra

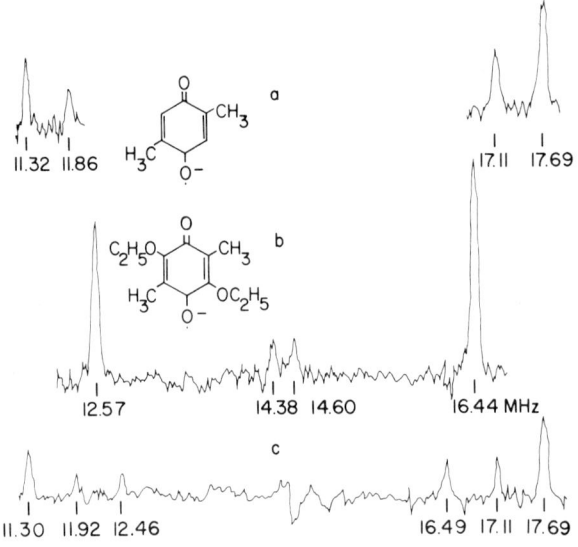

Figure 3-15. (a) ENDOR spectrum of 2,5-dimethyl-p-benzosemiquinone in ethanol at 253 K obtained by saturating line a in Fig. 3-14. (b) ENDOR spectrum of 3,6-diethoxy-2,5-dimethyl-p-benzosemiquinone in ethanol at 253 K obtained by saturating line b in Fig. 3-14. (c) ENDOR spectrum of both preceding radical anions obtained by saturating line c in Fig. 3-14. From N. M. Atherton et al., *J. Chem. Soc. Faraday II,* **68,** 470 (1972).

taken at these positions are shown in Fig. 3-15. It is clearly seen that the ENDOR spectrum taken on ESR line a is completely different from the ENDOR spectrum taken on ESR line b whereas the ENDOR spectrum taken on ESR line c seems to be a mixture of the preceding two spectra. Thus ESR lines a and b correspond to nonoverlapped lines of the two radicals in the mixture, whereas ESR line c corresponds to a magnetic field position where both radicals contribute to the ESR spectrum. In this particular case ESR line a is assigned to the 2,5-dimethyl-p-benzosemiquinone anion radical, which corresponds to the ESR spectrum seen originally when the quinone is added to the alkaline ethanol and is shown in Fig. 3-14A. Two coupling constants are obtained from the ENDOR spectrum and the assignments are 6.38 MHz for the six methyl protons and 5.22 MHz for the two protons at the 3,6 positions. The two different coupling constants obtained from ENDOR spectrum b in Fig. 3-15 are assigned to a secondary radical formed by reaction with ethanol to form a 3,6-diethoxy-2,5-dimethyl-p-benzosemiquinone anion with coupling constants of 3.89 MHz assigned to the six methyl protons in the 2,5 positions and 0.19 MHz assigned to the four ethoxy-methylene protons in the 3,6 positions. After about three days at room temperature, the mixture will gradually change to form the ethoxy-substituted anion radical exclusively, and the ESR spectrum correspondingly simplifies.[22] It also seems possible to sit on a nonoverlapped ENDOR line and obtain an ENDOR-induced ESR spectrum of each individual radical in the mixture. This technique has been applied to the following semiquinone anion system.

When 2,3,5,6,-tetramethylquinone (duroquinone) is reduced by potassium metal in 1,2-dimethoxyethane, the durosemiquinone anion is produced. The ENDOR spectrum of this radical is shown at 195 K in Fig. 3-16.[23] The free durosemiquinone anion is expected to have 12 equivalent protons; however three hyperfine couplings are indicated by the

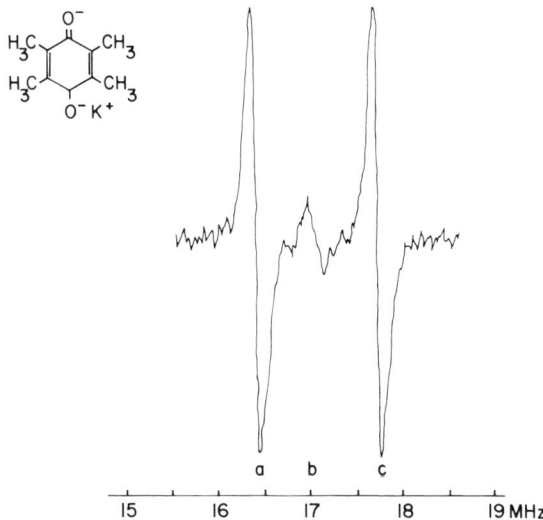

Figure 3-16. High frequency half ($\nu_p \approx 14.5$ MHz) of the ENDOR spectrum of durosemiquinone at 195 K formed by potassium reduction in 1,2-dimethoxyethane. Lines a and c are assigned to a tight ion pair between the durosemiquinone anion and potassium cation while line b is assigned to the free durosemiquinone anion. From R. D. Allendoerfer et al., *J. Amer. Chem. Soc.*, **92,** 6971 (1970).

ENDOR spectrum in Fig. 3-16. Thus at least two overlapping radicals must be present in the ESR spectrum and must contribute to the ENDOR spectrum. To assign the ENDOR lines and to separate the overlapping ESR spectra one may carry out ENDOR-induced ESR[8] in which one records the intensity of one particular ENDOR line while sweeping the magnetic field. Figure 3-17 shows that two distinctly different ESR spectra are obtained when this is done. The ENDOR-induced ESR spectrum in Fig. 3-17c is obtained when either ENDOR line a or c

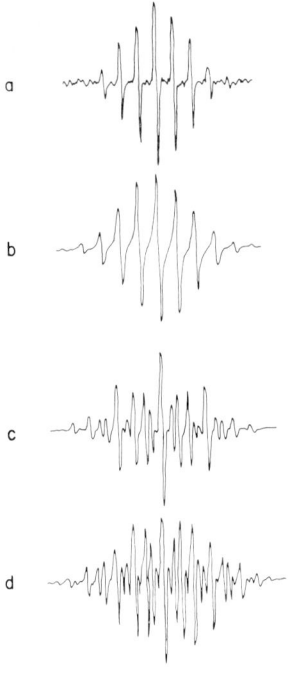

Figure 3-17. (a) The ENDOR-induced ESR spectrum of durosemiquinone at 195 K formed by potassium reduction in 1,2-dimethoxyethane when ENDOR line b in Fig. 3-16 is monitored. This spectrum is assigned to the free durosemiquinone anion. (b) The ESR spectrum of durosemiquinone at 353 K formed by potassium reduction in 1,2-dimethoxyethane. This spectrum is assigned largely to the free durosemiquinone anion; compare with the ESR spectrum at lower temperature in (d). (c) The ENDOR-induced ESR spectrum of durosemiquinone at 195 K formed by potassium reduction in 1,2-dimethoxyethane when ENDOR line a in Fig. 3-16 is monitored. This spectrum is assigned to a tight ion pair between durosemiquinone anion and potassium cation. (d) The ESR spectrum of durosemiquinone at 195 K formed by potassium reduction in 1,2-dimethoxyethane. This spectrum is assigned largely to the tight ion pair.

in Fig. 3-16 is monitored, whereas the ENDOR-induced ESR spectrum of Fig. 3-17a is obtained when ENDOR line b in Fig. 3-16 is monitored. This latter spectrum seems similar to that of the free durosemiquinone anion with coupling to 12 equivalent protons. Thus ENDOR line b is assigned to this coupling constant. ENDOR lines a and c are assigned to a tight ion pair between the durosemiquinone anion and potassium cation. This gives two sets of six nonequivalent protons whose hyperfine couplings are given by ENDOR lines a and c in Fig. 3-16. To the extent that the relative intensities can be compared it appears that the free durosemiquinone anion is only present to about 10% in the mixture at 195 K. If, however, one raises the temperature to 353 K, the ESR spectrum of the mixture (Fig. 3-17b) appears characteristic of the free durosemiquinone anion and is very much like the ENDOR-induced ESR spectrum in Fig. 3-17a. Note that when there are no nonoverlapped lines of one of the radicals in the ESR spectrum of a radical mixture, the ENDOR-induced ESR technique still serves to separate the ESR spectra of the two radicals, provided that one of them has a unique coupling constant and consequently a nonoverlapped ENDOR line. Unless the ESR spectrum is very well resolved, which is usually not the case in a radical mixture, one often finds it useful to overmodulate the ESR spectrum when recording the ENDOR spectrum so that contributions from all radicals appear with their maximum intensity in the ENDOR spectrum.

Finally it should be cautioned that ENDOR-induced ESR spectra may not always have the same relative intensities of the spectral lines as those that would be obtained in the directly detected ESR spectrum. Consider the case of an electron interacting with two equivalent protons. There are three symmetric nuclear spin states and one antisymmetric nuclear spin state. Since no magnetic dipole matrix elements connect the symmetric and antisymmetric spin states, the ENDOR-induced ESR transitions will only involve the symmetric spin states and would be expected to give a spectrum with a $1:1:1$ intensity ratio rather than the $1:2:1$ intensity ratio found in the directly detected ESR spectrum in which all spin states contribute. A demonstration of this behavior was found for the 2,5-di-*t*-butylsemiquinone anion prepared in alkaline ethanol.[8] At 243 to 253 K the ENDOR-induced ESR spectrum indeed shows the expected $1:1:1$ intensity ratios. However at higher temperature near 283 K the ENDOR-induced ESR spectrum shows the $1:2:1$ intensity ratios, implying that the radicals do not remember their spin wavefunction. This of course is possible if spin exchange occurs more rapidly than the ENDOR transitions. Spin exchange is favored by a higher temperature and provides an explanation for the change in intensity ratio noted. ENDOR-induced ESR spectra have not been utilized to a very great extent yet, but for complicated spectra the intensity anomalies do not seem so common. Of course this will depend on the temperature at which the ENDOR spectrum is obtained. To summarize, the relative intensities of the lines in ENDOR-induced ESR spectra may be different from directly detected ESR spectra, but in several complicated spectra investigated with more than two equivalent protons contributing to the observed ENDOR line, the relative intensity ratios of the two spectra seem to be about the same.

3.3 RATES OF INTRAMOLECULAR MOTION

Intramolecular motions affect ESR and ENDOR spectra when the motions occur at frequencies in the range of typical hyperfine couplings—10^5 to 10^7 Hz. Since hyperfine couplings are measured very accurately by ENDOR, small changes in these as a function of temperature, due to intramolecular motions, can be used to obtain quantitative information about the rates of the intramolecular motions.[24–27] In addition, the particular coupling constant that changes can often allow one to delineate the specific motion that causes the change in the ENDOR spectrum. Internal

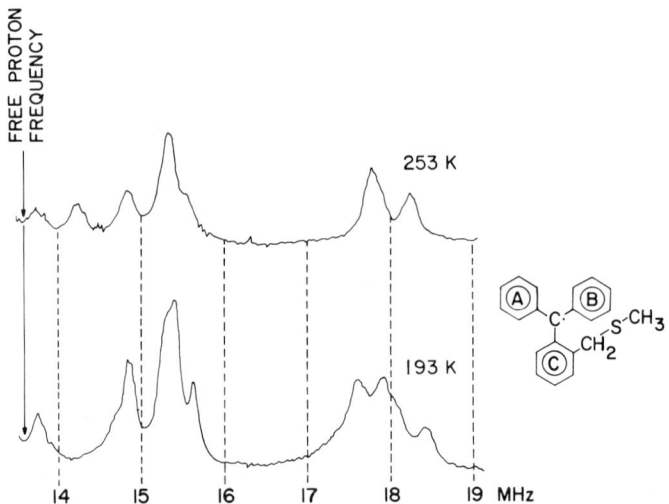

Figure 3-18. ENDOR spectra of the indicated substituted triphenylmethyl radical at $\sim 3 \times 10^{-4}$ M in ethylbenzene at two temperatures. Note the collapse of some of the lines at 193 K to a single average line at 253 K. From L. D. Kispert et al., *J. Phys. Chem.*, **72,** 4276 (1968).

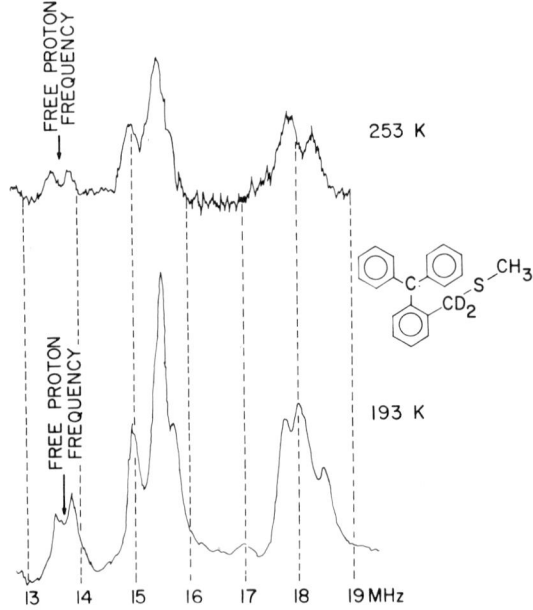

Figure 3-19. ENDOR spectra of the indicated substituted triphenylmethyl radical at $\sim 3 \times 10^{-4}$ M in ethylbenzene at two temperatures. The proton ENDOR lines from the deuterated position lie in the 13.5 to 15.0 MHz region; compare with Fig. 3-18. From L. D. Kispert et al., *J. Phys. Chem.*, **72,** 4276 (1968).

motions also affect the nuclear relaxation mechanisms and consequently the ENDOR intensities. However the analysis of such effects is rather subtle and has not yet been applied quantitatively.

An example of how intramolecular rates may be studied by ENDOR is illustrated by some ortho-substituted triphenylmethyl radicals. The structures of the radicals studied in the ENDOR spectra at two temperatures are given in Figs. 3-18 and 3-19. The couplings from the ENDOR spectra were assigned as shown in Table 3-3 on the basis of chemical analogy and computer simulation of the ESR spectra. The interesting point is that the number of couplings in the ENDOR spectrum is greater at 193 K than at 253 K. However it can be seen that ENDOR lines at about 17.9 and 17.7 MHz at 193 K seem to collapse to a single line at 17.8 MHz at 253 K. Likewise lines at 18.4 and 18.2 MHz at 193 K seem to collapse to a line at 18.3 MHz at 253 K. These lines are reasonably attributed to the ortho and para protons on the unsubstituted phenyl rings. The spectra at 193 K then show that the ortho protons on these two phenyl rings are not equivalent but that they become equivalent at 253 K. The same is true of the para protons, and it is clear that some intramolecular motion is being averaged out when the temperature is raised. This must be the motion of the ortho-substituted side chain in the radical. By deuterating the methylene group (see Fig. 3-19) the absence of a line at about 14.2 MHz at 253 K indicates that the methylene protons are inequivalent at 193 K and become equivalent at 253 K. Thus the intramolecular motion that is being examined is the rotation around the C—C bond between the phenyl ring and the ortho-substituted substituent. However since the ortho and para protons also become equivalent when the temperature is raised to 253 K, the intramolecular motion being examined is not simple rotation about a C—C bond but must involve a motion that interchanges the two unsubstituted rings to make them equivalent. This indicates that the motion is an interconversion of left-hand and right-hand propeller conformations of the radical.

The activation energy E_a and frequency factor ν_o of this process and a rate at a particular temperature can be obtained by observation of the change in the splitting of the two lines that collapse to a single line as a function of temperature.[24] These results can be analyzed in the same way as are NMR results.[27] The Arrhenius equation may be written as

$$\log \frac{1}{\tau \delta \omega} = \log \frac{2\nu_o}{\delta \omega} - \frac{E_a}{2.3\,RT} \qquad (3.2)$$

with

$$\frac{1}{\tau \delta \omega} = 2^{-1/2}\left[1 - \left(\frac{\delta \omega_e}{\delta \omega}\right)^2\right]^{1/2}$$

Table 3-3. ENDOR Couplings (MHz) of Mono (o-CH$_2$SCH$_3$)-triphenylmethyl Radical

ENDOR Coupling (193 K)	Number of Protons	Assignment[a]	ENDOR Coupling (253 K)
0.30	3	CH$_3$	0.03
0.50	1	CH$_2$ (one) ⎫	1.13
2.28	1	CH$_2$ (one) ⎭	
2.52	2	meta (C)	2.53
3.59	4	meta (A, B)	3.51
4.08	2	ortho, para (C)	4.02
8.21	2	ortho (A or B) ⎫	8.28
8.73	2	ortho (B or A) ⎭	
9.05	1	para (A or B) ⎫	9.12
9.62	1	para (B or A) ⎭	

From L. D. Kispert et al., *J. Phys. Chem.*, **72**, 4276 (1968)
[a] Refer to Fig. 3-18 for lettering of rings.

where $\delta\omega$ is the separation of the lines in the limit of slow exchange at low temperature, $\delta\omega_e$ is the experimentally observed line separation at various temperatures, and τ is the lifetime of a proton in a particular configuration. This equation assumes that the ENDOR linewidth is determined by $(T_{2e})^{-1}$ and is less than the line splitting. For the system in Fig. 3-18 a rate constant of $k = 10^{11} \exp(5.5 \text{ kcal}/RT) \text{ sec}^{-1}$ is obtained.

Another example of temperature dependent conformational changes resulting in temperature dependent collapse of two ENDOR lines is shown by the following dimethyl-substituted galvinoxyl.[25] The methide

proton is split at about 193 K in toluene and analysis of the decrease of this splitting corresponds to an activation energy of about 1 kcal mole^{-1} for the frequency of rotation of the ring about the bond to the methylene carbon.

One can also use the broadening of an ENDOR line as a function of temperature to analyze the rates of certain intramolecular motions in free radicals.[26] This is important when the two ENDOR lines corresponding to two different conformations overlap sufficiently so that the decrease in splitting as a function of temperature cannot be followed but only the decrease in overall linewidth can be followed. This is the case for substituted semiquinone anions. In particular, the ubisemiquinone anion gives an ENDOR spectrum as a function of temperature as shown in Fig. 3-20. The ENDOR line from the methyl protons at 15.2 MHz stays sharp over the temperature range in contrast to the ENDOR line from the methylene protons at 16.7 MHz. As the temperature is lowered, the methylene proton ENDOR line broadens and finally splits into two distinct lines corresponding to separate coupling constants for the two methylene protons. In this case the rotatory motion of the side chain on the ubisemiquinone anion has been slowed to a rate less than the time scale of the ENDOR experiment. Analysis of the ENDOR linewidth then gives a rate for the rotatory motion of this side chain and an activation energy of about 7 kcal mole^{-1} is obtained in dimethoxyethane and in ethanol solvents.[26]

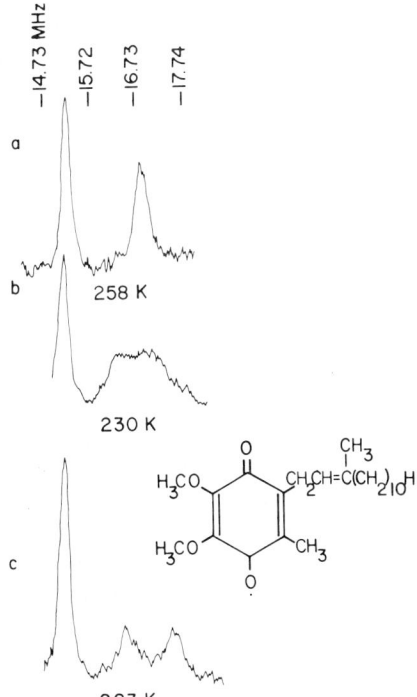

Figure 3-20. ENDOR spectra of ubisemiquinone anion in ethanol at various temperatures. The line at ~15.2 MHz is assigned to the ring methyl protons and the line at ~16.8 MHz is assigned to the methylene protons. Note that the methylene proton line broadens and splits as the temperature decreases. From M. R. Das et al., *J. Amer. Chem. Soc.*, **92**, 2258 (1970).

A theoretical analysis of ENDOR linewidths[28] gives the following expression for a two jump model of the rate process:

$$T_2^{-1}(\text{ENDOR}) = \tfrac{1}{64}\gamma_e^2 \tau_0 (A_1 - A_2)^2 \qquad (3.3)$$

In this expression the hyperfine constants A_1 and A_2 are those of the two methylene protons obtained at the lowest temperature in Fig. 3-20, γ_e is the gyromagnetic ratio of the electron, T_{2e}^{-1} is the ENDOR linewidth, full width at half height, and τ_0 is the rate of the process. This equation gives the contribution to the ENDOR linewidth from the intermolecular motion. The actual experimental ENDOR linewidth includes this contribution as well as other intrinsic contributions. Some measure of this intrinsic ENDOR linewidth must be obtained in order to carry out the analysis with eq. 3.3. In the ubisemiquinone anion case it was assumed that the methyl proton ENDOR line was an approximation to the intrinsic width, and the excess width was then attributed to the kinetic process and analyzed by eq. 3.3.

It has been seen that the rates of various types of intramolecular motion can be analyzed from temperature dependent ENDOR spectra. An important feature is that the ENDOR line itself, which shows such behavior characteristic of intramolecular motion, also helps to identify the location of the particular motion being studied.

3.4 APPLICATIONS TO ELECTRONIC STRUCTURE

A variety of radicals have been studied by liquid phase proton ENDOR. A summary of those reported through the end of 1973 is given in Table 3-4. Attention has focused on low symmetry radicals in which the profusion of coupling constants makes interpretation of the ESR spectrum ambiguous or impossible. The types of radicals studied can be classified as anions, cations, and neutrals. Among anions, semiquinones and substituted semiquinones have been most studied, together with a variety of aromatic anions. Only two cations have been studied, tetracene and rubrene. Many neutral radicals have been investigated, most of which fall into the categories of substituted galvinoxyls, substituted phenoxy radicals and substituted triphenylmethyl radicals. Almost all of the radical ions and neutral radicals studied have been hydrocarbons; only a few of the radicals have contained other atoms such as nitrogen, phosphorus, or arsenic, as shown in the last few entries in Table 3-4.

The objective of most of these studies has been to determine the hyperfine constants for various proton positions in the radical, to obtain "experimental" spin densities from the McConnell equation,

$$A_{CH}^{H} = Q_{CH}^{H} \rho_{C}^{\pi} \tag{3.4}$$

and to compare these spin densities with theoretical ones calculated generally by the McLachlan perturbation correction[29] to the Hückel LCAO-MO method. Satisfactory agreement between the experimental and calculated spin densities suggests that the delocalization of the π electrons in the radical is fairly well understood. The effect of various substituents on spin densities in radicals has been widely studied by this method. For example, Allendoerfer and Maki[30] studied the ENDOR spectra of a series of six methyl- and fluorine-substituted triphenylmethyl radicals. The complexity of the ESR spectrum of substituted triphenylmethyl radicals usually required ENDOR studies for interpretation. In this particular study they concluded that fluorine and methyl substitution in the meta and para positions had little effect on the spin density distribution, whereas a large effect was observed for ortho substitution. Table 3-4 indicates other studies of this type.

An interesting application of the comparison of experimental and calculated spin densities from ENDOR experiments involves the question of π-electron and σ-electron separability as studied by Möbius and co-workers.[20,31] In the 1-phenylnaphthalene and 2-phenylnaphthalene anions[20] there are large discrepancies between the experimental and calculated hyperfine constants, suggesting that the pure π-electron theories used to calculate the coupling constants are inappropriate and that there is some π-electron delocalization into the σ-electron system. Of course these anion radicals are nonplanar where this effect might be expected to be observed. Similar conclusions are also reached from studies of the negative and positive radical ions of rubrene (tetraphenyltetracene).[31] In this case the order of the phenyl proton coupling constants $A_H^{meta} > A_H^{para} = A_H^{ortho}$ is in contrast to the predictions of pure π-molecular orbital theories (i.e., $A^p > A^o > A^m$) and again suggests direct delocalization of the unpaired π-electron into the σ-electron system of the phenyl rings in these radical ions. On the other hand, no evidence for π-σ delocalization in the nonplanar pentaphenylcyclopentadienyl radical is found.[17]

Another interesting electronic structure study involves the lifting of ground state orbital degeneracy by methyl substituents in pentaphenylcyclopentadienyl radicals.[17] If the orbital ground state of a radical is twofold degenerate, methyl substitution may lower the symmetry and remove the degeneracy. An interesting example of this in which analysis is only possible by ENDOR occurs for methyl-substituted pentaphenylcyclopentadienyl radicals. The unsubstituted radical has D_5 symmetry and

Table 3-4 Summary of Liquid Phase Proton ENDOR Studies through 1974

Radical	Conditions	Objectives and Comments	References
Anions			
1,4-Naphthosemiquinone 2,3-Dimethyl-1,4-naphthosemiquinone 2-Methyl-1,4-naphthosemiquinone (menadione: vitamin K_3) 2-Methyl-3-phytyl-1,4-naphthosemiquinone (vitamin K_1 semiquinone) 2,3,5,6-Tetramethylsemiquinone (durosemiquinone) α-Tocopherol semiquinone (vitamin E semiquinone) Ubiquinone	ethanol, 223 K	To determine molecular electronic structure via spin densities and to determine geometry via β-H coupling constants and the equivalence of certain protons Some variable temperatures reported	M. R. Das, H. D. Connor, D. S. Leniart, and J. H. Freed, *J. Amer. Chem. Soc.*, **92**, 2258 (1970)
2,5-Dimethyl-*p*-benzosemiquinone 2,5-Di-*t*-butyl-*p*-benzosemiquinone 1,4-Naphthosemiquinone 2,3-Dichloro-1,4-naphthosemiquinone 9,10-Anthrasemiquinone 1,5-Dichloro-9,10-anthrasemiquinone 9,10-Phenanthrasemiquinone	ethanol methanol, 213–293 K, 10^{-3}–$10^{-4}\,M$	To assign coupling constants, to follow secondary reactions with alcohol solvent	N. M. Atherton and A. J. Blackhurst, *J. Chem. Soc. Faraday II*, **68**, 470 (1972)
Di-*t*-butylsemiquinone *p*-Benzosemiquinone		To demonstrate ENDOR feasibility	J. S. Hyde, *J. Chem. Phys.*, **43**, 1806 (1965)
p-Benzosemiquinone 1,4-Naphthasemiquinone 2,5-Di-*t*-butyl-*p*-benzosemiquinone *o*-Phenanthrasemiquinone		To measure coupling constants and to compare with calculated spin densities	R. J. Cook and D. J. Moss, *Proc. XVI Congress Ampere*, Romania Publishing House, Bucharest (1971), p. 1109.

2,5-Dimethyl-p-benzosemiquinone 9,10-Anthrasemiquinone 2,5-Di-t-butyl-p-benzosemiquinone	methanol, ethanol, and isopropanol, 193–273 K	To relate the temperature dependence of the ENDOR intensity to nuclear relaxation mechanisms	Y. Kotaka and K. Kuwata, *Bull. Chem. Soc. Japan*, **47**, 45 (1974)
2,3,5,6-tetramethylsemiquinone (durosemiquinone)	dimethoxyethane, 195 K, $\sim 10^{-3}$ M	To study ion pair equilibria with alkali metal cations and to separate spectra by ENDOR-induced ESR	R. D. Allendoerfer and R. J. Papez, *J. Phys. Chem.*, **76**, 1012 (1972); *J. Amer. Chem. Soc.*, **92**, 6971 (1970).
Naphthalene anion Anthracene anion Tetracene anion p-Terphenyl anion m-Terphenyl anion	dimethoxyethane, 204 K, 10^{-4}–10^{-3} M	To assign coupling constants and spin densities; to demonstrate ENDOR feasibility	A. Lagendijk et al., *Chem. Phys. Lett.*, **6**, 152 (1970).
Biphenyl anion o-Terphenyl anion m-Terphenyl anion p-Terphenyl anion	dimethoxyethane, K$^+$, 2-methyltetrahydrofuran, 175–185 K for DME, 150–220 K for *MTHF* $\sim 10^{-3}$ M	To assign coupling constants and to compare with calculated spin densities; to assess evidence for π-σ delocalization (none)	R. Biehl et al., *Chem. Phys. Lett.*, **10**, 605 (1971).
Tetraphenyltetracene anion (rubrene anion)	dimethoxyethane, K$^+$, 178 K	To demonstrate π-σ delocalization	R. Biehl et al., *Tetrahedron*, **29**, 363 (1973).
1-Phenylnaphthalene anion 2-Phenylnaphthalene anion	dimethoxyethane, K$^+$, 176 K	To measure couplings and compare with calculated spin densities; to demonstrate π-σ delocalization	K. P. Dinse et al., *J. Magn. Resonance*, **6**, 444 (1972).
1,2,3,6,7,8-Hexahydropyrene anion	dimethoxyethane, Li$^+$, 193 K	To measure coupling constants; to resolve couplings from axial and equatorial protons	A. I. Shain, *Mol. Phys.*, **22**, 733 (1971).

Table 3-4 *(Continued)*

Radical	Conditions	Objectives and Comments	References
Hexahelicene anion	dimethoxyethane, K^+, 193 K	To assign coupling constants (partially), to deduce geometry of complex with K^+	R. D. Allendoerfer and R. Chang, *J. Magn. Resonance*, **5**, 273 (1971).
4,4′-Diisopropylbiphenyl anion	dimethoxyethane, K^+, 188–213 K	To study the temperature dependence of the β-proton coupling constant to assess restricted rotation in the anion	F. Nemoto et al., *Chem. Lett.*, 693 (1974).
7,12-Dihydropleiadene anion 1-Methyl-7,12-dihydropleiadene anion 7,12-(o-Phenylene)-7,12-dihydropleiadene anion	dimethoxyethane, K^+, 193 K	To study spin densities and axial versus equatorial conformations of these anions	R. D. Allendoerfer et al., *J. Amer. Chem. Soc.*, **94**, 7702 (1972)
α-Phenylbenzylidene malononitrile anion	dimethoxyethane, K^+, 183 K	To compare coupling constants with calculated spin densities and to deduce conformation of the phenyl rings	R. Chang et al., *J. Phys. Chem.*, **76**, 3384 (1972).
m-Dibenzoylbenzene anion	hexamethylphosphoramide	To compare coupling constants with calculated spin densities and to distinguish syn and anti conformations	R. D. Allendoerfer, *J. Magn. Resonance*, **9**, 140 (1973).
Di-o-mesitoylbenzene anion · Li^+ Di-o-mesitoylbenzene anion · Na^+	2-methyltetrahydrofuran, 173–193 K	To deduce structure of complex from coupling constants, to observe Na and Li ENDOR, to assess relaxation mechanism for alkali metal nuclei	N. M. Atherton and B. Day, *J. Chem. Soc. Faraday Trans. II*, **69**, 1801 (1973).

System	Conditions	Purpose	Reference
Di-o-mesitoylbenzene anion · Rb^+ Di-o-mesitoylbenzene anion · Cs^+	2-methyltetrahydrofuran, 1,2-dimethoxyethane, diglyme, 150–220 K	Same as immediately above	H. van Willigen et al., *Mol. Phys.*, **26**, 793 (1973).
Cations			
Tetracene cation	concentrated H_2SO_4, 253–313 K, 10^{-3}–10^{-2} M	ENDOR feasibility, effect of temperature and concentration on signal intensity	J. S. Hyde, *J. Chem. Phys.*, **43**, 1806 (1965).
Tetraphenyltetracene cation (rubrene cation)	nitromethane ($AlCl_3$ oxidation), 190–250 K	To demonstrate π-σ delocalization	R. Biehl et al., *Tetrahedron*, **29**, 363 (1973).
Neutral Radicals			
Triphenylmethyl	toluene, 183 K, $\sim 10^{-3}$ M	ENDOR feasibility; to measure coupling constants	J. S. Hyde, *J. Chem. Phys.*, **43**, 1806 (1965).
Triphenylmethyl monosubstituted with o-CH_2SCH_3 o-CH_2OCH_3 o-$CH_2CH_2CH_3$ p-CH_2SCH_3	ethylbenzene, 193–253 K	To measure rates of conformational changes; to measure coupling constants and relate to intraradical interaction	J. S. Hyde et al., *J. Amer. Chem. Soc.*, **88**, 4763 (1966); L. D. Kispert et al., *J. Phys. Chem.*, **72**, 4276 (1968).
Substituted p-biphenyl-diphenyl-methyl (in Tschitschibabin's hydrocarbon solutions)	toluene, 211 K	To determine radical identity	J. S. Hyde et al., *Mol. Phys.*, **17**, 457 (1969).
Triphenylmethyl p-Monomethyl triphenylmethyl p,p',p''-Trimethyltriphenylmethyl (tritolylmethyl) p,p',p''-Tricyclopropyl triphenylmethyl	toluene, 183–300 K	To deduce preferred conformational forms from the temperature dependence of the β-proton coupling constants	N. L. Bauld et al., *J. Amer. Chem. Soc.*, **91**, 6667 (1969).

Table 3-4 (*Continued*)

Radical	Conditions	Objectives and Comments	References
Triphenylmethyl p-Biphenylyldiphenylmethyl Bis-(p-biphenylyl)phenylmethyl Tris-(p-biphenylyl)methyl	toluene, 193–213 K	To measure all hyperfine constants and to compare with MO calculations	A. H. Maki et al., *J. Amer. Chem. Soc.*, **90**, 4225 (1968).
Bis(m-fluorophenyl)phenylmethyl (p-Fluorophenyl)diphenylmethyl Tris(p-fluorophenyl)methyl (o-Fluorophenyl)diphenylmethyl (p-Tolyl)diphenylmethyl (o-Tolyl)diphenylmethyl	toluene, ~203 K ~10^{-3} M	To study substitutent effects on hyperfine constants and to compare with MO calculations	R. D. Allendoerfer and A. H. Maki, *J. Amer. Chem. Soc.*, **91**, 1088 (1969).
Perinaphthenyl	liquid crystal mixture, 320–360 K	To study coherence effects in ENDOR spectra	K. P. Dinse et al., *Z. Naturforsch.*, **28a**, 1069 (1973).
Pentaphenyl cyclopentadienyl 8-p-methyl substituted derivatives	octane, pentane, isopentane, 93–223 K	To study splitting of ground state energy level degeneracy	K. Mobius et al., *Mol. Phys.*, **20**, 289 (1971).
2,4,6-Triphenylphenoxy	benzene, 293 K ~8×10^{-5} M	To measure all coupling constants with aid of selective deuteration	J. S. Hyde, *J. Phys. Chem.*, **71**, 68 (1967).
2,4,6-Tri-t-butylphenoxy	mineral oil, 298 K; heptane, 183–253 K	To study effect of experimental parameters on ENDOR response	R. D. Allendoerfer and A. H. Maki, *J. Magn. Resonance*, **3**, 396 (1970).
4-Formyl-2,6-di-t-butylphenoxy	mineral oil, 298 K; hexane, 183–253 K	To study torsional oscillations of formyl group from temperature dependence of coupling constants and comparison with MO calculations	R. D. Allendoerfer and D. J. Eustace, *J. Phys. Chem.*, **75**, 2765 (1971).

Radical	Conditions	Purpose	Reference
4-Cyclohexyl-2,6-di-t-butylphenoxy	hexane, isopentane, 153–300 K, ~10^{-3} M	To measure coupling constants	R. F. Adams and N. M. Atherton, *Mol. Phys.*, **17**, 673 (1969).
4-Methyl-2,6-di-t-butylphenoxy 4-Ethyl-2,6-di-t-butylphenoxy 4-Isopropyl-2,6-di-t-butylphenoxy 4-Methoxy-2,6-di-t-butylphenoxy 4-Ethoxy-2,6-di-t-butylphenoxy 4-Amino-2,6-di-t-butylphenoxy 4-Dimethylamino-2,6-di-t-butylphenoxy	n-heptane, $\geq$180 K, 10^{-3}–10^{-4} M	To measure coupling constants	N. M. Atherton et al., *Trans. Faraday Soc.*, **67**, 2510 (1971).
Galvinoxyl (Coppinger's radical) N-galvinoxyl	n-heptane, 188–228 K; n-heptane, toluene, near 208 K	To demonstrate ENDOR feasibility	J. S. Hyde, *J. Chem. Phys.*, **43**, 1806 (1965).
Four galvinoxyls substituted with t-butyl, methyl, and methoxy groups	dichloromethane, toluene, 193 K	To obtain coupling constants and to compare them with MO calculations, to study conformational changes	C. Steelink et al., *J. Amer. Chem. Soc.*, **90**, 4354 (1968).
2,4,5-Triphenylimidazyl Tetraphenylpyrryl Tetrakis(p-tolyl)pyrryl Tetrakis(p-anisyl)pyrryl	toluene, xylene (pyrryls), ~298 K, ~5×10^{-5} M	To compare coupling constants with MO calculations, to study the twist angle of the phenyl with respect to the central N-containing ring	R. D. Allendoerfer and A. S. Pollock, *Mol. Phys.*, **22**, 661 (1971).
Bis(p-methoxyphenyl)nitroxide	toluene, 288 K, 5×10^{-4} M	To demonstrate proton ENDOR in aromatic nitroxides	R. D. Allendoerfer and J. H. Engelmann, *Mol. Phys.*, **20**, 569 (1971).
α,α'-Diphenyl-β-picrylhydrazyl (DPPH)	mineral oil, ~298 K, 10^{-2} M	Complete assignment of all proton couplings and comparison with MO theory	N. S. Dalal et al., *J. Chem. Phys.*, **59**, 3403 (1973).

Table 3-4 (*Continued*)

Radical	Conditions	Objectives and Comments	References
Picryl-N-aminocarbazyl α,γ-Bisdiphenylene-β-phenyl allyl	mineral oil, 298–340 K, 10^{-3}–10^{-2} M	Complete assignment of proton coupling constants	N. S. Dalal et al., *J. Chem. Phys.*, **61**, 1689 (1974).
1,3,5-Triphenylverdazyl and four methyl derivatives	toluene, 193–203 K	Effect of methyl substitution on coupling constants	K. Mukai et al., *Bull. Chem. Soc. Japan*, **47**, 1797 (1974).
N-(hydroxy-phenyl)-iminophosphorane (radicals from 18 derivatives) N-(hydroxy-phenyl)-iminoarsenane (radicals from two derivatives)	Nujol, ~308 K	Determination of proton coupling constants, concluded that conjugation across the heteroatoms seems prohibited	H. B. Stegmann et al., *Phosphorus*, **4**, 1 (1974).

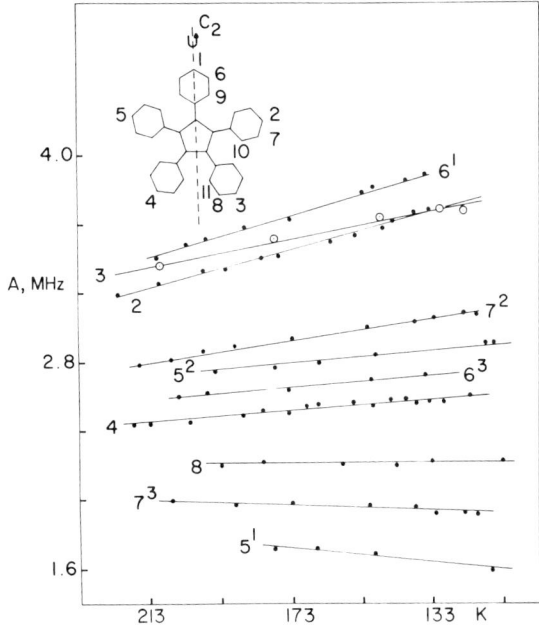

Figure 3-21. ENDOR-determined methyl coupling constants of methyl-substituted pentaphenylcyclopentadienyl (PPCPD) compounds (2) to (8) in isopentane as a function of temperature. Compound (2) 1-CH_3-PPCPD, (3) 2,5-CH_3-PPCPD, (4) 3,4-CH_3-PPCPD, (5) 1,2,5-CH_3-PPCPD, (6) 1,3,4-CH_3-PPCPD, (7) 2,3,4,5-CH_3-PPCPD, (8) 1,2,3,4,5-CH_3-PPCPD. The observed position for ENDOR is denoted by a superscript. From K. Möbius et al., *Mol. Phys.*, **20**, 289 (1971).

a doubly degenerate ground state for the unpaired electron. The symmetry is lowered to C_2 by partial p-methyl substitution, and thus the two degenerate states are split by an amount ΔE. If ΔE is greater than kT, the hyperfine splittings will reflect only the symmetry of the ground state, but if $\Delta E \sim kT$ the hyperfine splittings will be temperature dependent and will reflect an average of the ground state symmetry and the thermally accessible excited state symmetry. Figure 3-21 shows the various radicals studied and the temperature dependence of the methyl proton coupling constants as determined by ENDOR. Recall that the methyl proton ENDOR lines can be unambiguously assigned from the ENDOR spectrum because they broaden less than the ring proton lines when the temperature is lowered. The observed temperature dependence of the methyl proton couplings indicates that $\Delta E \sim kT$. Furthermore the ground state symmetry for each of the radicals studied can be determined on the basis of a simple electrostatic model of the methyl substitution. Since the methyl group is electron repelling, the preferred ground state should be

Table 3-5. Ground State Symmetry and Energy Gaps between the Symmetric and Antisymmetric States for Various Methyl-Substituted Pentaphenylcyclopentadienyl Radicals

Radical[a]	Ground State Symmetry	Experimental Energy Gaps (cm^{-1})
1-Methylpentaphenylcyclopentadienyl (0.053)	sym	115
2,5-Dimethylpentaphenylcyclopentadienyl (−0.086)	antisym	101
3,4-Dimethylpentaphenylcyclopentadienyl (0.033)	sym	89
1,2,5-Trimethylpentaphenylcyclopentadienyl (−0.033)	antisym	25
1,3,4-Trimethylpentaphenylcyclopentadienyl (0.086)	sym	136
2,3,4,5-Tetramethylpentaphenylcyclopentadienyl (−0.053)	antisym	58

Adapted from K. Möbius et al. *Mol. Phys.*, **20**, 289 (1971)
[a] Ring numbering system shown in Fig. 3-21. Sum of spin densities at substituent ring carbons shown in parentheses.

the one with the smallest π-charge density at the ring carbon to which the methyl is attached. On the basis of calculated spin densities the ground state symmetries of the radicals were assigned as shown in Table 3-5. A net positive (negative) spin density at the substituent carbons predicts a symmetric (antisymmetric) ground state. The temperature dependence of the measured methyl proton coupling A_m when the ground state is antisymmetric is given by $A_m = A_a + A_s \exp(-\Delta E/kT)/[1 + \exp(-\Delta E/kT)]$ where A_a and A_s are the coupling constants in the antisymmetric and symmetric states, respectively. For ground symmetric states the a and s subscripts are interchanged. The values of A_a and A_s are determined from the calculated spin densities. The ΔE values obtained are shown in Table 3-5. The sign of the temperature dependence is positive (negative) with increasing temperature for a given methyl proton coupling when the spin density at the substituent carbon is the opposite (same) as the net spin density on all the substituted ring carbons.

Another aspect of electronic structure that can be studied by ENDOR as well as by ESR is the preferred conformation of a radical. Again ENDOR is of aid in such studies when the ESR spectrum is too complicated to interpret. One example of a conformational result deduced by ENDOR occurs for the pentaphenylcyclopentadienyl radical.[17]

APPLICATIONS TO ELECTRONIC STRUCTURE   133

In this radical the conformational question concerns the twist angles of the phenyl rings with respect to the cyclopentadienyl plane. By comparison of the experimental spin densities deduced from the coupling constants measured by ENDOR with calculated spin densities for different twist angles, it is concluded that the average twist angle of the phenyl rings is about 40°.

Another type of conformational study concerns the conformation of protons attached to carbons β to π systems. The analysis is the same as in ESR where the relation between the β-proton hyperfine constant and the dihedral angle θ between the C—H$_\beta$ bond and the π orbital on the α carbon is assumed to be

$$A_H = \rho_\alpha (B_0 + B_2 \cos^2 \theta) \tag{3.5}$$

where B_0 and B_2 are empirical constants and ρ_α is the spin density on the adjacent carbon atom in the π system. Thus from the coupling constants deduced by ENDOR it is possible to determine the dihedral angle. The conformation of 7,12-dihydropleiadene radical anions was deduced by ENDOR in this way.[32] The temperature dependence of β-proton hyperfine constants deduced by ENDOR or ESR can also give information about preferred conformations.[33] Several other references to conformational studies by ENDOR are summarized in Table 3-4.

A final excellent example of an ENDOR contribution to the electronic structure of radicals is shown by the study of α,α'-diphenyl-β-picrylhydrazyl (DPPH).[34] DPPH has been studied a great deal by ESR but its ESR spectrum defied complete interpretation of all the proton coupling constants prior to ENDOR analysis. The structure of the radical and the approximate splitting constants determined by ENDOR are shown in Fig. 3-22. ESR and ENDOR spectra in mineral oil at room temperature are shown in Fig. 3-23. The five line ESR spectrum is due to coupling of the two nitrogens in the radical. It can be seen that the ENDOR spectrum reveals a tremendous amount of additional detailed information about the proton coupling constants. It is also worth noting that mineral oil is required as a solvent to obtain ENDOR spectra of DPPH. Earlier attempts using n-heptane as a solvent did not yield any ENDOR spectra.[8] Since the nuclear relaxation processes depend on the solvent viscosity, the relaxation rates are apparently optimum for ENDOR in mineral oil near room temperature for DPPH. Figure 3-22 indicates that the unpaired electron is delocalized over the entire DPPH molecule, but it also indicates some interesting nuances of the electronic structure of this molecule. For example, the ortho and meta protons in one phenyl ring are not equivalent to those protons in the other phenyl ring as expected from the molecular structure alone. Also the two meta

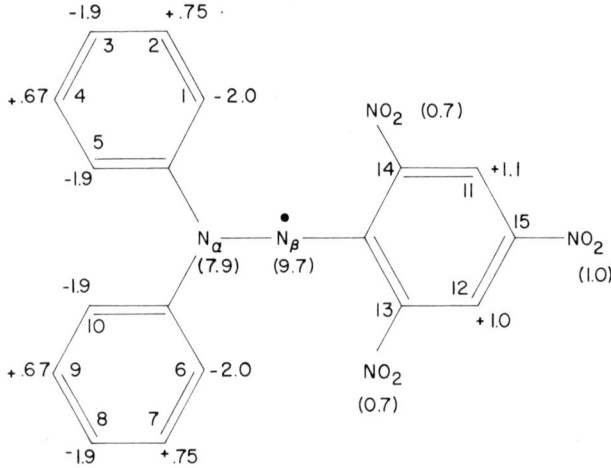

Figure 3-22. The ring numbering system and approximate hyperfine splittings in gauss for all the protons and nitrogens, as determined by ENDOR, for α,α'-diphenyl-β-picryl hydrazyl radical (DPPH). Data from N. S. Dalal et al., *J. Chem. Phys.*, **59**, 3403 (1973).

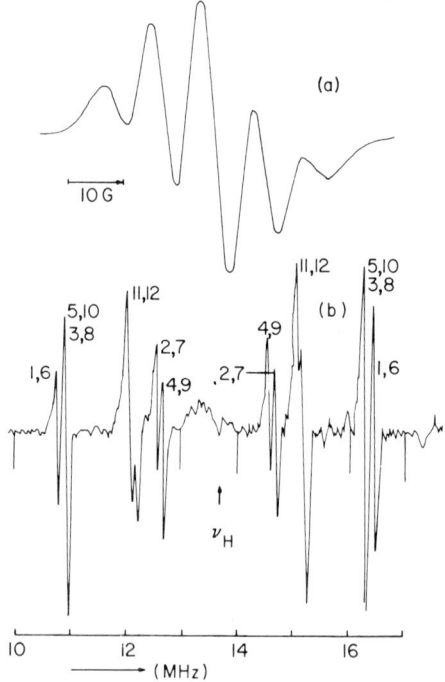

Figure 3-23. (*a*) ESR spectrum of DPPH radical in mineral oil as used for ENDOR. (*b*) ENDOR spectrum of DPPH in mineral oil at room temperature. The ENDOR lines are numbered according to the proton positions in Fig. 3-22 to which they are assigned. From N. S. Dalal et al., *J. Chem. Phys.*, **59**, 3403 (1973).

protons on the picryl ring are not quite equivalent. The theoretical calculations of spin densities and coupling constants for DPPH only give moderate agreement with experiment, and in this case the ENDOR results serve as a basis for improving the accuracy and validity of more refined calculations.[34]

3.5 NUCLEI OTHER THAN PROTONS

Except for ^{19}F the gyromagnetic ratio of most nuclei is much smaller than that for protons and the ENDOR intensity might be expected to be small with the available rf fields. However as explained in Section 1.4.3 the rf field at the nucleus is enhanced, particularly for larger coupling constants. Thus ENDOR is expected to be observable for a variety of nuclei if the isotropic coupling constant is about 10 G or more. Nevertheless there are only a few examples of ENDOR in the liquid phase from nuclei other than protons.[2-7]

We may take the ENDOR spectrum of ^{14}N from 1-oxyl-2,2,6,6-tetramethyl-4-piperidone (tanone) in n-heptane shown in Fig. 3-24 as an

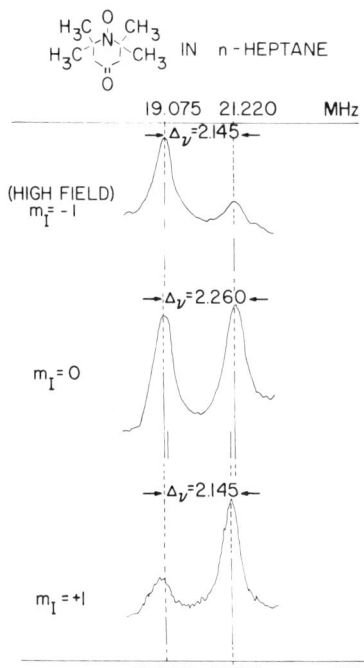

Figure 3-24. Nitrogen ENDOR signals for tanone in n-heptane at 213 K observed on each of the three ESR lines (denoted by m_I values) of this radical. The solid lines under the spectra are calculated intensities based on an idealized analysis and assumed relaxation parameters. From D. S. Leniart et al., *Chem. Phys. Lett.*, **6**, 637 (1970).

example. First we note from Table 1-1 that the nuclear frequency for ^{14}N at 3390 G is 1.04 MHz. Since twice the nuclear frequency is less than the hyperfine frequency of 40.15 MHz, the two ENDOR lines are centered at about half the hyperfine constant and are separated by twice the nuclear frequency. This is in contrast to the type of spectra we have encountered for proton ENDOR. This difference follows from eq. 1.6.

Although the separation is expected to be twice the nuclear frequency, it can be seen in Fig. 3-24 that the separation is slightly more than twice the nuclear frequency in a 3300 G field, which is 2.030 MHz. This difference is due to second order effects since the hyperfine constant to ^{14}N is relatively large.[2] The second order energy terms are proportional to the square of the hyperfine frequency divided by the microwave frequency. In general, the ENDOR frequencies corresponding to $m_I \to m_I + 1$ transitions are given to the second order by eq. 3.6. For $I = \frac{1}{2}$ and for $I = 1$ when the

$$\nu_{m_s}(m_I \to m_I + 1) = |m_s A + \nu_n| + \frac{m_s A^2}{\nu_e}(m_I + m_s + \tfrac{1}{2}) \qquad (3.6)$$

$m_I = 0$ ESR line is observed, the two ENDOR frequencies corresponding to the $\pm m_s$ nuclear manifolds are given by eq. 3.7a. It is seen that the separation between

$$\nu_\pm(I = \tfrac{1}{2} \text{ or } I = 1, m_I = 0) = \left|\frac{A}{2} \pm \nu_n\right| + \frac{A^2}{4\nu_e} \qquad (3.7a)$$

the ENDOR lines is not changed by the second order term, although the center of the two lines is shifted to a higher frequency. For $I = 1$ and observation of the $m_I = +1$ and $m_I = -1$ ESR lines the second order terms do change the ENDOR line separation as well as shifting the center of the two lines as shown by eqs. 3.7b and 3.7c.

$$\nu_\pm(m_I = 1) = \left|\frac{A}{2} \pm \nu_n\right| + \frac{A^2}{4\nu_e} \pm \frac{A^2}{4\nu_e} \qquad (3.7b)$$

$$\nu_\pm(m_I = -1) = \left|\frac{A}{2} \pm \nu_n\right| + \frac{A^2}{4\nu_e} \mp \frac{A^2}{4\nu_e} \qquad (3.7c)$$

For the spectrum in Fig. 3-24 the nitrogen hyperfine constant gives a second order shift between the ENDOR lines for the $m_I = \pm 1$ ESR lines of $A^2/2\nu_e = 0.087$ MHz, whereas the experimental value is $2.145 - 2.030 = 0.115$ MHz. This discrepancy occurs because for rapidly tumbling radicals in solution, the second order splitting also includes the mean square fluctuation of the hyperfine splitting constant δA^2.[35] This means that A^2 in eqs. 3.6 and 3.7 should be replaced by the mean square value $\langle A^2 \rangle = A^2 + \langle (\delta A)^2 \rangle$. Since δA^2 cannot be calculated without knowing details of the motion of the radical in solution, it is determined by difference from the experimental data and $A = 40.1$ MHz to be $\delta A^2 = (23.7 \text{ MHz})^2$. This is the same order of magnitude as the square of the isotropic hyperfine constant; this is also found to be so for ^{87}Rb ENDOR.[6]

We have seen that observation of nonproton ENDOR in solution typically depends on the enhancement of the rf field by a large hyperfine constant in order to increase the sensitivity enough for observation. The same large hyperfine constant that gives a favorable rf enhancement factor also produces second order shifts in the separation of high field and low field ENDOR lines. The static part of the second order shift can be calculated exactly but the dynamic part cannot. However the square of the dynamic part of the second order shift appears to be of the order of magnitude of the square of the isotropic hyperfine constant, so the separation of the two ENDOR lines of a nonproton nucleus in solution will typically be a little bit more than twice the free nuclear frequency. Nevertheless the quantitative details are understood well enough to identify unambiguously the nucleus producing the ENDOR transitions in most cases.

An additional feature of the spectra in Fig. 3-24 is the unequal intensity of the two ENDOR lines when the high field ($m_I = -1$) and low field ($m_I = +1$) ESR lines are observed. This is a consequence of the dominant nuclear relaxation mechanism. Figure 1-8 shows that when a cross-relaxation process is much faster than a nuclear spin-lattice relaxation process, one of the ENDOR transitions is much more intense than the other, depending on which ESR line is observed. Observation of an intensity ratio such as that shown for observation of the high field ESR line is not sufficient evidence to indicate dominance of cross relaxation, but when observation of the low field ESR line shows the reverse intensity ratio then cross relaxation is strongly indicated. (Nuclear relaxation mechanisms are discussed in more detail in Section 3.7.) It is interesting that for nonproton ENDOR the dominance of cross relaxation does seem to be somewhat general. The reverse intensity ratio for observation of high field and low field ENDOR lines is shown not only for ^{14}N (ref. 2), but also for ^{13}C (ref. 3), ^{23}Na (ref. 5), and ^{87}Rb (ref. 6).

3.6 LIQUID CRYSTAL SOLVENTS

Thus far the structural information available from ENDOR has been based on determination of isotropic coupling constants from analysis of the ENDOR spectrum. More information is of course available if the dipolar or anisotropic coupling constants of a radical are obtained, as is well known for radicals trapped in single crystals. In the liquid phase rapid tumbling of the radical averages out the anisotropic interaction so that this information is lost. This is true of both ESR and ENDOR spectra. However Luckhurst and others[36] have shown that if the molecular motion of a radical in solution can be restricted in a liquid crystal solvent, the position of the ESR lines will then depend on the anisotropic coupling. Many liquid crystals exhibit the transition from a disordered isotropic phase to a partially oriented nematic phase at a sharp transition temperature. The degree of alignment in the nematic phase depends on temperature and on the external magnetic field. In the nematic phase in the absence of a magnetic field large groups of perhaps 100 molecules are oriented along one axis but this axis slowly rotates randomly in the liquid. In the presence of a magnetic field all the axes of these "swarms" or groups of molecules are aligned in the same direction to give an ordered phase.

A radical produced in the nematic phase of the liquid crystal still has sufficient freedom of motion so that ESR spectral resolution is little impaired. It is then possible to measure the ESR spectrum in both isotropic and nematic phases of a liquid crystal solvent and to interpret the changes in the positions of the hyperfine lines in terms of the magnitude of the anisotropic interactions and the degree of radical alignment. To date the most important application of liquid crystal solvents in ESR measurements has been that under certain conditions it is possible to determine the signs of hyperfine coupling constants. Other information, such as the magnitude of the g tensor and the largest component of the hyperfine tensor, is also sometimes obtainable.[36] The sign of the hyperfine constant is important because it relates to the sign of the spin densities at different positions in a radical and serves as a test of the molecular wave functions used to calculate such spin densities.

The advantages of liquid crystal solvents are readily extendable to ENDOR, but the characteristics of the liquid crystal may strongly influence whether observation of ENDOR signals is possible or not. The strongest proton ENDOR signals are often seen in solvents of rather high viscosity, and since temperature is a very limited variable when dealing with liquid crystal solvents one must find a liquid crystal with a fairly viscous nematic phase. Möbius and co-workers[37,38] have performed successful ENDOR experiments in a liquid crystal mixture of two isomers of *p*-methoxy-*p'*-*n*-butylazoxybenzene, which exhibits its nematic phase between 289 and 349 K. They have shown how this liquid crystal solvent can be used to obtain information on the sign of isotropic coupling constants[37] and on quadrupole coupling constants.[38]

3.6.1 Sign of Isotropic Coupling Constants

The change in the average hyperfine constant of a radical measured in the isotropic and nematic phases of a liquid crystal is given by

$$A_{\text{nematic}} - A_{\text{isotropic}} = \Delta A = O_{33}A'_{33} + \tfrac{1}{3}(O_{11} - O_{22})(A'_{11} - A'_{22}) \quad (3.8)$$

where the O_{ii} equal the components of the traceless ordering tensor of the radical and the A'_{ii} are the components of the traceless hyperfine tensor. The A'_{ii} are thus the elements of the purely dipolar or anisotropic interaction. And the O_{ii} equal $\tfrac{1}{2}(3l_il_i - 1)$ where l_i is the direction cosine between the molecular axes i and the magnetic field direction. With this definition the component O_{33} is always negative. The axis system for both the ordering and anisotropic hyperfine tensors is a molecular axis system where direction 3 is typically the axis of highest symmetry passing through the molecule.

If either the ordering or anisotropic hyperfine tensor is axially symmetric, eq. 3.8 reduces to eq. 3.9.

$$\Delta A = O_{33}A'_{33} \quad (3.9)$$

Thus from the measured shift in average hyperfine constant either the ordering tensor component or the anisotropic hyperfine tensor component can be determined if the other is known. Since the sign of O_{33} is negative, it is always possible to determine the sign of the isotropic coupling constant if eq. 3.9 can be applied. It is usually assumed that the ordering tensor is axially symmetric,[37,38] since there is one preferred orientation axis in the liquid crystal solvent.

The ENDOR results for the perinaphthenyl radical (shown below) in the liquid crystal give negative ΔA for position 1 and positive ΔA for position 2. This means that the isotropic proton coupling for position 1 is

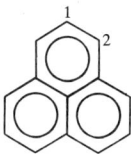

positive and the isotropic proton coupling for position 2 is negative in this radical. ΔA changes with temperature because the ordering parameter O_{33} changes with temperature.

Results on the tri-t-butylphenoxy radical in the isotropic and nematic phases of the liquid crystal are shown in Fig. 3-25. ΔA for all three

140 LIQUID PHASE ENDOR

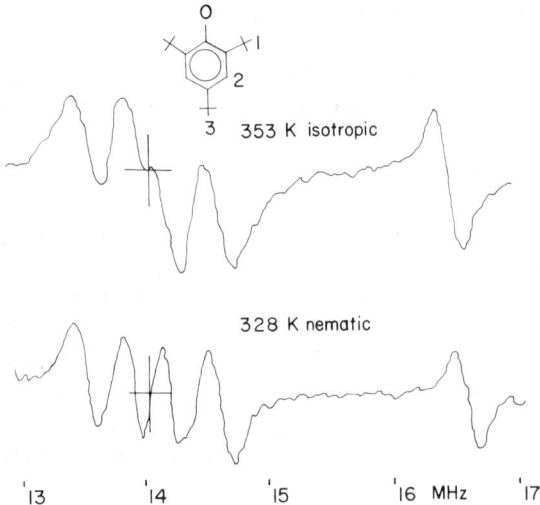

Figure 3-25. ENDOR spectra of tri-*t*-butylphenoxy radical in the isotropic and nematic phases of a liquid crystal mixture of two isomers of *p*-methoxy-*p'*-*n*-butylazoxybenzene. The measured proton splittings in the isotropic phase are $A_1 = 0.264$ MHz, $A_2 = 4.83$ MHz, and $A_3 = 1.07$ MHz; and in the nematic phase are $A_1 = 0.314$ MHz, $A_2 = 5.15$ MHz, and $A_3 = 1.10$ MHz. From K. P. Dinse et al., *Chem. Phys. Lett.*, **12,** 399 (1971).

couplings in this radical is positive so the isotropic coupling constants for all three positions are negative. The sign of the meta coupling at position 2 is of interest since Hückel molecular orbital theory predicts a rather large positive spin density at the meta position whereas the McLachlan self-consistent-field approach predicts a small negative spin density.[37]

One can also determine the ordering parameter if the anisotropic tensor component A'_{33} is calculated by McConnell and Strathdee's method.[39] By this method the meta proton tensor component is calculated to be -2.52 MHz, which gives an ordering parameter $O_{33} = -0.13$ at 328 K. It should be pointed out that the accuracy of the McConnell and Strathdee method for calculating anisotropic coupling constants has been questioned in this application.[36] However, ordering parameter components of -0.1 to -0.3 are typically found and do seem reasonable.

3.6.2 Quadrupole Coupling Constants

Quadrupole couplings may be important for radicals containing nuclei with $I \geq 1$. In organic compounds the ^{14}N nucleus is the most important one giving rise to observable quadrupole coupling effects. Thus organic nitroxide radicals seem to be appropriate systems for determining quadrupole splittings. The quadrupole coupling tensor does not depend on the magnetic spin quantum number of the electron so second order effects are necessary to enable their measurement by ESR in single crystals. In liquids, however, the quadrupole coupling information is lost in the ESR spectra of rapidly tumbling radicals. Even if the radicals are partially aligned in a nematic liquid crystal, the quadrupole interaction does not influence the positions of the ESR lines because the quadrupole coupling shifts all levels connected by ESR transitions by the same amount.[36] However, it turns out that the ENDOR spectra of a radical in a liquid crystal do give information about the quadrupole coupling.

The energy levels corresponding to the ENDOR transitions for a doublet radical with a nuclear spin $I = 1$ in the nematic phase of a liquid crystal are given by eqs. 3.10 to 3.13.

$$h\nu_{ENDOR}(m_I = -1) = \tfrac{1}{2}(A + \Delta A) \pm (\tilde{g}_I \beta_I H_0 + \overline{Q'}) + \tfrac{1}{2}C \quad (3.10)$$

$$h\nu_{ENDOR}(m_I = +1) = \tfrac{1}{2}(A + \Delta A) \pm (\tilde{g}_I \beta_I H_0 - \overline{Q'}) - \tfrac{1}{2}C \quad (3.11)$$

$$h\nu_{ENDOR}(m_I = 0) = \begin{cases} \tfrac{1}{2}(A + \Delta A) + \tilde{g}_I \beta_I H_0 \pm (\overline{Q' + \tfrac{1}{2}C}) \\ \tfrac{1}{2}(A + \Delta A) - \tilde{g}_I \beta_I H_0 \pm (\overline{Q' - \tfrac{1}{2}C}) \end{cases} \quad (3.12)$$

where

$$\overline{Q'} = Q'[O_{33} + \tfrac{1}{3}\eta(O_{11} - O_{22})] \quad (3.13)$$

$$Q' = \frac{3e^2 q'_{33} Q}{4I(2I-1)} \qquad \eta = \frac{q'_{11} - q'_{22}}{q'_{33}}$$

$$C = \frac{(A - \tfrac{1}{2}\Delta A)^2}{2g\beta H_0} \qquad \tilde{g}_I = g_I\left[1 + \frac{C}{2g_I \beta_I H_0}\right]$$

The q'_{ii} refers to the field gradient tensor at the nucleus and the primed components refer to the traceless parts of the various interactions. Each equation gives the two ENDOR frequencies observed by separately saturating the three different ESR hyperfine components corresponding to $m_I = -1$, 0, and +1.[38] The symbols and the equations are defined by the relations in eqs. 3.8 and 3.10. The quadrupole coupling constant is usually defined as e^2qQ/h in frequency units where the field gradient at the nucleus is denoted by the symbol eq and Q is the quadrupole moment of the nucleus. C is a second order shift as discussed in Section 3.5.

It can be seen that the two pairs of ENDOR lines for saturation of the $m_I = -1$ and $m_I = +1$ ESR components are separated by $2\tilde{g}_I \beta_I H_0 + 2\overline{Q'}$ and $2\tilde{g}_I \beta_I H_0 - 2\overline{Q'}$, respectively. Thus by measuring the difference between these two pairs of ENDOR lines the quantity $4\overline{Q'}$ is obtained which is related to the quadrupole coupling constant. Also from the

142 LIQUID PHASE ENDOR

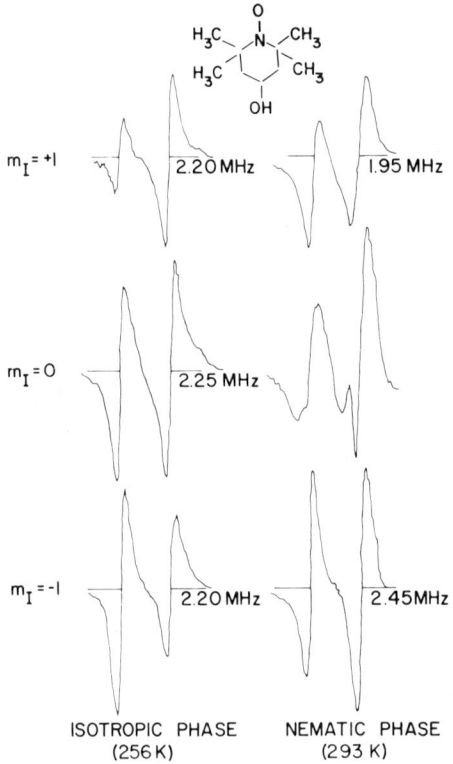

Figure 3-26. Nitrogen ENDOR spectra of 1-oxyl-2,2,6,6-tetramethyl-4-hydroxypiperidine (tanol) in the isotropic and nematic phases of a liquid crystal mixture of two isomers of p-methoxy-p'-n-butylazoxybenzene when observing each of the ESR lines denoted by m_I. From the shifts of the ENDOR lines between the isotropic and nematic phases when observing the $m_I = \pm 1$ ESR lines the nitrogen quadrupole coupling constant can be determined as explained in the text. From K. P. Dinse et al., *Chem. Phys. Lett.*, **14**, 196 (1972).

centers of gravity of the two pairs of ENDOR lines one can obtain the magnitude of the second order shift in the same way as discussed in Section 3.5.

Figure 3-26 shows nitrogen ENDOR spectra of 1-oxyl-2,2,6,6-tetramethyl-4-hydroxy-piperidine (tanol) in the isotropic and nematic phases of the same liquid crystal mixture described in Section 3.6.1. The results in the isotropic phase have already been discussed in Section 3.5. It can be seen that in the nematic phase the ENDOR lines for $m_I = +1$ and $m_I = -1$ are shifted in opposite directions by the quadrupole interaction as is predicted by eqs. 3.10 and 3.11. In addition, the mean frequency about which the ENDOR lines occur shifts from 19.67 MHz in the isotropic phase to 21.76 MHz in the nematic phase. This is just half of the shift ΔA, which was discussed in Section 3.6.1. The ENDOR spectrum for $m_I = 0$ in the nematic phase is both split by the quadrupole interaction and shifted by the second order constant C; the lineshape becomes complex and asymmetric and will not be discussed further here. It is also interesting that the relative intensities of the ENDOR lines for $m_I = +1$ and $m_I = -1$ are nearly equal in the nematic phase but are distinctly unequal in the isotropic phase. The inequality of the two lines has been discussed in terms of a cross-relaxation mechanism in Section 3.5. In the nematic phase it appears that the cross-relaxation mechanism is no longer dominant.

From the results in Fig. 3-26 one obtains $4\overline{Q'}/h = 0.50$ MHz. To go further with the interpretation one must assume that the ordering tensor of the radical is axially symmetric. Then one obtains the quadrupole coupling constant as given by eq. 3.14:

$$\frac{e^2 q'_{33} Q}{h} = \frac{4}{3} \frac{Q'}{h} = \frac{4}{3h} \frac{\overline{Q'}}{O_{33}} = \frac{4}{3} \frac{\overline{Q'}}{h} \frac{A'_{33}}{\Delta A} \qquad (3.14)$$

$\overline{Q'}$ and ΔA are given directly by the ENDOR experiment but A'_{33} must be determined separately. In some cases it can be determined from frozen solution ESR spectra if A'_{33} is large.[38] For the case at hand, $\overline{Q'}/h = 0.125$ MHz, $A'_{33} = -62.7$ MHz, and $\Delta A = 4.81$ MHz to give a quadrupole coupling constant of $e^2 q'_{33} Q/h = -2.5$ MHz. The ordering parameter for the radical turns out to be $O_{33} = -0.067$.

The analysis of the quadrupole coupling constant by this method is quite easy as long as one can assume axially symmetric ordering tensors in the liquid crystal system and can obtain the value of A'_{33}. If both the quadrupole and hyperfine tensors are axially symmetric, the ordering tensor does not have to be so for one to obtain the same results.

3.7 THEORY OF LIQUID PHASE ENDOR

3.7.1 Freed's Theory

The most detailed treatment of the steady state ENDOR response (and the ELDOR response) in liquid systems has been carried out by Freed and co-workers in a series of five papers.[19,28,40-42] They use a density matrix method[43] that may appear complex to many readers. This method is essentially a variant of time dependent perturbation theory and is a convenient way of computing thermal equilibrium properties of a system.

In Chapter 1 we consider saturation and double resonance responses in terms of populations of spin states. This neglects higher order, off-diagonal terms, which can be conveniently handled by a density matrix method. Also the microwave and rf fields can be added explicitly to the Hamiltonian, and steady state solutions of the power absorption of the spin system can be obtained for an arbitrary degree of saturation of each field. A detailed discussion of Freed's theory is beyond the scope of this book, so we only briefly describe some pertinent aspects.

Freed obtains detailed expressions for the ENDOR response and percent enhancement for the case when electron nuclear dipolar interactions are the only important nuclear spin dependent relaxation process.[28] He shows that this case applies to α protons. With this END mechanism the ENDOR effect is maximized when $T_{1e} \sim T_{1n}$; this confirms the simple approach to ENDOR in Chapter 1. Chemical exchange and Heisenberg spin-spin exchange among radicals reduce the ENDOR enhancements that result from other processes.[40] For most radicals with many magnetic nuclei, computer solutions of the general matrix expressions are required. In many cases for free radicals in liquids $T_{1e} \ll T_{1n}$ in the accessible experimental range, so that the ENDOR enhancement is small (0.01 to 1%). It is then possible to develop approximate analytical expressions for the general case of many nuclei by expanding in terms of T_{1e}/T_{1n}.[42] When the expansion is carried out only to the lowest order linear terms, it is possible to derive rather simple expressions for ENDOR enhancements that are called *average-ENDOR* responses. The average-ENDOR expressions agree fairly well with the exact results for $T_{1e}/T_{1n} < 0.025$. For spins of $I = \frac{1}{2}$ the average-ENDOR signal is predicted to be directly proportional to the number of equivalent nuclei contributing to the signal. This conclusion only applies if the END mechanism dominates the nuclear relaxation. Although the effects of spin-spin exchange still act to reduce the average-ENDOR response, the ENDOR signal is maximized by adjusting the spin concentration so that the rate of spin-spin exchange is approximately twice the electron spin-lattice relaxation rate.

3.7.2 Phenomenological Theory

We now give a simpler, more phenomenological treatment of the ENDOR response based on changes in the effective T_{1e}. This approach was introduced by Seidel[44] and has been explicitly applied to homogeneous ESR lines, as are often found in solution ENDOR, by Allendoerfer and Maki.[10]

3.7.2.1 H_1 Dependence of ENDOR Response

Spin relaxation is described qualitatively in Section 1.2. The relaxation process for homogeneously broadened ESR lines can be described phenomenologically by the Bloch equations, which give the rate of change of the Cartesian components of the magnetic moment.[45] M_o is the equilibrium magnetic moment in the presence of a steady magnetic field H_o and $\gamma_e H_o$ is the Larmor precession frequency of the electron spins.

$$\frac{dM_x}{dt} = \gamma_e H_o M_y - \frac{M_x}{T_{2e}}$$

$$\frac{dM_y}{dt} = -\gamma_e H_o M_x - \frac{M_y}{T_{2e}} \qquad (3.15)$$

$$\frac{dM_z}{dt} = -\frac{(M_z - M_o)}{T_{1e}}$$

To observe ESR we apply an oscillating microwave magnetic field of amplitude $2H_1$ that is equivalent to the sum of two counterrotating fields of strength H_1. Only the H_1 component rotating in the same direction as the Larmor precession is effective in inducing ESR transitions. The Bloch equations are modified by the presence of this H_1 and can be solved to give the steady state solutions.

The solution is most conveniently carried out in a coordinate system rotating at the Larmor frequency. In this rotating coordinate system u and v are the transverse components of the magnetic moment along the rotating x' and y' directions where H_1 is also in the x' direction. A relation between magnetic moment components in the fixed (M_x) and rotating coordinate system is given by

$$M_x = u \cos \omega t + v \sin \omega t. \qquad (3.16)$$

The steady state solutions are given by

$$u = \frac{M_o \gamma_e^2 H_1 T_{2e}^2 (H_o - H)}{1 + \gamma_e^2 T_{2e}^2 (H_o - H)^2 + \gamma_e^2 H_1^2 T_{1e} T_{2e}} \qquad (3.17)$$

$$v = \frac{M_o \gamma_e H_1 T_{2e}}{1 + \gamma_e^2 T_{2e}^2 (H_o - H)^2 + \gamma_e^2 H_1^2 T_{1e} T_{2e}} \qquad (3.18)$$

$$M_z = \frac{M_o + M_o \gamma_e^2 T_{2e}^2 (H_o - H)^2}{1 + \gamma_e^2 T_{2e}^2 (H_o - H)^2 + \gamma_e^2 H_1^2 T_{1e} T_{2e}} \qquad (3.19)$$

where $\omega = \gamma_e H$.

Both the u and v components can be experimentally detected. The u component is in phase with H_1 and corresponds to a dispersion signal whereas the v component is 90° out of phase with H_1 and corresponds to the commonly observed absorption signal. One often sees magnetic resonance signals written as proportional to the components of a complex spin susceptibility, $\chi = \chi' + \chi''i$. In these terms, $u = 2H_1\chi'$ and $v = 2H_1\chi''$.

Experimentally the first derivative of a magnetic resonance signal with respect to magnetic field is normally observed through phase sensitive detection (see Chapter 2). So the ESR absorption signal is given by

$$\frac{dv}{dH} = \frac{2M_o\gamma_e^3 T_{2e}^3 H_1(H_o - H)}{(1 + \gamma_e^2 T_{2e}^2(H_o - H)^2 + \gamma_e^2 H_1^2 T_{1e}T_{2e})^2}. \quad (3.20)$$

An ENDOR signal is typically observed by setting H at the maximum or minimum of the ESR derivative signal. To find this field, H_{max}, we set $d^2v/dH^2 = 0$ and find

$$H_o - H_{max} = \pm\left(\frac{1 + \gamma_e^2 H_1^2 T_{1e}T_{2e}}{3\gamma_e^2 T_{2e}^2}\right). \quad (3.21)$$

When eq. 3.21 is substituted into eq. 3.20, we have

$$\left.\frac{dv}{dH}\right|_{max} = \pm\frac{3\sqrt{3}}{8} \frac{M_o\gamma_e^2 H_1 T_{2e}^2}{(1 + \gamma_e^2 H_1^2 T_{1e}T_{2e})^{3/2}}. \quad (3.22)$$

We are considering that the ENDOR response arises from a change in T_{1e} so the enhancement E^A is given by

$$E^A = d\left(\left.\frac{dv}{dH}\right|_{max}\right) = \pm\frac{9\sqrt{3}}{16} \frac{M_o\gamma_e^4 T_{2e}^3 H_1^3}{(1 + \gamma_e^2 H_1^2 T_{1e}T_{2e})^{5/2}} \Delta T_{1e}. \quad (3.23)$$

This equation shows that the ENDOR signal height increases like H_1^3 at low microwave power, passes through a maximum, and decreases like H_1^{-2} at high microwave power. This behavior is indeed observed for the ENDOR lines of the tri-t-butylphenoxy radical as shown in Fig. 3-27. By setting $dE^A/dH_1 = 0$, we find that the maximum of E^A versus H_1 occurs at $\gamma_e^2 H_1^2 T_{1e}T_{2e} = \frac{3}{2}$. This may be compared with the condition for the maximum derivative ESR signal versus H_1, which is $\gamma_e^2 H_1^2 T_{1e}T_{2e} = \frac{1}{2}$. So the maximum ENDOR response is expected at a power three times higher (4.8 dB) than the maximum ESR signal height. This seems generally supported by experiment.

3.7.2.2 H_2 Dependence of ENDOR Response

To obtain a dependence of the ENDOR response on rf power we evaluate ΔT_{1e} for a particular relaxation pathway. It is convenient to deal with the maximum ENDOR response E^A_{max} versus H_1, which is found by substituting $\gamma_e^2 H_1^2 T_{1e}T_{2e} = \frac{3}{2}$ into eq. 3.23.

$$E^A_{max} = -0.181 M_o\gamma_e\left(\frac{T_{2e}}{T_{1e}}\right)^{3/2} \Delta T_{1e} \quad (3.24)$$

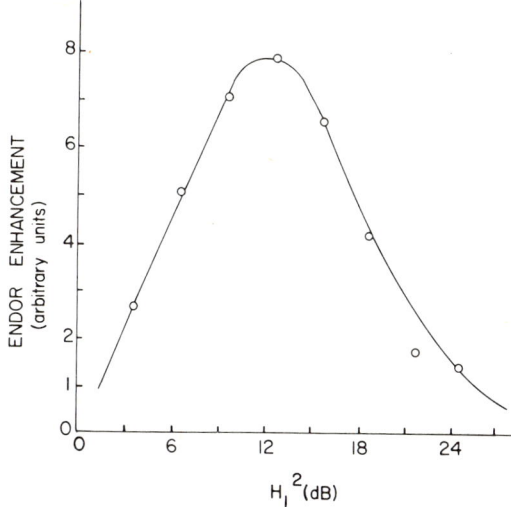

Figure 3-27. ENDOR signal height versus microwave power. The o's are experimental points for the 17-MHz ENDOR line for the 3,5 ring protons in the tri-t-butylphenoxy radical in mineral oil at room temperature. The solid line is calculated from eq. 3.23 and is normalized to fit the maximum observed intensity. From R. D. Allendoerfer and A. H. Maki, *J. Magn. Resonance*, **3**, 396 (1970).

The maximum fractional ENDOR enhancement F_{max} is obtained by dividing E_{max}^A by the ESR signal intensity $(dv/dH)_{max}$ at the same value of H_1.

$$F_{max} = -0.90 \frac{\Delta T_{1e}}{T_{1e}} \qquad (3.25)$$

To evaluate ΔT_{1e} we may consider the general relaxation pathways shown in Fig. 3-28. We will not need to specify the molecular mechanism

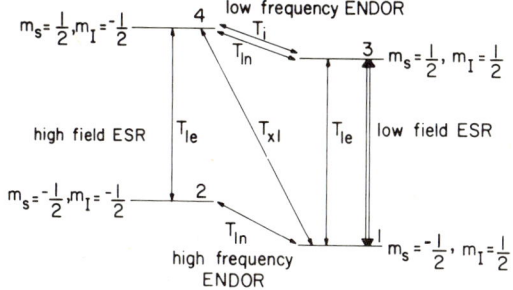

Figure 3-28. Energy levels and relaxation times for $S = I = \frac{1}{2}$ spin system with $A > 0$ and $A < 2\nu_n$.

of these relaxation pathways at this point. In Fig. 3-28 the 1–3 transition is saturated and the nuclear rf field induces 3–4 transitions at a rate T_i^{-1}. For spins in level 4 there are two pathways for relaxation to level 1. Pathway A involves the cross-relaxation process with a time T_{x1}, and B involves $T_{1e} + T_{1n}$. For ENDOR to occur we want $|\Delta T_{1e}| > 0$, so the induced transition rate must be equal to or greater than the rates of relaxation via pathways A or B. We must remember that ΔT_{1e} in eq. 3.26 is the change in effective relaxation time between the two levels of the observed ESR transition. With reference to Fig. 3-28 this might be more clearly designated as $(\Delta T_{1e})_{13}$ given by the difference between $(T_{1e})_{13}$ calculated in the absence of applied nuclear rf field $T_i^{-1} = 0$ and $(T_{1e})_{13}$ calculated in the presence of nuclear radiofrequency. If pathway A dominates B, we find

$$-(\Delta T_{1e})_{13}^A \approx \frac{T_{1e}^2}{T_{x1} + T_i} \tag{3.26}$$

and if pathway B dominates A with $T_{1n} \ll T_{1e}$, we have

$$-(\Delta T_{1e})_{13}^B \approx \frac{T_{1e}^2}{2T_{1n} + 4T_i}. \tag{3.27}$$

Both of these expressions involve T_i, which is dependent on nuclear rf power. Qualitatively T_i will decrease as the nuclear rf power increases. As long as $T_i \geq T_{x1}$ for A pathway domination or $T_i \geq \frac{1}{2}T_{1n}$ for B pathway domination expressions 3.26 and 3.27 will change with rf power. But at high rf power, when T_i becomes small enough to be neglected in the denominator of eqs. 3.26 and 3.27, the ENDOR response will reach a maximum and become independent of rf power.

For an explicit dependence of the ENDOR response on the rf power H_2^2, we assume a form for T_i suggested by Allendoerfer and Maki[10]

$$T_i^{-1} = \frac{\gamma_n^2 H_2^2 T_a}{1 + \gamma_n^2 H_2^2 T_a^2} \tag{3.28}$$

where $T_a = T_{x1}$ for dominance of the A relaxation pathway and $T_a = T_{1n}$ for dominance of the B relaxation pathway. The induced relaxation rate T_i^{-1} increases as H_2^2 at low H_2 and reaches a maximum value independent of the H_2 at high H_2. By using eqs. 3.26, 3.27, and 3.28 we obtain

$$E_{max}^A \text{ (A relaxation)} = 0.181 \frac{M_o \gamma_e T_{2e}^{3/2} T_{1e}^{1/2} \gamma_n^2 H_2^2 T_{x1}}{2\gamma_n^2 H_2^2 T_{x1}^2 + 1} \tag{3.29}$$

$$E_{max}^A \text{ (B relaxation)} = 0.181 M_o \gamma_e \frac{T_{2e}^{3/2} T_{1e}^{1/2} \gamma_n^2 H_2^2 T_{1n}}{6\gamma_n^2 H_2^2 T_{1n}^2 + 4}. \tag{3.30}$$

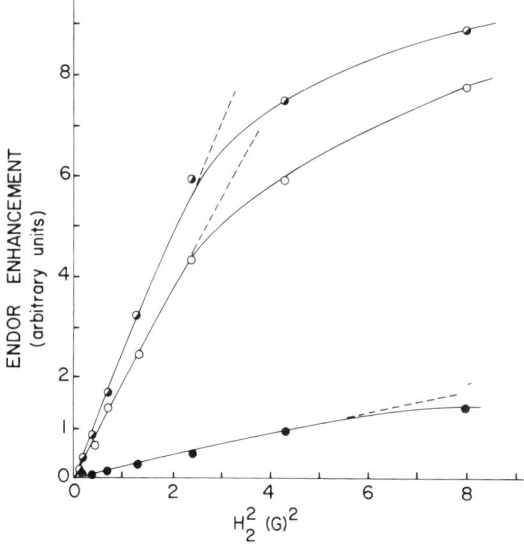

Figure 3-29. ENDOR signal height versus rf power for ENDOR lines of tri-t-butylphenoxy radicals in mineral oil at room temperature. ●'s are the data for the 2,6-t-butyl protons, ◐'s are for the 4-t-butyl protons, and ○'s are for the 3,5 ring protons. From R. D. Allendoerfer and A. H. Maki, *J. Magn. Resonance*, **3**, 396 (1970).

Figure 3-29 shows that this type of H_2 dependence seems to be approximately followed by the proton ENDOR response from tri-t-butylphenoxy radical in mineral oil at room temperature. If E_{max}^{-1} is plotted versus H_2^{-2} a linear plot results at low H_2 from which a value for T_{x1} or T_{1n}, depending on whether eq. 3.29 or eq. 3.30 applies, can be obtained from the ratio of the intercept to the slope.

3.7.2.3 Dependence of ENDOR Response on Hyperfine Coupling

As pointed out several times earlier in the chapter, the relative intensities of ENDOR lines are often not proportional to the number of protons contributing. This is partly due to different nuclear relaxation mechanisms for different kinds of protons. But it is also due to overlap of ESR transitions so that the saturating microwave field cannot saturate one without the other.[10] In this case the maximum ENDOR response cannot be attained because the nuclear rf field can create only a small population difference between the ESR levels of the observed saturated transition. In the limit of very small hyperfine coupling, both the 2-4 and 1-3 ESR transitions in Fig. 3-28 would be saturated equally by the microwave field and then no ENDOR response would be possible because the populations of levels 3 and 4 would be equal before application of a nuclear rf field.

150 LIQUID PHASE ENDOR

This effect may be treated quantitatively by the expression for the fractional ENDOR enhancement

$$F = F_{max} \frac{\Delta M_z(\Delta\omega_{obs})}{\Delta M_z(\Delta\omega \to \infty)} \quad (3.31)$$

where ΔM_z equals M_z for the observed, saturated ESR line minus M_z for another ESR line to be coupled by the nuclear rf field to obtain ENDOR and $\Delta\omega$ is the hyperfine coupling in hertz between the two ESR transitions.[10] M_z is the z component of the magnetization given by eq. 3.18. With $\gamma_e^2 H_1^2 T_{1e} T_{2e} = \frac{3}{2}$ for the maximum ENDOR response, the following useful expression is obtained. To apply this correction factor to F_{max}, $\Delta\omega$ is usually known but T_{2e} is often not. If the ESR line is homogeneously

$$F = F_{max} \frac{T_{2e}^2 \Delta\omega^2}{T_{2e}^2 \Delta\omega^2 + 2.5} \quad (3.32)$$

broadened with a Lorentzian shape, as has been implicitly assumed by using the Bloch equations in the derivation of eq. 3.32, then $T_{2e} = 2/\sqrt{3}\gamma_e \Delta H_{pp}$ where ΔH_{pp} is the peak-to-peak derivative width in gauss. But if the ESR line is inhomogeneously broadened, T_{2e} must often be estimated to be somewhat less than T_{1e}. An estimated value of about 2×10^{-7} sec has been used for T_{2e} in several applications of eq. 3.32 described earlier in this chapter.

It should be remembered that eq. 3.32 has been derived for a particular microwave field corresponding to the maximum ENDOR response. Also note that F_{max} depends on the particular nuclear relaxation mechanism of the protons observed by ENDOR. Nevertheless F_{max} seems to be about the same for many protons in aromatic radicals, and satisfactory intensity corrections using known $\Delta\omega$ and known or estimated T_{2e} have been made for many radicals.[12]

3.7.3 Nuclear Relaxation Mechanisms

Thus far we have discussed the ENDOR response in terms of generalized nuclear relaxation pathways. Now we consider specific nuclear relaxation mechanisms and how they relate to possible nuclear relaxation pathways and consequently to the ENDOR response. Finally we consider experimental methods to distinguish between mechanisms.

3.7.3.1 *Electron-Nuclear Dipolar Modulation*

In general, nuclear spin relaxation depends on the presence of time-varying magnetic fields at the nucleus. One of the easiest mechanisms to visualize for the nuclei in a radical in solution is the electron spin dipole–nuclear spin dipole (END) interaction, which creates an orientation dependent magnetic field at the nucleus (and at the electron). As the radical tumbles in solution, the magnitude of the magnetic field at the nucleus varies in time. This turns out to be one of the most important relaxation mechanisms for both nuclear spins and electron spins for α protons (ring protons) in aromatic radicals.[28,40,46]

The time dependence of the END mechanism will involve a correlation time for radical tumbling τ_c, and the nuclear transition probability can be written as

$$W_n^{END} = \frac{B\tau_c}{1+\omega_n^2\tau_c^2} \quad (3.33)$$

where ω_n is the Larmor frequency of the nucleus and B depends on the square of the magnitude of the anisotropic dipolar hyperfine interaction. The dipolar tensor may be calculated approximately by the theory of McConnell and Strathdee,[39] and τ_c can be obtained from the Stokes-Einstein hydrodynamic model for rotation of a sphere of radius a in a medium of viscosity η.

$$\tau_c = \frac{4\pi\eta a^3}{3kT} \quad (3.34)$$

If we examine Fig. 3-28, we see that to calculate the probability of the relaxation path from energy level 4 to 2 to 1, we need not only the nuclear relaxation probability (2–1 transition), but also the electron relaxation probability (4–2 transition). The electron relaxation probability for solution radicals depends on the END mechanism, but also on g anisotropy and on spin-rotation interaction. These mechanisms all have the same dependence on correlation time, so we may write

$$W_e = \frac{C\tau_c}{1+\omega_e^2\tau_c^2} \quad (3.35)$$

where ω_e is the Larmor frequency of the electron and C depends on the magnitude of the g and hyperfine anisotropy and of the spin-rotation interaction.

If we plot $T_{1e} = W_e^{-1}$ and $T_{1n} = W_n^{-1}$ versus τ_c, we obtain Fig. 3-30. The maximum ENDOR response for the 4–2–1 relaxation pathway in Fig. 3-28 is expected at $T_{1e} = T_{1n}$ (Section 1.4.2.2) and, in general, the ENDOR response is proportional to ΔT_{1e} or T_{1n}, at a given value of τ_c. Under typical experimental conditions in solution we have

$$\omega_e^2\tau_c^2 \gg 1 \quad (3.36)$$

$$\omega_n^2\tau_c^2 \ll 1 \quad (3.37)$$

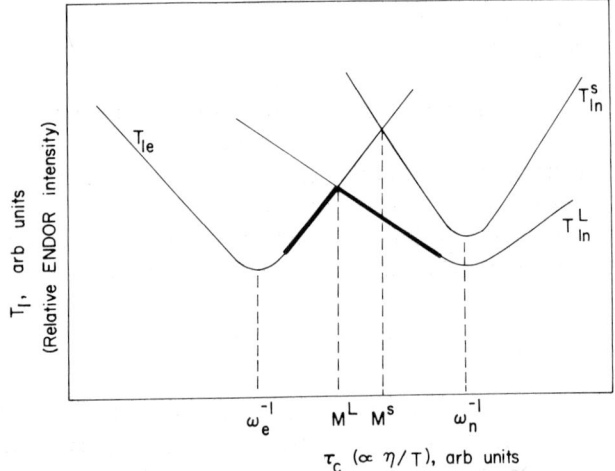

Figure 3-30. Schematic of the τ_c dependence of T_{1e} and T_{1n} where T_{1n} relaxation is dominated by large (T_{1n}^L) and small (T_{1n}^S) END terms. The optimum ENDOR response occurs when $T_{1e} = T_{1n}$ as shown by M^L and M^S for large and small END terms.

since $\omega_e \simeq 10^3 \omega_n$. If these inequalities hold we have

$$W_e = C\tau_c^{-1} \tag{3.38}$$

$$W_n^{END} = B\tau_c. \tag{3.39}$$

The heavy, dark line in Fig. 3-30 shows the expected τ_c or η/T dependence of the ENDOR response under these conditions; there is an optimum value of η/T for each type of proton dependent upon B/C. For two groups of protons in the same radical whose relaxation is dominated by the END mechanism, the C term cancels out and the ratio of optimum η/T values is

$$\frac{(\eta/T)_1}{(\eta/T)_2} = \left(\frac{B_2}{B_1}\right)^{1/2} \tag{3.40}$$

This is shown schematically in Fig. 3-30. So for the END mechanism, protons with larger END terms have a maximum ENDOR response at smaller η/T values, which occur at higher temperatures.

The validity of an η/T dependence for the ENDOR response is shown in Fig. 3-31 for the ring protons in 2,5-di-*t*-butyl-*p*-benzosemiquinone anion. Although the temperature dependence of the ENDOR response in different alcoholic solvents is different, the η/T dependence is the same for all solvents.

To ascertain whether the END mechanism dominates for particular classes of protons it is necessary to make detailed calculations. The fact

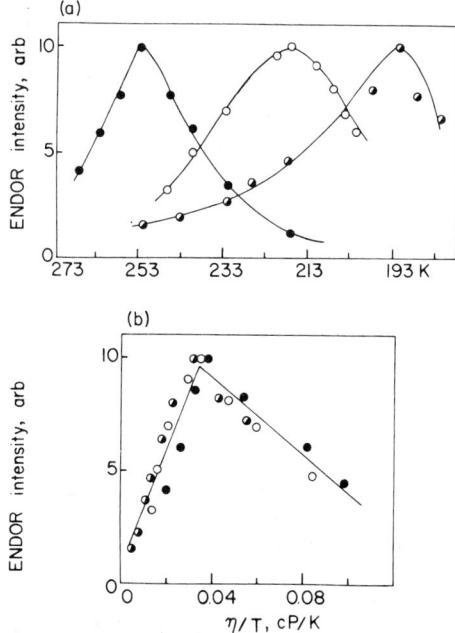

Figure 3-31. The (a) temperature and (b) viscosity to temperature dependence of the ENDOR intensity of the 3,6 ring protons in 2,5-di-t-butyl-p-benzosemiquinone anion, ◐ in methanol, ○ in ethanol, and ● in propanol. Note the comparison between (b) and the heavy dark line in Fig. 3-30. From Y. Kotake and K. Kuwata, *Bull. Chem. Soc. Japan*, **47**, 45 (1974).

that an η/T dependence is found is insufficient proof. In general, it appears that this mechanism does dominate for α protons in π radicals.[28,40,46,47] A simple way to test the END mechanism in such radicals is to note that the END terms of aromatic ring protons are approximately proportional to the square of the spin density on adjacent carbon atoms. Since the isotropic hyperfine coupling is also proportional to this spin density, we have

$$B_i \propto A_i^2 \qquad (3.41)$$

and eq. 3.40 becomes

$$\frac{(\eta/T)_1}{(\eta/T)_2} = \frac{A_2}{A_1}. \qquad (3.42)$$

Figure 3-32 shows a test of this equation for the 1 and 2 protons on the ring of 9,10-anthrasemiquinone anion radical in ethanol. As expected, the stronger coupled 2 proton ($A_2 = 2.73$ MHz) shows a maximum ENDOR

154 LIQUID PHASE ENDOR

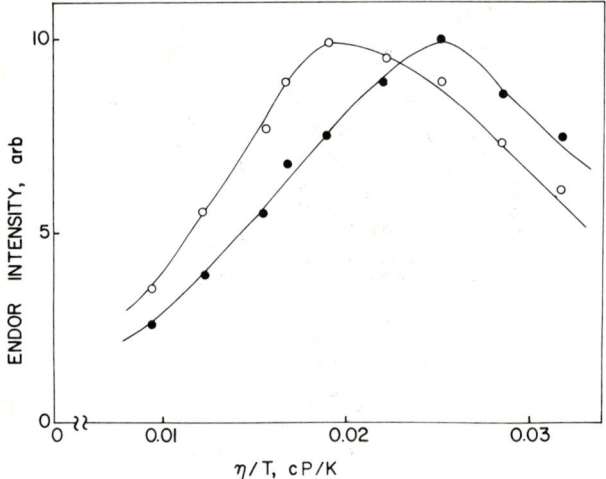

Figure 3-32. The viscosity to temperature dependence of the ENDOR intensity of the 1 proton (●) and 2 proton (○) in 9,10-anthrasemiquinone anion radical in ethanol. From Y. Kotake and K. Kuwata, *Bull. Chem. Soc. Japan*, **47**, 45 (1974).

intensity at a lower value of η/T than the weaker coupled 1 proton ($A_1 = 1.50$ MHz). Figure 3-32 gives $(\eta/T)_1/(\eta/T)_2 = 1.3$ to compare with $A_2/A_1 = 1.8$.

A more detailed comparison involves calculation of ΔT_{1e} for parameters characteristic of a particular radical and then calculation of the ENDOR enhancement by eq. 3.23 to compare experimental and theoretical results as a function of η/T. Reasonable agreement can be obtained for the single α proton on the central carbon of galvinoxyl radical[47] with assumption of a four level system as in Fig. 3-28 and neglect of coherence effects and rf field enhancement. The position of the maximum ENDOR response: (a) shifts to lower η/T (higher temperature) as the rf field is decreased; (b) is relatively insensitive to factor of two changes in H_1; (c) occurs at lower η/T (higher temperature) when the low field ESR transition is observed than when the high field transition is observed; (d) shifts to lower η/T if the spin-rotation term in the electron relaxation mechanism is neglected; (e) shifts to higher η/T as the effective molecular radius, which is essentially a parameter, decreases. Also, the ENDOR intensity is 25% greater for observation of the high field ESR line compared to the low field line.

3.7.3.2 Isotropic Hyperfine Modulation

A second possible nuclear relaxation mechanism of importance to ENDOR is modulation of the isotropic hyperfine (IH) coupling through internal motions of the radical.[47,48] An easily understood model for this mechanism comes from the angular dependence of β proton hyperfine constants. If the angle changes with time because of internal rotation about the C_α—C_β bond, the isotropic hyperfine constant can be written as

$$A_{iso}(t) = D_1 + D_2 \cos^2 \theta(t) \tag{3.43}$$

where D_1 and D_2 are orientation independent constants and θ is the dihedral angle defining the orientation of the C_β—H_β bond with respect to the axis of the p orbital containing the unpaired electron on C_α. The only relaxation caused by this type of modulation is a T_{x1} process in which both nuclear and electron spins are relaxed. As can be seen from Fig. 3-28 this is an excellent ENDOR mechanism when the 1–3 electron transition is saturated and the 3–4 nuclear transition is pumped. If we assume free rotational diffusion about the C_α—C_β bond, we find

$$W_{x1}^{IH} = \frac{b \langle A \rangle^2 \tau_r}{1 + \omega_{x1}^2 \tau_r^2} \tag{3.44}$$

where $\langle A \rangle$ is the observed average hyperfine coupling constant and b is a constant. τ_r is the correlation time for rotational diffusion given by

$$\tau_r = \frac{2\pi \eta a_r^3}{kT} \tag{3.45}$$

where a_r is the radius of the rotating group containing the β proton.

For small hyperfine constants $\omega_{x1} \approx \omega_e$ and for typical experimental conditions in liquids $\omega_{x1}^2 \tau_r^2 \gg 1$, so

$$W_{x1}^{IH} = b \langle A \rangle^2 \tau_r^{-1}. \tag{3.46}$$

This means that $T_{x1}^{IH} \propto \tau_r \propto \eta/T$ and according to Fig. 3-30 the ENDOR response should increase monotonically with η/T. If both END and IH nuclear relaxation mechanisms are important, then a maximum in the ENDOR response versus η/T is expected, but it will not necessarily correlate with that predicted from eq. 3.42. If we compare two proton ENDOR lines with nearly the same isotropic coupling constant, the proton relaxing by both END and IH mechanisms will show a maximum ENDOR response at a higher η/T than the proton relaxing by only an END mechanism. This can be understood by reference to Fig. 3-30, which illustrates an END mechanism. If an IH mechanism is added, the effective T_{1e} curve will drop so that the point at which $T_{1e} = T_{1n}$ moves to higher $\tau_c \propto \eta/T$.

Detailed calculations of the ENDOR response versus η/T for the single strongly coupled β proton in 2,6-di-t-butyl-4-cyclohexylphenoxy radical in hexane are shown in Fig. 3-33 and qualitatively support the importance

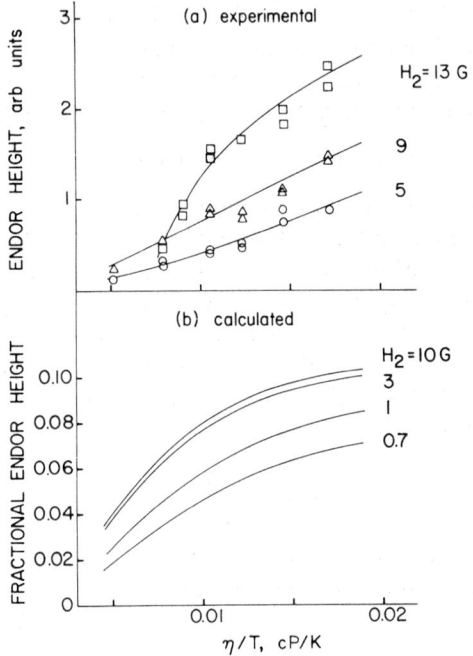

Figure 3-33. (a) ENDOR signal height of the high frequency ENDOR line (~19 MHz; see Fig. 3-34) from the single β proton in the 2,6-di-t-butyl-4-cyclohexylphenoxy radical in hexane when observing the high field ESR transition. (b) Calculated fractional ENDOR height for the same transition in a model β-proton system as described by N. M. Atherton and B. Day, *Mol. Phys.*, **27**, 145 (1974).

of the IH mechanism for strongly coupled β protons in aromatic radicals.[46] Both experiment and theory show a monotonic increase with η/T. Since the calculation involved both END and IH mechanisms, it appears that the IH mechanism dominates in this particular example where the β proton has a relatively large isotropic coupling (~9 MHz). For weakly coupled β protons, such as those in t-butyl groups attached to an aromatic radical, both END and IH mechanisms are weak and very likely neither greatly dominates.

3.7.3.3 Experimental Criteria to Distinguish END and IH Mechanisms

We have already indicated that detailed calculations of the η/T dependence of the ENDOR response for END and/or IH mechanisms can serve as reasonable criteria for distinguishing the relative importance of these mechanisms. However the calculations are complex even for a simplified four level system in the absence of coherence and rf enhancement effects, and the agreement with experiment is only qualitative or at best semiquantitative.

The best simple criterion for distinguishing these mechanisms appears to be the relative intensity of high and low frequency ENDOR lines and/or the intensity change in an ENDOR line when high and low field ESR lines are monitored. This can be seen by reference to Fig. 3-28. For a $T_{1e} + T_{1n}$ relaxation pathway the intensity of the ENDOR lines is predicted to be unchanged for the different observations indicated. This is independent of the particular mechanism as long as the $T_{1e} + T_{1n}$ relaxation pathway dominates. However we have found that the END mechanism is a principal mechanism for this pathway. Actual calculations for the END mechanism for α protons suggest that the high frequency ENDOR line is about 25% more intense than the low frequency ENDOR line.

For the T_{x1} relaxation pathway, which we will consider dominated by the IH mechanism, large intensity differences are expected. From Fig. 3-28 we see that when observing the saturated low field ESR line, the low frequency ENDOR line should be strong and the high frequency ENDOR line zero. Analogously, when observing the saturated high field ESR line, the high frequency ENDOR line should be strong and the low frequency one zero. These conclusions are true for either positive or negative coupling constants. Actual calculations of the relative intensities of the ENDOR lines for saturating high and low field ESR lines for a model four level system including both END and IH mechanisms for β protons give a typical ratio of 300:1.[47]

Experimental results qualitatively confirming the ENDOR intensity ratios expected for END mechanism dominant (α protons) or IH mechanism dominant (β protons) are shown in Fig. 3-34 by the ENDOR spectrum of 2,6-di-t-butyl-4-cyclohexylphenoxy radical. The ESR spectrum of this radical is dominated by the large β-proton coupling, which gives an ENDOR line at ~19 MHz. ENDOR spectra a and b correspond to observation of the high and low field components of the β proton doublet in the ESR spectrum, respectively. The 19 MHz ENDOR line shows a ratio of 3.5:1 between a and b, which is much less than the 300:1 calculated ratio but is characteristically greater than the ratio of 1.2:1 for the 16.6 MHz ENDOR line due to the α protons on the aromatic ring. Also note that the weaker proton couplings due to the t-butyl protons and other cyclohexyl protons generally show an intensity ratio between a and b and between corresponding high and low frequency ENDOR lines characteristic of a dominant IH mechanism. These γ protons are in rotating groups attached to the aromatic ring and will be modulated by the isotropic hyperfine coupling just as β protons are.

158 LIQUID PHASE ENDOR

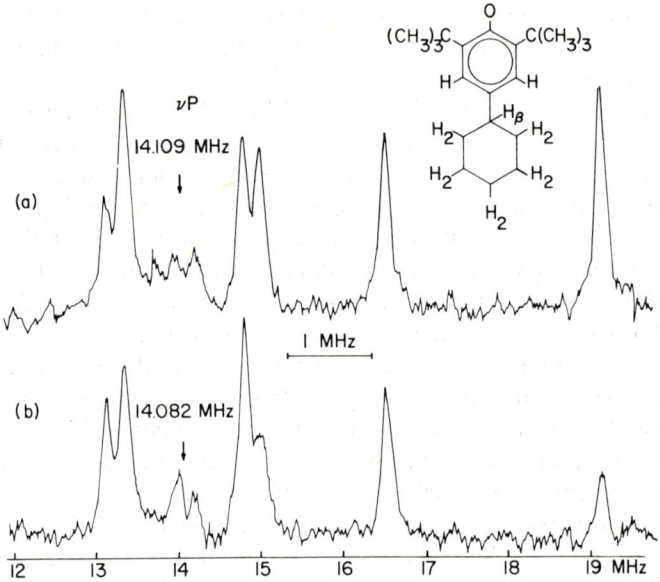

Figure 3-34. ENDOR spectra from 2,6-di-*t*-butyl-4-cyclohexylphenoxy radical in hexane when the high field (*a*) and low field (*b*) components of the β-proton doublet in the ESR spectrum are observed. Note the difference in the intensities of corresponding ENDOR lines between the two spectra. From N. M. Atherton and B. Day, *Chem. Phys. Lett.*, **15**, 428 (1972).

We caution that the intensity criteria really only distinguish between dominance of T_{x1} versus $T_{1e} + T_{1n}$ relaxation pathways without characterizing the nuclear relaxation mechanism of these relaxation pathways. But it appears that the most important relaxation mechanisms for these pathways are known.

3.7.4 RF Coherence Effects

Up to this point we have considered a four-level system for a radical in which each energy level is characterized by one electron spin quantum number and one nuclear spin quantum number, m_s and m_I. However, in the presence of sufficiently strong microwave or rf fields this description is inadequate; the energy levels become mixed and depend on more than one value of m_s and one value of m_I. In a vector diagram this means that the electron spin becomes quantized along the resultant of the applied, hyperfine, and H_1 fields (see Fig. 1-22) while the nuclear spin becomes quantized along the applied, hyperfine, and H_2 fields. The physical effects of such quantization may be called coherence effects because the spin precesses coherently with H_1 and H_2. The observed effect is a splitting of the ENDOR line, but there are three mechanisms that can give rise to such splitting.[19,49]

The first mechanism depends on the intensity of the microwave field. Essentially the strong microwave field mixes and shifts the energy levels shown in Fig. 3-28 and makes transitions between all levels allowed. This results in a splitting of the NMR line observed by ENDOR and consequently broadens and eventually splits the ENDOR line. The amount of the splitting equals the H_1 field and provides a handy calibration of the H_1 field intensity. An example of this effect is shown in Fig. 3-35 for the

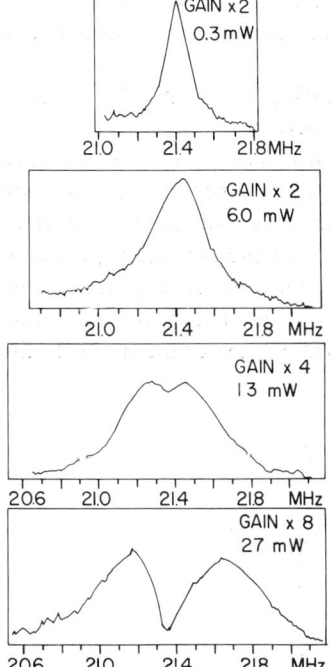

Figure 3-35. The ENDOR line from the methyenyl proton in $\sim 3 \times 10^{-4}\,M$ Coppinger's radical in n-heptane at 188 K versus microwave power. The incident microwave powers and relative gains are given. The ENDOR line splits because of coherence effects as discussed in the text. From J. H. Freed et al., *J. Chem. Phys.*, **47**, 2762 (1967).

methylenyl proton in Coppinger's radical. It is seen that considerable broadening is observed before any actual splitting can be ascertained. At 27 mW the observed splitting of 470 kHz agrees rather well with the 523 kHz expected from an independent calibration of H_1.[19] In practice, the symmetry of the split ENDOR line depends rather sensitively on the field position observed on the ESR line, a consequence of observing a first derivative peak of the ESR line rather than the line center.[19]

160   LIQUID PHASE ENDOR

A second mechanism leading to ENDOR line splitting depends on the rf field intensity and is parallel to the first mechanism described. The strong rf field mixes and shifts the energy levels shown in Fig. 3-28 and makes all transitions allowed. This results in a splitting of the ESR line observed and should be observable in the ESR spectrum alone at the proper rf frequency. The ENDOR line will split because the peak of the observed ESR line decreases as the ESR line splits. This mechanism requires rather high rf fields (≥ 20 G) for most radicals and appears to be difficult to observe.[49]

Both the first and second mechanisms described are due to partial uncoupling of the hyperfine interaction. A strong microwave field perturbs the electron spins, making it difficult for the nucleus to distinguish between electron spin up or down. Likewise a strong rf field perturbs the nuclear spins and makes it difficult for the electron to distinguish between nuclear spin up or down.

The third mechanism of ENDOR line splitting also depends on the rf field intensity but is different from the first two mechanisms, depending on the simultaneous absorption of two rf quanta. The probability for such a process depends on $(\Delta - 2\omega_{rf})^{-1}$ where Δ is the energy of the transition and so is very sharply peaked at exact resonance. A real energy level does not have to exist at ω_{rf} above the lowest level but the transition probability is maximized if one does. Consider the energy level diagram in Fig. 3-36 for a radical with two equivalent $I = \frac{1}{2}$ nuclei. If the nondegenerate 6–3 ESR transition is saturated in an ENDOR experiment, both the

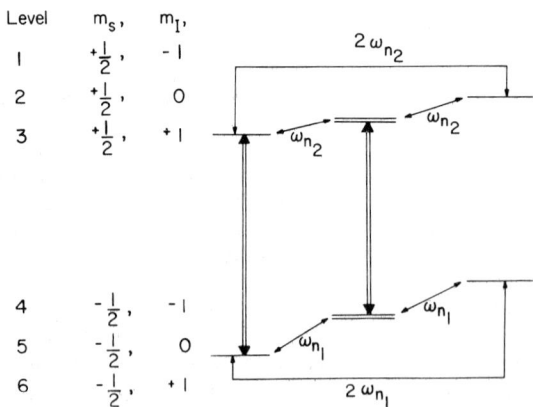

Figure 3-36. Energy level diagram for a radical with hyperfine coupling to two equivalent $I = \frac{1}{2}$ nuclei showing single ($\omega_{n_1}, \omega_{n_2}$) and double ($2\omega_{n_1}, 2\omega_{n_2}$) rf quantum transitions. The double horizontal lines indicate energy level degeneracy and the double vertical lines indicate saturated transitions.

single quantum ENDOR transition ω_{n_1} and the double quantum transition $2\omega_{n_1}$ will add spins to level 6 to decrease the saturation and lead to ENDOR enhancement. But if the degenerate 5–2 ESR transition is saturated, the double quantum transition $2\omega_{n_1}$ partially opposes ENDOR enhancement by the ω_{n_1} transitions. This effect sharply peaks at exact resonance $\Delta_{64} = 2\omega_{n_1}$, and splits the ENDOR line by decreasing its enhancement in the absence of double quantum transitions at the very center of the line. This physical description is oversimplified but it should serve for qualitative understanding.

This double quantum coherence effect allows one to distinguish between degenerate and nondegenerate ENDOR lines and can be most helpful in the assignment of spectra (see Section 3.2.5). An example was seen in Fig. 3-12 for degenerate and nondegenerate lines in Coppinger's radical. The observed splitting should give a measure of the H_2 field intensity, but it is difficult to develop high enough H_2 fields to obtain well resolved splittings. For the same reason this double quantum splitting can only be seen with rather narrow ENDOR lines.

Both the decoupling mechanism two and the double quantum mechanism three depend on the rf field intensity. However they appear to be distinguishable because the decoupling mechanism seems to require higher rf fields to observe a splitting than does the double quantum mechanism. The decoupling mechanism is expected to significantly broaden the ENDOR line before any splitting is observed as shown for the microwave field decoupling mechanism in Fig. 3-35. However the double quantum mechanism does not cause much broadening before line splitting is detectable because of its sharply resonant nature (see Fig. 3-12).

3.7.5 Dispersion Mode ENDOR

The phenomenological picture of the ENDOR response in Section 3.7.2 was limited to absorption mode signals because they are most commonly observed. It is interesting, however, that detection of the magnetization in-phase with the microwave field or the dispersion mode signal gives somewhat greater ENDOR sensitivity. This is shown by the same phenomenological treatment used in Section 3.7.2.[50]

From the Bloch equations the u component of the magnetization (dispersion mode) is given by eq. 3.9. The normally detected ESR signal is a first derivative of the magnetic field, which is

$$\frac{du}{dH} = \frac{M_o \gamma_e^2 H_1 T_{2e}^2 [\gamma_e^2 T_{2e}^2 (H_o - H)^2 - (1 + \gamma_e^2 H_1^2 T_{1e} T_{2e})]}{[1 + \gamma_e^2 T_{2e}^2 (H_o - H)^2 + \gamma_e^2 H_1^2 T_{1e} T_{2e}]^2}. \quad (3.47)$$

The u-mode signal has its maximum absolute amplitude at $H = H_o$, so this is the optimum field for ENDOR, which gives

$$\left.\frac{du}{dH}\right|_{max} = \frac{-M_o \gamma_e^2 H_1 T_{2e}^2}{1 + \gamma_e^2 H_1^2 T_{1e} T_{2e}}. \tag{3.48}$$

We again consider the ENDOR response to arise from a change in T_{1e} so the enhancement of the dispersion signal E^D is given by

$$E^D = d\left(\left.\frac{du}{dH}\right|_{max}\right) = \frac{M_o \gamma_e^4 H_1^3 T_{2e}^3}{(1 + \gamma_e^2 H_1^2 T_{1e} T_{2e})^2} \Delta T_{1e}. \tag{3.49}$$

If we compare the dispersion mode (eq. 3.49) with the absorption mode (eq. 3.23) signals, we have

$$\frac{E^D}{E^A} = 1.03(1 + \gamma_e^2 H_1^2 T_{1e} T_{2e})^{1/2} \tag{3.50}$$

so the dispersion mode ENDOR response will always be larger, and especially so at larger H_1.

The maximum dispersion mode ENDOR enhancement versus H_1 is found by substituting $\gamma_e^2 H_1^2 T_{1e} T_{2e} = 3$ into eq. 3.49:

$$E_{max}^D = 0.32 M_o \gamma_e \left(\frac{T_{2e}}{T_{1e}}\right)^{3/2} \Delta T_{1e} \tag{3.51}$$

This occurs at twice the optimum microwave power for the absorption mode ENDOR response. If we compare E_{max}^D with E_{max}^A (eq. 3.24), we find $E_{max}^D / E_{max}^A = 1.8$. This theoretical prediction has been semiquantitatively confirmed experimentally for 1×10^{-3} M galvinoxyl radical in mineral oil at room temperature.[50]

REFERENCES

1. J. S. Hyde and A. H. Maki, *J. Chem. Phys.*, **40**, 3117 (1964).
2. D. S. Leniart, J. C. Vedrine, and J. S. Hyde, *Chem. Phys. Lett.*, **6**, 637 (1970).
3. K. P. Dinse, K. Möbius, R. Biehl, and M. Plato, *Magnetic Resonance and Related Phenomena*, Proc. XVII Congress Ampere, V. Hovi, ed., North-Holland, Amsterdam, 1973, pp. 419–422.
4. H. B. Stegmann, K. Scheffler, G. Bauer, R. Grimm, S. Hieke, and D. Sturner, *Phosphorus*, **4**, 1 (1974).
5. M. N. Atherton and B. Day, *J. Chem. Soc., Faraday Trans. II*, **69**, 1801 (1973).
6. H. van Willigen, M. Plato, R. Biehl, K. P. Dinse, and K. Möbius, *Mol. Phys.*, **26**, 793 (1973).
7. R. D. Allendoerfer and A. H. Maki, *J. Amer. Chem. Soc.*, **91**, 1088 (1969).
8. J. S. Hyde, *J. Chem. Phys.*, **43**, 1806 (1965).

9. A. H. Maki, R. Allendoerfer, J. C. Danner, and R. T. Keys, *J. Amer. Chem. Soc.*, **90**, 4225 (1968).
10. R. Allendoerfer and A. H. Maki, *J. Magn. Resonance*, **3**, 396 (1970).
11. R. D. Allendoerfer and J. H. Engelmann, *Mol. Phys.*, **20**, 569 (1971).
12. R. D. Allendoerfer and E. J. Eustace, *J. Phys. Chem.*, **75**, 2765 (1971).
13. L. D. Kispert, J. S. Hyde, C. DeBoer, D. LaFollette, and R. Breslow, *J. Phys. Chem.*, **72**, 4276 (1968).
14. H. M. McConnell, C. Heller, T. Cole, and R. W. Fessenden, *J. Amer. Chem. Soc.*, **82**, 766 (1960).
15. J. R. Morton and A. Horsfield, *J. Chem. Phys.*, **35**, 1142 (1961).
16. J. S. Hyde, G. H. Rist, and L. E. G. Eriksson, *J. Phys. Chem.*, **72**, 4269 (1968).
17. K. Möbius, H. van Willigen, and A. H. Maki, *Mol. Phys.*, **20**, 289 (1971).
18. J. S. Hyde, *J. Phys. Chem.*, **71**, 68 (1967).
19. J. H. Freed, D. S. Leniart, and J. S. Hyde, *J. Chem. Phys.*, **47**, 2762 (1967).
20. K. P. Dinse, R. Biehl, K. Möbius, and M. Plato, *J. Magn. Resonance*, **6**, 444 (1972).
21. N. M. Atherton and A. J. Blackhurst, *J. Chem. Soc. Faraday Trans. II*, **68**, 470 (1972).
22. Y. Kotake and K. Kuwata, *Bull. Chem. Soc. Japan*, **45**, 2663 (1972).
23. R. D. Allendoerfer and R. J. Papez, *J. Amer. Chem. Soc.*, **92**, 6971 (1970).
24. J. S. Hyde, R. Breslow, and C. DeBoer, *J. Amer. Chem. Soc.*, **88**, 4763 (1966).
25. C. Steelink, J. D. Fitzpatrick, L. D. Kispert, and J. S. Hyde, *J. Amer. Chem. Soc.*, **90**, 4354 (1968).
26. M. R. Das, H. D. Connor, D. S. Leniart, and J. H. Freed, *J. Amer. Chem. Soc.*, **92**, 2258 (1970).
27. H. S. Gutowsky and C. H. Holm, *J. Chem. Phys.*, **25**, 1228 (1956).
28. J. H. Freed, *J. Chem. Phys.*, **43**, 2312 (1965).
29. A. D. McLachlan, *Mol. Phys.*, **3**, 233 (1960).
30. R. D. Allendoerfer and A. H. Maki, *J. Amer. Chem. Soc.*, **91**, 1088 (1969).
31. K. P. Dinse, K. Möbius, and R. Biehl, *Z. Naturforsch.* **28a**, 1069 (1973).
32. R. D. Allendoerfer, P. E. Gallagher, and P. T. Lansbury, *J. Amer. Chem. Soc.*, **94**, 7702 (1972).
33. N. L. Bauld, J. D. McDermed, C. E. Hudson, Y. S. Rim, J. Zoeller, R. D. Gordon, and J. S. Hyde, *J. Amer. Chem. Soc.*, **91**, 6666 (1969).
34. N. S. Dalal, D. E. Kennedy, and C. A. McDowell, *J. Chem. Phys.*, **59**, 3403 (1973).
35. G. K. Fraenkel, *J. Phys. Chem.*, **71**, 139 (1967).
36. H. R. Falle and G. R. Luckhurst, *J. Magn. Resonance*, **3**, 161 (1970).
37. K. P. Dinse, R. Biehl, K. Möbius, and H. Haustein, *Chem. Phys. Lett.*, **12**, 399 (1971).
38. K. P. Dinse, K. Möbius, M. Plato, R. Biehl, and H. Haustein, *Chem. Phys. Lett.*, **14**, 196 (1972).
39. H. M. McConnell, and J. Strathdee, *Mol. Phys.*, **2**, 129 (1959).
40. J. H. Freed, *J. Phys. Chem.*, **71**, 38 (1967).
41. J. H. Freed, *J. Chem. Phys.*, **50**, 2271 (1969).
42. J. H. Freed, D. S. Leniart, and H. D. Connor, *J. Chem. Phys.*, **58**, 3089 (1973).

43. [For an introduction to density matrices in magnetic resonance see] C. P. Slichter, *Principles of Magnetic Resonance*, Harper & Row, New York, 1963, pp. 127–159.
44. H. Seidel, *Z. Phys.*, **165,** 239 (1961).
45. [For an introductory description see] A. Carrington and A. D. McLachlan, *Introduction to Magnetic Resonance*, Harper & Row, New York, 1967, Chapter 1.
46. Y. Kotake and K. Kuwata, *Bull. Chem. Soc. Japan*, **47,** 45 (1974).
47. N. M. Atherton and B. Day, *Mol. Phys.*, **27,** 145 (1974).
48. N. M. Atherton and B. Day, *Chem. Phys. Lett.*, **15,** 428 (1972).
49. N. M. Atherton, *Electron Spin Resonance*, Halsted, New York, 1973, pp. 390–393.
50. R. D. Allendoerfer, *J. Magn. Resonance*, **9,** 226 (1973).

4. ENDOR in Solids

4.1 Introduction
4.2 Anisotropic Hyperfine Interaction
    4.2.1 Energy Levels
    4.2.2 Single Crystal Analysis—General Case
    4.2.3 Ionic Crystal Analysis—Special Case
    4.2.4 Signs of Hyperfine Constants
    4.2.5 Spin Density Determination
    4.2.6 Second Order Effects
4.3 Quadrupole Interaction
4.4 Organic Single Crystals
    4.4.1 Interpretation of Hyperfine Tensors
    4.4.2 Radical Identification and Orientation
    4.4.3 Reaction Mechanisms of Radical Formation
    4.4.4 Intramolecular Motion: Methyl Group Tunneling
    4.4.5 Distant ENDOR
    4.4.6 Triplet State ENDOR
        4.4.6.1 General Features
        4.4.6.2 Structural Studies
4.5 Molecular Inorganic Single Crystals
4.6 ENDOR in Disordered Matrices
    4.6.1 Anisotropic ENDOR
    4.6.2 Matrix ENDOR
        4.6.2.1 Lineshape Models
        4.6.2.2 Analysis of Unpaired Electron Distribution
        4.6.2.3 Analysis of Motional Processes
        References

4.1 INTRODUCTION

ENDOR in solids is a somewhat broader field than ENDOR in liquids. A much wider variety of nuclei and of chemical systems has been studied by solid phase ENDOR. This is at least partly due to the fact that the experiments are easier to do. But, as we shall see, they are often more involved to interpret. In the solid phase one can always lower the temperature so that the relaxation times that make ENDOR possible can be short-circuited by the available microwave and nuclear rf power. For low power ENDOR, which we may define as 1 W or less of rf power, the ENDOR rf coil can often simply be a few turns of wire about the sample or sample holder placed in the ESR cavity. Of course high power ENDOR is still useful in many solid studies, particularly if one wants to study radicals in solids at higher temperatures where the relaxation times are shorter. In addition, high power ENDOR is often desirable for studying disordered solids.

In the solid phase the interactions are more complex and consequently more information at the expense of a complex analysis is often available. In the liquid phase except for special phases such as in liquid crystal studies the basic information available from the ENDOR spectrum is the isotropic hyperfine coupling constant as well as the nuclear g factor. In solids we also obtain information about the dipolar or anisotropic hyperfine coupling constant in addition to the isotropic one. Since the anisotropic hyperfine interaction is orientation dependent, single crystal studies are clearly desirable. It also turns out that quadrupole interactions are observable in a first order ENDOR spectrum. This is not true of a first order ESR spectrum. The quadrupole interaction is also orientation dependent, and hence by orientation studies both the anisotropic hyperfine tensor and the quadrupole interaction tensor can be determined.

The variety of systems that have been studied by ENDOR in solids can be roughly classified into four categories: (*a*) transition metal ions in ionic crystals, (*b*) defect centers in ionic crystals, (*c*) molecular crystals (mainly organic), and (*d*) polycrystalline and amorphous solids. In keeping with the orientation toward chemistry in this book the last two areas are emphasized in this chapter. The ENDOR of transition metal ions in ionic crystals has recently been comprehensively discussed[1] as have the ENDOR studies of defect centers in ionic crystals.[2,3] These areas have traditionally been of most interest to physicists and we only cite a few examples where they are particularly appropriate. In this chapter we describe how to use solid phase ENDOR to study anisotropic hyperfine and quadrupole interactions and their use for identification and electronic structure determination of free radicals. As in the liquid phase we mainly concentrate on proton ENDOR since it has been most widely used to study a variety of radicals in organic single crystals of both chemical and biochemical interest. This also includes the study of triplet states by ENDOR, which is a more recent development. Finally we discuss the rather new area of ENDOR in disordered solid systems since many systems of chemical and biochemical interest cannot be obtained as single crystals. Although the information content from ENDOR is generally less for disordered systems as compared to single crystals, new developments are leading to surprisingly detailed information from such disordered systems.

4.2 ANISOTROPIC HYPERFINE INTERACTION

An anisotropic or dipolar hyperfine interaction always exists between two magnetic dipoles. Here we are concerned with the electron dipole–nuclear dipole interaction. This interaction is orientation dependent just as is the interaction between two bar magnets. In the liquid phase where radical rotation is fast the dipolar hyperfine interaction averages out on the ESR or ENDOR time scales so it does not enter in the spectra. If the motion is partially arrested as in liquid crystals (Section 3.6), then we encounter anisotropic hyperfine effects involving one principal axis in the ENDOR spectra. If the radical motion is completely arrested, except for vibration and some internal motion, as in a solid, we must understand the anisotropic hyperfine interaction to analyze the ENDOR spectra.

4.2.1 Energy Levels

We consider the typical case for organic radicals in single crystals where g is assumed isotropic but A is not. Then the spin Hamiltonian can be written

$$\mathcal{H} = g\beta \mathbf{H} \cdot \mathbf{S} - g_n\beta_n \mathbf{H} \cdot \mathbf{I} + h\mathbf{S} \cdot \mathbf{A} \cdot \mathbf{I} \quad (4.1)$$

where $\mathbf{A}$ is a tensor consisting of nine Cartesian components that represent the coupling between two three-component vectors, $\mathbf{S}$ and $\mathbf{I}$. If we use a set of laboratory axes $x'y'z'$ and take the magnetic field to be in the z' direction, and again use the strong field approximation in which the electron Zeeman interaction dominates, we have

$$\mathcal{H} = g\beta H_{z'}S_{z'} - g_n\beta_n H_{z'}I_{z'} + h(S_{z'}A_{z'x'}I_{x'} + S_{z'}A_{z'y'}I_{y'} + S_{z'}A_{z'z'}I_{z'}) \quad (4.2)$$

All the $S_{x'}$ and $S_{y'}$ terms in the hyperfine interaction drop out because $S_{z'}$ is aligned along the magnetic field H_o. Then for $S = \tfrac{1}{2}$ we have ENDOR frequencies given by

$$\nu_\pm = \left| \nu_n \pm \frac{R}{2} \right| \quad (4.3)$$

which is analogous to eq. 1.6, and where

$$R = (A_{z'x'}^2 + A_{z'y'}^2 + A_{z'z'}^2)^{1/2}. \quad (4.4)$$

When the crystal is oriented so that the tensor is diagonal in the laboratory $x'y'z'$ axis system, then $R = A_{z'z'}$. R is an effective hyperfine coupling for a particular orientation of the magnetic field with respect to the axes of the radical or of the crystal. R will vary with orientation and involve contributions of other components of the hyperfine tensor in general. From a complete study of the effective hyperfine splitting versus angle for rotation of the magnetic field around three mutually perpendicular axes of a single crystal, all the components of the A tensor can be obtained.

4.2.2 Single Crystal Analysis—General Case

Single crystal analysis by ESR or ENDOR is similar in principle but is usually somewhat easier for ENDOR. The advantage of ENDOR is simply that the resolution is better, either in terms of spectral density or absolutely (Section 1.4.5.2), so the angular variation of the hyperfine lines is easier to follow, which allows more definitive assignment of the lines.

First you orient the crystal by its external morphology or by x-ray analysis. Then you pick three orthogonal crystal axes; call them xyz. For molecular crystals one generally must pick orthogonal axes that are not symmetry axes of the radical or the molecules in the crystal. However at least one crystallographic axis is usually chosen if known. The direction of the external magnetic field relative to the xyz axes is given by the direction cosines: l_x, l_y, l_z.

Experimentally R is measured from the ENDOR frequencies given by eq. 4.3. In general, R is given by[3]

$$\begin{aligned}
R = [\, & l_x^2(A_{xx}^2 + A_{xy}^2 + A_{xz}^2) + l_y^2(A_{yx}^2 + A_{yy}^2 + A_{yz}^2) \\
& + l_z^2(A_{zx}^2 + A_{zy}^2 + A_{zz}^2) + 2l_xl_y(A_{xx}A_{xy} + A_{xy}A_{yy} + A_{zx}A_{zy}) \\
& + 2l_xl_z(A_{xx}A_{xz} + A_{xy}A_{zy} + A_{xz}A_{zz}) \\
& + 2l_yl_z(A_{xy}A_{xz} + A_{yy}A_{yz} + A_{yz}A_{zz})\,]^{1/2} \quad (4.5)
\end{aligned}$$

which can be rewritten as

$$R = [l_x^2 T_{xx} + l_y^2 T_{yy} + l_z^2 T_{zz} + 2l_xl_y T_{xy} + 2l_xl_z T_{xz} + 2l_yl_z T_{yz}]^{1/2}. \quad (4.6)$$

It can be recognized that the T_{ij} elements form a symmetric tensor that is the square of the hyperfine tensor; this can be verified by matrix multiplication. Thus if we determine the T_{ij} elements, we can obtain the A_{ij} elements.

The T_{ij} elements are obtained by taking data with $x \perp H_o$ and rotation in the yz plane with θ defined as the angle between the z axis and H_o. Then the direction cosines of H_o are (0, sin θ, cos θ) and eq. 4.6 gives

$$R(\theta) = (\sin^2 \theta\, T_{yy} + \cos^2 \theta\, T_{zz} + 2 \sin \theta\, T_{yz})^{1/2}. \quad (4.7)$$

Then $T_{yy}^{1/2} = R(90°)$, $T_{zz}^{1/2} = R(0°)$, and T_{yz} is determined by a least squares fit. Similarly rotation about the y and z axes gives the other T_{ij}. The 3×3 T matrix must then be rotated to a new coordinate system, XYZ, in which it is diagonal. Since the T matrix is symmetric, it can always be diagonalized. Diagonalization is performed by finding the roots to det $\mathbf{T} - \lambda\mathbf{1}) = 0$ where $\mathbf{1}$ is the unit matrix. Expansion gives a cubic equation in λ and the three roots are the principal values of the diagonalized T matrix in a new coordinate system. In diagonal form $T_{XX} = A_{XX}^2$ so the principal values of the diagonalized hyperfine tensor in the XYZ coordinate system are now determined except for an ambiguity in sign. In most cases the signs of all the principal values of the A tensor are the same; however, exceptions can occur when the isotropic coupling is small.

We now are in a position to separate the total hyperfine coupling tensor into its isotropic and anisotropic components. The isotropic component is given by

$$A_{iso} = \tfrac{1}{3}(A_{XX} + A_{YY} + A_{ZZ}) \quad (4.8)$$

and the anisotropic components are given by

$$\begin{aligned} B_{XX} &= A_{XX} - A_{iso} \\ B_{YY} &= A_{YY} - A_{iso} \\ B_{ZZ} &= A_{ZZ} - A_{iso}. \end{aligned} \quad (4.9)$$

Note that the anisotropic components add to zero so the trace of the dipolar part of the total hyperfine interaction is zero. This means that the dipolar interaction goes to zero when averaged over all directions with respect to the magnetic field as occurs for radicals in liquids. The dipolar tensor **B** is called axial when two of its components are equal. This will occur for appropriate molecular symmetry.

To relate the principal axes of the total hyperfine tensor **A** in the XYZ coordinate system to the hyperfine tensor **A** in our original xyz coordinate system which we know from the laboratory, we must determine the direction cosines of the principal axes relative to the xyz axes. The direction cosines for the kth principal value axis where T_k is the kth principal value are given by

$$\sum_{j=x}^{z} T_{ij} l_{kj} = T_k l_{ki} \quad \text{for } i = x, y, z \text{ and } k = X, Y, Z \quad (4.10)$$

where l_{kj} for $j = x, y, z$ are the direction cosines. Usually the principal values, A_k, and their direction cosines, l_{kj}, which are the same as for T_k, are given in the scientific literature. The transformation to obtain the A_{ij} components in the xyz coordinate system is

$$\begin{vmatrix} l_{xX} & l_{xY} & l_{xZ} \\ l_{yX} & l_{yY} & l_{yZ} \\ l_{zX} & l_{zY} & l_{zZ} \end{vmatrix} \begin{vmatrix} A_{XX} & & \\ & A_{YY} & \\ & & A_{ZZ} \end{vmatrix} \begin{vmatrix} l_{xx} & l_{xy} & l_{xz} \\ l_{Yx} & l_{Yy} & l_{Yz} \\ l_{Zx} & l_{Zy} & l_{Zz} \end{vmatrix} = \begin{vmatrix} A_{xx} & A_{xy} & A_{xz} \\ A_{yx} & A_{yy} & A_{yz} \\ A_{zx} & A_{zy} & A_{zz} \end{vmatrix}$$

(4.11)

Then from the A_{ij} and eqs. 4.6 and 4.3 the ENDOR spectra can be calculated to check for self-consistency.

To obtain the most detailed picture of the electronic structure of a radical in a single crystal one needs to know the crystal structure. Then the orientation of the principal values of the hyperfine tensor can be related to the molecules in the crystal and to the expected symmetry of the radical. The hyperfine tensor for a particular nucleus can then be used to locate that particular nucleus in the crystal. It is usually found that organic radicals produced in single crystals by ultraviolet or ionizing radiation are oriented nearly the same as the undamaged molecules.

Defect centers and transition metal ions are usually studied in ionic crystals for which the structure is known and for which the orientation of the paramagnetic center in the crystal is known or at least is simply related to the crystal axes. In this case one does not have to start with an arbitrary axis system and can often choose the crystal axes coincident with the principal axes of the paramagnetic center. Furthermore axial symmetry often exists. This makes the analysis somewhat simpler.

4.2.3 Ionic Crystal Analysis—Special Case

Manifold ENDOR studies have been carried out on transition metal ions and defect centers in ionic single crystals. In many cases the principal axes of the hyperfine tensors are coincident with the crystal axes, which can be selected experimentally from the external morphology of the crystal. Thus one can choose a laboratory coordinate system in which the hyperfine tensor is diagonalized. The spin Hamiltonian of eq. 4.1 can still be used along with the general analysis in the previous section. However it has become common to separate the isotropic and anisotropic parts of the hyperfine tensor in the spin Hamiltonian.[4] So that the reader can easily follow the scientific literature we review this approach here.

In the principal axis system of the anisotropic hyperfine tensor all off-diagonal terms vanish and the spin Hamiltonian can be written as

$$\mathcal{H} = g\beta \mathbf{H} \cdot \mathbf{S} - g_n\beta_n \mathbf{H} \cdot \mathbf{I} + A_{iso}\mathbf{I} \cdot \mathbf{S} + B_{xx}I_xS_x$$
$$+ B_{yy}I_yS_y + B_{zz}I_zS_z. \quad (4.12)$$

Then in the strong field approximation, the observed hyperfine splitting is given by

$$R = A_{iso} + B_{xx}l_x^2 + B_{yy}l_y^2 + B_{zz}l_z^2 \quad (4.13)$$

where l_x, l_y, l_z are the direction cosines of the magnetic field with respect to the xyz principal axis system of the hyperfine tensor. In the strong field approximation ($g\beta H \gg A_{iso}$) both **S** and **I** are quantized along the field and hence have the same direction cosines as **H**. This is the origin of the squared direction cosines in eq. 4.13.

For the common case of axial symmetry where the nucleus lies on an axis that is at least a threefold symmetry axis of the electron distribution, we can simplify R. Let z be the symmetry axis so that $B_{zz} = -2B_{xx} = -2B_{yy}$. Then if the external magnetic field is perpendicular to the x axis and the angle θ is measured from z to H_o in the yz plane, we have $l_x = 0$ $l_y = \sin\theta$, and $l_z = \cos\theta$. This gives

$$R = A_{iso} + \tfrac{1}{2}B_{zz}(3\cos^2\theta - 1). \quad (4.14)$$

Let us now consider the ENDOR spectrum of excess electrons trapped in a bromide ion vacancy site in single crystal KBr (F centers).[4] The excess electron wavefunction interacts with several shells of surrounding matrix nuclei so many ENDOR lines are possible. Figure 4-1 shows the relative locations of the nuclei assigned to various shells out to shell VIII with respect to the excess electron. One may anticipate that the closest shells will have large enough overlap with the electron wavefunction to make A_{iso} large and consequently $R/2 > \nu_n$. Thus the ENDOR lines from these closest shells will occur at $R/2$ split by $2\nu_n$. Also one expects the more distant shells to have $R/2 < \nu_n$ so that ENDOR lines from these shells occur at ν_n split by R. Figure 4-2 shows an ENDOR spectrum for trapped electrons in KBr with the magnetic field parallel to the 100 crystal direction. It is seen that ENDOR lines are observed from about 0.5 to 26 MHz.

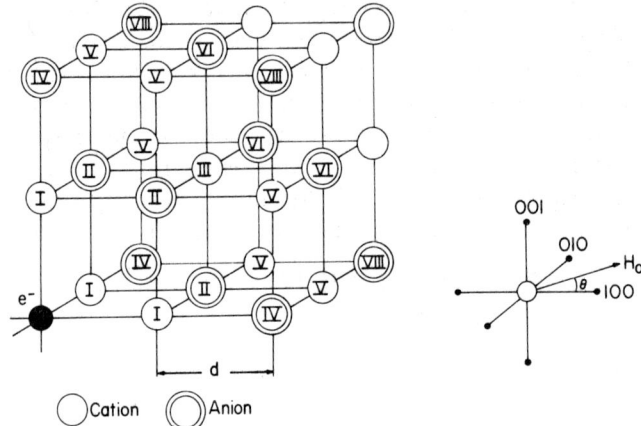

Figure 4-1. Environment of an excess electron (F center) in a cubic alkali halide crystal showing the positions of surrounding shells of nuclei. The definitions of crystal directions are also shown.

The assignment of all the lines in Fig. 4-2 to nuclei in the first through eighth shells is no mean task but can be unambiguously accomplished by considering (1) the dependence of the lines as the angle between the field direction and a crystal axis is varied, (2) the pairwise appearance of lines about the free nuclear frequency, (3) the pairwise appearance of lines separated by $2\nu_n$, (4) the repeated appearance of lines with a frequency ratio equal to the ratio of nuclear g factors of isotopes present, and (5) additional splitting due to quadrupole or second order hyperfine interactions. Assignments based on these considerations are indicated in Fig. 4-2.

The most important guide is the angular dependence of the ENDOR lines. Figure 4-3 shows how nuclei in different shells may have characteristically different angular dependencies. However some shells will have the same angular dependence, as, for example, shells I and IV. This can be seen from Fig. 4-1. In this case the distinction can usually be made from the magnitude of the hyperfine constants since the more distant nuclei have smaller hyperfine constants. Deviations from axial symmetry, which we have assumed here, will be revealed by departures from the idealized plots in Fig. 4-3.

Figure 4-3 also illustrates site splitting. For shell I at $\theta = 0°$ there are two distinct sites for equivalent nuclei with hyperfine constants of $A_{iso} + B_{zz}$ and $A_{iso} - \frac{1}{2}B_{zz}$. As θ is increased three sites corresponding to nuclei in the 100, 010, and 001 directions are observed. Although this adds to the number of ENDOR lines and serves to complicate the spectra, site splitting also may help to assign certain ENDOR lines.

ANISOTROPIC HYPERFINE INTERACTION   173

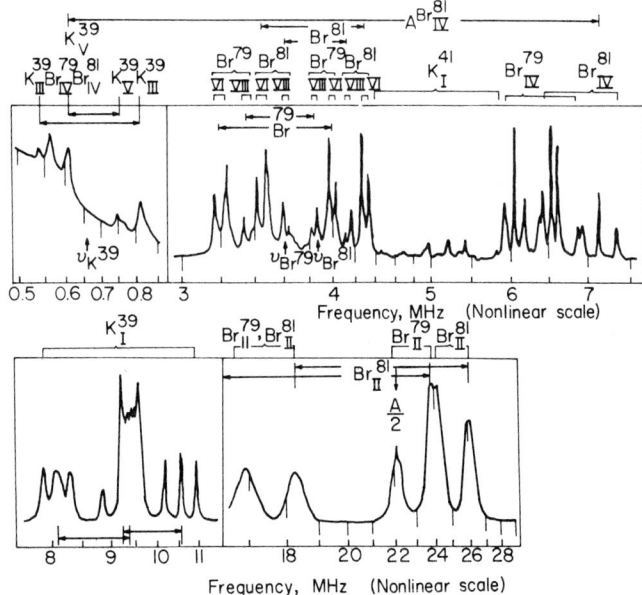

Figure 4-2. ENDOR spectrum of a trapped electron (F center) in KBr at 90 K for the magnetic field parallel to the 100 crystal direction (see Fig. 4-1). The lines are assigned to the various nuclei shown subscripted with the shell to which they belong (see Fig. 4-1). For the close shells I and II A_{iso} is large and the ENDOR lines occur at half the hyperfine frequency split by $2\nu_n$. In addition, there are two sites for nuclei in these shells at this orientation, so for Br_{II}^{81} there are four ENDOR lines, one pair from each site, as indicated in the 16 to 28 MHz region. For K_I^{39} there are also two sites, and the four line positions are shown in the 8 to 11 MHz region. Each of those lines is further split into a triplet by a quadrupole interaction and the center two triplets overlap. For the more distant shells the ENDOR lines occur at ν_n split by the hyperfine frequency. Site splitting complicates the clarity of the spectrum. Adapted from H. Seidel, Z. Physik., **165**, 239 (1961).

The final result of a structural ENDOR study is usually the isotropic and anisotropic hyperfine constants for various nuclei. (Quadrupole constants will be discussed in Section 4.3.) Table 4-1 summarizes these constants for a trapped electron in KBr. The experimental hyperfine constant measured is R given by eq. 4.14 for axial symmetry. The isotropic and anisotropic components can be obtained from R from its angular dependence. Also if two ENDOR lines corresponding to the same shell are known at a given angle, then A_{iso} and B_{zz} can be obtained.

Let us consider assignment of some of the lines in Fig. 4-2. Except for shells I and II the other ENDOR lines are centered about ν_n and split by R. The free nuclear frequency for K^{39} for $H_o = 3347$ G is 0.66 MHz, and pairs of ENDOR lines in the range 0.5 to 0.85 MHz seem to be centered around this frequency. Cations occur in shells I, III, and V and since shell

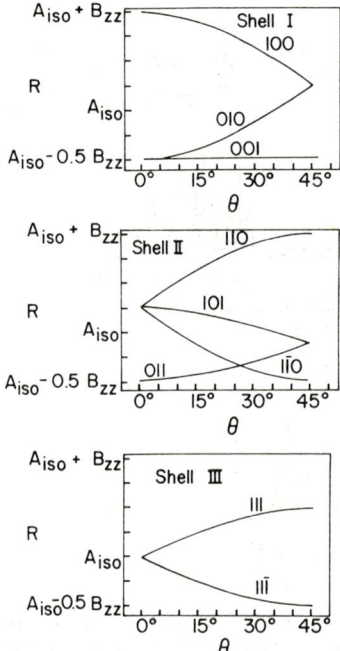

Figure 4-3. Angular dependence of the hyperfine splitting R (see eq. 4.14) for shells I to III of nuclei about a trapped electron (F center) in a cubic alkali halide structure. The positions of the nuclei and the rotation axis for θ are shown in Fig. 4-1; at $\theta = 0°$, H_o is parallel to the 100 axis. The different curves are for different sites for equivalent nuclei and are identified by the crystal axis direction in which the nuclei are located in relation to the trapped electron.

Table 4.1. Hyperfine Interaction Constants of the F Center in KBr Measured with ENDOR[a]

Shell	Nucleus	ν_n^b (MHz)	A_{iso} (MHz)	B_{aniso} (MHz)	T (K)
I	K^{39}	0.67	18.8	0.74	300
			18.3	0.77	90
II	Br^{81}	3.90	42.8	2.8[c]	90
III	K^{39}		0.27	0.022	90
IV	Br^{81}		5.70	0.41	90
V	K^{39}		0.16	0.02	90
VI	Br^{81}		0.84	0.086[c]	90
VIII	Br^{81}		0.54	0.07	90

[a] H. Seidel, *Z. Physik*, **165**, 718 (1961).
[b] At 3990 G.
[c] Measurable deviation from axial symmetry.

I is expected to have a large hyperfine coupling centered around $\frac{1}{2}R$, these two pairs of lines can be assigned to K_{III}^{39} for the larger coupling and to K_V^{39} for the smaller coupling. Furthermore, for shell III at $\theta = 0°$ there is no site splitting and $R = A_{iso}$, which gives A_{iso} directly. Site splitting is expected for shell V and is probably the source of the distorted ENDOR line at 0.75 MHz. The free nuclear frequency for K^{41} is 0.36 MHz so ENDOR lines from shells III and V associated with this nucleus are beyond the experimental spectral range. Likewise, pairs of ENDOR lines including site splitting about the nuclear frequencies of both bromine isotopes can be assigned to bromide ions in shells IV, VI, and VIII. Note that the Br_{IV}^{81} and K_V^{39} low frequency lines overlap.

The prominent triplet structure centered around 8.1 and 10.6 MHz is due to quadrupole coupling by the potassium nucleus. This interaction will be discussed in Section 4.3. These two triplets correspond to the 010/001 and 100 sites, respectively, and illustrate how much site splitting can alter the spectrum. The other two components of these two sites overlap in the 8.9 to 9.9 MHz region.

4.2.4 Signs of Hyperfine Constants

Only magnitudes of hyperfine constants are normally determined by either ESR or ENDOR. The sign of the hyperfine constant is important because it relates to the sign of the unpaired electron spin density and consequently to the electronic structure of the radical. In Section 3.6 it was shown that the sign of isotropic hyperfine constants could be determined by ENDOR for some radicals in liquid crystal solvents. Here we describe a method that is independent of a special solvent in which relative signs of two different hyperfine constants can be determined in a "double" ENDOR experiment involving two simultaneous rf fields.[5]

Figure 4-4a shows an energy level diagram for an electron coupled to two inequivalent protons. Thus there are four possible ENDOR transitions associated with each ESR line. In a "double" ENDOR experiment an electron transition and one nuclear transition are saturated to give the level populations shown in Fig. 4-4a. The intensity of an ENDOR transition is roughly proportional to the population difference between the two nuclear levels involved. In an ordinary ENDOR experiment this difference is ε, but in the double ENDOR experiment, in which a second rf field is applied, this difference can be increased to $4\varepsilon/3$ as for the 7–8 ENDOR transition or decreased to $2\varepsilon/3$ as for the 2–4 ENDOR transition. In general, it turns out that two simultaneous ENDOR transitions reduce each other's intensity if they both occur in the same subset of

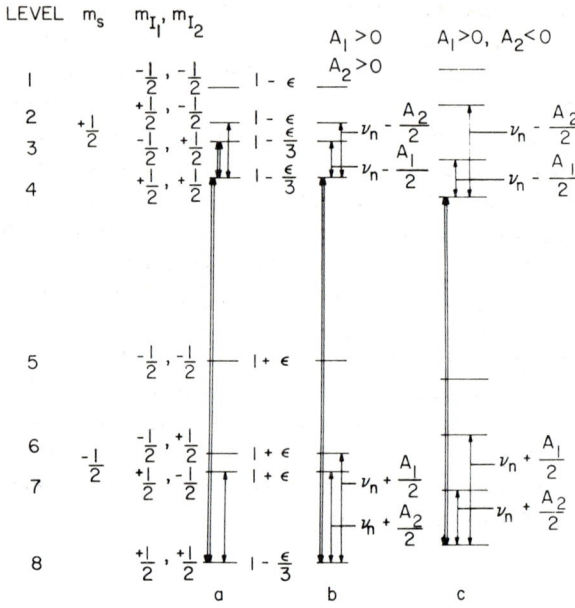

Figure 4-4. Energy level diagram for $S=\frac{1}{2}$, $I_1=\frac{1}{2}$, $I_2=\frac{1}{2}$ system with $\nu_n > A_1/2$, $A_1 > A_2$, $A_1 > 0$, and $A_2 > 0$. (a) Level populations when the 4–8 electron transition and the 4–3 nuclear transition are saturated. In this case the 4–2 ENDOR transition intensity is decreased and the 7–8 ENDOR transition intensity is increased in comparison to when the 4–3 transition is not saturated. The four ENDOR transitions associated with saturation of the 4–8 electron transition are shown for (b) $A_1 > 0$ and $A_2 > 0$ and for (c) $A_1 > 0$ and $A_2 < 0$. By comparison with the "double" ENDOR experiment in (a), it can be seen that the two hyperfine constant sign cases of (b) and (c) can be distinguished. See text for additional explanation.

electron spin states (e.g., $m_s = +\frac{1}{2}$) and they enhance each others intensity if they occur in different subsets of electron spin states. This difference can be used to determine the relative signs of two coupling constants.

Consider Fig. 4-4b in which the two coupling constants have the same sign. If the 3–4 ENDOR transition is observed and the second rf field is frequency swept, both of the higher frequency ENDOR transitions, 6–8 and 7–8, will enhance the observed 3–4 transition and two positive peaks will be seen. However if the two coupling constants have opposite signs, the energy level diagram is changed to that in Fig. 4-4c. Then when the 3–4 ENDOR transition is observed and the second rf field is swept, only the 6–4 higher frequency ENDOR transition is enhanced, whereas the other transition (2–4) is reduced. Thus one positive and one negative peak will be seen, which is diagnostic of coupling constants of opposite signs.

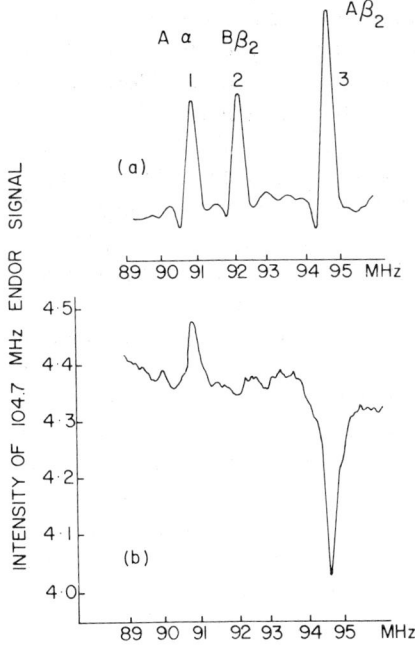

Figure 4-5. (a) ENDOR signals at 35 GHz from HOOCĊHCH$_2$COOH radical in x-irradiated succinic acid crystals at 77 K. α and β refer to protons near the radical site and A and B refer to magnetically distinguishable sites. (b) Double ENDOR signals obtained while observing the 104.7 MHz ENDOR line and sweeping a second rf oscillator. From R. J. Cook and D. H. Whiffen, *Proc. Phys. Soc.*, **84**, 845 (1964).

This method of relative hyperfine constant sign determination[5] is demonstrated in Fig. 4-5 for the major radical in x-irradiated succinic acid single crystal. The radical site has the structure —ĊH—CH$_2$— so that there are one α and two β protons. Part of the higher frequency ENDOR spectrum is shown in Fig. 4-5a for a spectrometer operating at 35 GHz. For this particular orientation there are two magnetically inequivalent sites. Lines 1, 2, and 3 refer to the α proton coupling in site A, the β_2 proton coupling in site B, and the β_2 proton coupling in site A. In Fig. 4-5b the intensity of the β_1 proton coupling in site A at 104.7 MHz is observed while a second rf field is swept. It is seen that line 1 is enhanced, line 2 is unaffected because it corresponds to a different radical site, and line 3 is reduced. Thus the α and β_2 proton coupling constants have different signs as expected. Furthermore since the high frequency ENDOR line of the β_1 proton is being observed and the high frequency ENDOR lines of the α and β_2 protons are being pumped, it is clear that the β_1 and β_2 protons have coupling constants of the same sign and the α and β_1 protons have coupling constants of opposite sign.

The preceding method only gives relative signs of pairs of hyperfine constants involving the same nucleus, but this is often sufficient to deduce the absolute signs if other structural evidence is taken into account. Cook and Whiffen[6] have also described a method of absolute sign determination utilizing ENDOR in which the signs of the hyperfine constants are related to those of the nuclear–nuclear dipolar coupling. However the method is somewhat tedious to apply and has not been used much.

The preceding application of double ENDOR to the known succinic acid radical illustrates not only that relative signs of hyperfine constants are obtained, but also that ENDOR lines belonging to magnetically distinct radical sites can be distinguished. Note that pumping line 2 in Fig. 4-5b did not produce a double ENDOR effect. This identifies that line as belonging to a radical in a different site from the radical being observed. This aspect can be quite useful in assigning the ENDOR lines of an unknown radical in a single crystal. Both of these advantages of double ENDOR have been utilized by Hampton and Alexander[7] to study the radical produced in x-irradiated cytidine single crystal at room temperature. They found three proton coupling constants and showed by double ENDOR that they all had the same sign. Since at least one proton coupling is likely to be due to an α proton, they concluded that the unpaired electron is largely localized on two carbon atoms and couples to three α protons with two of the protons on one atom. This helped them to assign a probable structure to the radical and to locate it in the ribose sugar group.

Although little exploited thus far, it appears that the double ENDOR method has considerable potential for the study of radicals in organic single crystals of complex compounds. It should be cautioned, however, that the model in Fig. 4-4 only applies to transient or effectively transient ENDOR signals.[8] This can be seen by recalling from Chapter 1 that the steady state ENDOR signal intensity depends on ΔT_{1e} produced by the observed ENDOR transition. If a second ENDOR transition in *either* electron spin substate is pumped, it will provide another relaxation path between the two levels of the ESR transition and shorten the effective T_{1e} of the ESR transition. This will decrease the ΔT_{1e} produced by the observed ENDOR transition. Since this occurs for pumping in either electron spin substate, the information on which relative hyperfine sign determinations is based is lost but the distinguishability of ENDOR lines from radicals in different sites is not necessarily lost. So it is necessary to observe transient ENDOR or at least ENDOR in which the transient component is more intense than the steady state component. Operationally if one observes an increase of the observed ENDOR signal in a double ENDOR experiment, one can conclude that one is observing ENDOR with a dominant transient component. Transient ENDOR is favored by longer relaxation times and higher field or rf modulation frequencies. It appears that for many organic radicals in solids at room temperature and below with typical modulation frequencies >100 Hz, the observed ENDOR does have a dominant transient component. Thus double ENDOR is still practically useful for hyperfine sign determination.

However in systems containing paramagnetic ions with short relaxation times, the double ENDOR may not work for hyperfine sign determination. An example is CaF_2 doped with Tm^{2+} in which relative sign determination of the ^{169}Tm and ^{19}F hyperfine constants was attempted.[8]

Another method for relative hyperfine sign determination from ENDOR has been described for $S = \frac{1}{2}$ systems having one or more nuclei with a twofold or higher symmetry axis strongly coupled to the electron spin and a set of weakly coupled nuclei.[9] ENDOR measurements are made on the weakly coupled nuclei for an orientation of the external magnetic field along the symmetry axis of the strongly coupled nuclei. The method depends on the hyperfine coupling of the strongly coupled nuclei being large enough compared to the nuclear Zeeman energy so that the effective field seen by the weakly coupled nuclei depends on the strongly coupled spins. Then the relative signs of the weakly and strongly coupled nuclei can be obtained from the dependence of the hyperfine couplings of the weakly coupled nuclei, measured by ENDOR, on the different hyperfine multiplets of the strongly coupled nuclei. This method has been demonstrated for the AsO_4^{4-} radical in KH_2AsO_2 in which As is the strongly coupled nucleus and matrix protons are the weakly coupled nuclei.[9]

Whereas hyperfine sign determination in $S = \frac{1}{2}$ systems often requires special conditions, this is not true for $S \geq 1$ systems where the sign can be determined from the ESR spectrum. However if one can put an $S = \frac{1}{2}$ radical into an $S \geq 1$ environment, it is then possible to obtain absolute sign information. This can be done in the special case of radical pair systems $(S - 1)$ in which there is a strong electron-electron dipolar interaction.[10] The sign of the hyperfine constant relative to this dipolar interaction is determined by ENDOR. If the absolute sign of the dipolar interaction is known, as is the case in single crystals from the geometry, then absolute hyperfine signs are determined.

In an $S = 1$ radical pair system there will be at least two interacting magnetic nuclei, one from each radical of the pair, which will have different coupling constants for an arbitrary orientation. The dipolar interaction D separates the ESR transitions into two groups separated by $2D$ and given by

$$\nu_{ESR} = \nu_e \pm D + (m_{I_1}A_1 + m_{I_2}A_2). \quad (4.15)$$

Only half of the possible ENDOR transitions occur when one of the groups of ESR transitions is saturated. Thus when either the low field or high field ESR transitions of the radical pair are saturated, only two ENDOR lines are observed, and these correspond to selecting a particular electron spin substate. By analogy to the double ENDOR method (Fig. 4-4) this contains at least relative hyperfine sign information.

Specifically, if D is positive the upper sign in eq. 4.15 corresponds to the low field (high frequency) ESR transitions and when these transitions are saturated, the observed ENDOR transitions are

$$\nu_1 = |A_1 - \nu_n| \qquad (4.16)$$

$$\nu_2 = |A_2 - \nu_n|. \qquad (4.17)$$

Likewise when the high field (low frequency) ESR transitions are saturated, the ENDOR transitions are

$$\nu_3 = |A_1 + \nu_n| \qquad (4.18)$$

$$\nu_4 = |A_2 + \nu_n|. \qquad (4.19)$$

When $A_1 > 0$ and $A_2 > 0$, ν_1 and ν_2 are the two lower frequency ENDOR transitions, and when $A_1 < 0$ and $A_2 < 0$, they are the two higher frequency ENDOR transitions. When $A_1 < 0$ and $A_2 > 0$ or vice versa, and the low field ESR transitions are saturated, the ENDOR transitions ν_1 and ν_2 will correspond to one of the two lower frequency ENDOR transitions (ν_2) and to one of the two higher frequency ENDOR transitions (ν_1). The various possibilities are summarized in Table 4-2. It is seen that relative sign information between A_1 and A_2 is readily obtained and that if the

Table 4-2 Hyperfine Sign Determination from ENDOR of Radical Pairs

Signs of Coupling Constants			ENDOR Seen When Observing	
D	A_1	A_2	Low Field ESR	High Field ESR
+	+	+	The two lower frequency ENDOR lines	The two higher frequency ENDOR lines
+	−	−	The two higher frequency ENDOR lines	The two lower frequency ENDOR lines
+	+	−	One lower (A_1) and one higher (A_2) frequency ENDOR line	One lower (A_2) and one higher (A_1) frequency ENDOR line
+	−	+	One lower (A_2) and one higher (A_1) frequency ENDOR line	One lower (A_1) and one higher (A_2) frequency ENDOR line
−	+	+	The two higher frequency ENDOR lines	The two lower frequency ENDOR lines
−	−	−	The two lower frequency ENDOR lines	The two higher frequency ENDOR lines
−	+	−	One lower (A_2) and one higher (A_1) frequency ENDOR line	One lower (A_1) and one higher (A_2) frequency ENDOR line
−	−	+	One lower (A_1) and one higher (A_2) frequency ENDOR line	One lower (A_2) and one higher (A_1) frequency ENDOR line

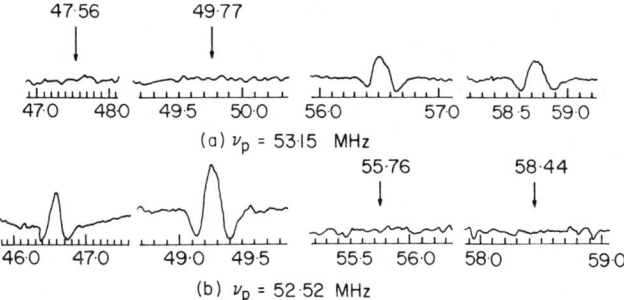

Figure 4-6. Proton ENDOR transitions at 35 GHz from radical pairs in x-irradiated dimethylglyoxime single crystals at 77 K: (a) H_o set to the center of the high field ESR spectrum. (b) H_o set to the center of the low field ESR spectrum. From R. J. Cook, *Colloque Ampere XV*, North-Holland, Amsterdam, 1969, p. 269.

sign of D is known, the absolute signs are known. Since D is determined by a purely dipolar interaction its sign is known from the geometry of the crystal.

An example of this kind of analysis is shown for radical pairs in dimethylglyoxime single crystals in Fig. 4-6. The sign of D is negative for this orientation and by analogy to Table 4-2 it is seen that A_1 and A_2 are both negative.

4.2.5 Spin Density Determination

In Chapter 3 it was mentioned that isotropic hyperfine couplings determined by ENDOR and ESR on liquid phase radicals are used to determine experimental spin densities, which may in turn be used to check the validity of theoretical predictions of spin densities. For π-electron radicals the experimental spin densities at ring carbon atoms are determined from the measured σ proton hyperfine couplings via the McConnell relation (eq. 3.4). The accuracy of such determinations depends on the constancy and value of the proportionality constant Q, which is in fact known to vary somewhat with radical electronic structure.

It is independently possible to determine experimental spin densities in π-electron radicals from the anisotropic hyperfine couplings, although this method is only beginning to be explored.[11,12,13] In the liquid state these interactions average to zero so they must be measured in solids. From ESR alone it has seldom been possible to determine accurate anisotropic hyperfine tensors of σ protons in π-electron radicals in solids because of linewidth considerations. However, as we have pointed out in the present section, the higher resolution of ENDOR makes this possible.

Ngo, Budzinski, and Box[12] have proposed the following relationship for anisotropic coupling, which is analogous to the McConnell relationship for isotropic couplings.

$$A_{max} - A_{min} = D\rho \qquad (4.20)$$

In this equation ρ is the spin density on the atom to which the α proton is bonded and the proportionality factor D is analogous to McConnell's Q

Table 4-3 Calculations of Spin Densities (ρ) on Ring Atoms of π-Electron Radicals from Anisotropic and Isotropic Hyperfine Couplings and Comparison with Hückel Molecular Orbital Theory

σ Proton	ρ_{aniso}	ρ_{iso}^a	$\rho_{Hückel}$
Histidine · HCl cation (ref. 12)[b]			
C_5—H	0.32	0.40	0.33
C_6—H	0.33	0.35	0.30
Histidine · HCl H adduct (ref. 12)[b]			
N_2—H	0.26	0.28	0.21
N_3—H	0.32	0.31	0.21
C_6—H	0.24	0.24	0.22
1,2,4-Triazole H adduct (ref. 11)[c]			
N_1—H	0.3	0.36	0.19
$N_2 \cdots$ H	0.3	–	0.31
C_3—H	0.03	0.03	0.03
$N_4 \cdots$ H	0.2	–	0.3
C_5—H	0.08[d]	0.11[d]	0.08[d]
C_5—H'	0.08[d]	0.11[d]	0.08[d]
Imidazole H adduct (ref. 13)			
N_1–H	0.20	0.23	0.14
N_3—H	0.25	–	0.33
C_4—H	0.08	0.08	0.09
C_5—H	0.28	0.28	0.29
C_2—H	0.07[d]	0.10[d]	0.07[d]
C_2—H'	0.07[d]	0.09[d]	0.07[d]

[a] Calculated with $Q_C = -83.7$ MHz and $Q_N = -66.9$ MHz.
[b] ρ_{aniso} calculated from eq. 4.20.
[c] ρ_{aniso} calculated from all possible dipole-dipole contributions. The dotted bonds are H bonds.
[d] Proton spin densities.

and is given by[14]

$$D = \frac{3gg_n\beta\beta_n}{R^3}\left[1 - \frac{30}{K^2R^2} + \left(\frac{K^3R^3}{12} + \frac{3K^2R^2}{4} + 4KR + 14 + \frac{30}{KR} + \frac{30}{K^2R^2}\right)e^{-KR}\right]$$
(4.21)

where R is the dipole-dipole coupling distance between a σ proton and an atom bearing an unpaired electron in a $2p\pi$ orbital and K is a parameter of the Slater function used to describe the $2p\pi$ orbital. The formulation in eq. 4.20 assumes that dipole-dipole coupling of the σ proton with other orbitals may be neglected. This is not strictly true but may be a good approximation for many aromatic radicals. In the more general case[11] a consistent molecular coordinate system must be defined and dipole-dipole contributions from unpaired spin density in nearest and next nearest orbitals to a given proton must be calculated.

Table 4-3 shows four radicals for which the spin densities have been calculated from both the anisotropic and isotropic couplings of σ protons. The agreement is not perfect, but it appears that both the anisotropic and isotropic couplings are equally reliable for spin density determinations. Where possible, both should be used to test the validity of theoretical calculations. For the radicals shown, the Hückel molecular orbital calculations are not bad. For the 1,2,4-triazole H-adduct radical INDO molecular orbital calculations were also carried out but they gave completely unsatisfactory spin densities.[11] Also for the imidazole H-adduct radical, both McLachlan and INDO molecular orbital calculations give rather poor results.[13]

4.2.6 Second Order Effects

Second order effects on the hyperfine couplings measured by ENDOR have been treated in Section 3.5. Since the second order effects vary as $A^2/4\nu_e$, they can generally only be detected for $A \geq 30$ MHz. In liquids proton couplings of this magnitude have seldom been investigated by ENDOR because they are usually resolvable from the ESR spectrum. However, in solids large proton couplings are investigated in order to obtain accurate dipolar tensors. Neglect of second order effects for α and β protons in alkyl-type radicals can typically lead to errors as large as 1 MHz in the elements of the hyperfine tensor.[15] Inclusion of second order effects is also necessary to identify correctly some ENDOR transitions[16] and to account for splittings of some ENDOR lines.[17]

For example, the methyl protons in the $CH_3\dot{C}HCOOH$ radical produced in x-irradiated succinic acid at room temperature show second order splitting in their ENDOR spectra. For three equivalent protons the low frequency ENDOR transitions for $m_s = -\frac{1}{2}$ are given to the second order by

$$\nu_1 = \tfrac{1}{2}A + \nu_H + \frac{3A^2}{4\nu_e}$$

$$\nu_2 = \tfrac{1}{2}A + \nu_H + \frac{A^2}{4\nu_e} \qquad (4.22)$$

$$\nu_3 = \tfrac{1}{2}A + \nu_H - \frac{A^2}{4\nu_e}$$

These second order splittings are ~ 0.25 MHz but are readily observable in the ENDOR spectrum of CH$_3$ĊHCOOH. When the ESR line corresponding to $\sum m_I = +\tfrac{3}{2}$ or $-\tfrac{3}{2}$ only ν_3 or ν_1 is observed, respectively, but when $\sum m_I = +\tfrac{1}{2}$ or $-\tfrac{1}{2}$, two ENDOR lines are resolved corresponding to ν_2 and ν_3 or ν_1 and ν_2.[17]

4.3 QUADRUPOLE INTERACTION

Quadrupole interaction occurs in radicals with nuclei with $I > \tfrac{1}{2}$, for example, nitrogen nuclei. As discussed in Section 3.6.2 for radicals in liquid crystals, the quadrupole interaction does not affect ESR spectra to the first order, but it does lead to additional splitting in ENDOR spectra.

The spin Hamiltonian can be written analogously to eq. 4.1 as

$$\mathcal{H} = g\beta \mathbf{H} \cdot \mathbf{S} - g_n\beta_n \mathbf{H} \cdot \mathbf{I} + h\mathbf{S} \cdot \mathbf{A} \cdot \mathbf{I} + h\mathbf{I} \cdot \mathbf{Q} \cdot \mathbf{I} \qquad (4.23)$$

where $\mathbf{Q}$ is the quadrupole coupling tensor. The general analysis of this spin Hamiltonian is rather complex.[18–20] For illustrative purposes we will treat the simple case in which the $\mathbf{A}$ and $\mathbf{Q}$ tensors have the same principal axes, $|A| \gg |Q|$ and the magnetic field is aligned along a principal axis. Then we have

$$\frac{\mathcal{H}}{h} = \nu_s S_z - \nu_n I_z + A_{zz} S_z I_z + Q_{zz} I_z^2 \qquad (4.24)$$

and for the common case of $I = 1$ the ENDOR frequencies are given by

$$\nu(\text{ENDOR}) = \left| \frac{A_{zz}}{2} \pm \nu_n \pm Q_{zz} \right|. \qquad (4.25)$$

Figure 4-7 shows the effect of a quadrupole interaction on the energy levels and the resulting four ENDOR frequencies for $I = 1$. Note that when there is negligible quadrupole interaction the same two ENDOR transitions are observed for each ESR line. However with an observable

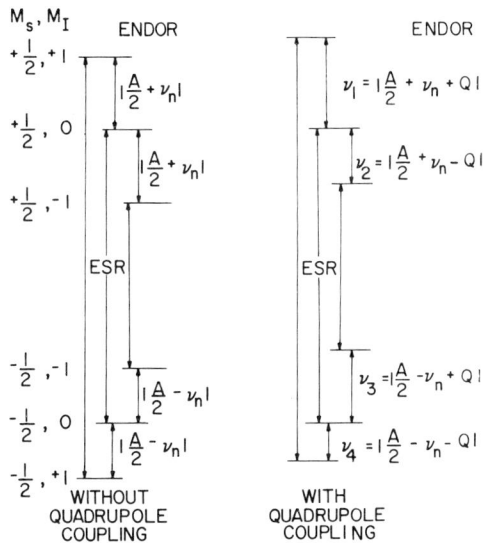

Figure 4-7. Energy level diagram for $S=\frac{1}{2}$, $I=1$ system showing ESR and ENDOR transitions in the absence and presence of quadrupole coupling.

quadrupole interaction two ENDOR lines are observed for the $m_I = 1$ ESR line, two different ENDOR lines are observed for the $m_I = -1$ ESR line, and all four ENDOR lines are observed for the $m_I = 0$ ESR line.

The fact that observation of different ESR lines separates the ENDOR frequencies into two groups allows one to obtain relative signs of the quadrupole and hyperfine interactions.[21] Refer to Fig. 4-7. If the signs of A and Q are the same, saturation of the low field ($m_I = +1$) ESR line gives the highest and lowest frequency ENDOR lines, ν_1 and ν_4. But if the signs of A and Q are opposite, saturation of the low field ESR line gives the intermediate frequency ENDOR lines, ν_2 and ν_3. For nitrogen centers in diamond it was found that A and Q have opposite signs.[21]

It is also possible to assign ENDOR lines to particular radical sites if several exist within a given crystal by using field swept ENDOR,[21] which is ENDOR-induced ESR as described in Section 3.1. One sets the rf oscillator on an ENDOR frequency and sweeps the magnetic field. An ENDOR-induced ESR spectrum results that will correspond to ESR lines belonging only to one radical site. For example, if ENDOR frequency ν_1 for one radical site (Fig. 4-7) is pumped, the $m_I = +1$ and 0 ESR transitions will be observed, and if ENDOR frequency ν_4 for the same radical site is pumped, the $m_I = -1$ and 0 ESR transitions will be observed. This is a method of separating overlapping ESR spectra where the overlapping spectra correspond to the same radical located in magnetically inequivalent sites. It has been used successfully to assign the ENDOR lines to nitrogen atoms in four different sites in diamond crystals.[21,22]

From the expressions for the ENDOR frequencies in Fig. 4-7 it is seen that the average of the ENDOR frequencies associated with a high field or low field ESR line depends only on the hyperfine coupling. This provides a quick and convenient way to obtain the hyperfine tensor alone.[23] However it is only valid when the hyperfine and quadrupole tensors have the same principal axes. This cannot, in general, be assumed,[19,20] although it often has been. General methods for obtaining the hyperfine and quadrupole tensors from ENDOR measurements independent of any assumption about common principal axes have been described.[19,20]

Most examples of quadrupole coupling tensors for radicals in molecular crystals have dealt with nitrogen nuclei. Results have been reported for N atoms in diamond,[22] NO_3^{2-} and NO_2 (ref. 23), and copper-8-hydroxyquinolinate substituted into single crystals of phthalimide and of 8-hydroxyquinoline.[24] The Na quadrupole coupling ($I = \frac{3}{2}$) with CO_2^- in sodium formate crystals has also been detected[18] as has the Cl quadrupole coupling ($I = \frac{3}{2}$) with H atoms in KCl crystals.[25] Physically the quadrupole coupling is sensitive to the total electron density at the nucleus, in contrast to the hyperfine coupling, which is sensitive to only the unpaired spin density at the nucleus. Thus quadrupole couplings are more directly related to chemical bond strengths.

4.4 ORGANIC SINGLE CRYSTALS

The application of ENDOR to radicals in organic single crystals has focused mainly on carboxylic acids, amino acids, and some constituents of nucleic acids. Although many of these compounds are of biological importance, they are also well characterized molecular systems. In Chapter 7 we deal with radicals in real biological systems such as various proteins. Table 4-4 summarizes most of the ENDOR studies on organic single crystals through 1974. The analysis of the ENDOR spectra has been directed toward radical identification, radical orientation in the lattice, and radical formation and transformation mechanisms. Such analysis depends largely on the interpretation of hyperfine tensors, which will be considered in a separate section. Hyperfine tensors together with the molecular crystal structure constitute the most important method for

Table 4-4. Summary of ENDOR Studies on Organic Single Crystals through 1974

System	Radicals	Irradiation Temperature (K)	Objectives	References
CARBOXYLIC ACIDS				
Malonic acid $CD_2(COOD)_2$	$\cdot CD(COOD)_2$	4	To demonstrate distant ENDOR of neutral molecules	R. C. McCalley and A. L. Kwiram, *Phys. Rev. Lett.*, **24**, 1279 (1970).
Methylmalonic acid $CH_3CH(COOH)_2$	$CH_3\dot{C}(COOH)_2$	300	To study methyl tunneling	S. Clough et al., *J. Phys. C: Solid State Phys.*, **5**, 518 (1972).
$CD_3CH(COOH)_2$	$CD_3\dot{C}(COOH)_2$	300	To study methyl tunneling	S. Clough et al., *J. Phys. C: Solid State Phys.*, **6**, 2357 (1973).
Succinic acid $HOOCCH_2CH_2COOH$	$HOOCCH_2CH_2\dot{C}(OH)_2$	77	To determine two OH and two CH proton coupling tensors; to study mechanism of protonation	H. Muto et al., *J. Chem. Phys.*, **61**, 1075 (1974).
	$HOOCCH_2CH_2COOH^-$	4	To determine the two CH proton coupling tensors	J. Wells, *J. Chem. Phys.*, **52**, 4062 (1970).
	$HOOCCH_2\dot{C}HCOOH$	300	To determine relative and absolute signs of α-H and β-H coupling constants	R. J. Cook et al., *Proc. Phys. Soc.*, **84**, 845 (1964); *J. Chem. Phys.*, **43**, 2908 (1965).
	$CH_3\dot{C}HCOOH$	300	Radical identification and study of methyl rotation	S. F. J. Read et al., *Mol. Phys.*, **12**, 159 (1967).

Table 4-4 (*Continued*)

System	Radicals	Irradiation Temperature (K)	Objectives	References
CARBOXYLIC ACIDS (*Continued*)				
Glutaric acid HOOCCH$_2$CH$_2$CH$_2$COOH	HOOCCH$_2$CH$_2$ĊHCOOH	300	To determine α-H and β-H coupling tensors	A. L. Kwiram, *J. Chem. Phys.*, **55**, 2484 (1971).
Adipic acid HOOC(CH$_2$)$_4$COOH	HOOC(CH$_2$)$_3$ĊHCOOH	300	To demonstrate room temperature ENDOR	A. L. Kwiram et al., *J. Chem. Phys.*, **42**, 791 (1965).
1,1-Cyclobutane-dicarboxylic acid (CH$_2$)$_3$C(COOD)$_2$	CH(CH$_2$)$_2$C(COOD)$_2$	300	To determine D and H hyperfine tensors and D quadrupole tensor of neutral molecule by distant ENDOR	L. R. Dalton et al., *J. Amer. Chem. Soc.*, **94**, 6930 (1972).
Thiodiglycollic acid HOOCCH$_2$SCH$_2$COOH	HOOCCH$_2$ṠCH$_2$COOH	4	To identify radical, four H$_\beta$ couplings seen	H. C. Box et al., *J. Chem. Phys.*, **49**, 3974 (1968).
	HOOCCH$_2$SCH$_2$C$\begin{smallmatrix}\diagup O^- \\ \diagdown OH\end{smallmatrix}$	4	To determine both H$_\beta$ coupling tensors	J. Wells, *J. Chem. Phys.*, **52**, 4062 (1970).

Compound	Radical	T (K)	Description	Reference
Disodium tartrate (Rochelle salt) NaOOCCHOHCHOHCOONa	$CHCO_3^{2-}$ (?)	300	To determine hyperfine tensors of some 11 matrix protons; these were assigned to CH or OH protons by deuteration	I. Suzuki, *J. Phys. Soc. Japan*, **37**, 1379 (1974).
Potassium hydrogen malonate $KOOCCH_2COOH$	Carboxyl anion	4	To measure two methylene proton coupling tensors	H. C. Box et al., *J. Chem. Phys.*, **55**, 315 (1971).
Sodium formate HCOONa	$CO_2^- \cdots Na$	77	Na^{23} ENDOR analyzed to give Na^{23} hyperfine and quadrupole tensors	R. J. Cook et al., *J. Phys. Chem.*, **71**, 93 (1967).
Sodium oxalate $NaHC_2O_4 \cdot H_2O$	CO_2^-	300	Hyperfine tensors determined for three H-bonded protons	O. Edlund et al., *J. Magn. Resonance*, **10**, 7 (1973).
AMINO ACIDS				
Glycine	$H_3\overset{+}{N}\dot{C}HCO_2^-$	77	Measured three proton tensors of non-rotating NH_3	M. A. Collins et al., *Mol. Phys.*, **10**, 317 (1966).
			Measured all four proton tensors at 77 and 300 K but only reported isotropic values	M. Welter et al., *Proc. XVI Colloque Ampere*, Publ. House of Romania, Bucharest, 1971, p. 435.
			Measured all four proton tensors and nitrogen hyperfine and quadrupole tensors	M. F. Deigen et al., *Biofizika*, **18**, 235 (1973).
	$H_3\overset{+}{N}CH_2CO_2^{2-}$ (anion)	77	Deduced location of four matrix protons from their dipolar tensors; measured proton tensors for two CH and two NH protons in the anion	M. Iwasaki et al., *J. Chem. Phys.*, **61**, 5315 (1974).

Table 4-4 (*Continued*)

System	Radicals	Irradiation Temperature (K)	Objectives	References
AMINO ACIDS (*Continued*)				
Glycine · HCl Cl$^-$(NH$_3$)$^+$CH$_2$COOH	Anion	4	The two β-H tensors were determined. Electron transfer between deuterated and protonated carboxyl groups seen	E. E. Budzinski et al., *J. Chem. Phys.*, **59**, 2899 (1973).
	CH$_2$ĊOOH	4 warm to 110	Two α-H tensors given	H. C. Box et al., *J. Chem. Phys.*, **50**, 2880 (1969).
N-acetylglycine CH$_3$CONHCH$_2$COOH and deuterated analogs	CD$_3$CONDĊH$_2$COOD$^-$ (carboxyl anion)	4	Identification of radicals; two β-H tensors are given for two different radical conformations	H. C. Box et al., *J. Chem. Phys.*, **57**, 4295 (1972).
	CH$_3$CO$^-$NDCD$_2$COOD (carbonyl anion)		Three β-H tensors given for methyl group	
	CD$_3$CONDĊH$_2$		Two α-H tensors given	
N-acetylglycine CH$_3$CONHCH$_2$COOH	CH$_3$CONHĊHCOOH (?)	300	Hyperfine tensor for rotating methyl group found	R. E. Piazza et al., *Mol. Phys.*, **17**, 213 (1969).
	CH$_3$CONHĊHCOOH (?) ⋯H$^+$	300	Although complete or partial proton tensors were found for 13 protons including matrix protons, radical identification remains uncertain	H. A. Helms et al., *J. Chem. Phys.*, **59**, 5055 (1973).

Compound	Radical	T (K)	Notes	Reference
Glycylglycine · HNO₃ $NO_3^- NH_3^+ CH_2 CONH$ $\quad\quad HOOC-CH_2$	NO_3^{2-}	4	Nitrogen hyperfine and quadrupole tensors found	S. N. Rustgi et al., *J. Chem. Phys.*, **59**, 4763 (1973).
	NO_2 (on warming)			
Glycylglycine · HCl $Cl^- NH_3^+ CH_2 CONH$ $\quad\quad HOOC-CH_2$ and deuterated analogs	Carboxyl anion	4	Two β-H tensors found	J. Y. Lee et al., *J. Chem. Phys.*, **61**, 428 (1974).
	Carbonyl anion $ND_3^+ CH_2 CONDĊH_2$		Two β-CH tensors found Two α-H tensors found	
L-alanine $CH_3 ĊHNH_3^+ CO_2^-$	$CH_3 CHNH_3^+ COOH$ (protonated carboxyl anion)	77	Proton transfer mechanism studied; three proton tensors for CH_β, OH_β, and one NH found plus two matrix proton tensors.	H. Muto et al., *J. Chem. Phys.*, **59**, 4821 (1973).
Chloroacetyl-DL-alanine $CH_2 ClCONHCHC_3 COOH$	$CH_2 ClCONHĊCH_3 COOH$	300(?)	Rotating methyl group proton tensor determined	J. W. Wells et al., *J. Chem. Phys.*, **48**, 2542 (1968).
DL-valine $(CH_3)_2 CHCHNH_3^+ COO^-$	$(CH_3)_2 CHĊHCOOH$	77	α-H and β-H tensors determined	H. C. Box et al., *J. Chem. Phys.*, **46**, 4470 (1967).
	$(CH_3)_2 ĊCHNH_3^+ CO_2^-$ (after warming)	77	Four β-H tensors for methyl protons with one methyl rotating and one not were found; nitrogen tensor also found	
L-valine · HCl · H₂O $(CH_3)_2 CHCHNH_3^+ Cl^- COOH$	Protonated carboxyl anion	77	Proton transfer mechanism studied; two OH proton tensors given	H. Muto et al., *J. Chem. Phys.*, **61**, 5311 (1974).
α-Amino isobutyric acid $(CH_3)_2 CHNH_3^+ CO_2^-$	$(CH_3)_2 ĊCOOH$ (on warming)	77	Three conformations are observed from the methyl proton tensors; two correspond to rotation of both methyls but the third corresponds to one methyl rotating and the other fixed	J. W. Wells et al., *J. Chem. Phys.*, **46**, 2935 (1967).

Table 4-4 (Continued)

System	Radicals	Irradiation Temperature (K)	Objectives	References
AMINO ACIDS (Continued)				
α-Amino isobutyric acid $(CH_3)_2CHNH_3^+CO_2^-$	Carboxyl anion	77	NH proton tensor determined for one NH proton in anion and three NH H-bonded matrix protons	M. Iwasaki et al., J. Chem. Phys., **61**, 5315 (1974).
L-glutamic acid · DCl $DOOCCH_2CH_2CHND_3^+$·Cl^-COOD	$DOOC\dot{C}HCH_2CHND_3^+$-Cl^-COOD	300	Hyperfine tensors determined for one α-H and two β-H	D. J. Whelan, J. Chem. Phys., **49**, 4734 (1968).
DL-serine $HOCH_2CHNH_3^+CO_2^-$ and deuterated analogs	Protonated anion $DOCH_2\dot{C}HND_3^+$ (oxidation product) · $OCH_2CHNH_3^+CO_2^-$ (decays at 4 K)	4	Radical identification; hyperfine tensor for one β-H in anion is given; tensors for one α-H and two β-H in oxidation product are given; two β-H tensors for the third radical are given	J. Y. Lee et al., J. Chem. Phys., **59**, 2509 (1973).
DL-serine	Protonated anion, about five other radicals produced on warming	77	Radical identification; hyperfine tensors are given for protons in three different radicals	B. W. Castleman et al., J. Chem. Phys., **57**, 2762 (1972).

Compound	Radical		Description	Reference
L-cysteic acid · H_2O $SO_3^-CH_2CHNH_3^+COOH$	Carboxyl anion $SO_3^-CH_2\dot{C}HNH_3^+$ (oxidation product) Protonated anion	4	Radical identification; hyperfine tensor for one β-H is given for anion; three CH and two NH proton tensors given for oxidation product; one CH and one OH proton tensors given for protonated anion	H. C. Box et al., *J. Chem. Phys.*, **60**, 3337 (1974).
histidine · HCl $\underset{HN}{\overset{H}{\underset{\|}{C}}}\overset{NH}{\underset{\|}{C}}\ Cl^-$ $CH_2CHNH_3^+CO_2^-$	Protonated carboxyl anion $RCH_2\dot{C}HND_3^+$ Imidazole cation H adduct at the apical ring carbon (on warming)	4	Radical identification; β-CH and OH tensors are given for anion; α-H and one β-H tensors are given for $RCH_2\dot{C}HND_3^+$. Two ring C-H tensors are given for the cation. Two NH and two CH ring proton tensors are given for the H-adduct radical	F. Q. H. Ngo et al., *J. Chem. Phys.*, **60**, 3373 (1974).
Tyrosine · HCl $HO-\underset{HC_2^{\ 6}CH}{\overset{HC_3^{\ 4\ 5}CH}{\underset{\|}{C}}}-CH_2$ $Cl^-NH_3^+CHCOOH$	Ring cation, H loss from OH, Carboxyl anion	4	Radical identification; three H tensors from C_3H, C_5H and one of the CH_2 protons are given for the cation; the C_3H and C_5H tensors are found for the OH scission radical; two CH and one OH proton tensors are given for the anion	H. C. Box et al., *J. Chem. Phys.*, **61**, 2222 (1974).

NUCLEIC ACIDS

Compound	Radical		Description	Reference
Barbituric acid · $2H_2O$	Loss of H atom from NH (oxidation product) Anion	4	Radical identification; two proton tensors for the methylene protons in the anion are given	H. C. Box et al., *J. Chem. Phys.*, **59**, 1588 (1973).

Table 4-4 (*Continued*)

System	Radicals	Irradiation Temperature (K)	Objectives	References
NUCLEIC ACIDS (*Continued*)				
Methyl cytosine	Two radicals corresponding to H addition to both C's of the C=C bond	4	Radical identification; one α-H and two β-H tensors are found for each radical	S. N. Rustgi et al., *J. Chem. Phys.*, **60**, 3343 (1974).
Thymidine		300	Hyperfine tensors for the two CH_2 protons at carbon 6 and the methyl group rotational splitting constant are determined	H. C. Box et al., *J. Chem. Phys.*, **61**, 1136 (1974).
Thymidine	Anion formed by electron attachment	4	The hyperfine tensor for the C_6 α-H is given	H. C. Box et al., *J. Chem. Phys.*, **62**, 197 (1975).
	Oxygen radical formed by loss of H from OH bonded to $C_{5'}$		The tensors for the two β-H bonded to $C_{5'}$ are found	

Compound	Structure	Conditions (K)	Observations	Reference
1-Methyl uracil 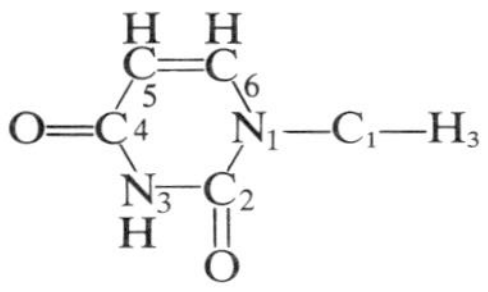	(structure shown)	77 or 300	Radical I formed by H abstraction from methyl group. Radical II formed by H addition at C_5. Radical structure; in radical I the hyperfine tensors are given for the two C_1—H_2 protons, C_5—H and C_6—H protons as well as for four matrix protons; tensors in radical II are given for two C_5—H_2, C_6—H and methyl group protons (equivalent) as well as for two matrix protons. Matrix protons are assigned specifically from their dipolar tensors	J. N. Herak et al., *J. Chem. Phys.*, **61**, 1129 (1974).
Cytidine 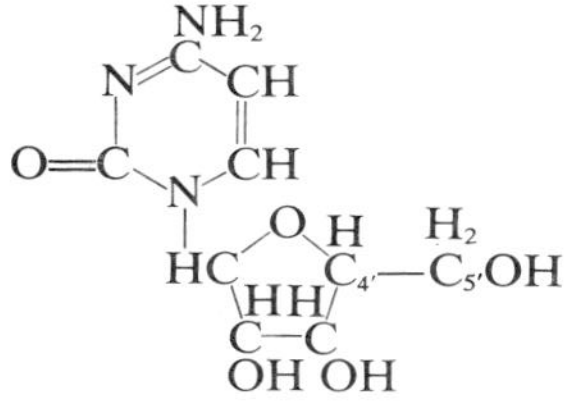	(structure shown)	300	Radical I is stable at 300 K and has the unpaired spin density localized on C_4 and $C_{5'}$; exact identity unknown. Three α-H tensors for the protons on C_4 and $C_{5'}$ are given for radical I	D. A. Hampton et al., *J. Chem. Phys.*, **58**, 4891 (1973).
			Unknown radical II is unstable at 300 K. One β-H tensor is found for unknown radical II	D. L. Allison et al., *J. Magn. Resonance*, **14**, 366 (1974).

AROMATICS

Compound	Structure	Conditions (K)	Observations	Reference
1,2,4-Triazole 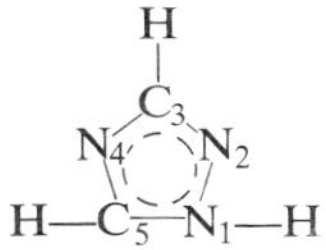	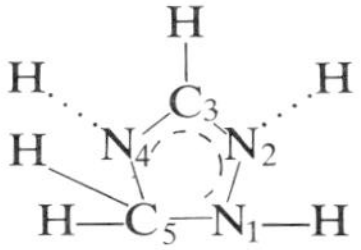 (structure shown)	300	Radical identification; six proton tensors are determined and assigned to all protons shown in the radical including the two H-bonded matrix protons	P. Gloux et al., *Mol. Phys.*, **25**, 161 (1973).

Table 4-4 *(Continued)*

System	Radicals	Irradiation Temperature (K)	Objectives	References
AROMATICS *(Continued)*				
Imidazole		300	Radical identification; six proton tensors are determined and assigned to all protons shown in the radical including the H-bonded matrix proton	B. Lamotte et al., *J. Chem. Phys.*, **59**, 3365 (1973).
4-Methyl-2,6-di-*t*-butyl phenol		300	To study CH$_3$ group tunneling; tunneling splitting and hyperfine tensors of CH$_3$ protons are determined	S. Clough et al., *J. Chem. Phys.*, **51**, 2076 (1969).
Naphthalene	α-Hydronaphthyl	253	Spin density distribution; all nine proton tensors are determined but not given	U. R. Böhme et al., *Chem. Phys. Lett.*, **17**, 582 (1972).

Compound	Structure	T (K)	Purpose	Reference
Anthracene				
Dibenzocyclohexadienyl		300	Spin density distribution and radical confirmation; all eleven proton tensors are given	U. R. Böhme et al., *Chem. Phys. Lett.*, **3**, 329 (1969).

MISCELLANEOUS

Compound	Structure	T (K)	Purpose	Reference
Dimethylglyoxime	Radical pairs of $H_3C-C=NO \cdot$ $H_3C-C=NOH$	77	To demonstrate hyperfine sign determination of the dipolar interaction for both proton and nitrogen ENDOR lines	R. J. Cook, *Proc. Colloque Ampere XV*, North-Holland, Amsterdam, 1969.
Copper-8-hydroxy quinolinate in phthalimide and 8-hydroxyquinoline crystals			To measure N hyperfine and quadrupole tensors and H hyperfine tensor of the two equivalent protons shown	G. H. Rist et al., *J. Chem. Phys.*, **50**, 4532 (1969).
Bis (salicylaldoximato) Cu (II) in bis (salicylaldoximato) Ni (II) crystals			To measure hyperfine tensors for the two equivalent nitrogens and the protons indicated; ^{63}Cu ENDOR is also observed	A. Schweiger et al., *Chem. Phys. Lett.*, **31**, 48 (1975)

assignment of a particular ENDOR line to a particular nucleus. Nevertheless deuteration, especially of exchangeable protons, is often used to aid assignment. Other methods used in liquids such as ESR spectral simulation, relative ENDOR line intensities, temperature dependence of ENDOR linewidths and intensities, and coherence effects have been little used in single crystals.

The occurrence of overlapping radical spectra is perhaps more common in single crystals than in liquids. First, in crystals one has the additional problem of site splitting. For a given orientation of the crystal in the magnetic field there will generally be two or more magnetically inequivalent radical orientations. Although the radicals are chemically identical, they are not identical magnetically. Second, high energy radiation is generally used to produce radicals in single crystals. In general, there will be at least two different primary radicals formed corresponding to the cation (oxidized form) and the anion (reduced form) if the undamaged molecule was neutral. Subsequent reactions of these primary radicals may lead to one dominant radical, but often there are two or more radical spectra superimposed. Mitigating the greater occurrence of overlapping radical spectra in single crystals is the fact that the angular dependence of the ESR and ENDOR lines often allows separation of the spectra. In addition, the uniqueness of observed ENDOR lines associated with different ESR lines and the technique of ENDOR-induced ESR (Section 3.2.6) allow spectral separation.

An example of the first method is shown in Fig. 4-8.[26] The ESR spectrum of x-irradiated methyl cytosine is shown in Fig. 4-8a. ENDOR

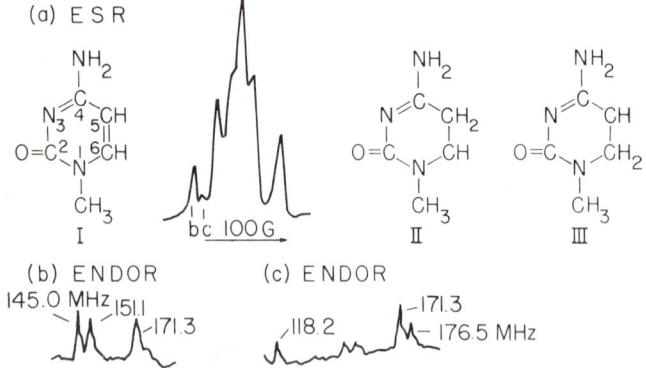

Figure 4-8. Single crystal N-methyl cytosine (I) x-irradiated to 80 Mrad at room temperature: (a) ESR spectrum at 70 GHz, with the magnetic field parallel to the c axis of the crystal, (b) ENDOR at 4 K at the field indicated in (a) where the indicated ENDOR lines are assigned to radical II, (c) ENDOR at 4 K at the field indicated in (a) where the labeled ENDOR lines are assigned to radical IV. From H. C. Box, *J. Magn. Resonance*, **14**, 323 (1974).

spectra associated with the two low field ESR lines are different and indicate chemically different radicals or magnetically inequivalent radicals. In this case analysis shows that the radicals are chemically different, as illustrated in the figure. This method will only work when some of the ESR lines are unique to one radical. The best probability for this occurs with the extreme high or low field ESR lines. This is perhaps why the best ENDOR signals in single crystals are generally obtained when observing the outermost ESR lines.[27] A second reason is probably minimization of spin-spin cross relaxation for these lines.

The use of ENDOR-induced ESR or field swept ENDOR to assign ENDOR lines corresponding to magnetically inequivalent sites for N atoms in diamond crystals was described in Section 4.3. These two methods for separating overlapping spectra are the same as for liquids (Section 3.2.6); no new principles are involved.

Intramolecular motion in organic single crystals has not been much studied. The main examples involve methyl group rotation, which has been studied in some detail and will be described in a separate section.

One interesting special application of ENDOR is selection of twinned crystals from single crystals.[28] In some crystals, such as valine, twinning is common and difficult to detect by optical or ESR measurements. However the higher resolution of ENDOR easily reveals twinning because more ENDOR lines are seen than in a true single crystal.

4.4.1 Interpretation of Hyperfine Tensors

Hyperfine tensors are interpreted first in terms of the signs and magnitudes of their components; next they are interpreted in terms of the direction cosines for the principal axes of the hyperfine tensor relative to the crystal axes. We will initially consider proton hyperfine tensors. They can be roughly classified into three groups based on the magnitude of the anisotropy and on the ratio of dipolar hyperfine components to isotropic components. These groups correspond to α protons, β protons, and more distant protons, including matrix protons. It is convenient to separate out the isotropic and anisotropic components (eqs. 4.8 and 4.9).

The α proton dipolar tensors exhibit large, often nearly axial, anisotropy amounting to 30 to 40 MHz for unit spin density on the adjacent carbon. The maximum anisotropy $A_{max} - A_{iso}$ is about 50% of the isotropic coupling. As the spin density on the adjacent carbon decreases, as in aromatic radicals, both the isotropic and anisotropic components decrease proportionately. A selection of α proton tensors is shown in Table 4-5. The origin of the anisotropy can be understood in terms of an

Table 4-5. Selection of α-Proton Tensors Determined by ENDOR

Radical	Proton	A_1 (MHz)	A_2 (MHz)	A_3 (MHz)	A_{iso} (MHz)	Reference
HOOCCH$_2$CH$_2$ĊHCOOH	CH	−27.4	−54.9	−89.2	−57.2	A. L. Kwiram, *J. Chem. Phys.*, **55**, 2484 (1971)
·CH$_2$COOH	CH(1)	−30.0	−58.8	−93.0	−60.6	H. C. Box et al., *J. Chem. Phys.*, **50**, 2880 (1969)
	CH(2)	−26.2	69.8	91.8	59.3	
CH$_3$CONDĊH$_2$	CH(1)	−22.6	−47.4	−80.2	−50.1	H. C. Box et al., *J. Chem. Phys.*, **57**, 4295 (1972).
	CH(2)	−11.2	−38.0	−72.4	−40.5	
(CH$_3$)$_2$CHĊHCOOH	CH	−23	−71	−92	−62	H. C. Box et al., *J. Chem. Phys.*, **46**, 4470 (1967).
H, H, HN$_2$, N$_3$H Cl$^-$, C$_6$, C=CH	N$_2$H	−0.6	−23.2	−33.2	−19.0	F. Q. H. Ngo et al., *J. Chem. Phys.*, **60**, 3373 (1974).
	N$_3$H	0.6	−24.8	−38.8	−21.0	
CH$_2$CHNH$_3^+$CO$_2^-$	C$_6$H	−7.5	−22.0	−21.2	−20.2	

electron dipole–nuclear dipole interaction.[14] If the signs of the hyperfine tensor components are determined, α protons may also be characterized by their negative isotropic coupling.

The β proton dipolar tensors exhibit relatively small anisotropy amounting to <10 MHz for unit spin density on the α carbon. The maximum anisotropy is often ~10% of the isotropic coupling for unit spin density on an aliphatic or aromatic α carbon. However even for unit spin density the isotropic coupling to a β proton varies approximately as $A_{iso} \propto \cos^2 \theta$ where θ is the dihedral angle between two planes both of which contain the α carbon–β carbon bond axis. The anisotropy does not vary in this way. For neutral radicals formed by irradiated carboxylic acids, the maximum anisotropy remains about constant for β proton isotropic couplings ranging from 20 to 140 MHz.[29] On the other hand, for radical anions formed by addition of an electron to the carbonyl oxygen of a carboxylic acid where the unpaired electron is localized primarily in a $2p\pi$ orbital on the carboxyl carbon, it appears that the maximum anisotropy of the two β protons is somewhat larger (11 versus 7 MHz) for the β proton having the smaller isotropic coupling.[29] In the case of the radical anion in potassium hydrogen malonate the maximum anisotropy and the isotropic coupling are comparable (~11 MHz). Thus β proton tensors always have small anisotropy but this is not always small compared to the isotropic coupling. A selection of β proton tensors is shown in Table 4-6. If the signs of the hyperfine tensor components are determined, β protons may also be characterized by their positive isotropic coupling.

More distant protons, including protons on adjacent molecules to the radical (matrix protons), generally exhibit a nearly pure dipolar coupling in which the maximum anisotropy is small (<10 MHz) but is greater than the isotropic coupling. Here the sign of the isotropic coupling is not characteristic. It is only through ENDOR that dipolar tensors for such weakly coupled protons have been measured. Table 4-7 gives a selection of distant proton tensors.

In general, the hyperfine tensors of protons bonded to other atoms such as nitrogen and oxygen are somewhat analogous to protons bonded to carbon. A large anisotropy for α protons bonded to nitrogen is expected. This is observed in the 1,2,4-triazole H-adduct radical,[11] and few other examples have been reported. Protons bonded to oxygen generally show small anisotropy because the protons are often β to the site of primary spin density.[30]

A few ENDOR studies of nitrogen hyperfine tensors have been made but it is difficult to make any secure generalizations yet. The studies deal with inorganic radicals, N atoms,[22] NO_3^{2-} and NO_2 (ref. 23), organocopper complexes,[24] and amino acid radicals.[28] In the inorganic radicals

Table 4-6. Selection of β-Proton Tensors Determined by ENDOR

Radical	Proton	A_1 (MHz)	A_2 (MHz)	A_3 (MHz)	A_{iso} (MHz)	Reference
HOOCCH$_2$CH$_2$Ċ(OH)$_2$	OH(1)	15.9	−9.0	−11.1	−1.4	H. Muto et al. *J. Chem. Phys.*, **61**, 1075 (1974).
	OH(2)	19.9	−5.3	−7.5	−2.4	
	CH(1)	83.6	73.8	71.9	76.4	
	CH(2)	34.2	18.7	17.4	23.4	
HOOCCH$_2$CH$_2$ĊHCOOH	CH(1)	129.0	131.4	142.2	134.2	A. L. Kwiram, *J. Chem. Phys.*, **55**, 2484 (1971).
	CH(2)	38.0	38.9	50.0	42.3	
H$_3$ṄCH$_2$CO$_2^{2-}$	CH(1)	82.7	74.6	71.4	76.2	M. Iwasaki et al., *J. Chem. Phys.*, **61**, 5315 (1974).
	CH(2)	23.0	8.6	6.6	12.7	
Cl$^-$(NH$_3$)$^+$CH$_2$COOH$^-$	OH	54.6	26.4	21.8	34.3	E. E. Budzinski et al., *J. Chem. Phys.*, **59**, 2899 (1973).
	CH(1)	85.0	76.8	74.6	78.8	
	CH(2)	43.0	27.2	26.0	32.1	
(CH$_3$)CHĊHCOOH	CH	98	73	67	79	H. C. Box et al., *J. Chem. Phys.*, **46**, 4470 (1967).

Table 4-7. Selection of Matrix Proton Tensors Determined by ENDOR

Radical	Proton	A_1 (MHz)	A_2 (MHz)	A_3 (MHz)	A_{iso} (MHz)	Reference
$H_3\overset{+}{N}CH_2CO_2^-$	CH	11.0	8.1	7.2	8.8	M. Iwasaki et al., *J. Chem. Phys.*, **61**, 5315 (1974).
	NH(1)	18.2	−0.6	−4.8	4.2	
	NH(2)	9.3	−10.1	−13.4	−4.7	
	NH(3)	8.1	−3.6	−3.8	0.2	
$CH_3CHNH_3^+COOH^-$	NH(2)	11.9	−2.7	−3.0	2.1	H. Muto et al., *J. Chem. Phys.*, **59**, 4821 (1973).
	NH(3)	9.7	−4.5	−5.2	0.0	
$HOOCCH_2CH_2COOH^-$	OH	19.9	−5.3	−7.5	2.4	H. Muto et al., *J. Chem. Phys.*, **61**, 1075 (1974).

the maximum anisotropy is large with typical values of 20 to 50 MHz, compared to 90 to 180 MHz isotropic couplings. In the organo-copper complexes the maximum anisotropy is typically 6 MHz, compared to isotropic couplings of 30 to 45 MHz. In a secondary radical in irradiated valine[28] the maximum anisotropy is 5 MHz, compared to an isotropic coupling of 20 MHz.

The direction cosines of the hyperfine tensors allow one to locate a particular atom (generally protons) in the radical. It is generally found for complex organic molecules that the resulting radicals produced by irradiation are located in the crystal lattice with the same orientation as the undamaged molecules. Thus the hyperfine tensors relative to the crystal axes can generally be related to the molecular axes. This is aided by some general characteristics of the hyperfine tensors. The axis between the proton and the nearest atom bearing unpaired spin density is often near to a principal hyperfine tensor axis and corresponds to the largest dipolar tensor component. The α protons in π-electron radicals are all located in the molecular plane and the unpaired electron spin distribution shows this planar symmetry. Thus another principal direction for these protons is perpendicular to the plane, and all the ring protons will have one set of direction cosines nearly identical. This direction will correspond to the smallest dipolar tensor component. Matrix protons in undamaged molecules adjacent to the radical may also be located as in or out of the molecular plane by comparing their direction cosines with those of protons in the radical.

The distance to matrix protons from the radical can be calculated from their dipolar tensor components and compared with the crystal structure if the unpaired electron distribution can be reasonably well located on different atoms of the radical. In the simple case where the bulk of the spin density is located on one closest atom of the radical, the dipolar distance r can be calculated from the dipolar principal value A_{ii} by

$$A_{ii} \text{ (MHz)} = g_e \beta_e g_n \beta_n (3 \cos^2 \theta - 1)/\hbar r^3 \qquad (4.26)$$

where θ is the dihedral angle between r and the principal axis direction i. Equation 4.26 has been applied to calculate proton-copper distances in organo-copper complexes where the unpaired electron is largely located on the copper atom.[31]

4.4.2 Radical Identification and Orientation

To illustrate the approach to radical identification from hyperfine tensors we will consider several example systems where ENDOR has made a major contribution. First we consider the radicals in N-acetylglycine x-irradiated at 4 K.[32] In general, more than one radical is expected. In the simplest case we might expect anion and cation radicals if the temperature is low enough to trap the primary ionic species. The structure of N-acetylglycine is shown below.

$$CH_3-C(\!=\!O)-N(H)-CH_2-C(\!=\!O)-OH$$

The ESR spectrum only shows a partially resolved doublet; however, ENDOR reveals nine different proton couplings. Specifically, deuterated molecules were used to help assign these nine proton couplings.

For $CD_3CONDCH_2COOD$ six proton couplings are observed and the tensors for these protons are given as 1 to 6 in Table 4-8. Proton tensors 1–4 have small anisotropy and are assigned to β protons. The significant isotropic hyperfine coupling indicates that these are not matrix protons. Proton tensors 5–6 have large anisotropy and are assigned to α protons. Since there are only two protons in this deuterated molecule, it is obvious that these proton tensors must belong to at least two different radicals. Furthermore, since both protons are located on the same carbon in the undamaged molecule it appears that one radical contains two α protons and another radical contains two β protons. Table 4-8 shows the radical structures suggested. The radical with two α protons is identified as the N-acetylglycine cation followed by loss of H^+ and CO_2 to give $CD_3CONDĊH_2$. It could also be assumed that the C—N bond breaks to give $\cdot CH_2COOD$, but the former is favored on chemical grounds. This uncertainty could be removed by nitrogen ENDOR but it is not observed. Recall that lack of an ENDOR signal does not prove the absence of that nucleus since the relaxation processes may be unfavorable. The CH_2 group in the radical forms a plane and the perpendicular to this plane should be a principal axis of the hyperfine tensor of both protons. This is confirmed by finding that the direction cosines of one axis do coincide for both the α proton tensors.

The radical with two β protons is assigned to the N-acetylglycine anion with the electron added to the carboxyl group. This produces a radical with most of the unpaired spin on the carboxyl carbon and one strongly coupled and one weakly coupled β proton. Since there are two sets of these protons, it is concluded that this radical anion is produced in two different conformations.

For $CH_3CONDCD_2COOD$ three proton couplings are seen and the tensors for these protons are given as 7 to 9 in Table 4-8. This molecule

Table 4-8. Proton Hyperfine Tensors and Assigned Structures of Radicals Formed in N-Acetylglycine x-Irradiated at 4 K

Proton	Isotropic Hyperfine (MHz)	Anisotropic Hyperfine (MHz)	Radical Structure
1	76.4	+6.0 −1.8 −4.2	
2	77.4	+6.4 −1.6 −4.8	$CD_3-C(=O)-N(D)-CH_2-C(=O)(OD)$ (O⁻) (anion) (two conformations)
3	19.7	+10.1 −4.5 −5.7	
4	13.6	+9.6 −4.2 −5.4	
5	−50.1	−30.1 +2.7 +27.5	$CD_3-C(=O)-N(D)-\dot{C}H_2$
6	−40.5	−31.9 +2.5 +29.3	(cation product)
7	85.3	+6.7 −2.7 −3.9	$CH_3-C(O^-)-N(D)-CD_2-C(=O)(OD)$ (anion)
8	15.8	+9.6 −4.4 −5.2	
9	7.5	+9.5 −4.1 −5.5	

From H. C. Box, E. E. Budzinski, and K. T. Lilga, J. Chem. Phys., **57**, 4295 (1972).

only has three protons so the proton tensors 7 to 9 must be assigned to the three methyl protons. The anisotropies are all small (<10 MHz), so these tensors are characteristic of β protons and the spin density is localized on the carbonyl carbon. The radical is assigned to the molecular anion formed by electron addition to the carbonyl oxygen. No coupling to the α nitrogen was seen; therefore it is suggested that almost all the spin density is on the carbonyl carbon. This was supported by determination of the ^{13}C tensor of this carbon by ESR in an isotropically enriched sample.

Irradiation at room temperature often produces a single dominant radical, which is rarely an ion. An example of radical identification under these conditions where the structure is deduced almost entirely by ENDOR without appreciable chemical intuition is the radical formed in 1,2,4-triazole.[11]

There are three protons in the parent molecule, but the ENDOR spectra show six proton lines for a single crystallographic site. Table 4-9 shows these tensors and the assigned radical structure. Protons 2 and 4 have nearly zero isotropic coupling and may be assigned to matrix protons on molecules adjacent to the radical. This leaves four protons to be assigned to the radical, so it looks as though the radical is formed by H atom addition to the parent molecule. This could occur at C_3 or C_5 to form a methylene group. The two large couplings 5 and 5' are assigned to these two protons. Their tensors are characteristic of β protons; therefore it may be concluded that the π electrons are not delocalized over the methylene group. The two large couplings 5 and 5' are assigned to these is planar. Thus the methylene protons should be symmetrically oriented on both sides of this plane; this is what is found. It remains to be determined whether the methylene carbon is C_3 or C_5. This was resolved by deducing that the H_3 proton tensor directions were consistent only with bonding to C_3.

The 1 proton tensor has large anisotropy and is clearly an α proton bonded to a ring atom. The 3 proton tensor could also correspond to an α proton bonded to a ring atom with low spin density, although this is not so obvious. However both the 1 and 3 proton tensors have one principal axis direction perpendicular to the molecular plane. This identifies these protons as aromatic α protons. Furthermore the large isotropic coupling

Table 4-9. Proton Hyperfine Tensors and Assigned Structure for the Radical Formed in 1,2,4-Triazole γ-Irradiated at 300 K

Proton	Isotropic Hyperfine (MHz)	Anisotropic Hyperfine (MHz)	Structure
1	−23.83	27.82	
		−22.52	
		−5.30	
2	0.06	5.66	
		−3.14	
		2.52	
3	−2.65	5.94	
		−2.18	
		−3.76	
4	0.16	6.61	
		−3.64	
		−2.97	
5	159.58	6.08	
		−1.84	
		−4.24	
5′	154.99	7.08	
		−2.22	
		−4.86	

From P. Gloux and B. Lamotte, *Mol. Phys.*, **25**, 161 (1973).

of proton 1 means that there is considerable spin density on the ring atom to which it is bonded. Thus its dipolar interaction will be due largely to this nearest spin density and another principal direction for it will be nearly along the bond direction. The direction cosines for proton tensor 1 then show that it must correspond to the N_1—H bond.

Now all four ring protons on the radical have been unambiguously assigned. We will return to location of the positions of the matrix protons on adjacent molecules. A point dipole model for the dipolar interaction is axially symmetric along the direction between the two point dipoles, with the largest principal component of the dipolar tensor lying along this bond direction. Note that the two dipolar tensors for matrix protons 2 and 4 are nearly axially symmetric. This implies a large spin density on the nearest radical atom in each case and the approximate validity of a point dipole model for the dipolar tensor. The direction cosines of the largest tensor component for these two protons then define directions that are close to those for protons H-bonded to atoms N_4 and N_2 in the radical. Thus the structure of this radical has been quite completely elucidated by the proton dipolar tensors determined by ENDOR. Additional information would be available from nitrogen ENDOR but none was observed at 100 K where these measurements were done.

Finally we mention one additional case of radical identification in an aromatic hydrocarbon system. When single crystals of naphthalene are x-irradiated at room temperature, one predominant radical is formed, which is unambiguously identified by ENDOR as the α-hydronaphthyl radical[33] shown in Fig. 4-9. The radical is formed by H atom addition to

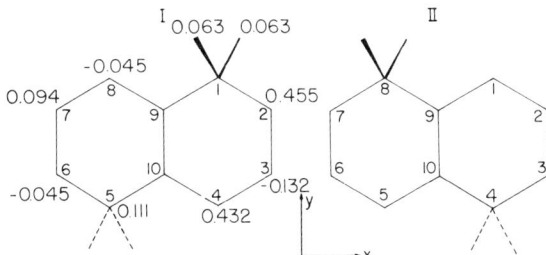

Figure 4-9. α-Hydronaphthyl radicals with mirror image symmetry. The calculated spin densities by McLachlan's SCF MO method are also shown. Adapted from U. R. Bohme and H. C. Wolf, *Chem. Phys. Lett.*, **17**, 582 (1972).

position 1 or 8. There are two different radicals in the crystal structure that are related by reflection in their yz planes. ENDOR lines from all nine protons are observed. Since there are two magnetically inequivalent molecules per unit cell of the monoclinic crystal and two different radicals, there are a total of 36 different high frequency ENDOR lines. A careful angular analysis gives a set of nine hyperfine tensors for each radical, I and II. Two of the protons have large isotropic couplings and are situated symmetrically out of the radical plane; these can be uniquely assigned to the methylene 1 and 1′ protons in radical I. The other seven protons all have one principal axis of their hyperfine tensor in common, which is perpendicular to the radical plane within 3°; this is characteristic of aromatic ring protons. A second principal axis of each tensor is expected to coincide with the direction of the C—H bonds in the crystal and can be used to identify the hyperfine tensors with specific protons. This is quite precisely true for the 2, 4, and 7 protons, but deviations of the largest tensor axes from the crystallographic bond directions of ~18° are observed for protons 5 and 8 and of ~9° for protons 3 and 6. These deviations suggest departures from a point dipole interaction for these protons with the spin density on the carbons to which they are bonded.

The calculated spin densities based on the McLachlan SCF MO method, as shown in Fig. 4-9, indicate the origin of these departures. Carbons bonded to protons 3, 6, and 8 have negative spin densities resulting from polarization of the σ electrons in the C—C bonds, so the dipolar contributions from these σ electrons must be included. Proton 5 is bonded to a carbon with a much smaller spin density than on the nearby carbon 4; the direction of the maximum dipolar tensor of proton 5 can be quantitatively understood if the dipolar interaction from both carbons 5 and 4 is included.

In general, the preceding principles involving the values of the hyperfine tensor components and their direction cosines have been used along with chemical knowledge to assign the radical structures summarized in Table 4-4. Although mistakes in assignment can still be made, the use of ENDOR data is much more reliable than use of ESR data alone.

4.4.3 Reaction Mechanisms of Radical Formation

The high resolution of ENDOR allows the direct study of radical formation and radical transformation mechanisms. But first, the experimental conditions must be chosen to optimize trapping of the primary radical species. With ionizing radiation molecular cations and electrons are primary species, although neutral radicals could also be formed as primary species by excited molecule decomposition. In carboxylic acids, amino acids, and aromatic molecules the electron can be trapped on a C=O group or an aromatic ring to produce a molecular anion. In order to trap and observe primary cations and anions it is necessary to irradiate at as low a temperature as possible, typically 4 K. Even then the primary ions (especially cations) may not be observed. At higher temperatures than 4 K the charges are eventually neutralized to form primary neutral radicals. As the temperature is increased further these neutral radicals may react to form secondary neutral radicals. Those final neutral radicals are often identical to the radicals formed by irradiation at room temperature. This detailed sequence of radical formation and transformations has rarely been followed in all details because of the complexity of overlapping spectra. However ENDOR is a great aid toward making such studies possible. Here we will describe several different types of radical transformations and specific electron and proton transfer reactions that have been followed by ENDOR.

In glycine · HCl, $Cl^-(NH_3)^+CH_2COOH$, radiolysis at 4 K produces a cation or hole localized on the Cl^- to give Cl.[34] This rapidly reacts with a nearby Cl⁻ to yield Cl_2^-, which is identified by ESR. The electron is captured by the carboxyl oxygen to form the molecular anion. This anion is identified by two tensors with small anisotropy characteristic of β

$$Cl^-(NH_3)^+ - CH_2 - C \begin{array}{c} O^- \\ \diagdown \\ OH \end{array}$$

protons ($A_{iso(1)} = 81$ MHz, $A_{iso(2)} = 31$ MHz) and a splitting due to the hydroxyl proton ($A_{iso} = 34$ MHz). Most of the spin density is on the carboxyl carbon, as is typical for this type of anion. The advantage of using the hydrochloride salt is that the hole species Cl_2^- is stable on warming, so any changes can be attributed to transformations of the anion.

On warming the irradiated crystal to 110 K the anion ESR spectrum disappears and is replaced quantitatively by a new spectrum. By ENDOR two new proton hyperfine tensors are determined that have large anisotropy characteristic of α protons. This suggests that the reaction involves breaking of the C—N bond to form ·CH₂COOH. The overall reaction may be represented by

$$Cl^-(NH_3)^+ - CH_2COOH^- \rightarrow Cl^- + NH_3 + \cdot CH_2COOH. \quad (4.27)$$

In glycine itself radiolysis at 77 K produces the same ·CH₂COOH radical.

A second example of radical transformations on warming is provided by radiolysis of valine at 77 K;[28] valine has apparently not yet been studied after radiolysis at 4 K. The structure of valine is

$$\begin{array}{c} CH_3 \\ \diagdown \\ CH_3 \end{array} \begin{array}{c} H \quad H \\ C-C \end{array} \begin{array}{c} NH_3^+ \\ \diagup \\ COO^- \end{array} \qquad (I)$$

The ESR signal at 77 K is complex and is attributed to superimposed cations and anions; no ENDOR on this signal has been reported. After warming to 225 K the ESR spectrum changes and a radical with two proton hyperfine tensors is produced. One of these tensors is characteristic of an α proton and the other of a β proton, so the radical is assigned as

$$\begin{array}{c} CH_3 \\ \diagdown \\ CH_3 \end{array} \begin{array}{c} H \quad H \\ C-\overset{\cdot}{C}-COOH. \end{array} \qquad (II)$$

This neutral radical corresponds to loss of NH_3 from valine and may be produced by proton transfer to the molecular anion followed by loss of NH_3. Upon further warming to 300 K radical II transforms to a new radical identified as III, which is formed by hydrogen abstraction by II from I.

$$\begin{array}{c} CH_3 \\ \diagdown \\ \dot{C}_1-C_2 \\ \diagup \\ CH_3 \end{array} \begin{array}{c} HNH_3^+ \\ \diagup \\ \diagdown \\ COO^- \end{array} \qquad (III)$$

The final product radical III was identified from its proton and nitrogen ENDOR at 4 K. Four high frequency ENDOR lines are seen, all having small anisotropy upon crystal rotation; these are attributed to β protons from one rotating methyl group giving one ENDOR line and one stationary methyl group (the ENDOR is observed at 4 K) giving three ENDOR lines. This assignment is supported by the facts that the average isotropic coupling of the three protons in the stationary methyl group (63 MHz) agrees fairly well with the isotropic coupling for the rotating methyl group (69 MHz) and that the anisotropic hyperfine tensor for the rotating methyl protons is in good agreement with that for the similar radical $(CH_3)_2\dot{C}$—COOH. It is rather surprising that no ENDOR line is found for the C_2—H proton in III. This must be a consequence of the particular orientation of this bond to the unpaired electron in the $2p\pi$ orbital on carbon C_1 (i.e. $\cos \theta \sim 0$). Nitrogen ENDOR is also seen near 11 MHz, which confirms the existence of N in radical structure III. The isotropic coupling of this β—N is rather large (19.5 MHz) so it seems to be oriented favorably (i.e. $\cos \theta \sim 1$) so as to produce a large coupling at the expense of the β—H on C_2. Since the full hyperfine tensor and direction cosines of the β—N were measured, it would seem possible to define the interesting orientation around carbon C_2 in more detail if the crystal structure of valine were known.

A special radical transformation is shown by observation of the interesting electron transfer reaction (4-28) in glycine ·HCl crystals.[35] When either the protiated or partially deuterated compound is x-irradiated at

$$Cl^-(NH_3)^+ - CH_2 - C\begin{array}{c} O^- \\ \diagup \\ \diagdown \\ OH^+ \end{array} + Cl^-(ND_3)^+ - CH_2 - C\begin{array}{c} O \\ \diagup \\ \diagdown \\ OD \end{array} \longrightarrow$$

IV

$$Cl^-(NH_3)^+ - CH_2 - C\begin{array}{c} O \\ \diagup \\ \diagdown \\ OH \end{array} + Cl^-(ND_3)^+ - CH_2 - C\begin{array}{c} O^- \\ \diagup \\ \diagdown \\ OD \end{array} \qquad (4.28)$$

V

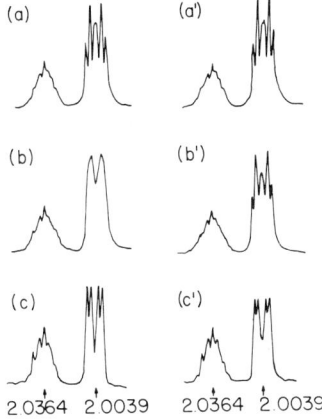

Figure 4-10. The ESR spectrum obtained from single crystals of glycine hydrochloride x-irradiated and measured at 4.2 K. The magnetic field was parallel to the a axis where $a^* = b \times c$. (a) Undeuterated crystal, (b) crystal with 50% of the exchangeable hydrogen atoms replaced by deuterium, (c) crystal with substantially all the exchangeable hydrogen atoms replaced by deuterium. After warming to 77 K and subsequently recooling to 4.2 K these crystals yielded the spectra shown in Figs. 1a' to 1c'. Adapted from E. E. Budzinski, K. T. Lilga, and H. C. Box, *J. Chem. Phys.*, **59**, 2899 (1973).

4 K it produces the molecular anion IV or V, respectively, along with Cl_2^- as described earlier.[34] When the pure protiated or partially deuterated crystals are warmed to 77 K and then recooled to 4 K, there is little change in their characteristic ESR or ENDOR spectra as shown in Fig. 4-10a and c. However when mixtures of the protiated and partially deuterated crystals are studied, warming to 77 K produces a distinct change in the ESR spectra (Fig. 4-10b) indicative of the electron transfer reaction in eq. 4.28. This reaction is irreversible, since it is observed after recooling to 4 K. The ENDOR spectra of IV and V are slightly different and confirm this reaction. The hyperfine tensor components of the methylene β protons in the protiated anion IV are each about 0.5 MHz larger than the analogous components for the partially deuterated anion V.

A common reaction in irradiated polar compounds is proton transfer. This is often deduced indirectly from the final product radical. By ENDOR in L-cysteic acid monohydrate (VI) it is possible to observe the proton transfer reaction directly.[36] When this crystal is x-irradiated at 4 K

$$SO_3^- - CH_2 - \underset{\underset{NH_3^+}{|}}{CH} - C\underset{OH}{\overset{O}{\diagup}} \qquad\qquad (VI)$$

the ESR spectrum shown in Fig. 4-11a is observed. The ENDOR spectra at the high and low field lines of this ESR spectrum are not shown but are different and allow identification of an oxidation product $SO_3^- - CH_2 - \dot{C}(NH_3^+)H$ and the anion reduction product VII. The high frequency

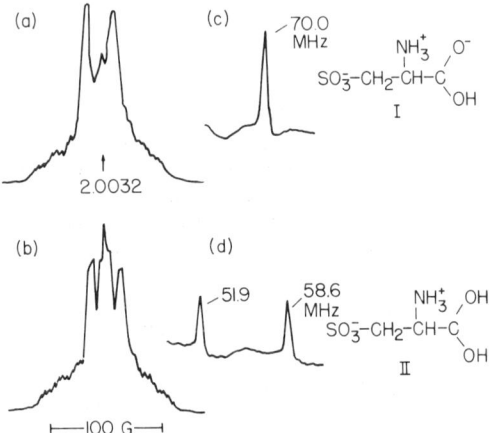

Figure 4-11. The ESR absorption and ENDOR resonances from a single crystal of L-cysteic acid monohydrate with the magnetic field parallel to the *a* axis: (*a*) ESR from a crystal irradiated and observed at 4.2 K, (*b*) after warming to 48 K for 5 min and recooling to 4.2 K. The absorption component that becomes prominent after warming can also be discerned as a weak absorption before warming. (*c*) ENDOR resonance corresponding to species I. (*d*) ENDOR resonance corresponding to species II. From H. C. Box and E. E. Budzinski, *J. Chem. Phys.*, **60**, 3337 (1974).

ENDOR line in Fig. 4-11*c* corresponds to the anion. This proton tensor

$$SO_3^- - CH_2 - \underset{(2)}{CH} - \underset{(1)}{C} \overset{NH_3^+}{\underset{OH}{\diagup}} \overset{O^-}{\diagdown} \quad \quad \text{(VII)}$$

has low anisotropy characteristic of a β proton with $A_{iso} = 68.6$ MHz and is assigned to the $C_{(2)}$ proton in VIII. An ENDOR line is also seen for the hydroxyl proton, but it could not be followed for all crystal orientations so its tensor was not determined. After warming to 48 K for 5 min and recooling to 4 K, the ESR spectrum changed to that shown in Fig. 4-11*b*. ENDOR of the new central component gives the ENDOR lines in Fig. 4-11*d*. Their tensors serve to identify the product of proton transfer VIII. One proton ENDOR line remains after exchange of the original crystal

$$SO_3^- - CH_2 - \underset{(2)}{CH} - \underset{(1)}{C} \overset{NH_3^+}{\underset{OH}{\diagup}} \overset{OH}{\diagdown} \quad \quad \text{(VIII)}$$

with D_2O, so it is assigned to the β proton at $C_{(2)}$ with $A_{iso} = 48.7$ MHz.

The second proton ENDOR line, which disappears after D_2O exchange, is assigned to one of the OH protons with $A_{iso} = 35.3$ MHz. The other OH proton has a small isotropic coupling of 3.9 MHz. The proton tensors support these assignments; although the isotropic coupling of the $C_{(2)}$ proton is reduced from 68.6 MHz in VII to 48.7 MHz in VIII, the principal axes of the CH coupling tensors are not much changed. It is clear from Fig. 4-11 that little could have been deduced about this proton transfer reaction from the ESR spectra alone.

Although the previous example demonstrates proton transfer to a carboxyl anion, the full exploitation of the detailed structural information from ENDOR can delineate the particular proton transferred from a neighboring molecule. This is impressively shown by an elegant ENDOR study by Muto and Iwasaki[37] on L-alanine. Alanine has structure IX in an undamaged crystal in which there are three H bonds to the carboxyl oxygens; the three-dimensionality of this structure is not shown. The H-bonded protons arise from NH_3^+ groups in three adjacent molecules.

$$\begin{array}{c} H_1 \\ | \\ CH_3-C-C \\ | \\ H_4-N^+-H_2 \\ | \\ H_3 \end{array} \begin{array}{c} O \cdots H_1' \\ \\ \\ O \cdots H_2' \\ | \\ H_3' \end{array}$$ (IX)

After radiolysis at 77 K a single radical dominates whose structure is deduced as X:

$$\begin{array}{c} H_1 \\ | \\ CH_3-\overset{\cdot}{C_2}-\overset{\cdot}{C_1} \\ | \\ H_4-N^+-H_2 \\ | \\ H_3 \end{array} \begin{array}{c} O-H_1' \\ \\ \\ O^- \cdots H_2' \\ | \\ H_3' \end{array}$$ (X)

in which the H_1' H-bonded proton has been transferred to the radical. By now we know that a main radical produced at low temperature in carboxylic acids is the molecular anion. So it appears that X is formed by proton transfer to the molecular anion.

The great amount of potential information available from the ENDOR spectra of this radical is shown by the region near the free proton frequency in Fig. 4-12. In Fig. 4-12b the N—H protons have been removed by exchange with D_2O. The angular variation of many of these lines can be measured to obtain hyperfine tensors; however, to emphasize the proton

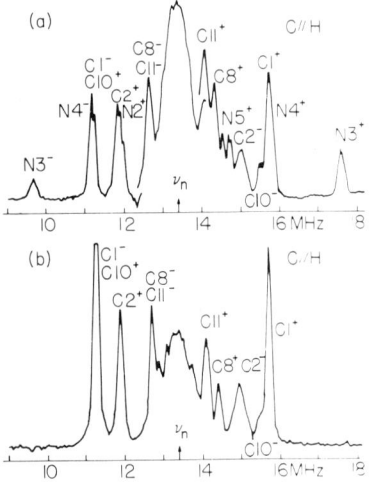

Figure 4-12. ENDOR spectra at 77 K near the free proton frequency (ν_n) of the anions of (a) L-alanine and (b) L-alanine-d_3. The symbols NX and CX represent the ENDOR lines for the couplings to the N—H and C—H protons, respectively. The plus and minus signs correspond to ν_+ and ν_-, respectively, where ν_+ is designated as the higher frequency line observed in the orientation that gives the maximum coupling throughout the measured angular variations. N2, N3, and N4 were assigned to the couplings to the H_2', H_3' protons in the neighboring molecules and H_2 in the radical molecule, respectively. (see structure X in text). From H. Muto and M. Iwasaki, *J. Chem. Phys.*, **59**, 4821 (1973).

transfer process we will only discuss the N—H proton tensors measured and the tensor of the β—H attached to C_2. The lines marked N_2, N_3, N_4 in Fig. 4-12 could be analyzed, as could line N_1, which occurs at frequencies higher than 18 MHz. Table 4-10 gives the hyperfine tensors and their assignments to particular protons. These assignments were based on a comparison of the principal axes of the hyperfine tensors with expected directions from the crystal structure. Since the unpaired electron is largely localized on the carboxyl carbon, the point dipole approximation may be made and the direction of the largest positive anisotropic tensor component is taken as the direction from the C_1 atom to the

Table 4-10. Isotropic Hyperfine Constants (A) and Anisotropic Hyperfine Tensors (B) Assigned to Various Protons in the Protonated Radical anion of *l*-Alanine (X)

Proton[a]	A	B_{max}	B_{int}	B_{min}
H_1'	14.23G	6.54G	−2.45G	−4.09G
H_2'	0.74	3.51	−1.71	−1.80
H_3'	−0.05	3.47	−1.62	−1.85
H_2	−0.23	2.54	−0.83	−1.72
H_1	19.19	2.75	−1.05	−1.69

Taken From H. Muto and M. Iwasaki, *J. Chem. Phys.*, **59**, 4821 (1973).

[a] See structure X in text for proton locations.

Table 4-11. Protonated Radical Anion in *l*-Alanine: Comparisons of the Direction Cosines of the Maximum Dipolar Tensor Elements (Observed) with the C_1—H Bond Directions from the Crystal Structure (Expected)

Proton[a]	Observed			Expected			Angular Difference
	l_x	l_y	l_z	l_x	l_y	l_z	
H_1'	0.651	−0.744	0.151	0.583	−0.785	0.206	6°
				(0.486	−0.855	0.181)[b]	11.5°
H_2'	−0.678	0.718	0.158	−0.586	0.737	0.337	11.5°
H_3'	0.319	0.083	0.944	0.090	0.040	0.996	14°
H_2	0.400	0.178	−0.899	0.491	0.180	−0.852	6°
H_1	−0.257	0.600	−0.758	−0.351	0.592	−0.726	5°

From H. Muto and M. Iwasaki, *J. Chem. Phys.*, **59**, 4821 (1973).
[a] See structure X in text for proton locations.
[b] Direction cosines for H_1' assuming this proton was not transferred to protonate the anion.

coupling proton. Table 4-11 shows how good the agreement is for the particular protons assigned. This analysis uniquely assigns the H-bonded protons and the N—H_2 proton in the radical itself. Note that all these remote protons, including the H_2 proton in the radical itself, have very small isotropic couplings, as expected.

Table 4-11 suggests that the H_1' proton is the one transferred to the radical, since the directional agreement is better in the transferred position and since it has a large isotropic coupling. However the isotropic coupling alone does not yield the position of this proton. This information is carried by the anisotropic coupling. Assuming the point dipole approximation, which implies neglect of the deviation from axial symmetry in the hyperfine tensor, the distance between the unpaired electron on C_1 and the coupling proton can be calculated from eq. 4.26. The results are given in Table 4-12 and clearly support the assignment of H_1' as the transferred proton.

The transferred H_1' proton is in a direction which is out-of-plane to the plane of the COO group. This is consistent with the large positive isotropic coupling to this proton, which can be interpreted as a typical β proton coupling dependent upon $\cos^2 \theta$. For the out-of-plane direction $\theta > 90°$ so $\cos^2 \theta > 0$. It is interesting that if the H_3' had been transferred, it would have been nearly in the COO plane and a small isotropic coupling would be predicted.

The transfer of specific H-bonded protons to form neutral radicals has also been demonstrated by ENDOR in other systems, including succinic acid,[38] L-valine · HCl,[39] glycine,[40] α-amino isobutyric acid,[40] and imidazole.[13] In all these cases except imidazole the proton transfer is

Table 4-12. Distances from the Radical Carbon Atom C_1 to Various N—H Protons in the Protonated Anion of *l*-Alanine

Proton[a]	Calculated Distances from the Dipolar Tensor with Point-Dipole Approximation (Å)	Calculated Distances from Crystal Structure	
		Far[b] (Å)	Close[b] (Å)
$C_1 \cdots H_1'$	2.05	2.97	1.97
$C_1 \cdots H_2'$	2.52	2.99	1.97
$C_1 \cdots H_3'$	2.53	2.56	1.97
$C_1 \cdots H_2$	2.82	2.56	—

From H. Muto and M. Iwasaki, *J. Chem. Phys.*, **59**, 4821 (1973).
[a] See structure X in text for proton locations.
[b] Far and close refer to the H-bonded proton position and transferred proton position in the H bond, respectively.

stereospecific. In imidazole the proton transfer apparently occurs along an H bond, but the transferred proton can occupy either of two geometrical positions in the neutral radical.[13] In carboxylic acids it appears that two factors control the proton transfer: first, the parallelism of the H-bond direction with the unpaired electron orbitals, and second, the shorter H-bond distances.[40] In glycine and in α-amino isobutyric acid the ENDOR results indicate that two H-bonded protons, one to each carboxyl oxygen, tend to protonate the molecular anion.[40] The competition makes transfer of these protons incomplete and the calculated dipolar distances place the protons in the middle of their hydrogen bonds. These are average positions and both protons may be jumping between the close and far positions of the hydrogen bond.

4.4.4 Intramolecular Motion: Methyl Group Tunneling

The ESR spectrum of the methyl group in the radical type, CH_3—$\dot{C}R_1R_2$, is a well known $1:3:3:1$ quartet even in solids at 77 K. This spectrum corresponds to three equivalent methyl protons and arises from the rapid rotation of the methyl group. The corresponding ENDOR spectrum is a single pair of lines with small anisotropy characteristic of β protons. At sufficiently low temperatures one expects to be able to stop the rotation of the methyl group. Then the three protons would be inequivalent and give an eight line ESR spectrum and three pairs of ENDOR lines. This situation is observed at 4 K for one methyl group in the radical XI:

$$\underset{O}{\overset{HO}{>}}C-\dot{C}\underset{CH_3}{\overset{CH_3}{<}} \qquad \text{(XI)}$$

formed in α-aminoisobutyric acid x-irradiated at 77 K and warmed to produce a particular conformation before cooling to 4 K.[27] In addition to a classically stationary methyl group at low temperature one can envision a quantum mechanical tunneling process that exchanges the methyl protons. Two successive proton pair exchanges correspond to rotation of the methyl group through $2\pi/3$; this is called tunneling rotation. Whereas classical rotation is spin independent, tunneling rotation is spin dependent because it is correlated with exchanges of proton spin states. Thus the tunneling rotational motion of the methyl group affects the energies of the spin states and leads to an additional term in the spin Hamiltonian. This term introduces a so-called tunneling splitting.[41]

A methyl group has C_3 symmetry and two rotational energy states corresponding to the symmetric, nondegenerate A and antisymmetric, doubly degenerate E irreducible representations of the C_3 group. The energy difference of the A and E spatial functions is the tunneling splitting. This splitting shows up in the spin Hamiltonian because the A and E spatial functions can only be combined with A and E spin functions, respectively, to give total eigenfunctions consistent with the exclusion principle. This is seen as follows. The exclusion principle requires that eigenfunctions be antisymmetric with respect to exchange of space and spin coordinates of any pair of protons. Rotation of a methyl group through $2\pi/3$ is equivalent to two successive proton pair exchanges, so the eigenfunctions for this motion must be symmetric. The products $A_{spin}A_{spatial}$ or $E_{spin}E_{spatial}$ are symmetric, but the product $A_{spin}E_{spatial}$ or vice versa is not.

Classically one can envision the A and E spatial functions as arising from linear combinations of three nonorthogonal harmonic oscillator states representing the methyl group oscillating near each one of three equivalent orientations constrained by a hindering barrier. The A function represents an oscillating methyl group in one orientation with periodic tunneling rotational jumps through $2\pi/3$ without change in the phase of oscillation, whereas a change in the phase of oscillation occurs for the E function.

The spin Hamiltonian may be written as[42]

$$\mathcal{H}h^{-1} = \nu_e S_z - \nu_n \sum_j I_{jz} + \sum_j S \cdot A_j \cdot I_j - 2J \sum_{j>k} I_j \cdot I_k \qquad (4.29)$$

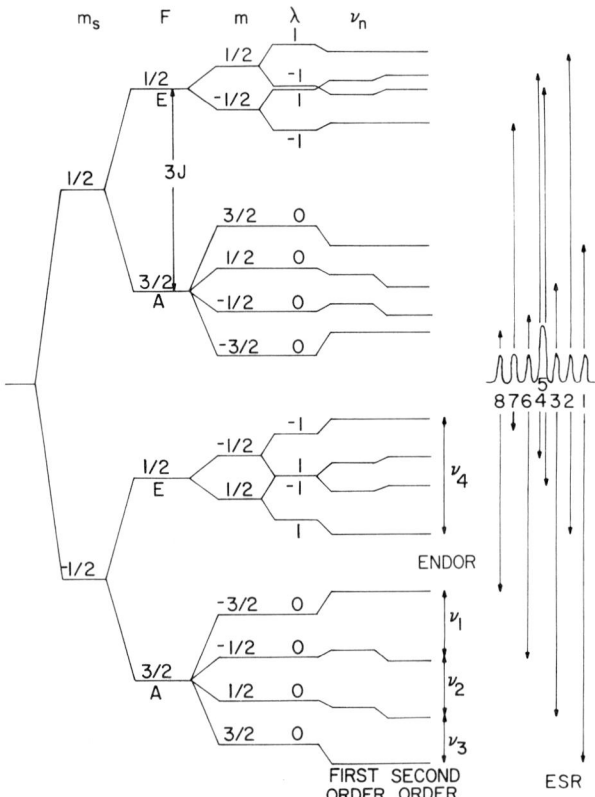

Figure 4-13. Schematic energy level diagram for a methyl group undergoing rapid tunneling rotation at low temperature where classical rotation is frozen out. The diagram corresponds to the successive energy terms in eq. 4.30 plus second order interaction. From left to right we have the electron Zeeman splitting, the tunneling splitting $= 3J$, the hyperfine splitting of the A rotational state, the hyperfine splitting of the E rotational state, the nuclear Zeeman shift, and the second order shift. The quantum numbers correspond to the symbols at the top of each column and are defined by eq. 4.30 in the text. The high frequency ENDOR transitions are given by ν_1 to ν_4; ν_1 and ν_3 carry information about the tunneling splitting $3J$ (see eq. 4.31) whereas the ESR transitions do not. The ESR spectrum is shown at the right. ESR transitions 1,3,6, and 8 are associated with the A rotational state and the others with the E state. As the system is warmed so that classical rotation begins to occur, lines 7 and 5 move toward line 6 and likewise lines 4 and 2 more toward line 3 to eventually give the familiar 1:3:3:1 spectrum of a classically rotating methyl group.

where the terms on the right-hand side are, respectively, the electron Zeeman, the nuclear Zeeman, and the hyperfine and the nuclear exchange interactions. The last term gives a splitting of $3J$ in the energy level diagram, which is equivalent to the tunneling splitting or the energy separation of the A and E states. The solution of this Hamiltonian is somewhat involved when both the electron Zeeman and nuclear exchange interaction are large, which is the case of interest for rapid tunneling. The energy levels are given to first order by eq. 4.30:

$$E(m_s, F, m, \lambda)h^{-1} = \nu_e m_s - J[F(F+1) - \tfrac{9}{4})] + \tfrac{1}{3}mm_s(A_{zz}^A + A_{zz}^E) - \nu_n m \quad (4.30)$$

where $m_s = \pm\tfrac{1}{2}$, the electron spin quantum number; $F = \tfrac{3}{2}$ (A state) or $\tfrac{1}{2}$ (E state), the total proton angular momentum quantum number; $m = F$, $F - 1, \ldots, -F$, the z component of the total proton angular momentum; and $\lambda = \pm 1$ for $F = \tfrac{1}{2}$ and 0 for $F = \tfrac{3}{2}$. The two hyperfine tensors A^A and A^E are related to A_j in eq. 4.29. Figure 4-13 shows the energy level shifts for each term in eq. 4.30. The eight ESR transitions are those for which $\Delta m_s = \pm 1$ with the other quantum numbers unchanged. The central pair of transitions almost coincide so a seven line ESR spectrum with relative intensities of $1:1:1:2:1:1:1$ is typically observed. Note that ESR transitions between A and E states are not allowed. This ESR spectrum is characteristic of a rapidly tunneling methyl group, but as seen in Fig. 4-13, it is independent of the tunneling splitting, $3J$. However the ENDOR transitions can give the tunneling splitting when the energy levels are calculated to second order.

Four high frequency ENDOR transitions are shown in Fig. 4-13 corresponding to $\Delta m = \pm 1$. The frequencies ν_1, ν_2, and ν_3 are equal in the first order treatment illustrated. But the second order shift is significant and lowers the center two levels in the lowest quartet of energy levels to make $\nu_1 \neq \nu_2 \neq \nu_3$. Note that the ESR frequencies and the ENDOR frequencies ν_2 and ν_4 are not affected by the second order shift. But ENDOR frequencies ν_1 and ν_3 contain information about J. Since A^A and E^E are roughly equal and isotropic, ν_1 is given to a good approximation by

$$\nu_1 = \nu_n + \frac{1}{6}A_{zz}^A + \frac{|A_{zz}^E|^2}{216J} \quad (4.31)$$

where the A_{zz} components are determined independently and the last term on the right-hand side is the second order shift. Different ENDOR lines can be selected by observing different ESR lines as seen from Fig. 4-31. Also ENDOR-induced ESR can be done.[42]

The preceding treatment and predicted ESR and ENDOR spectra hold for rapid tunneling rotation where the tunneling splitting is larger than the proton hyperfine splitting. When the tunneling and hyperfine splittings are nearly equal, the ESR spectra may give information on J. And when the hyperfine splitting is at least several times greater than the tunneling splitting, we have the case of an effectively stationary methyl group, as discussed originally.

Clough and co-workers have made several detailed studies of methyl tunneling by ESR and ENDOR.[41-43] For the 4-methyl-2,6-di-t-butylphenoxy radical in the corresponding phenol at 4.2 K they find a methyl group tunneling frequency of 3600 MHz, which corresponds to a 2.7 kJ mole^{-1} tunneling barrier height.[41] However, the methyl tunneling frequency is only 192 MHz for the $CH_3\dot{C}(COOH)_2$ radical in the methylmalonic acid at 4.2 K and just barely falls into the rapid tunneling category.[42] If the methyl group is deuterated as in $CD_3\dot{C}(COOH)_2$, the analysis becomes much more complex, but a tunneling frequency of ~1 MHz is expected if the tunneling barrier height is unaffected by deuteration.[43] Instead a deuteron tunneling frequency ≥ 10 MHz is deduced in the deuterated crystal, which implies a lower barrier than in the protiated crystal. As mentioned earlier, one methyl group in radical XI appears effectively stationary so its tunneling frequency is much less than its hyperfine frequency. Thus the tunneling frequency of a methyl group varies greatly from radical to radical. It still remains to correlate such differences to specific effects of molecular or crystal structure.

Types of intramolecular motion other than tunneling have not been much studied by ENDOR. However ENDOR should be uniquely useful for studying molecular motions whenever freezing out of the motion is revealed by the inequivalence of small hyperfine couplings. One such example is provided by the inversion of nonplanar ring compounds. The cyclobutyl-1-carboxylic acid radical (XII) is formed by x-irradiation of the

$$H_2C\text{———}\dot{C}\text{—COOH}$$
$$H_2C\text{———}CH_2$$
(XII)

dicarboxylic acid at room temperature.[44] ENDOR at 4 K on this radical shows two sets of β-proton axial and equatorial couplings, indicating that the ring exists in a static pucker relative to the hyperfine frequency. However at 77 K this radical shows equivalent β-proton couplings, indicating rapid inversion relative to the hyperfine frequency. In contrast, in the five-membered ring acid radical analogous to (XII), ENDOR indicates that the conformation is static at 77 K and rapidly inverting at 300 K.

4.4.5 Distant ENDOR

The occurrence of ENDOR from distant nuclei in matrix molecules via a nuclear depolarization mechanism was described in Section 1.4.2.4. This type of ENDOR signal gives NMR information about the neutral molecules in the matrix with a much greater sensitivity (typically 10^2 to 10^3) than is possible by direct detection of NMR. Application to organic crystals has been made by Kwiram and co-workers, to partially deuterated 1,1-cyclobutane-dicarboxylic acid, $(CH_2)_3C(COOD)_2$ (ref. 44), and to deuterated malonic acid, $CD_2(COOD)_2$ (ref. 45) to obtain structural information about the neutral molecules. Paramagnetic centers are introduced into the single crystals by x-irradiation, but the distant ENDOR spectra are independent of the type of radicals formed. Both deuteron and proton distant ENDOR spectra have been analyzed. The deuteron spectra are of more interest because they give ENDOR lines as narrow as 2.5 kHz, which permit determination of quadrupole coupling tensors for different deuterons. Figure 4-14 shows deuteron lines from

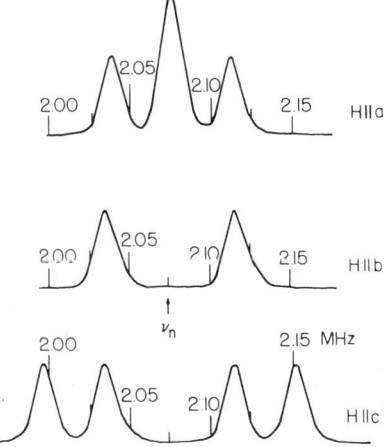

Figure 4-14. Deuteron distant ENDOR spectra at 4.2 K in single crystals of $(CH_2)_3C(COOD)_2$ with the magnetic field parallel to orthogonal crystal axes a, b, and c^*. The free deuteron frequency is 2.07 MHz. From L. R. Dalton and A. L. Kwiram, *J. Amer. Chem. Soc.*, **94**, 6930 (1972).

$(CH_2)_3C(COOD)_2$ crystals centered around the free deuteron frequency of 2.07 MHz. Since these spectra are effectively pure NMR spectra detected by ENDOR, there is no hyperfine splitting, only nuclear quadrupole splitting. The two deuterons in $(CH_3)_2C(COOD)_2$ give different quadrupole splittings for different orientations. Two pairs of lines corresponding to both splittings are shown for $H_o \parallel c^*$ axis, whereas the two splittings are equivalent for the $H_o \parallel b$-axis orientation. Proton lines are observed near the free proton frequency, but their resolution is generally poor. The proton distant ENDOR lines give the proton nuclear dipole tensor and the distance between two protons.

It should be noted that a nuclear polarization mechanism for distant ENDOR implies a signal response time characteristic of nuclear spin-lattice relaxation. For deuterons and protons in organic crystals at 4 K this appears typically to be ≥ 1 sec, so magnetic field and rf modulation are precluded, although the signal-to-noise of the distant ENDOR signal can be increased by averaging repetitive sweeps with a computer. Thus the modulation frequencies in commercial ENDOR spectrometers will discriminate against distant ENDOR signals.

Analysis of the angular dependence of the proton and deuteron distant ENDOR lines yields the dipolar and quadrupole coupling tensors and their direction cosines. These data in turn allow determination of the molecular structure and the orientation of the molecules to the external morphology of the crystal. Comparisons with x-ray crystallographic results indicate that molecular conformations determined by the two methods agree to within 5°. Since distant ENDOR experiments can be easily carried out at 4 K and below, this method appears to be a useful complement to x-ray crystallography, which is often difficult to carry out at low temperatures. The generality of the distant ENDOR method has yet to be explored, however.

4.4.6 Triplet State ENDOR

4.4.6.1 General Features

ENDOR offers particular advantages for looking at hyperfine interactions in molecular triplet states because the hyperfine structure is rarely revealed in the ESR spectrum. The predicted ENDOR spectrum of a triplet may be seen from the spin Hamiltonian with isotropic electron g factor for $S = 1$ in eq. 4.32 and the energy level diagram in Fig. 4-15. The symbols D and E

$$\mathcal{H} = g\beta H \cdot S + DS_z^2 + E(S_x^2 - S_y^2) - g_n\beta_n H \cdot \sum_k I_k + \sum_k S \cdot A_k \cdot I_k$$

(4.32)

in eq. 4.32 are the fine structure splitting constants, which are independent of field (so-called zero field splitting) and arise from the electron dipole–electron dipole interaction within the triplet molecule. For the electron Zeeman term alone (first term in eq. 4.32) one expects a single ESR line for the triplet state corresponding to degenerate $-1 \rightarrow 0$ and $0 \rightarrow +1$ transitions. However because of the electron dipolar interaction these

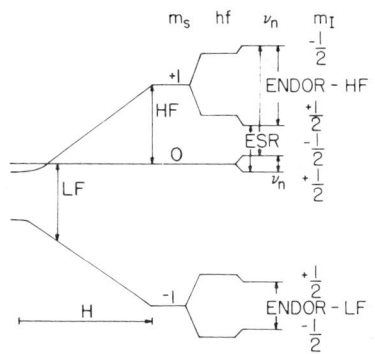

Figure 4-15. Energy level diagrams for a triplet state molecule ($S=1$) interacting with one proton ($I=\frac{1}{2}$). At zero magnetic field, at extreme left, the triplet energy levels are nondegenerate because of electron dipolar interaction. As the field is increased, low field (LF) and high field (HF) ESR transitions are observed. The splitting of the electron Zeeman energy levels (denoted by m_s) is shown for the higher field ESR transition. In this case we have taken the hyperfine splitting (hf) to be larger than the nuclear Zeeman splitting (ν_n). The high field and low field ENDOR transitions are shown together with the ν_n ENDOR transition.

two transitions are split by D in the special case of an axially symmetric (i.e., $E = 0$) dipolar or fine structure interaction. In general, the fine structure interaction is a tensor determined by ESR. For the energy level diagram shown in Fig. 4-15, observation of the high field ESR line will give an ENDOR line at the free nuclear frequency and another ENDOR line for each set of equivalent nuclei. If we neglect the ENDOR line at the free nuclear frequency, we expect for each set of equivalent nuclei one ENDOR line for triplet states in contrast to two ENDOR lines for doublet states. Also, for $A < g_n\beta_n H$ the ENDOR lines will be split from the free nuclear frequency, $g_n\beta_n H$, by A for triplet states in contrast to $A/2$ for doublet states. The general expression for the ENDOR frequencies is

$$\nu_{\text{triplet ENDOR}} = |A \pm \nu_n| \qquad (4.33)$$

where either the plus or minus sign, but not both, is used when observing a single ESR triplet transition.

A proton ENDOR spectrum of triplet fluorene[46] (see Table 4-13 for structure) is shown in Fig. 4-16. Because of transitions due to matrix protons the ENDOR transition at the free nuclear frequency is not prominent. Thus it is often necessary to measure ν_n separately with a proton gaussmeter. The well resolved ENDOR lines above 10 MHz correspond to all the protons in the molecule where the 2,2′,3,3′, etc., proton pairs are equivalent. Proton 7B is also seen by ENDOR but is off this frequency scan.

Theoretically no ENDOR lines should appear at low field, but lines do appear below the free proton frequency. This must be due to some specific, rapid relaxation pathways between the ESR levels. The fact that ENDOR transitions not allowed by the energy level diagram of Fig. 4-15 can be observed is clearly shown for triplet naphthalene.[47] With H_o

Table 4-13 Summary of ENDOR Studies on Triplet Molecules through 1974[a]

Triplet Molecule	Matrix Crystal	ENDOR Temperature (K)	ENDOR Results	References
GROUND STATE TRIPLETS				
1. Fluorenylidene	Diazofluorene	4.2	Determined hyperfine tensors of protons 3, 4, 5, and 6. Protons 3 and 3', etc., were equivalent. Determined spin densities on all carbons from dipolar proton tensors.	C. A. Hutchison, Jr., and G. A. Pearson, *J. Chem. Phys.*, **47**, 520 (1969)
2a. Diphenylmethylene	1,1'-Diphenylethylene	4.2	Proton pairs 3,3' and 7,7' were equivalent; other pairs were not. Determined hyperfine tensors for all protons and spin densities on all carbons from the dipolar proton tensors. Determined twist (54°) and bend (16.2°) angles of rings around C_1 carbon.	C. A. Hutchison, Jr., and B. E. Kohler, *J. Chem. Phys.*, **51**, 3327 (1969).
2b. Diphenylmethylene	1,1'-Diphenylethylene	4.2	Determined hyperfine tensors for 6 matrix protons and deduced distortion of matrix molecules adjacent to triplet from dipolar proton tensors.	D. C. Doetschman and C. A. Hutchison, Jr., *J. Chem. Phys.*, **56**, 3964 (1972).
EXCITED STATE TRIPLETS				
3. Benzene-h_6	Benzene-d_6	1.8	Three ENDOR lines assigned to 1,1'; 2,2'; and 3,3' proton pairs. Tensor for 1,1' pair determined and indicated that spin density on 1,1' carbons is less than at other carbons. Molecule is nonplanar and elongated.	A. M. Ponte Goncalves and C. A. Hutchison, Jr., *J. Chem. Phys*, **49**, 4235 (1968).

#	Compound	Structure	D (cm⁻¹)·10²	Comments	Reference
4.	Naphthalene-h_8, d_2, d_1	Durene	4.2	Hyperfine tensors determined for α and β protons and α deuterons. All ENDOR lines were slightly split into doublets indicating that only a center of symmetry existed; i.e., 1,5 and 4,8 α proton pairs were equivalent. Spin densities determined from isotropic hyperfine with assumed Q value.	P. Ehret and H. C. Wolf, Z. Naturforsch., **23a**, 1740 (1968).
5.	Naphthalene-h_8 Pairs	Naphthalene-d_8	1.9	Proton ENDOR showed that all the hyperfine tensor values were one-half those for the isolated triplet molecule indicating strong spin exchange between the pairs.	C. A. Hutchison Jr. and J. S. King Jr., J. Chem. Phys., **58**, 392 (1973).
6.	Diphenyl-h_{10}	Diphenyl-d_{10}	1.9	ENDOR lines seen for 4,4'; 2,2'; and 6,6' pairs indicating that only a center of symmetry exists in the triplet.	H. C. Brenner, C. A. Hutchison, Jr., and M. D. Kemple, J. Chem. Phys., **60**, 2180 (1974).
7.	Anthracene	Phenazine	1.5	Hyperfine tensors determined for the proton pairs: 9,10; 1,5; 4,8; 2,6; and 3,7: Hence only a center of symmetry exists in the triplet. Spin densities at all carbons were deduced from the dipole proton tensors.	R. H. Clarke and C. A. Hutchison, Jr., J. Chem. Phys., **54**, 2962 (1971).
8.	Phenanthrene-d_{10}	Diphenyl	1.7	Hyperfine tensors were determined for the deuteron pairs: 9,10; 3,6; 1,8; 2,7; and 4,5 and spin densities on all carbons were deduced from the dipolar tensors.	C. A. Hutchison, Jr., and V. H. McCann, J. Chem. Phys., **61**, 820 (1974).

Table 4-13 (*Continued*)

Triplet Molecule	Matrix Crystal	ENDOR Temperature (K)	ENDOR Results	References
EXCITED STATE TRIPLETS (*Continued*)				
9a. Fluorene	Fluorene	4.2	Hyperfine tensors were obtained for the 7A and 7B protons and for the proton pairs: 2,2′; 3,3′; 4,4′; and 5,5′. Spin densities at corresponding carbons were determined from isotropic hyperfine coupling with an assumed Q value.	V. Zimmermann, M. Schwoerer, and H. C. Wolf, *Chem. Phys. Lett.*, **31**, 401 (1975).
9b. Fluorene	Fluorene	4.2	Hyperfine tensors were obtained for five matrix protons and their dipolar tensor was used to assign them to particular positions in matrix molecules.	V. Zimmermann, H. C. Wolf, and M. Schwoerer, *Chem. Phys. Lett.*, **31**, 406 (1975).

[a] Only triplets detected by microwave absorption are included.

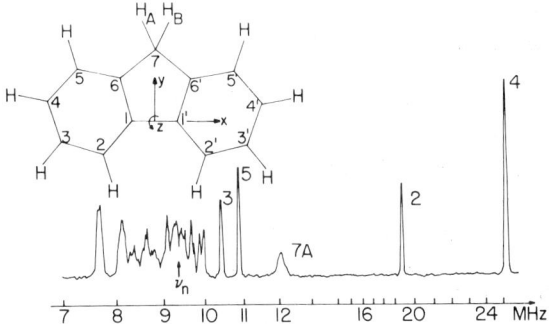

Figure 4-16. Proton ENDOR spectrum of triplet state fluorene at 4.2 K in a single crystal. The external field is directed along the z axis. The free proton frequency is 9.36 MHz. The numbers of the high frequency ENDOR lines refer to the corresponding proton positions in the molecule. The 2,2′,3,3′ etc., protons are equivalent. The 7B proton can also be observed at higher frequency. Many additional lines near the free proton frequency are assigned to matrix protons. From V. Zimmermann, M. Schwoerer, and H. C. Wolf, *Chem. Phys. Lett.*, **31**, 401 (1975).

parallel to the y axis of the molecule only half of the possible ENDOR transitions are seen when observing a given ESR line in accordance with the simple model presented earlier. However when H_o is parallel to the x or z axes of the molecule, all ENDOR transitions corresponding to both signs in eq. 4.33 are observed with roughly equal intensity when only a single ESR transition is saturated. The dynamics of ENDOR transitions in triplet states appear to present some interesting theoretical problems that have not yet been investigated.

To determine proton hyperfine tensors of triplets by ENDOR it is necessary to carry out angular measurements with respect to the magnetic field. For arbitrary orientation of the crystal, ENDOR is often not seen, in contrast to doublet state studies. In general, it appears that ENDOR lines of triplets are observable only when H_o is nearly perpendicular to a principal axis of the hyperfine tensor.[48] Although these principal axes are not known *a priori*, they are often parallel to the principal axes of the electron dipolar tensor. Thus triplets are first studied by ESR to determine the electron dipolar tensor, and then ENDOR measurements are made with the magnetic field initially oriented perpendicular to the various dipolar tensor axes. If ENDOR for a particular proton is seen only for one axis perpendicular to H_o, it probably implies that the dipolar and hyperfine tensors are only parallel along this one axis. It may then not be possible to determine the entire hyperfine tensor. Different situations may obtain for different protons in the same triplet molecule. For example, the anthracene triplet in phenazine crystals shows ENDOR for the 9,10, and α protons (see Table 4-13 for structural numbering) along all three axes of the dipolar tensor but only along one dipolar axis for β protons.[48]

Since, in the ideal case, only one ENDOR line above or below the free nuclear frequency is observed for each set of equivalent protons, the sign of the hyperfine component is determined if the sign of the dipolar tensor is known. The sign of the dipolar tensor can be found by ESR and thus the identity of the states between which the electron transition occurs $(0 \leftrightarrow \pm 1)$ gives $(\nu_{ENDOR} - \nu_n) > 0$ for positive A_i and $(\nu_{ENDOR} - \nu_n) < 0$ for negative A_i whereas the low field ESR transition gives the opposite signs of $(\nu_{ENDOR} - \nu_n)$. Note, however, that the sign determination method will not work if ENDOR transitions corresponding to both signs in eq. 4.33 are observed when one ESR line is monitored, as is seen in some systems.[47]

4.4.6.2 Structural Studies

Typical structural studies of triplet molecules carried out by ENDOR are summarized in Table 4-13. All the triplets have been produced by photolysis. Stable ground state triplets such as fluorenylidene[49] and diphenylmethylene[50] may be produced at 77 K and the ENDOR detected at lower temperatures after photolysis. Excited state triplets require observation during photolysis. One objective of ENDOR is to simply determine proton hyperfine tensors of intramolecular nuclei in triplets that are unobtainable by ESR. Even deuteron ENDOR has been detected in triplet molecules.[47] From the hyperfine tensors both spin density and geometrical information can be obtained.

Spin density information has been obtained in two ways. The easiest, but perhaps more inaccurate, way is to use the isotropic proton coupling constant and McConnell's relation (eq. 3.4) with some Q value.[47] However, as is well known, the Q value may differ for different protons. An independent method for determining spin densities is via the anisotropic or dipolar hyperfine interaction, as discussed in Section 4.2.5. This method must be used with some model for positioning point spin densities in order to simulate the dipolar components. This method has been used extensively by Hutchison and co-workers.[48-51] They have shown that generally the best selection of spin densities to agree with *all* the hyperfine tensor components does not imply a constant Q for the various aromatic protons. In fact, for the diphenylmethylene triplet the dipolar tensors imply a spin density on carbon-6 that implies $Q_{CH} = -118.4$ MHz compared with a standard "constant" value of $Q_{CH} = -66.9$ MHz.[50]

The geometry of triplet molecules is also revealed by the proton hyperfine constants. Often protons are inequivalent that would be equivalent for planar geometry; hence the triplet state often induces nonplanarity. Benzene,[52] napthalene,[47] and anthracene[48] triplets have only a center of symmetry and are nonplanar, as shown by ENDOR. For example, the benzene triplet has three observable ENDOR lines corresponding to three pairs of nonequivalent protons. Some geometrical information is also obtainable indirectly by allowing geometry to be a variable in finding the best fit to all the dipolar hyperfine tensors. This approach was used for diphenylmethylene where the ground state triplet is clearly not constrained to be planar.[50] The best fit was found for a twist angle between the two ring planes of 54° and a bending angle of 16.2°.

Although most ENDOR studies of triplets have dealt with intramolecular protons or deuterons, in two investigations proton ENDOR from matrix molecules has been successfully analyzed.[53,54] The matrix proton ENDOR was assigned to protons at specific positions in the crystal lattice from a point spin density model of the spin distribution determined by ENDOR in the triplet molecule itself. Since the matrix proton tensors were almost purely dipolar, this model could be used to calculate their entire hyperfine tensors. The very detailed information obtainable about the matrix molecule geometry is illustrated by Table 4-14.[53] There the crystal coordinates of three matrix protons in molecules surrounding a triplet molecule are compared with the coordinates of the same protons in

Table 4-14. Comparison of Coordinates for Protons in 1,1-Diphenylethylene Molecules Surrounding a Diphenylmethylene Triplet Molecule with the Analogous Protons in 1,1-Diphenylethylene in the Undistorted Crystal Lattice (origin fixed at origin of crystallographic axis system)

Proton Number	Crystal Coordinates	Distorted Lattice (Å)	Undistorted Lattice (Å)	Distance Differences (Å)
1	a	+0.389	+0.609	0.2
	b	+0.144	−0.037	0.2
	c	+4.491	+4.389	0.1
2	a	+3.781	+2.728	1.1
	b	−2.022	−2.860	0.8
	c	−0.232	−0.105	0.1
3	a	+0.458	+0.589	0.1
	b	−2.520	−2.730	0.2
	c	−1.316	−1.342	0.0

Adapted from D. C. Doetschman and C. A. Hutchison, Jr., J. Chem. Phys., 56, 3964 (1972).

the undisturbed bulk crystal lattice. It is seen that some coordinates are changed by as much as 1 Å but that the typical changes are more like 0.2 Å. This example is for the ground state triplet diphenylmethylene in which a molecule of nitrogen is lost in forming the triplet. We may expect this to disrupt the lattice much more than for an excited state triplet. Matrix protons surrounding the excited state triplet fluorene[54] do seem to be little distorted from the bulk crystal lattice. It is clear that ENDOR is a powerful method for studying the structural details of the intermediate stages of solid state radical or triplet reactions.

4.5 MOLECULAR INORGANIC SINGLE CRYSTALS

Little ENDOR work has been done on molecular inorganic single crystals. Here we exclude all ENDOR studies of transition metal ions, since these have been comprehensively discussed,[1] and only describe some typical studies. The most comprehensive investigations have dealt with hydrogen bonding of radical centers in the ferroelectric crystal KH_2AsO_4 and the antiferroelectric crystal $NH_4H_2AsO_4$.

In KH_2AsO_4 (ref. 55), x-irradiated at room temperature, an AsO_4^{4-} paramagnetic center is formed. ENDOR at 4 K reveals two sets of lines arising from protons in two equilibrium positions along the hydrogen bonds to the AsO_4 tetrahedra. These positions can be designated "close" and "far," corresponding to a near chemically bonded proton and a more distant hydrogen-bonded proton. The proton ordering in these two positions presumably corresponds to the two ferroelectric domains existing at low temperature. The tensors for these two types of protons show that there is little distortion of the lattice around the paramagnetic center. Both types of protons exhibit significant negative isotropic coupling. This can be understood by positive spin density on the oxygens and a spin polarization mechanism operating through a partially covalent $O \cdots H$ bond.

Somewhat similar results are found for the $HAsO_3^-$ radical formed by room temperature irradiation in $NH_4H_2AsO_4$.[56] ENDOR at 1.5 K allows determination of three proton hyperfine tensors, which correspond to protons H-bonded to the three oxygens of the radical. One proton has a larger isotropic coupling than the other two and more nonaxial symmetry and is assigned to a "close" proton to give a radical of formula $HAsO_3^-$ instead of AsO_3^{2-}. The $HAsO_3^-$ species could be simply formed by breaking an As—OH bond in $H_2AsO_4^-$ to give $HAsO_3^- + OH$. The "far" protons have nearly axially symmetric tensors and are assigned to protons H-bonded to the other two oxygens. However they do show a finite negative isotropic coupling that can be attributed to some covalent bonding and a spin polarization mechanism as described earlier. The two "far" protons are oriented along different crystal axes and presumably correspond to an antiferroelectric ordering scheme.

As a last example we consider OH radicals produced in x-irradiated single crystal ice.[57] ENDOR at 4 K gives three different proton hyperfine tensors, which correspond to OH radicals produced in three different environments. The differences in the tensor components are typically 1 to 2 MHz, which could only be distinguished by ENDOR. From the orientation of the principal axes of the three hyperfine tensors it is possible to assign them to OH radicals formed by three possible modes of dissociation of the ice lattice.

4.6 ENDOR IN DISORDERED SOLIDS

Many radicals cannot be studied in single crystals because insufficiently large or no crystals can be obtained. This is particularly true of biological systems, as we see in Chapter 7. Also single crystal studies are time-consuming and it is sometimes useful to be able to obtain less detailed information more rapidly. Hence ENDOR in disordered solids, polycrystalline, glassy, and amorphous media is an area of increasing interest. Extraction of information from ESR spectra in disordered solids is, in general, difficult, but we shall see that the analogous problem is somewhat simpler for ENDOR spectra.

The type of ENDOR spectra to be expected in disordered solids is illustrated by Fig. 4-17. In the liquid phase the triphenylmethyl radical in

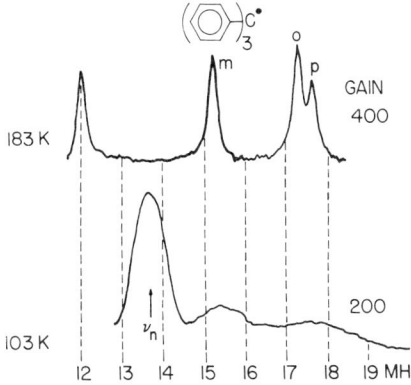

Figure 4-17. Proton ENDOR spectra of triphenylmethyl radical in the liquid (183 K) and glassy (103 K) phases of toluene. The three high frequency peaks are assigned as indicated to the meta (m), ortho (o), and para (p) protons, respectively. A matrix ENDOR line at the free proton frequency ν_n appears when the solution is frozen. From J. S. Hyde, G. H. Rist, and L. E. G. Eriksson, *J. Phys. Chem.*, **72**, 4269 (1968).

toluene shows three narrow ENDOR lines above the free proton frequency corresponding to the meta, ortho, and para ring protons. In the frozen glassy matrix two things occur. First, the liquid phase ENDOR lines broaden and become very weak, often undetectable. This is due to an average of absorptions from different orientations of radicals with respect to the magnetic field, which depends on the magnitude of the hyperfine anisotropy. For α protons this anisotropy is about half of A so that principal values for α protons occur near $A/2$, A, and $3A/2$. Thus the ENDOR spectra are expected to be spread out over this range but with some buildup of intensity at the three values corresponding to those molecules with their respective principal axes oriented along the magnetic field. β protons have considerably less anisotropy than α protons and generally exhibit much stronger ENDOR lines in disordered solids. In particular, β protons in rotating methyl groups show quite strong lines, as shown for the tritolylmethyl radical in Fig. 3-9.

The second feature of Fig. 4-17 is the appearance in the solid of a strong ENDOR line at the free nuclear frequency. This line has been called both a distant ENDOR line[58] and a matrix ENDOR line.[59] The distinction has been discussed in Chapter 1. We believe that observations of this line at high rf power and with some sort of high frequency modulation in the ENDOR detection system are probably best identified as matrix ENDOR lines. These lines are due to almost purely dipolar coupling of the unpaired electron with surrounding (i.e., "matrix") magnetic nuclei.

It is convenient to consider separately the information available from the anisotropic ENDOR lines (i.e., those occurring away from the free nuclear frequency) and from the matrix ENDOR lines in disordered solids.

4.6.1 Anisotropic ENDOR

We may consider two different cases of anisotropic ENDOR. In one case it is possible to select only certain orientations of radicals in the magnetic field. It is then possible to obtain spectra from disordered solids that are *single-crystal-like*. In the second case, all orientations contribute to the ENDOR spectra, and one has powder-type ENDOR.

Single-crystal-like ENDOR spectra can be obtained by setting the magnetic field at so-called turning points in the ESR spectra where g or hyperfine anisotropy is evident. A turning point refers to a magnetic field at which one orientation of a g or hyperfine tensor dominates sufficiently to cause a significant change in shape of an idealized Gaussian or

Lorentzian ESR line. In general, the larger the anisotropy, the better the selection of one orientation of radicals.

There are several cases where strong magnetic anisotropy can lead to single-crystal-like ENDOR spectra. (a) The anisotropy of the hyperfine tensor of one nucleus is larger than for all other nuclei and larger than the g anisotropy. This occurs for nitroxide radicals where the nitrogen anisotropy dominates the ESR spectrum. It may then be possible to determine the hyperfine tensors of protons in the radical, providing their tensors are parallel to the nitrogen tensor. (b) The g anisotropy dominates all hyperfine interactions. One can then set the magnetic field at $g_\parallel$ or $g_\perp$ to obtain $A_\parallel$ and $A_\perp$ for various magnetic nuclei if the g and A tensors have parallel axes. Even if the axes are not quite parallel it is sometimes possible to deduce the angle of rotation between the two tensors in one plane by doing simulations of the ESR spectra. In many metal ion complexes, particularly iron and cobalt complexes, g anisotropy dominates. This is the case in ferrimyoglobin and hemoglobin, and examples of such analysis will be given in Chapter 7. (c) Even when the hyperfine anisotropy of one nucleus and the g anisotropy are the same order of magnitude, if their axes of largest anisotropy coincide it is possible to obtain hyperfine tensors for other nuclei. This case is shown by copper complexes where the g-tensor and copper hyperfine tensor axes coincide, and hyperfine tensors of ligand nitrogen and proton nuclei can often be determined. (d) The anisotropy of the electron spin–electron spin interaction is larger than the g or hyperfine anisotropies. This results in a triplet state spectrum dominated by the electron dipolar coupling tensor D. By setting the magnetic field at $D_\parallel$ or $D_\perp$ positions one may be able to determine hyperfine tensors by ENDOR.

An example of case a is provided by the 1,3,6,8-tetra-t-butyl carbazyl radical in perdeuterated toluene at 77 K whose structure and ESR spectrum is shown in Fig. 4-18.[60] The ESR spectrum is dominated by the parallel component of the nitrogen hyperfine anisotropy ($A_\parallel$ = 20.52 G and $A_\perp$ = 0.08 G). By setting the magnetic field at the high field turning point marked a, the molecules with the magnetic field parallel to the nitrogen p-orbital and perpendicular to the molecular plane are selected. ENDOR then shows a single-crystal-like spectrum shown in Fig. 4-19a. The two outer lines of the ENDOR spectrum are assigned to the 2,7 protons and the inner lines are assigned to rotating t-butyl protons by analogy to isotropic couplings determined in solution. This gives $A_\parallel$ = A_z = 2.7 MHz for the 2,7 protons. The $A_\perp$ proton hyperfine component cannot be clearly determined like $A_\parallel$ because there is no well defined turning point for the nitrogen perpendicular component in the ESR spectrum. When the magnetic field is set on the center ESR line, a

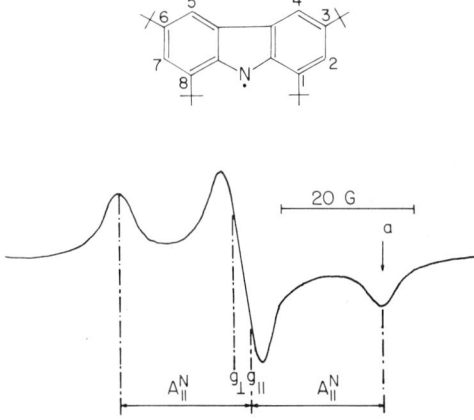

Figure 4-18. The 1,3,6,8 tetra-*t*-butyl carbazyl radical and its ESR spectrum in per-deuterotoluene at 77 K. Field *a* denotes the field for a parallel ENDOR spectrum. From R. D. Allendoerfer, *Chem. Phys. Lett.*, **17,** 172 (1972).

powder ENDOR spectrum is obtained that contains contributions from all orientations of the radical. However at the particular field $g_\perp$ the ENDOR spectrum in Fig. 4-19*b* is obtained that shows additional weak lines near 13.6 and 15.0 MHz. These lines are assigned to $A_y = 1.4$ MHz for the 2,7 protons. Then from the isotropic coupling of 2.53 MHz measured for the 2,7 protons in solution the remaining tensor component, $A_x = 3.5$ MHz, is obtained. So the complete proton hyperfine tensor is determined.

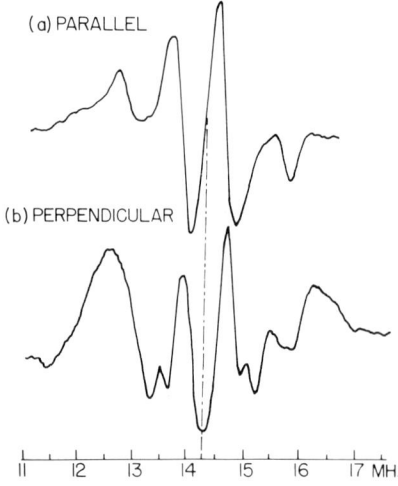

Figure 4-19. The ENDOR spectrum of the 1,3,6,8 tetra-*t*-butyl carbazyl radical with (*a*) magnetic field set at position *a* in Fig. 4-18 to select those molecules oriented with their nitrogen *p* orbital parallel to the magnetic field, (*b*) magnetic field set at $g_\perp$. The dashed line indicates the free proton frequency. From R. D. Allendoerfer, *Chem. Phys. Lett.*, **17,** 172 (1972).

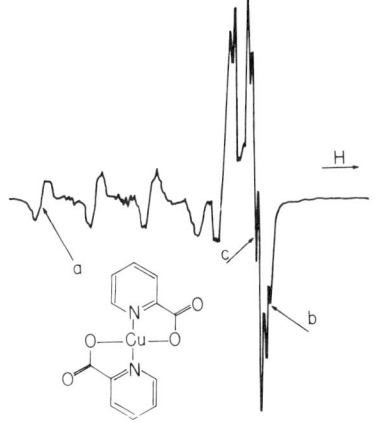

Figure 4-20. Second derivative ESR powder spectrum of copper picolinate in zinc picolinate tetrahydrate at 10 to 20 K. The shape is characteristic of an axially anisotropic g factor with the $g_\perp$ component of copper at low field. This component is split into four lines by the $A_\perp$ copper splitting. ENDOR spectra in Fig. 4-21 were taken at the magnetic fields indicated by the letters. From G. H. Rist and J. S. Hyde, *J. Chem. Phys.*, **52**, 4633 (1970).

As one more example we will consider a copper complex that exemplifies case c.[61] Figure 4-20 shows the ESR spectrum and structure of copper picolinate doped into zinc picolinate tetrahydrate. It is a typical copper spectrum showing g anisotropy with the $g_\perp$ component clearly split into a quartet by the $A_\perp$ component of the hyperfine interaction due to the $I = \frac{3}{2}$ spin of copper. The $A_\perp$ coupling of the ligand nitrogen is revealed in a single-crystal-like ENDOR spectrum obtained at position *a* in Fig. 4-20; see Fig. 4-21. The selection of one orientation of molecules is quite specific and a well resolved spectrum is found. The four lines between 12.5 and 18 MHz are due to nitrogen as described in Section 4.3. The high and low frequency pairs are split by $2\nu_N \sim 2$ MHz, and the frequency separation of the centers of these two pairs is the perpendicular component of the quadrupole coupling constant $Q_\perp^N = 1.35 \pm 0.1$ MHz. The center of the four lines is at $\frac{1}{2}A_\perp^N$. In addition, some proton couplings are seen near the matrix ENDOR line at the free proton frequency. When the observing magnetic field is moved to points *b* or *c* in Fig. 4-20, the ENDOR spectra broaden and new lines appear at higher frequency. This seems to be a typical powder ENDOR spectrum in which all orientations contribute. The higher frequency lines near 22.2 and 24.2 MHz can be assigned to the pair of lines at $\frac{1}{2}A_\| + Q \pm \nu_N$. If Q is taken as isotropic, $A_\| \sim 43.7$ MHz, which completes determination of the nitrogen hyperfine tensor.

The radicals formed in irradiated polycrystalline carboxylic acids do not show any strong, characteristic hyperfine anisotropy so their ENDOR spectra are expected to be of the powder type. In addition at 4 K the cross-relaxation times T_x are shorter than the electron spin-lattice relaxation times, so one expects the ENDOR spectrum to be the same regardless of which part of the ESR spectrum is saturated.[62] To analyze such

238 **ENDOR IN SOLIDS**

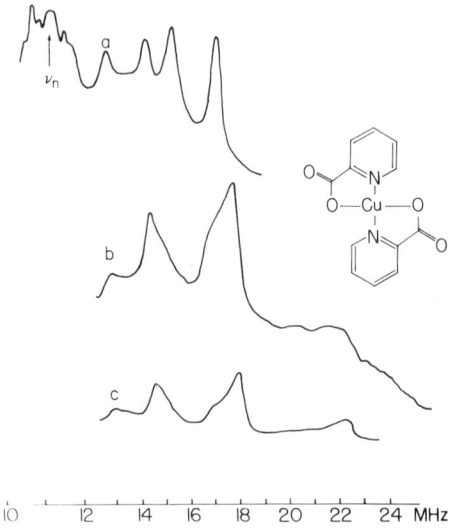

Figure 4-21. ENDOR spectra in a polycrystalline sample of copper picolinate in zinc picolinate tetrahydrate at 10 to 20 K. The letters indicate the magnetic field position in the ESR spectrum as shown in Fig. 4-20. The lines above 12.5 MHz are due to nitrogen and those at lower frequencies in the range shown are due to protons. Trace a is a single crystal type spectrum in which molecules oriented with the magnetic field perpendicular to the plane of the molecule predominate. Traces b and c correspond to contributions from molecules in many orientations. Adapted from G. H. Rist and J. S. Hyde, *J. Chem. Phys.*, **52**, 4633 (1970).

ENDOR spectra it is necessary to simulate the powder ENDOR spectra and to obtain the coupling constants from the best fit.

A simulation method has been developed by Dalton and Kwiram that seems quite successful.[62] First the ENDOR transition frequencies are calculated to second order, assuming certain hyperfine parameters. Second, the relative ENDOR amplitudes from given hyperfine interactions are calculated, partly phenomenologically, by considering various relaxation pathways and calculating transition moments with the second order wavefunctions. Third, powder ENDOR spectra are simulated by summing spectra from different orientations at 0.3 to 1° intervals. The relative signal amplitude for a given proton hyperfine interaction is given by

$$\chi''(\theta, \phi) = \frac{S[1 \mp B'(\theta, \phi)/2\nu_p]^2 R}{1 + S[1 \mp B'(\theta, \phi)/2\nu_p]^2} \quad (4.34)$$

where $S = 0.25 \gamma_p H_2^2 T_{1n} T_{2n}$ is taken as an isotropic constant, ν_p is the frequency at which a proton ENDOR line is observed, $R = 0.5(1 - \alpha_\pm)$ is also taken as an isotropic constant with $\alpha_\pm$ a relaxation parameter that

ENDOR IN DISORDERED SOLIDS

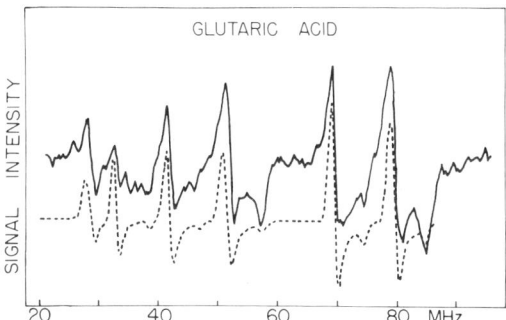

Figure 4-22. The first derivative proton ENDOR spectrum at 4.2 K of the HOOCĊHCH$_2$COOH radical in polycrystalline glutaric acid x-irradiated at room temperature. The solid line is the observed spectrum and the dashed line is a computer simulated spectrum based on eq. 4.34. From L. R. Dalton and A. L. Kwiram, *J. Chem. Phys.*, **57**, 1132 (1972).

depends on electron, nuclear, and cross-relaxation transition probabilities, and B' is the S_xI_x coefficient in the hyperfine Hamiltonian, which equals A_{iso} for purely isotropic hyperfine interactions. S and R are parameters whereas B' and ν_p depend upon the ENDOR frequencies. The simulations are quite good for β protons. Figure 4-22 shows simulated and experimental spectra for the radical in irradiated glutaric acid. Both the positions and the relative intensities are reproduced rather well by the simulation. Analysis gives both parallel and perpendicular hyperfine components for radicals of two different conformations, so rather detailed information can be obtained. In the general case where both α and β protons are present, the ENDOR features due to the α protons are suppressed because of their larger anisotropy.

Analysis of powder ENDOR spectra by simulation is easier than for powder ESR spectra. The ENDOR transition frequencies associated with a given hyperfine interaction are independent of the other magnetic interactions, whereas this is not true for ESR spectra. The spectral density is less for powder ENDOR, as described in Chapter 1. The ENDOR linewidths are less than ESR linewidths. Forbidden transitions complicate the ESR but not the ENDOR spectra.

4.6.2 Matrix ENDOR

The most prominent ENDOR line in most solid disordered systems is the matric ENDOR line occurring at the free nuclear frequency (see Fig. 3-9). This line has been interpreted as being due to a purely dipolar interaction between an unpaired electron and surrounding magnetic nuclei in the matrix.[59] In liquids this line is averaged to zero by the rapid

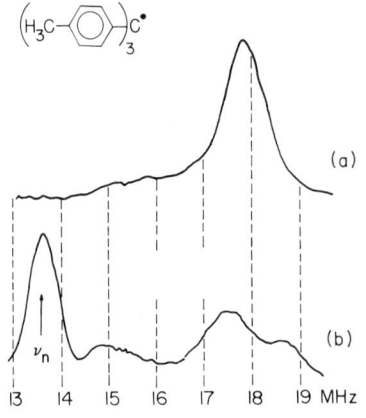

Figure 4-23. The proton ENDOR spectra of tritolylmethyl radical at 143 K in the (a) glassy and (b) polycrystalline phases of toluene. The arrow marks the free proton frequency. The strong line in (a) at ~17.7 MHz is assigned to the rotating methyl groups. From J. S. Hyde, G. H. Rist, and L. E. G. Eriksson, *J. Phys. Chem.*, **72**, 4269 (1968).

tumbling of the radical. So matrix ENDOR can be used to probe the amount of molecular motion as a function of temperature and to compare the amount of molecular motion in different phases and different matrices at the same temperature. As an example, consider Fig. 4-23 where proton matrix ENDOR associated with the tritolylmethyl radical is not seen in glassy toluene at 143 K but is quite prominent in polycrystalline toluene at the same temperature. Thus the amount of molecular motion appears to be considerably greater in the glassy phase. Qualitatively matrix ENDOR will be observed when the tumbling frequency of the radical or matrix molecules becomes comparable with the ENDOR linewidth. A typical linewidth is 1 MHz, which corresponds to molecular motions of 10^{-6} sec.

The occurrence of matrix ENDOR also depends on whether there are magnetic nuclei in the local environment of the unpaired spin, typically within 5 to 6 Å. For example, proton matrix ENDOR is seen for stable radicals in toluene but the proton matrix ENDOR line disappears in the deuterated matrix. If the radical site is located in a large complex molecule such as a protein, contributions to the proton matrix ENDOR line will arise from protons in the protein itself as well as from the solvent molecules. If the proton matrix ENDOR line does not change when the solvent is deuterated, it means that the radical site is inaccessible to solvent molecules. This is a very useful qualitative application of matrix ENDOR, particularly in biological systems, and examples will be given in Chapter 7.

Matrix ENDOR seems to be rather generally observed for protons. Fluorine matrix ENDOR has also been observed,[63] but it is not as generally observable for different radicals in different fluorinated matrices as is proton matrix ENDOR. When both protons and fluorines occur in

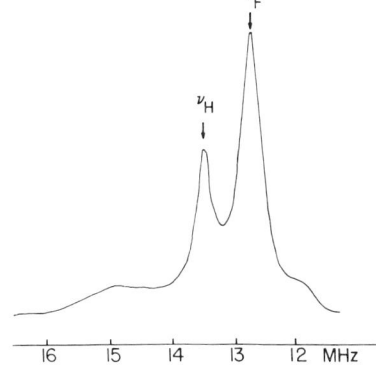

Figure 4-24. ENDOR spectrum of di-*t*-butylnitroxide in 1H,1H-heptafluor-1-butanol glass at 48 K showing resolved proton and fluorine matrix ENDOR lines. From R. N. Schwartz, M. K. Bowman, and L. Kevan, unpublished work.

the matrix, resolution is sufficiently good that both matrix ENDOR lines may be distinguished, as in Fig. 4-24.[64]

To understand how various physical parameters determine the matrix ENDOR quantitatively as a probe of the unpaired electron delocalization of radicals over nearby matrix molecules and the weak interactions of stable radicals with their molecular surroundings it is necessary to have a lineshape model for matrix ENDOR. Only a very simplified approach to this problem has yet been made, but it has produced a variety of interesting semiquantitative applications of matrix ENDOR.

4.6.2.1 Lineshape Models

Matrix ENDOR lines contain information about the magnetic nuclear environment of a radical. For specificity we consider that these magnetic nuclei are protons. It is convenient to divide the protons into two groups: near protons on which there is appreciable spin density from the unpaired electron wavefunction and matrix protons that are farther away and on which there is negligible unpaired electron spin density. The electron spin–nuclear spin interaction involving the near protons, which "see" the electron wavefunction, will involve an isotropic part (Fermi contact interaction) and an anisotropic part (dipolar interaction). The Fermi contact interaction with these near protons gives rise to ENDOR lines at $\nu_p \pm A_p/2$ unless broadened beyond detection by the dipolar interaction or by some other mechanism, where ν_p is the free proton resonance frequency in the magnetic field used and is typically 13 to 14 MHz at X-band fields of 3300 G. The electron spin–nuclear spin interaction with the matrix protons consists only of the dipolar interaction, since there is little or no electron spin density on these protons. This dipolar interaction produces a matrix ENDOR line centered at ν_p.

We will write the general lineshape of a matrix ENDOR signal as

$$f(\nu) = k \int_{\bar{a}}^{r} \int_{0}^{\pi} \int_{0}^{2\pi} R(r, \theta, \phi) g(\nu - \nu_o(r, \theta, \phi)) r^2 \sin\theta \, dr \, d\theta \, d\phi \quad (4.35)$$

where k is a constant that affects the amplitude but not the shape of the line, R is a function of various relaxation times that determine the ENDOR intensity, and $g(\nu - \nu_o)$ is the nuclear spin packet lineshape centered at the resonant frequency ν_o. The lower limit of the radial integral $\bar{a}$ represents an effective distance at which the "matrix" nuclei begin for which only a dipolar interaction is considered. The ϕ dependence of R and $g(\nu - \nu_o)$ can be eliminated by considering the magnetic moments to be aligned along the external magnetic field.

If the frequency dependence of $g(\nu - \nu_o)$ is determined mainly by the electron-nuclear dipolar interaction, as has been assumed, the matrix ENDOR lineshape will depend on the nuclear relaxation processes that determine the form of R. In the more general case both T_{1n} and T_x processes should be considered, but here we only consider the dominance of T_{1n} processes[65] for which the ENDOR intensity is proportional to T_{1n}^{-1}.

For the simplest case we consider T_{1n} to be independent of angle. An example of this is nuclear relaxation by time dependent fluctuations in the isotropic hyperfine interaction. The angular dependence of the ENDOR lineshape then depends only on the electron-nuclear dipolar interaction, which determines the frequency dependence of $g(\nu - \nu_o)$. The frequency ν is given by $\sum_i g_e \beta_e g_n \beta_n (3\cos^2\theta - 1) m_s I_{z_i} r_i^{-3}$ where the sum is over the i nuclei at distances r_i. The two values of m_s mean that a doublet lineshape is expected. Simulations show that the matrix ENDOR lineshape is relatively insensitive to Gaussian or Lorentzian functional forms for $g(\nu - \nu_o)$. Figure 4-25a shows the doublet matrix lineshape predicted. However most experimental observations of matrix ENDOR do not show a doublet but rather a singlet lineshape. This leads to the consideration of alternative nuclear relaxation mechanisms.

The electron-nuclear dipolar relaxation mechanism (END) has already been implicated in Chapter 3 as the dominant ENDOR active mechanism for aromatic radicals in solution. In disordered solids where the unpaired electron and the nuclei are fixed in position, nuclear relaxation may occur by (a) the fluctuating magnetic field at the nucleus that is caused by relaxation of the electron spin, or (b) changes in the magnitude of the electron-nuclear dipolar interaction caused by unusual motion that modulates the radial interaction distance.[65] In general, the END interaction can be written in terms of five spherical tensor components; the $I_z S_z$ term

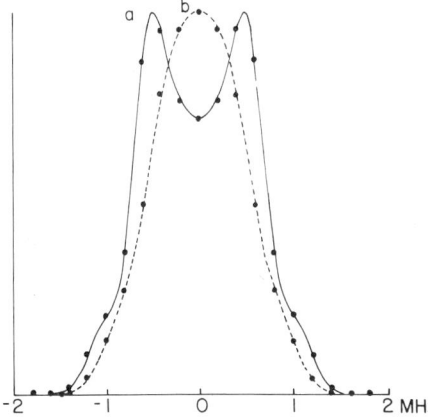

Figure 4-25. A comparison of simulated matrix ENDOR lineshapes resulting from two different types of nuclear relaxation based on eq. 4.35 with $R = T_{1n}^{-1}$, a Gaussian nuclear spin packet lineshape of width 200 kHz and a dipolar interaction of the electron with the matrix nuclei of 600 kHz. The solid line (a) is for the assumption that T_{1n} is independent of angle. The dashed line (b) is for the assumption that $T_{1n}^{-1} \propto \sin^2 \theta \cos^2 \theta$ as given by eq. 4.36. From D. S. Leniart, J. S. Hyde, and J. C. Vedrine, *J. Phys. Chem.*, **76**, 2079 (1972).

will be denoted by superscript (0), the two $S_z I_\pm$ terms by superscript (± 1), and the two $S_\pm I_\pm$ terms by superscript (± 2).

We can write the contributions of these various components, to T_{1n} for a $S = \frac{1}{2}$, $I = \frac{1}{2}$ system as follows:

$$(T_{1n}^{(0)})^{-1} = \frac{1}{16} \gamma_e^2 \gamma_n^2 \hbar^2 \frac{(1 - 3\cos^2 \theta)^2}{r^6} \frac{T_{1e}}{1 + \omega_e^2 T_{1e}^2} \quad (4.36a)$$

$$(T_{1n}^{(\pm 1)})^{-1} = \frac{9}{16} \gamma_e^2 \gamma_n^2 \hbar^2 \frac{\sin^2 \theta \cos^2 \theta}{r^6} \frac{T_{1e}}{1 + \omega_n^2 T_{1e}^2} \quad (4.36b)$$

$$(T_{1n}^{(\pm 2)})^{-1} = \frac{9}{16} \gamma_e^2 \gamma_n^2 \hbar^2 \frac{\sin^4 \theta}{r^6} \frac{T_{1e}}{1 + \omega_e^2 T_{1e}^2} \quad (4.36c)$$

where γ_n is the magnetogyric ratio of the proton and ω_e and ω_n are electronic and proton angular frequencies. In general, these contributions must be summed to calculate the matrix ENDOR lineshape, but for mechanism a only eq. 4.36b is important. This is seen from the last factor in the preceding equations: $(T_{1e}/(1 + \omega_n^2 T_{1e}^2) \sim (\omega_n^2 T_{1e})^{-1}$ is much larger than $(T_{1e}/(1 + \omega_e^2 T_{1e}^2) \sim (\omega_e^2 T_{1e})^{-1}$. The matrix ENDOR lineshape for mechanism a is calculated from eqs. 4.36b and 4.35 assuming a Gaussian nuclear spin packet lineshape and is shown in Fig. 4-25b. A single line is now found that is similar to that observed experimentally. The angular dependence of T_{1n} has changed the doublet in Fig. 4-25a to a singlet in Fig. 4-25b.

The nuclear relaxation is dominated by motional processes when either the radical or the matrix nuclei undergo random motion in a time $\tau_c \ll T_{1e}$.[65] Nuclear relaxation via motional processes is then faster than by the fluctuating field of the END interaction. When $\omega_e \tau_c \sim 1$ the magnitudes of all three components in eq. 4.36 become comparable. This leads to a matrix ENDOR lineshape with a maximum at the free proton frequency and one or two sets of shoulders on both sides. Trapped hydrogen atoms in zeolite matrices exhibit this type of matrix ENDOR lineshape and are discussed in more detail later.[66]

4.6.2.2 Analysis of Unpaired Electron Distribution

Kevan and co-workers have used matrix ENDOR to determine average sizes of unpaired electron wavefunctions.[63,67-72] They have used the lineshape model of eq. 4.35 with the assumption that the ENDOR intensity is dominated by T_{1n} processes in which T_{1n}^{-1} is given by eq. 4.36b. The nuclear spin packet lineshape $g(\nu)$ is taken as Lorentzian with a half width at half height of α. The matrix ENDOR lineshape is essentially insensitive to the choice of either Gaussian or Lorentzian shapes for $g(\nu)$. After the preceding substitutions, the lineshape expression becomes

$$f(\nu) = N \int_0^\pi \int_{\bar{a}}^\infty \frac{\cos^2 \theta \sin^3 \theta}{r^4} x \left[\frac{1}{\alpha^2 + [\nu - (q/r^3)]^2} + \frac{1}{\alpha^2 + [\nu + (q/r^3)]^2} \right] d\theta \, dr$$

(4.37)

where $q = (4\pi)^{-1} \gamma_e \gamma_n h (3\cos^2 \theta - 1)$. Integration to $r = \infty$ yields results comparable to a finite upper limit because the very distant protons make small dipolar contributions. Empirically it is found that good fits with the experimental data are obtained for $r \sim 10$ Å as an upper limit. The integration of r implies that the matrix nuclei are in a uniform continuous distribution.

Equation 4.37 for the lineshape contains two parameters, α and $\bar{a}$. By comparing various experimental spectra to simulated ones from numerical integration of eq. 4.37, it was found that the shape fit is much more sensitive to α than to $\bar{a}$ and that the best fit is obtained with $\alpha \sim 80$ kHz. The ENDOR linewidth, full width at half height, can then be simulated with a particular value of $\bar{a}$, the lower limit of the r integral. The $\bar{a}$ value can be considered to represent the average size of the unpaired electron wavefunction.

This type of analysis has been applied to a variety of different systems as summarized in Table 4-15. A particularly interesting example is the use of matrix ENDOR to study the wavefunction of excess electrons trapped in glassy matrices of varying polarity.[67] These were the first measurements of the average spherical size of the trapped electron wavefunctions. As the matrix polarity decreases from aqueous matrices to

Table 4-15. Matrix ENDOR Linewidths ($\Delta\nu$) and Effective Unpaired Electron Radii ($\bar{a}$) of Various Radicals in Disordered Matrices

Radical	Matrix	D_s^a	$\Delta\nu$(MHz)	$\bar{a}$(Å)	Comment
$(CH_3O\phi)_2NO$	methanol	32.6	0.51	5	polyxline[b]
	95% methanol + 5% H_2O	~33	0.55	4.3	
	ethanol	24.3	0.78	3.3	
	isopropanol	18.3	0.78	3.3	
	methyltetra-hydrofuran	4.6	0.81	3.2	
$(NO_2\phi)_2NO$	95% methanol + 5% H_2O	~33	0.82	3.1	
	ethanol	24.3	0.90	3.0	
Ag^o	H_2O	78.5	0.76	3.3	polyxline
	methanol	32.6	1.63	2.0	
	isopropanol	18.3	2.0	1.7	
	methyltetra-hydrofuran	4.6	2.2	1.5	
e_t^-	10 M NaOH	~78	1.31	2.3	2.1 Å theory
	95% methanol + 5% H_2O	~33	1.21	2.5	2.3 Å theory
	methyltetra-hydrofuran	~4.6	1.00	2.8	2.9 Å theory
H_t	14.9 M H_3PO_4/H_2O	–	0.72	3.6	
	7.0 M H_2SO_4/H_2O	–	0.73	3.6	
	2.7 M $KHSO_4/H_2O$	–	1.49	2.6	polyxline
	2.4 M KH_2PO_4/H_2O	–	1.77	2.3	polyxline
Polyenyl	poly(vinyl fluoride)	–	0.74	3.8	amorphous
	poly(vinylidene fluoride)	–	0.50	4.3	amorphous
			0.39 (F)	4.7 (F)	F-matrix ENDOR
	poly(vinyl chloride)	–	0.41	4.6	amorphous
	poly(methyl methacrylate)	–	0.44	4.5	amorphous

[a] Static dielectric constant of matrix at 298K.
[b] All matrices are glassy unless otherwise noted.

alcohol matrices to ether matrices, the matrix ENDOR analysis indicates that the spatial extent of the trapped electron wavefunction increases in good agreement with independent theoretical calculations based on an assumed trapping potential, dependent on matrix properties, for the electron.

It is also possible to use specifically deuterated matrix molecules to infer how the unpaired electron wavefunction overlaps these molecules.[70] A portion of the molecule that overlaps strongly with the unpaired electron wavefunction will have sufficient isotropic coupling to shift the ENDOR response away from the free proton frequency. If this portion is deuterated there will be little change in the matrix ENDOR response. But if a portion of the molecule that has mainly a dipolar interaction with the unpaired electron is deuterated, these deuterons will not contribute to the matrix proton ENDOR signal and the average distance deduced to the nearest "matrix" protons will increase. This kind of study has been made for trapped electrons in methanol glass at 77 K where it was shown that the trapped electron wavefunction is mainly localized on the O—H bonds and not over the entire molecule of the first solvation shell methanols.

The molecular details of solvation can also be studied by matrix ENDOR if the solvation process can be arrested at different stages.[72] For example, excess electrons are stabilized in a partially solvated state in ether (2-methyltetrahydrofuran) and alcohol (50% ethylene glycol–50% water by volume) glasses when the electrons are generated at 4 K. When the matrix temperature is raised to 77 K the first solvation shell molecules change their orientation around the electron toward an equilibrium configuration. The change in matrix ENDOR linewidth between the partially and more completely solvated states gives an indication of the distance changes to the matrix protons as the solvation process proceeds. In this case the matrix molecules appear to reorient so that the negative end of the average CH bond dipole moves 0.2 to 0.4 Å further away from the excess electron as solvation becomes more complete at higher temperatures.

For trapped electrons in organic and aqueous glasses it is deduced that the electron wavefunction increases in average radius as the matrix polarity decreases. This is a consequence of the decreasing depth of the trapping potential for the excess electron as the matrix polarity decreases. However for a radical that does not depend primarily on the matrix for its stability, we might expect that more polar matrices would tend to perturb and delocalize the unpaired electron distribution more than less polar matrices. This appears to be demonstrated by the data in Table 4-15 on silver atoms and nitroxide radicals.[69]

We may consider the electron distribution in Ag° to be spherically symmetric since it has a 5s electronic configuration. The single bond covalent radius of Ag° is 1.34 Å and the tetrahedral covalent radius of Ag° is 1.52 Å as derived by Pauling.[73] The smallest derived $\bar{a}$ value from the ENDOR linewidth measurements is 1.5 Å in 2-methyltetrahydrofuran (MTHF). It thus appears that the Ag° electron distribution is nearly unperturbed in the relatively nonpolar MTHF matrix. However as the polarity of the matrix, as measured by the static dielectric constant at 298 K, D_s, increases, the $\bar{a}$ value for Ag° steadily increases; until in ice $\bar{a}$ has increased by more than a factor of 2. This indicates that the more polar matrices interact with the unpaired electron in Ag° to delocalize it.

In $(CH_3O\phi)_2NO$ the unpaired electron is somewhat delocalized over the aromatic rings and the overall electron distribution is expected to be crudely spherical. A clear correlation of $\bar{a}$ with matrix polarity is seen for this radical also. The unpaired electron radius, as measured by $\bar{a}$, is distinctly larger than for Ag°, as is expected. It is interesting that the fractional increase in $\bar{a}$ on going from MTHF to methanol glass (MeOH) is 1.33 for both $(CH_3O\phi)_2NO$ and Ag°. It appears that the extent of matrix interaction with the unpaired electron is similar for both silver atoms and this aromatic nitroxide. In $(CH_3O\phi)_2NO$ the $\bar{a}$ value seems larger than for $(NO_2\phi)_2NO$ in the same matrix. This may reflect specific matrix interaction effects at the NO site. The electron withdrawing character of the NO_2 group tends to delocalize unpaired spin density into the aromatic rings and thus decrease the net matrix interaction. The electron donating character of the CH_3O group acts in just the opposite way.

It may be concluded that matrix ENDOR linewidths do serve as effective probes of weak interactions between radicals and their molecular environment in solid disordered matrices. For simple radicals with a spherical unpaired electron distribution and for some more complex radicals, the matrix ENDOR linewidth can be analyzed in terms of an effective radius of the unpaired electron distribution, which increases monotonically with increasing matrix polarity.

In certain systems matrix ENDOR may be of aid in radical identifications.[63] Polyenyl radicals are produced in some γ-irradiated polymers such as poly(vinyl chloride) aad poly(vinyl fluoride) at high irradiation doses. The formula for a polyenyl radical is $—CH_2—\dot{C}H(—CH=CH—)_n-CH_2—$ where n is unknown. Matrix ENDOR can yield a measure of n from the average unpaired electron delocalization radius and the C—C bond length. For the polymers mentioned earlier and the two others shown in Table 4-15, n is determined to be 5 to 7.

4.6.2.3 Analysis of Motional Processes

Matrix ENDOR signals can yield information about molecular or lattice motion if the motion has a cycle time shorter than electron relaxation times. In the simplest case one can consider "lattice" vibrations modulating the dipolar interaction to weakly coupled protons. This may then give rise to a temperature dependent ENDOR linewidth. Too few cases have been studied to make any generalizations, but one example may be given. If partially deuterated polycrystalline sucrose is γ-irradiated at room temperature, it produces an intense matrix ENDOR signal characterized by a strongly temperature dependent ENDOR linewidth between 100 and 300 K, although the ESR linewidth does not vary in this temperature range.[74] This was interpreted by fitting the ENDOR width to a hyperbolic cotangent function given by eq. 4.38

$$\Delta\nu(T) = \Delta\nu(0) \coth(\hbar\omega/kT) \tag{4.38}$$

where $\Delta\nu(T)$ and $\Delta\nu(0)$ are the ENDOR widths at temperature T and 0 K, respectively, and ω is a vibration frequency responsible for the modulation. By fitting to experiment ω and $\Delta\nu(0)$ are determined. The frequency ω is then identified with some particular lattice motion and $\Delta\nu(0)$ can be interpreted by eq. 4.37 to give a dipolar distance to protons at a specific distance. In the case of sucrose radicals, the matrix ENDOR line is interpreted as a superposition of broad and narrow components. The temperature dependence gives $\omega_1 = 532$ cm^{-1} and $\omega_2 = 50.5$ cm^{-1} together with $R_1 = 3.3$ Å and $R_2 = 6.5$ Å for the protons contributing to these two components. Previous ESR data suggest that the radical in sucrose, which is composed of pyranose and furanose rings, is located on the pyranose ring, so R_1 is associated with protons on the pyranose ring and ω_1 seems typical of ring breathing frequencies. R_2 is assigned to protons on the furanose ring and ω_2 to the oscillation of the furanose ring with respect to the pyranose ring. These results seem physically reasonable and are compatible with x-ray crystallographic data on sucrose, but the applicability of eq. 4.38 has yet to be theoretically justified for purely dipolar interactions.

Molecular motion may also manifest itself in matrix ENDOR by affecting the nuclear relaxation mechanism to give rise to additional structure in the matrix ENDOR line.[66] As discussed at the end of Section 4.6.2.1, nuclear relaxation is dominated by motional processes characterized by time τ when $\tau \ll T_{1e}$. Then τ replaces T_{1e} in eqs. 4.36, and since $\tau \sim \omega_e$ the last factors in eqs. 4.36 all approximate τ. The $\sin^4\theta$ and $\sin^2\theta\cos^2\theta$ terms (eqs. 4.36b and 4.36c) are then the most important. The $\sin^4\theta$ tends to give an overall doublet structure to the matrix

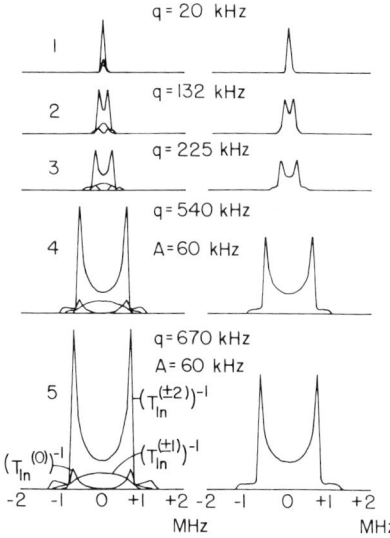

Figure 4-26. Simulated matrix ENDOR lineshapes involving all five dipolar components that contribute to $(T_{1n}^{(m)})^{-1}$ and consequently to the ENDOR intensity when the characteristic motional modulation time $\tau \ll T_{1e}$. The left side shows the separate contributions (see eqs. 4.36) for $m = 0, \pm 1, \pm 2$ for matrix protons interacting at different distances from the paramagnetic center as indicated by the dipolar constant $q = g_e \beta_e g_n \beta_n / 2r^3$ and with a isotropic interaction A. The right side shows the summations of all terms at the left and corresponds to the simulated ENDOR for interacting matrix protons at a single distance. Adapted from J. C. Vedrine, J. S. Hyde, and D. S. Leniart, J. Phys. Chem., **76**, 2087 (1972).

ENDOR lineshape if the dipolar coupling is larger than the nuclear spin packet width as shown in Fig. 4-26. Of course it is difficult to tell from an experimental spectrum showing doublet structure near the free proton frequency whether the structure is due to purely dipolar coupling dominated by motional processes or to weak isotropic coupling. This judgment must usually be made on chemical and physical grounds.

Trapped hydrogen atoms produced by γ irradiation in several different matrices appear to exemplify both cases. Trapped hydrogen atoms in H_2SO_4/H_2O and H_3PO_4/H_2O glassy matrices at 77 K show a proton ENDOR lineshape in Fig. 4-27 with prominent sideband structure.[68] The trapped hydrogen atoms appear to be surrounded by four nearest neighbor protons at distances of 2.6 Å (H_2SO_4) and 2.41 Å (H_3PO_4) from an analysis of spin-flip satellite lines.[75] This is a small enough trapping site

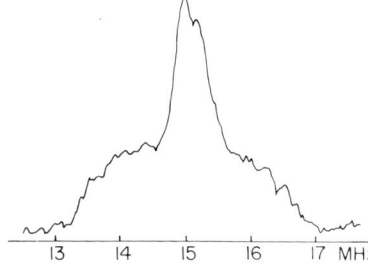

Figure 4-27. Proton matrix ENDOR line at 73 K for trapped hydrogen atoms in 7.0 M H_2SO_4 ice γ-irradiated to 2.0 Mrad. The high field ESR line was observed. Note the prominent shoulders on the center line. Results of J. Helbert and L. Kevan.

250 ENDOR IN SOLIDS

that rapid motional modulation of the dipolar interaction seems improbable. Thus the prominent sideband structure is assigned to weak isotropic coupling of 0.75 G to the nearest neighbor protons. This magnitude of coupling seems consistent with the geometry of the trapping site. Somewhat similar results and conclusions have been reached for the ENDOR lineshape observed for hydrogen atoms trapped in aluminum hydroxide powders where the cages that serve as probable trapping sites have diameters of 3 to 4 Å.[76] In these cases the central part of the matrix ENDOR line can be analyzed by eq. 4.37 to give distances to the more weakly coupled protons. It has also been suggested that the effect of high spin concentration, brought about by added paramagnetic ions or by high irradiation dose, on the ENDOR lineshape can serve to distinguish sidebands due to isotropic coupling and due to purely dipolar coupling.[68] At high spin concentration it appears that sidebands due to isotropic coupling are more prominent.

In contrast to the preceding cases, the ENDOR lineshape from trapped

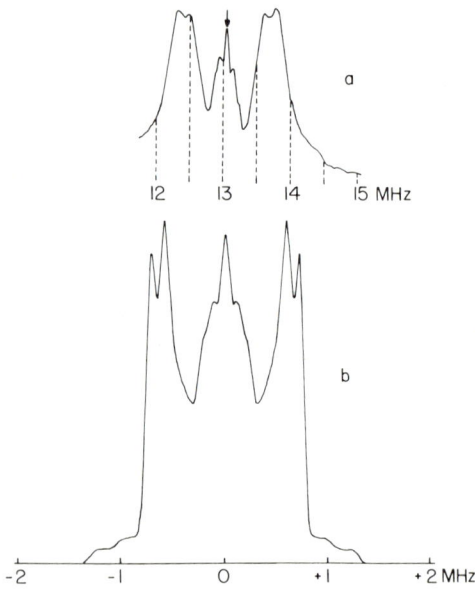

Figure 4-28. (a) Proton ENDOR spectrum at 15 K of trapped hydrogen atoms in γ-irradiated NH$_4$ Y-type zeolite activated at 673 K. The arrow indicates the free proton frequency. (b) Simulated proton ENDOR spectrum for trapped hydrogen atoms in zeolite obtained by adding the five right-hand lines in Fig. 4-26. Note that the vertical and horizontal scales are different from the spectrum in (a). From J. C. Vedrine, J. S. Hyde, and D. S. Leniart, *J. Phys. Chem.*, **76**, 2087 (1972).

Table 4-16. Deduced Coupling Parameters and Comparison of Distances Obtained by Matrix ENDOR with x-ray Structural Data for Hydrogen Atoms Trapped in Y-Type Zeolites

Proton	Relative Number of Protons	Isotropic Coupling A^H(kHz)	Dipolar Coupling q(kHz)	Distance from H_t to Proton by ENDOR (Å)	Estimated Distance from H_t to Proton from x-Ray Data (Å)
1	60	0.0	20	–	–
2	3.4	0.0	132	3.91	3.81
3	1.3	0.0	225	4.20	4.29
4	0.9	60.0	540	5.62	6.16
5	1.0	60.0	670	6.72	7.14

From J. C. Vedrine, J. S. Hyde, and D. S. Leniart, *J. Phys. Chem.*, **76**, 2087 (1972).

hydrogen atoms in Y-type zeolite powders has been attributed to motional modulation.[66,77] These zeolites are composed of SiO_4 and AlO_4 tetrahedra in the ratio of 2.4 to 1. These tetrahedra are arranged to form cubo-octahedral sodalite cages of diameter 6 to 7 Å. The sodalite cages are joined together via their hexagonal faces forming small hexagonal prismatic cages. ESR studies of trapped hydrogen atoms produced by γ-irradiation of zeolites activated to ~673 K indicate that the H atoms are trapped in the larger sodalite cages; this is based on an analysis of the matrix effects on the H-atom hyperfine constants and g factors. An ENDOR spectrum at 15 K is shown in Fig. 4-28a. A great deal of structure is exhibited but it is quite temperature dependent. This spectrum can be simulated by assuming several isotropic coupling constants together with a central matrix ENDOR line, but the larger, required, coupling constants (1.8 MHz) seem too large for interactions with protons that are ≥4 Å away as indicated by the sodalite cage structure. Thus a motional modulation mechanism was suggested based on a two jump model of the trapped hydrogen atom between two positions in the large sodalite cage. Dipolar interactions with protons at four specific distances were considered to account for the four sets of peaks surrounding the central line in Fig. 4-28a. This model satisfactorily simulated the observed ENDOR spectrum as shown by Table 4-16 and indicate a remarkable correlation between distances deduced from the ENDOR simulation and those deduced from x-ray structural data, assuming that any of the cage oxygens can be protonated.

REFERENCES

1. A. Abragam and B. Bleaney, *Electron Paramagnetic Resonance of Transition Ions*, Oxford University Press, London, 1970, Chapter 4.
2. (a) H. Seidel and H. C. Wolf, in *Physics of Color Centers*, W. B. Fowler, ed., Academic, New York, 1968, Chapter 8; (b) H. Seidel, *Proc. Colloq. Ampere XV*, North-Holland, Amsterdam, 1969, pp. 141–156.
3. N. M. Atherton, *Electron Spin Resonance*, Halsted, London, 1973, Chapter 4.
4. H. Seidel, *Z. Physik*, **165**, 218 (1961).
5. R. J. Cook and D. H. Whiffen, *Proc. Phys. Soc.*, **84**, 845 (1964).
6. R. J. Cook and D. H. Whiffen, *J. Chem. Phys.*, **43**, 2908 (1965).
7. D. A. Hampton and C. Alexander, *J. Chem. Phys.*, **58**, 4891 (1973).
8. J. M. Baker and W. B. J. Blake, *J. Phys. C: Solid State Phys.*, **6**, 3501 (1973).
9. J. A. R. Coope, N. S. Dalal, C. A. McDowell, and R. Srinivasan, *Mol. Phys.*, **24**, 403 (1972).
10. R. J. Cook, *Colloq. Ampere XV*, North-Holland, Amsterdam, 1969, pp. 269–273.
11. P. Gloux and B. Lamotte, *Mol. Phys.*, **25**, 161 (1973).
12. F. Q. Ngo, E. E. Budzinski, and H. C. Box, *J. Chem. Phys.*, **60**, 3373 (1974).
13. B. Lamotte and P. Gloux, *J. Chem. Phys.*, **59**, 3365 (1973).
14. H. M. McConnell and J. Strathdee, *Mol. Phys.*, **2**, 129 (1958).
15. A. L. Kwiram, *J. Chem. Phys.*, **55**, 2484 (1971).
16. P. Gloux, *Mol. Phys.*, **21**, 829 (1971).
17. S. F. J. Read and D. H. Whiffen, *Mol. Phys.*, **12**, 159 (1967).
18. R. J. Cook and D. H. Whiffen, *J. Phys. Chem.*, **71**, 93 (1967).
19. K. A. Thuomas and A. Lund, *J. Magn. Resonance*, **18**, 12 (1975).
20. M. Iwasaki, *J. Magn. Resonance*, **16**, 417 (1974).
21. R. J. Cook, *J. Sci. Instrum.*, **43**, 548 (1966).
22. R. J. Cook and D. H. Whiffen, *Proc. Roy. Soc.*, **295A**, 99 (1966).
23. S. N. Rustgi and H. C. Box, *J. Chem. Phys.*, **59**, 4763 (1973).
24. G. H. Rist and J. S. Hyde, *J. Chem. Phys.*, **50**, 4532 (1969).
25. J. M. Spaeth and M. Sturm, *Phys. Stat. Sol.*, **42**, 739 (1970).
26. H. C. Box, *J. Magn. Resonance*, **14**, 323 (1974).
27. J. W. Wells and H. C. Box, *J. Chem. Phys.*, **46**, 2935 (1967).
28. H. C. Box, H. G. Freund, and E. E. Budzinski, *J. Chem. Phys.*, **46**, 4470 (1967).
29. H. C. Box, H. G. Freund, and E. E. Budzinski, *J. Chem. Phys.*, **57**, 4290 (1972).
30. J. W. Wells, *J. Chem. Phys.*, **52**, 4062 (1970).
31. A. Schweiger, G. Rist, and H. H. Günthard, *Chem. Phys. Lett.*, **31**, 48 (1975).
32. H. C. Box, E. E. Budzinski, and K. T. Lilga, *J. Chem. Phys.*, **57**, 4295 (1972).
33. U. R. Böhme and H. C. Wolf, *Chem. Phys. Lett.*, **17**, 582 (1972).
34. H. C. Box, E. E. Budzinski, and H. G. Freund, *J. Chem. Phys.*, **50**, 2880 (1969).
35. E. E. Budzinski, K. T. Lilga, and H. C. Box, *J. Chem. Phys.*, **59**, 2899 (1973).
36. H. C. Box and E. E. Budzinski, *J. Chem. Phys.*, **60**, 3337 (1974).
37. H. Muto and M. Iwasaki, *J. Chem. Phys.*, **59**, 4821 (1973).
38. H. Muto, K. Nunome, and M. Iwasaki, *J. Chem. Phys.*, **61**, 1075 (1974).

39. H. Muto, K. Nunome, and M. Iwasaki, *J. Chem. Phys.*, **61,** 5311 (1974).
40. H. Muto and M. Iwasaki, *J. Chem. Phys.*, **61,** 5315 (1974).
41. S. Clough and F. Poldy, *J. Chem. Phys.*, **51,** 2076 (1969).
42. S. Clough, J. Hill, and F. Poldy, *J. Phys. C.: Solid State Phys.*, **5,** 518 (1972).
43. S. Clough and F. Poldy, *J. Phys. C.: Solid State Phys.*, **6,** 2357 (1973).
44. L. R. Dalton and A. L. Kwiram, *J. Amer. Chem. Soc.*, **94,** 6930 (1972).
45. R. C. McCalley and A. L. Kwiram, *Phys. Rev. Lett.*, **24,** 1279 (1970).
46. V. Zimmermann, M. Schwoerer, and H. C. Wolf, *Chem. Phys. Lett.*, **31,** 401 (1975).
47. P. Ehret and H. C. Wolf, *Z. Naturforsch.*, **23a,** 1740 (1968).
48. R. H. Clarke and C. A. Hutchison, Jr., *J. Chem. Phys.*, **54,** 2962 (1971).
49. C. A. Hutchison, Jr., and G. A. Pearson, *J. Chem. Phys.*, **47,** 520 (1967).
50. C. A. Hutchison, Jr., and B. E. Kohler, *J. Chem. Phys.*, **51,** 3327 (1969).
51. C. A. Hutchison, Jr., and V. H. McCann, *J. Chem. Phys.*, **61,** 820 (1974).
52. A. M. Ponte Goncalves and C. A. Hutchison, Jr., *J. Chem. Phys.*, **49,** 4235 (1968).
53. D. C. Doetschman and C. A. Hutchison, Jr., *J. Chem. Phys.*, **56,** 3964 (1972).
54. V. Zimmermann, H. C. Wolf, and M. Schwoerer, *Chem. Phys. Lett.*, **31,** 406 (1975).
55. N. S. Dalal, C. A. McDowell, and R. Srinivasan, *Mol. Phys.*, **24,** 417 (1972).
56. J. Gaillard, P. Gloux, and B. Lamotte, *Mol. Phys.*, **27,** 1441 (1974).
57. H. C. Box, E. E. Budzinski, K. T. Lilga, and H. G. Freund, *J. Chem. Phys.*, **53,** 1059 (1970).
58. M. Decaillot and J. Uebersfeld, *Compt. Rend. Acad. Sci. Paris*, **265,** B155 (1967).
59. J. S. Hyde, G. H. Rist, and L. E. G. Eriksson, *J. Phys. Chem.*, **72,** 4269 (1968).
60. R. D. Allendoerfer, *Chem. Phys. Lett.*, **17,** 172 (1972).
61. G. H. Rist and J. S. Hyde, *J. Chem. Phys.*, **52,** 4633 (1970).
62. L. R. Dalton and A. L. Kwiram, *J. Chem. Phys.*, **57,** 1132 (1972).
63. J. N. Helbert, B. E. Wagner, E. H. Poindexter, and L. Kevan, *J. Poly. Sci. (Phys.)*, **13,** 825 (1975).
64. R. N. Schwartz, M. K. Bowman, and L. Kevan, unpublished work.
65. D. S. Leniart, J. S. Hyde, and J. C. Vedrine, *J. Phys. Chem.*, **76,** 2079 (1972).
66. J. C. Vedrine, J. S. Hyde, and D. S. Leniart, *J. Phys. Chem.*, **76,** 2087 (1972).
67. J. Helbert, L. Kevan, and B. L. Bales, *J. Chem. Phys.*, **57,** 723 (1972).
68. J. Helbert and L. Kevan, *J. Chem. Phys.*, **58,** 1205 (1973).
69. B. L. Bales, R. N. Schwartz, and L. Kevan, *Chem. Phys. Lett.*, **22,** 13 (1973).
70. R. N. Schwartz, M. K. Bowman, and L. Kevan, *J. Chem. Phys.*, **60,** 1690 (1974).
71. B. L. Bales, R. N. Schwartz, and L. Kevan, *Ber. Bunsenges. Phys. Chem.*, **78,** 194 (1974).
72. H. Hase, F. Q. H. Ngo, and L. Kevan, *J. Chem. Phys.*, **62,** 985 (1975).
73. L. Pauling, *Nature of the Chemical Bond*, 3rd ed., Cornell University Press, Ithaca, N.Y., 1960, pp. 246, 256.
74. E. G. Derouane and J. C. Vedrine, *Chem. Phys. Lett.*, **29,** 222 (1974).
75. M. Bowman, L. Kevan, and R. N. Schwartz, *Chem. Phys. Lett.*, **30,** 208 (1975).
76. J. C. Vedrine, B. Imelik, and E. G. Derouane, *J. Magn. Resonance*, **16,** 95 (1974).
77. J. C. Vedrine, D. S. Leniart, and J. S. Hyde, *Ind. Chim. Belg.*, **38,** 397 (1973).

5. Liquid Phase ELDOR

5.1 Introduction
5.2 Field Swept ELDOR Spectra
    5.2.1 Temperature and Concentration Variations
    5.2.2 Microwave Power Dependence
    5.2.3 Applications to Molecular Motion Studies
    5.2.4 Application to Magnetic Relaxation
    5.2.5 Modulation Frequency Influence on R Factors
5.3 Frequency Swept ELDOR Spectra
    5.3.1 Conditions for Setting the Observing Field
    5.3.2 Hyperfine Lines and Combination Lines
5.4 Separation of Overlapping Spectra
5.5 Comparison of ELDOR and ENDOR Measurements in Solution
References

5.1 INTRODUCTION

The previous chapters on ENDOR have dealt with the response of a magnetic spin system to constant microwave and magnetic fields in addition to an intense variable rf field. In this chapter on liquid phase ELDOR we deal with the response of the spin system of a radical in solution to the same constant microwave and magnetic fields. However we add a second microwave frequency in place of the rf field. The relaxation conditions necessary for the observations of ELDOR spectra in solution are notably different from those required for the detection of solution ENDOR spectra. Moreover, solution ELDOR studies have been primarily involved with radicals containing nitrogen.[1-11]

Although ELDOR in the solid phase was first carried out in 1962, it

INTRODUCTION

was not until 1968 that the first ELDOR study of free radicals in solution was reported by Hyde, Chien, and Freed.[1] This lag was due (as in ENDOR) in part to the lack of commercial frequency swept ELDOR spectrometers and in part to a lack of interest in liquid phase ELDOR. ELDOR studies in liquids reported so far have not been as numerous as those reported for ENDOR, therefore limiting the number of ELDOR applications that can be covered. Nevertheless we outline in this chapter the use of ELDOR to study relaxation mechanisms of radicals in liquids such as electron-nuclear dipolar interactions,[1-5] Heisenberg and chemical exchange,[1,2,6] spectral diffusion (rotational and translational),[8-11] and spin exchange in polyradicals.[7] From an examination of these relaxation mechanisms, one will be able to explain several features of the ELDOR spectra. For instance, it will be possible to show that largely because of the magnitude of the electron-nuclear dipolar interaction, the ELDOR spectra observed for dilute solutions of nitrogen-centered radicals are more intense than those observed for protonated radicals.[1] On the other hand, one will note that in concentrated solutions, where Heisenberg exchange dominates, the difference in the spin-lattice relaxation between a protonated and a nitrogen-centered radical results in more intense ELDOR spectra for the protonated radical.[1]

Spectroscopically we show in this chapter that ELDOR techniques are ideally suited for the determination of large hyperfine splittings associated with radicals where a number of weakly coupled nuclei give rise to poorly resolved ESR spectra.[3] In general, weakly coupled nuclei (often protons) do not contribute to the ELDOR spectrum. Furthermore we show that ELDOR techniques are ideally suited for the study of rotational diffusion of paramagnetic probes (such as spin labels) in glasses and liquids and have made possible the detection of very slowly tumbling spin labels in human oxyhemoglobin.[9]

As stated in Chapter 2, there are two common modes in which ELDOR spectra are recorded: field swept and frequency swept. A number of theoretical equations have been derived that permit relaxation mechanisms to be deduced[1,4] from the ELDOR intensity of a field swept ELDOR spectrum. Because of this and the fact that several field swept studies have been reported,[1,2,5,11] the analysis of a field swept ELDOR spectrum is discussed in detail in Sections 5.2.1 to 5.2.4, using as the primary example the 4-N-maleimido-2,2,6,6-tetramethylpiperidine nitroxide radical studied by Hyde, Chien, and Freed.[1]

In Sections 5.2.1 to 5.2.4 the magnitude of the reduction factors are treated as if the modulation frequency has been chosen sufficiently low (270 Hz) that the modulation frequency dependence of the reduction factors is insignificant. In Section 5.2.5 we show that at high modulation frequency (10^4 to 10^5 Hz) the absolute magnitude of the reduction factors can be quite dependent on the modulation frequency. In fact, to deduce quantitative relaxation parameters from the reduction factors, a theoretical formulation of the reduction factors must be performed to deduce the modulation frequency dependence for a given modulation amplitude, spin-lattice relaxation time (T_{1e}), spin-spin relaxation time (T_{2e}), microwave saturation, energy transfer processes, the pumping to observing power ratio, the type of ESR lineshape, inhomogeneity, and the mode of ESR detection.

Spectroscopically, frequency swept ELDOR spectra have a considerable advantage over field swept ELDOR spectra in solving certain problems. Included among these are the separation of overlapped ESR spectra resulting from several simultaneously occurring radicals and the deduction of certain hyperfine splittings from a poorly resolved spectrum. Because such information is essential to the understanding of free radical reactions, a detailed analysis of the frequency swept ELDOR spectra of DPPH in solution is given[3] in Section 5.3.

5.2 FIELD SWEPT ELDOR SPECTRA

Before we can give an analysis of the field swept ELDOR spectra of a nitroxide radical, it is necessary briefly to describe the ESR spectrum. The ESR spectrum of the nitroxide radical in solution studied by Hyde, Chien, and Freed[1] consists of three well resolved, equally intense lines 44 MHz apart due to the hyperfine splitting of the ^{14}N nucleus ($I = 1$). Each of these three lines is inhomogeneously broadened (fine structures can be detected on each nitrogen line at low modulation amplitude and low concentrations) by weak couplings with the protons in the molecule. Because of imperfect averaging of the anisotropic interactions, the low field ESR line $M_I = +1$ is more intense (narrower) and saturates more readily than the high field line $M_I = -1$. Analysis of the saturation behavior shows that the transverse relaxation time T_{2e} does not change significantly over the temperature range employed. On the other hand, the longitudinal relaxation time T_{1e} decreases by a factor of 2 as the temperature is increased. In addition, it is difficult to saturate the samples at high concentration, and if the samples are not degassed, no saturation is observed.

In order to analyze a field swept ELDOR spectrum, one must first identify the pumped and observed transitions. To determine this an energy diagram is given in Figs. 5-1A and 5-1B for a ^{14}N nucleus of spin $I = 1(M_I = +1, 0, -1)$ interacting with an electron $S = \frac{1}{2}$ in an applied

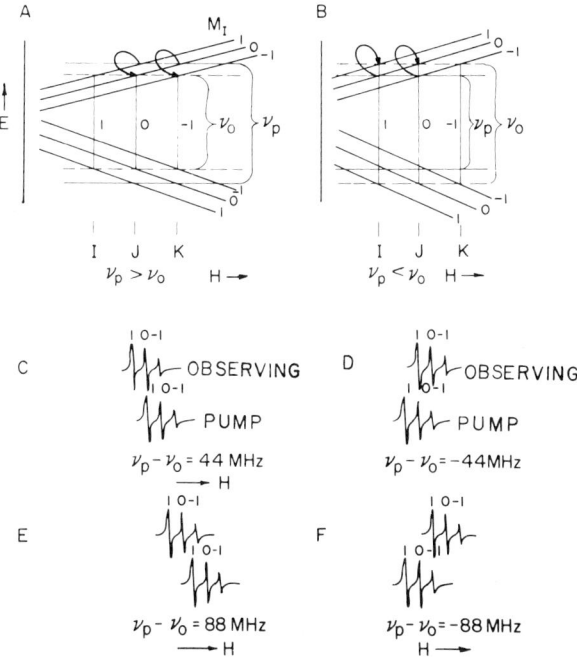

Figure 5-1. Energy diagram for a ^{14}N nucleus ($I = 1$) interacting with a magnetic field. (A) The pump frequency (ν_p) is greater than the observing frequency (ν_o) by the hyperfine splitting A_N. The curved arrow indicates a possible route for transfer of spin population. (B) $\nu_p - \nu_o = -A_N$; only the low field lines are affected by the pumping transition. In the lower half of the figure is given the relative magnetic field position of the observed (upper) and pumped (lower) ESR spectrum for a nucleus with $I = 1$ when (C) $\nu_p - \nu_o = 44$ MHz. (D) $\nu_p - \nu_o = -44$ MHz, (E) $\nu_p - \nu_o = +88$ MHz, and (F) $\nu_p - \nu_o = -88$ MHz.

magnetic field. Three ESR transitions I, J, and K are observed for a constant microwave frequency ν_o and varying magnetic field H. We obtain the field swept ELDOR spectrum by sweeping the magnetic field while the pumping (ν_p) and observing (ν_o) microwave frequencies are each set to a predetermined value. If the difference between the observing and pumping frequencies is set equal to either A_N (the nitrogen hyperfine splitting) or $2A_N$, the resulting change in the ESR signal height is a maximum.

The reason for this is given in Figs. 5-1A and 5-1B. When the pumping frequency exceeds the observing frequency by $A_N = +44$ MHz (Fig. 5-1A), a pumped ESR transition (bound by the horizontal solid lines) will occur between the upper and lower $M_I = 1$ levels at the same magnetic field (position J) that an observed transition occurs (bound by the horizontal dashed lines) between the upper and lower $M_I = 0$ levels. A portion (dependent on the ratio T_{1e}/T_{1n}) of the spin population from the upper pumped level ($M_I = 1$) can be transferred at this magnetic field (indicated by the arrow) to the upper observed $M_I = 0$ level by a nuclear spin-flip. We then see an ELDOR effect as a decrease in the ESR intensity at position J. Similarly spins are transferred at position K from the pumped $M_I = 0$ to the observed $M_I = -1$ level (as indicated by the arrow) resulting in a decrease in the ESR intensity. Note that it is not possible to transfer saturation to the upper observed $M_I = 1$ level at magnetic field position I because no pumped transition occurs at this field. Thus the ESR spectrum at position I remains unchanged in height.

Somewhat similar effects occur in Fig. 5-1B, where $\nu_p - \nu_o = -44$ MHz. In this case saturation is transferred at position I from the upper pumped $M_I = 0$ level to the upper observed $M_I = +1$ level, and at position J from the pumped $M_I = -1$ level to the observed $M_I = 0$ level, resulting in a change in the intensity of lines I and J. However instead of considering an energy level diagram of this sort each time to determine the M_I value of the pumped and observed transition, it is more convenient to note the relative positions of the ESR lines at a given pumping and observing microwave frequency difference. Figures 5-1C to 5-1F illustrate the respective positions of the ESR spectra in the observing and pumping modes when $\nu_p - \nu_o$ equals +44, −44, +88, and −88 MHz, respectively. By referring to Fig. 5-1A, one can see that the M_I value of the pumping and observing ESR lines located at the same magnetic field in Fig. 5-1C represents the pump transition from which the spins are transferred to the observing transition. For instance, in Fig. 5-1C the $M_I = 1$ ESR line of the pumped line is located at the same magnetic field as the $M_I = 0$ line of the observed line. This corresponds to the same M_I values as those of position J in Fig. 5-1A. Therefore the assignment of the M_I values can be obtained immediately from the matched ESR lines after the ESR spectra have been shifted to account for the microwave frequency differences.

Once we determine the M_I values of the pumped and the observed ESR lines for a given microwave frequency difference, we can predict the field swept ELDOR spectral intensity. For example, when the pump power is set to approximately 300 mW and the pump frequency is set to either one hyperfine frequency below the observer (i.e., $\nu_p - \nu_o = -44$ MHz) or to one hyperfine frequency above the observer ($\nu_p - \nu_o = +44$ MHz), the spectral intensity of an ESR spectrum of a solution of 10^{-4} M nitroxide radical in ethylbenzene (Fig. 5-2a) is changed to that in Fig. 5-2b. This is as predicted in that only two low field ESR lines or two high field lines are affected when $\nu_p - \nu_o = -44$ MHz or $\nu_p - \nu_o = +44$ MHz, respectively.

This is more clearly seen in Fig. 5-2c by the appearance of two lines at

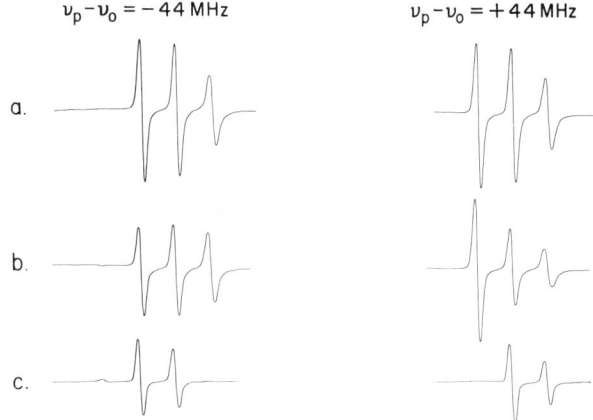

Figure 5-2. (a) The ESR spectrum of 10^{-4} M nitroxide radical (4-N-maleimido-2,2,6,6-tetramethylpiperidine nitroxide radical) in ethylbenzene at 193 K. (b) The ESR spectra at the same conditions as (a) but with the pump frequency set first to one hyperfine separation below and then to one hyperfine separation above the observing microwave frequency. (c) The field swept ELDOR spectrum that is the difference between spectra (a) and (b). The maximum pump and observing power available was used. From J. S. Hyde et al., *J. Chem. Phys.*, **48**, 4211 (1968).

lower ($\nu_p - \nu_o = -44$ MHz) or higher ($\nu_p - \nu_o = 44$ MHz) magnetic field depending on the pump frequency when the difference is taken between the spectral intensity of Fig. 5-2a and that of Fig. 5-2b.

On the other hand, when the frequency difference ($\nu_p - \nu_o$) is set to either -88 MHz (two hyperfine frequency intervals) or $+88$ MHz, only the low field or the high field ESR line is affected (Fig. 5-3b), respectively. The field swept ELDOR spectrum difference (Fig. 5-3c) is then composed of only one line at either low ($\nu_p - \nu_o = -88$ MHz) or high ($\nu_p - \nu_o = +88$ MHz) magnetic field.

If the frequency differs by $(44 \pm \Delta)$ MHz where Δ is the full width at half height of the ESR line, the ELDOR effect has been found[1] to be diminished by half. In fact, when the frequency difference is not set to a hyperfine interval, the difference lineshapes observed in Figs. 5-2c and 5-3c resemble dispersion curves. It has been suggested[1] that the lineshape in this difference mode can be used to determine a more accurate value of the hyperfine splitting constant when only a field swept ELDOR presentation is available.

Once we obtain a value for the ESR height reduction, we measure the ELDOR intensity in terms of a reduction factor R that is defined as:

$$\frac{\text{(ESR signal with pump off)} - \text{(ESR signal with pump on)}}{\text{ESR signal with pump off}} = R$$

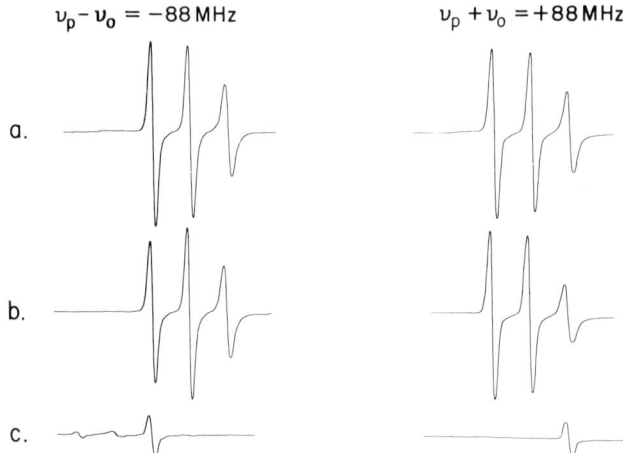

Figure 5-3. The same conditions as in Fig. 5-2 except the frequency difference between observer and pump equals −88 MHz (two hyperfine separations below the observing frequency) and +88 MHz (two hyperfine separations above the observing frequency). From J. S. Hyde et al., *J. Chem. Phys.*, **48**, 4211 (1968).

or equivalently, $R = 1 - (I/I_o)$ where I = intensity of ESR line with pump and I_o = intensity of ESR line without pump. All field swept ELDOR spectra are reported in terms of this reduction factor, which is dependent on sample temperature, concentration, microwave power, molecular motion, magnetic relaxation, and modulation frequency and phase. An analysis of these dependencies in the next few sections shows how the relaxation mechanism responsible for the ELDOR spectrum is obtained.

5.2.1 Temperature and Concentration Variations

First we must determine the variation of the reduction factor with temperature and concentration. As an example, a plot of R versus the reciprocal of temperature is given in Fig. 5-4 for the 4-N-maleimido-2,2,6,6-tetramethylpiperidine nitroxide radical[1] where the pumping and observing powers equal 300 mW and 200 mW, respectively. The reason for plotting the reduction factors versus the reciprocal of the temperature is given in Section 5.2.3. The plot is constructed from data obtained when the central ($M_I = 0$) line of the nitroxide radical is pumped and the low field line ($M_I = +1$) is observed. The same situation was depicted in Fig. 5-1B for observation of line I. The break in the curve indicates that at least two relaxation mechanisms are responsible for the observed ELDOR spectrum. At the lowest temperatures all samples from 3×

10^{-5} M (□) to 10^{-2} M (○) result in approximately the same R values. As the temperature is increased, the reduction factor R decreases and for the weakest sample (3×10^{-5} M) no ELDOR signals are observed above 273 K. However for higher concentrations, 10^{-4} (△) to 10^{-2} M (○), observable reductions are found to increase with increasing concentration and the reductions are independent of temperature above 273 K. Furthermore as the concentration increases, R is found to be independent of temperature at lower temperatures. These results will be shown in Section 5.2.4 to be consistent with an intermolecular or concentration dependent relaxation mechanism at high concentration and temperatures and with an intramolecular relaxation mechanism at the lowest concentrations and temperatures.

We can also obtain reduction factors when the microwave frequencies are separated by $2A_N$. The R values resulting under these conditions at

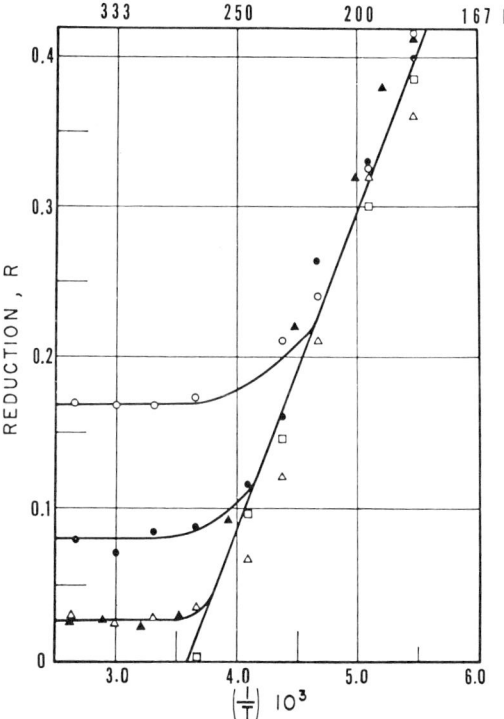

Figure 5-4. A plot of the reduction factor R as a function of $1/T$ where T is the temperature at (○) 10^{-2} M, (●) 10^{-3} M, (△) 3×10^{-4} M, (▲) 10^{-4} M, and (□) 3×10^{-5} M 4-N-maleimido-2,2,6,6-tetramethylpiperidine nitroxide radical in ethylbenzene. The central ($M_I = 0$) line is pumped and the low field ($M_I = +1$) line is observed. From J. S. Hyde et al., *J. Chem. Phys.*, **48**, 4211 (1968).

low concentrations and temperatures are smaller by a factor of nearly 1.5 than those obtained at A_N.[1] However R values found at high concentration and temperature are observed to be independent of the hyperfine interval separating the two microwave frequencies.

Further experiments with a sample of $10^{-4} M$ (193 K) TCNE anion[1] radicals show that R decreases by a factor of approximately 1.5 for each increase in separation of the two klystron frequencies by one hyperfine interval. In an investigation of a $10^{-4} M$ sample of DPPH at 193 K the value of R decreases by a factor of approximately 1.8 for each hyperfine interval. On the other hand, the observed reductions for concentrated samples of ($10^{-2} M$) of DPPH and TCNE at 298 K are independent of the temperature and the number of hyperfine intervals separating the two frequencies. This observed M_I independence of R at high concentrations is shown in Section 5.2.4 to be characteristic of intermolecular relaxation; conversely the appearance of an R value dependent on the hyperfine interval separating the two frequencies and independent of concentration is shown to be characteristic of intramolecular nuclear relaxation mechanisms.

5.2.2 Microwave Power Dependence

When one measures reduction factors, one also finds that the reduction factors depend to a small degree on the observing microwave power and to a significant degree on the pump microwave power.[1,2,6] An example of the dependence on observing microwave power is given in Fig. 5-5 for a $10^{-4} M$ sample of the nitroxide radical (given in Section 5.2.1) in ethylbenzene at 193 K with the pump power near the maximum available. Only a 10 to 15% decrease in the reduction factor was observed over a variation of 200 mW in the observing microwave power. On the other hand, the dependence of the reduction factor on the pumping microwave power level is considerably larger. In Fig. 5-6 a plot of $(1/R)$ versus the reciprocal of the pump power is given for the same nitroxide sample at the same temperature as in Fig. 5-5 with the observing power near maximum. A linear relationship is observed.

Such a linear relationship can be derived theoretically[12] by considering the time rate of change (dn/dt) of the excess number of spins (n) in the lower Zeeman level of the pumped (for instance, line 1 of Fig. 1-28) and observed (for instance, line 2 of Fig. 1-28) transitions due to relaxation processes. For both the pumped and observed transitions, one can set up expressions for dn/dt that include the time rate of change of excess spin population via T_{1e} relaxation processes, via the applied microwave

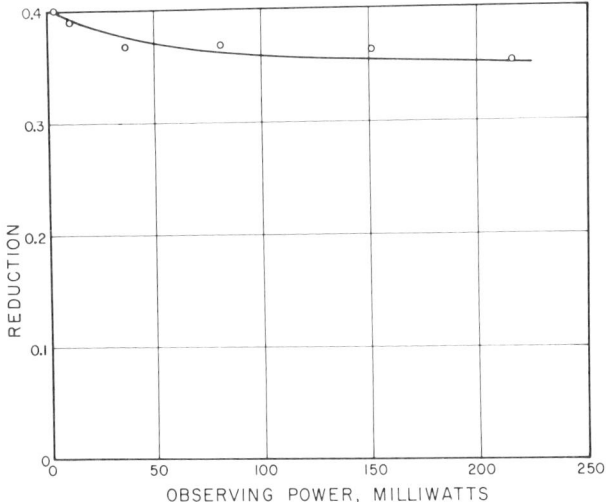

Figure 5-5. A plot of the ELDOR reduction factor R versus the observing microwave power level for a $10^{-4}\,M$ solution of nitroxide (4-N-maleimido-2,2,6,6-tetramethylpiperidine nitroxide radical) in ethylbenzene at 193 K with a strong saturated pump level. The low field ($M_I = +1$) line is observed and the central ($M_I = 0$) line is pumped. From J. S. Hyde et al., *J. Chem. Phys.*, **48**, 4211 (1968).

source, and via the cross-relaxation processes (T_{x1} and T_{x2}). Furthermore if we only consider ELDOR experiments carried out under steady state conditions, then $dn_o/dt = dn_p/dt = 0$ where the subscripts o and p denote observed and pumped spins, respectively. From such expressions the ratios n_o/n_o^o, and n_p/n_p^o (the excess spin populations relative to those at thermal equilibrium) can be obtained and are given by eqs. 5.1 and 5.2 for the four level scheme depicted in Fig. 1-28.

$$\frac{n_o}{n_o^o} = \left(1 + \frac{T_{1e}}{2T_{x2}} \frac{n_p}{n_p^o}\right)\left(1 + 2W_{so}T_{1e} + \frac{T_{1e}}{2T_{x2}}\right)^{-1} \quad (5.1)$$

$$\frac{n_p}{n_p^o} = \left(1 + \frac{T_{1e}}{2T_{x1}} \frac{n_o}{n_o^o}\right)\left(1 + 2W_{sp}T_{1e} + \frac{T_{1e}}{2T_{x1}}\right)^{-1} \quad (5.2)$$

In eqs. 5.1 and 5.2 the superscript o denotes thermal equilibrium populations, W_{so} and W_{sp} are the stimulated transition probabilities induced by the observing and pumping microwave frequency, respectively, and are proportional to microwave power, $N_o/n_o^o \simeq N_p/n_p^o$ since cross relaxation requires that the o and p energy level differences be similar, and N denotes the total number of spins. Equations 5.1 and 5.2 can be made more general[12] for any observed (o) and pumped (p) transitions by setting T_{1e} in eq. 5.1 equal to T_{1o}, $T_{po} = T_{x2}$, $T_{op} = T_{x1}$, and T_{1e} in eq. 5.2

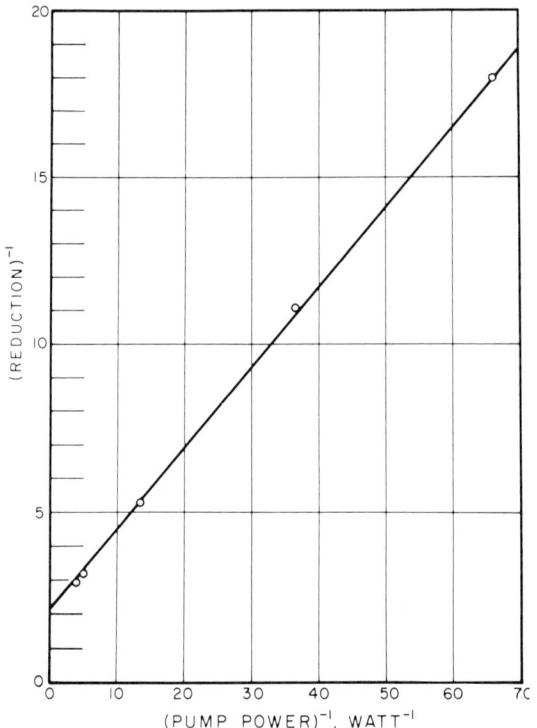

Figure 5-6. A plot of the reciprocal of the ELDOR reduction factor R versus the reciprocal of the pumping microwave power level for a $10^{-4}\,M$ solution of nitroxide radical (4-N-maleimido-2,2,6,6-tetramethylpiperidine nitroxide radical) in ethylbenzene at 193 K with the observing power near the maximum available (~ 800 mW). The low field ($M_I = +1$) line is observed and the central ($M_I = 0$) line is pumped. From J. S. Hyde et al., J. Chem. Phys., **48**, 4211 (1968).

equal to T_{1p}. The resulting equations are useful for describing the reduction dependence with power when intermolecular relaxation between different spin systems dominates.

In any event, assuming that the observing microwave is small, $2W_{so}T_{1c} \ll 1$ and thus the $2W_{so}T_{1e}$ term can be dropped from the denominator of eq. 5.1. Then substituting eq. 5.2 into eq. 5.1, we obtain

$$\frac{n_o^o}{n_o^o - n_o} = 1 + \frac{2T_{x2}}{T_{1e}} + (2W_{sp}T_{1e})^{-1}\left(1 + \frac{2T_{x2}}{T_{1e}} + \frac{T_{x2}T_{1e}}{T_{1e}T_{x1}}\right). \tag{5.3}$$

Since $1/R = (n_o^o)/(n_o^o - n_o)$, eq. 5.3 predicts that a plot of R^{-1} versus $W_{sp}^{-1} = $ (pump power)$^{-1}$ will give a linear plot with intercept $1 + 2T_{x2}/T_{1e}$.

Because of this dependence on the pump power level, it has been shown that values of R should be extrapolated to infinite pump power[1,6] and a value R_∞ deduced, that is, the value $1/R$ at the intercept of the straight line with the $(1/R)$ axis. From a plot of R_∞ versus $1/T$, we can make a quantitative evaluation of relaxation mechanisms, providing the effects of modulation frequency are taken into account (see Section 5.2.5). Benderskii et al.[7] have measured R_∞ as a function of temperature and concentration for the nitroxide radical 2,2,6,6-tetramethyl-4-oxopiperidine-1-oxide. Qualitatively a dependence (Fig. 5-7) similar to that in

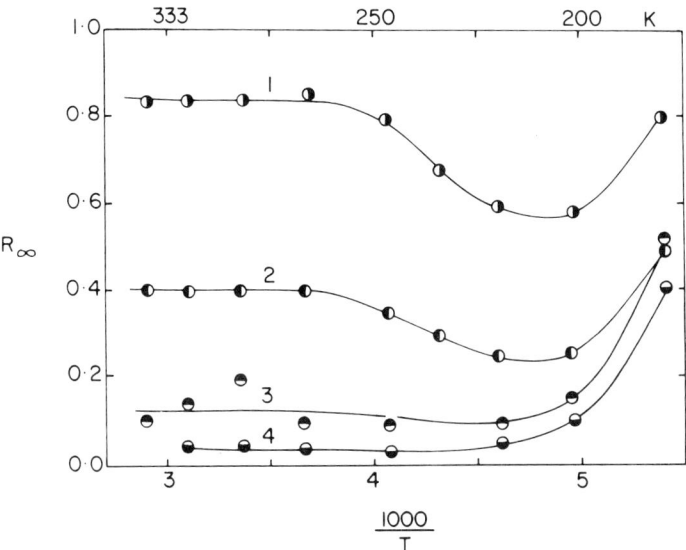

Figure 5-7. A plot of the ELDOR reduction factor R extrapolated to infinite pumping power (R_∞) at (1) 3×10^{-3} M, (2) 1×10^{-3} M, (3) 3×10^{-4} M, and (4) 1×10^{-4} M of the 2,2,6,6-tetramethyl-4-oxopiperidine-1-oxide radical in toluene. The low field $(M_I = +1)$ line is observed and the central $(M_I = 0)$ line is pumped. From V. A. Benderskii et al. *Mol. Phys.*, **24**, 449 (1972).

Fig. 5-4 was found; quantitatively, however, the shape of the curves is different. Although qualitatively Hyde, Chien, and Freed[1] agree with the results of Benderskii,[7] the differences in the curves result in different values for the relaxation times (T_{1e}).

As mentioned in the introduction, we only can obtain quantitative relaxation times from the reduction factors by including the modulation frequency in the theoretical analysis of the R factors. However, approximate parameters can be deduced directly from the R factors by recording the ELDOR spectra at low modulation frequencies[10,11] (270 Hz or below) where the modulation frequency dependence is minimal. If this is done, two major results can be obtained. First the rotational correlation time τ_c (the average time for a radical to rotate) as well as the type of the rotational motion undergone by the radical can be deduced for dilute samples ($\leq 10^{-3}$ M). Second, a test of the theoretical model for a given relaxation mechanism can be obtained by carrying out a careful measurement of the reduction factors for a given set of experimental conditions. Examples of these results are given in Sections 5.2.3 and 5.2.4, respectively. Unfortunately the reduction factors given as examples were obtained using 100 kHz field modulation, so errors as large as 50 to 100% in the reduction factors must be taken into account when considering the magnitude of the derived τ_c values.

5.2.3 Application to Molecular Motion Studies

As noted in Section 3.7.3.1, the single most important relaxation mechanism for both nuclear spins and electron spins is that caused by the radical tumbling in solution. This is because the tumbling motion of the radical causes a time dependent averaging of the anisotropic intramolecular electron-nuclear dipolar interaction[13,14] (anisotropic hyperfine coupling), a time dependent averaging of the anisotropic spectroscopic splitting factor (g_x, g_y, g_z), a time dependent averaging of the spin-rotational interaction, and a time dependent averaging of any existing quadrupole interaction. This averaging process causes the magnitude of the magnetic field at the electron to vary with time; this is reflected by a change in the spin-lattice relaxation time T_{1e} and a corresponding change in the observed ELDOR reduction factor. In a similar manner, pure anisotropic nuclear spin-flip interactions can be averaged[15,16] producing a change in the nuclear spin-lattice relaxation time T_{1n}.

Theoretically, values for the electron spin-flip transition probability W_e and the nuclear spin-flip transition probability W_n, or alternatively T_{1e}^{-1} and T_{1n}^{-1}, can be calculated from an exact solution of the time dependent Hamiltonian for a radical system undergoing a tumbling motion characterized by a rotational correlation time τ_c. From expressions for W_e and W_n a theoretical reduction factor can be calculated for each possible tumbling motion. A comparison of the theoretical and experimental reduction factors enables one to determine not only the rotational correlation time, but also the form of the tumbling motion exhibited by the radical. A difficulty with derivation of theoretical reduction factors is the nontrivial effort needed to solve the time dependent Hamiltonian. In some cases simplifying assumptions can be made. For instance, a first order perturbation treatment of the time dependent Hamiltonian is valid if $\omega_e\tau_c \gg 1$ and $\omega_n\tau_c \ll 1$. Since $\omega_e \simeq 6 \times 10^{10}$ Hz rad (the electron Zeeman frequency) and $\omega_n \simeq 8.7 \times 10^7$ Hz rad (nuclear Zeeman frequency) at X band frequencies; τ_c must be longer than approximately 10^{-11} sec but shorter than 10^{-8} sec. Fortunately this is the typical range of correlation times found for a number of free radicals in solution such as nitroxide radicals in reasonably nonviscous solvents like ethylbenzene. It is also fortunate for this range of τ_c that cross terms involving both electron and nuclear dipolar frequencies[13] can also be neglected, which further simplifies the calculation. In general, this is known as the intermediate tumbling region.

Expressions for W_e and W_n based on a perturbation calculation were given previously in eqs. 3.35 and 3.33 in which $W_e = C\tau_c(1+\omega_e^2\tau_c^2)^{-1}$ and $W_n^{END} = B\tau_c(1+\omega_n^2\tau_c^2)^{-1}$. To evaluate W_e and W_n^{END}, the functional relationship of the constant C to the g anisotropy and the spin-rotational interaction,[1,13] and the functional relationship of the constant B to the anisotropic dipolar terms, as well as τ_c must be known.

Specifically the electron spin probability (W_e^G) from rotational averaging of the g tensor is given by[13,14]

$$W_e^G = \left[\sum_{i=1}^{3} \frac{(g_i - g_s)^2}{40}\right]\left[\frac{\omega_e^2\tau_c}{1+\omega_e^2\tau_c^2}\right] \quad (5.4)$$

and the electron spin probability (W_e^{SR}) from the spin-rotational interaction, is expressed as[1,13]

$$W_e^{SR} = \sum_{i=1}^{3} \frac{(g_i - g_e)^2}{18\tau_c} \quad (5.5)$$

where the g_i's are the g_x, g_y, and g_z components of the g tensor,

$$g_s = \tfrac{1}{3}(g_x + g_y + g_z), \quad (5.6)$$

g_e is the free electron g value, ω_e is the angular microwave frequency at X band, and τ_c is the isotropic rotational correlation time defined from the Stokes–Einstein relation given in eq. 3.34.

Spin-rotational interaction arises because the electron cannot rigidly follow the moment of the nuclear framework as the radical rotates. This imbalance of the rotating charge generates an angular momentum that can interact with the electron spin. Since both the spin rotation and the rotational angular momentum depend on lattice position and orientation, they can give rise to a relaxation mechanism. The intramolecular spin-rotational relaxation interaction is independent of changes in concentrations and solvent[16] and is observed as an ESR linewidth contribution that is independent of the anisotropy of the hyperfine tensors.

Note that the ratio of these mechanisms (eq. 5.4 and 5.5) is

$$\frac{W_e^G}{W_e^{SR}} = 0.45\left(\frac{\omega_e^2 \tau_c}{1+\omega_e^2\tau_c^2}\right) X \left[\frac{\sum_i (g_i - g_s)^2}{\sum_i (g_i - g_e)^2}\right]. \qquad (5.7)$$

For most organic radicals in solution the last bracket term will be close to unity as $g_s \simeq g_e = 2.0023$. Then when $\omega_e\tau_c > 1$ we have

$$\frac{W_e^G}{W_e^{SR}} \propto \frac{\omega_e^2\tau_c^2}{\omega_e^2\tau_c^2} \sim 1. \qquad (5.8)$$

Since both W_e^{SR} and W_e^G are inversely proportional to τ_c when $\omega_e\tau_c \gg 1$, W_e can be redefined to reflect this dependence by eq. 3.38. Using the relationship that $\tau_c \propto \eta/T$ eq. 3.34 results in

$$W_e = \frac{CT}{\eta}. \qquad (5.9)$$

Note that W_e can be approximated for a radical in solution by measuring the viscosity of the solution as a function of temperature, providing that the anisotropic g values are known.

W_n^{END} can be evaluated from

$$W_n^{END} = \tfrac{1}{10}\gamma_e^2\gamma_n^2\hbar^2 \sum_m (D_n^{(m)} D_n^{(-m)})\tau_c \qquad (5.10)$$

where γ_n and γ_e are the nuclear and electron magnetogyric ratios and the $D_n^{(\pm m)}$ are electron-nuclear dipolar terms that must be calculated. Typically the value of W_n^{END} for a nitrogen nucleus in nitroxide radicals is approximately an order of magnitude larger than that for protons since the electron density lies on adjacent carbon atoms for α protons whereas the ^{14}N nucleus interacts with its own $2p\pi$ unpaired electron density. As before $\tau_c \propto \eta/T$ can be substituted into eq. 3.39 to give

$$W_n^{END} = \frac{B\eta}{T} \qquad (5.11)$$

so that W_n^{END} can be approximated experimentally given the value of B from the leading terms in eq. 5.10.

Although an experimental value of τ_c could be obtained according to eq. 3.34 ($\tau_c \propto \eta/T$), a large error will result if the tumbling of the radical in solution does not behave as a sphere of radius a in a medium of viscosity η. Therefore to obtain experimental values of τ_c it is necessary to express the R factors in terms of the relaxation parameters W_e, W_n, etc. This requires that the appropriate transition probability matrix be

Table 5-1. ELDOR Reduction Factor R for Strongly Saturated Observing Transitions of a Single $I = 1$ Nucleus[a]

Line Pumped	Line Observed		
	+1	0	−1
+1	–	$b/(1+3b)$	$b^2/(1+3b+2b^2)$
0	$(b+2b^2)/(1+4b+3b^2)$	⋯	$(b+2b^2)/(1+4b+3b^2)$
−1	$b^2/(1+3b+2b^2)$	$b/(1+3b)$	–

[a] The table gives the results for END mechanisms only where $b = W_n/W_e$. For Heisenberg chemical exchange only, replace all nonzero elements in the table by $b''/(1+2b'')$ where $b'' = W_{ex}/6W_e$ and $W_{ex} = W_{HE} + W_{CE}$, where W_{HE} and W_{CE} are the Heisenberg and chemical exchange frequencies, respectively. From J. S. Hyde et al., *J. Chem. Phys.*, **48**, 4211 (1968).

evaluated according to procedures outlined in Section 1.5.2.2 (see eqs. 1.20 to 1.26 for the case where $I = \frac{1}{2}$ and $S = \frac{1}{2}$). The results of such a calculation where the observing transitions of a dilute nitroxide sample are strongly saturated[1] are given in Table 5-1 in terms of the parameter b where $b = W_n/W_e$. It must be pointed out that these expressions are valid for $b \ll 1$ if an END mechanism predominates. Note that when the $M_I = 0$ nitrogen line is observed and the $M_I = +1$ line (low field) is pumped, $R = b/1 + 3b$, and with $b \ll 1$, $R \simeq b$. On the other hand, if the pumped and observed intervals are separated by two hyperfine intervals, that is, $M_I = -1$ is observed and $M_I = +1$ is pumped, then $R = b^2/(1+3+2b^2)$ and with $b \ll 1$, $R \simeq b^2$. Thus a significant decrease is predicted in the ELDOR intensity with increasing separation of the pumped and observing microwave frequencies. This dependence was previously shown in Section 5.2.1 to be true experimentally for the nitroxide radical. Note also that if b is calculated in terms of the redefined magnitudes of W_n (eq. 5.11) and W_e, (eq. 5.9), then $b \equiv W_n/W_e = (B/A)(\eta/T)^2$. Since $R \simeq b$ when the END mechanism predominates, it is possible to explain why the functional form of the R factor as a function of $1/T$ shown in Fig. 5-7 below 230 K appears as a parabolic curve.

Once the expressions of R in terms of W_e, W_n^{END}, etc., are obtained, and experimental values of R measured, values of τ_c can be calculated from expressions such as those given in Table 5-1 and the definition of W_e and W_n in eqs. 5.4, 5.5, and 5.10.

Values of the anisotropic g and D terms can usually be obtained by independent measurements or calculations. However keep in mind that a number of assumptions have been made. For instance, one must assume that W_e is composed of only W_e^{SR} and W_e^G, that the ELDOR reduction factors have been measured under strongly saturating conditions, that the proper detecting mode and modulation frequency have been used, and that R values have been extrapolated to infinite pumping power.[1,6-8] Let us estimate τ_c for nitroxide radicals.[1] The anisotropic D and g values have been measured by McConnell et al.[17] so W_e^{SR}, W_e^G, and W_n^{END} can be evaluated in terms of τ_c. Here the total W_e is just the sum of the two separate contributions since this is like adding rates of various channels to get the total rate. Then for $\omega_e \tau_c > 1$ with the D and g values of McConnell et al. $W_e \simeq 3.7 \times 10^{-6} \tau_c^{-1}$ sec^{-1} and $W_n^{END} \simeq 3.55 \times 10^{15} \tau_c$ sec^{-1} so $b = W_e/W_n \simeq 9.6 \times 10^{20} \tau_c^2$. From experimental values of R at 193, 223 and 253 K; $b = 1, 0.39$, and 0.14 for which $\tau_c = 3.2, 2.0$, and 1.2×10^{-11} sec, respectively.[1]

Even though the preceding calculation is adequate for radicals with rotational correlation times shorter than 10^{-8} sec, a number of examples exist for which τ_c is longer. In these cases the condition $|H_1(t)|\tau_c \ll 1$ required in the perturbation treatment[14,18] is no longer valid[19,20] and we must turn to another method of calculating τ_c. The function $H_1(t)$ mentioned here includes terms that are randomly changed (modulated) by the tumbling motion of the radical and lead to line broadening and relaxation. An example of this is the electron-nuclear dipolar term (the anisotropic hyperfine coupling) for nitrogen, which may have a magnitude as large as 10^8 Hz and thus $H_1(t)\tau_c \sim 1.0$ for $\tau_c = 10^{-8}$ sec. This violates the $|H_1(t)| \tau_c < 1$ condition needed for a valid perturbation calculation and eqs. 5.4, 5.5, and 5.11 used for calculating τ_c in ethylbenzene are no longer valid.

A method valid for calculating spectral lineshapes for all τ_c is Kubo's stochastic Liouville method.[21,22] The stochastic Liouville method is a time dependent probability treatment of the random motions undergone by a radical in a viscous medium. Freed[19] has expanded Kubo's stochastic Liouville method by starting from the density matrix equations of motion (a mathematically calculable form of the time dependent spin Hamiltonian) so that the microwave field can be included and saturation effects studied. Excellent agreement between the theoretical and experimental ESR lineshapes has been found[19,20] for nitroxides and for the peroxylamine disulfonate radical. It has been found that the off-diagonal terms in the density matrix (pseudosecular dipolar terms) make significant contributions to the slow tumbling ESR lineshapes. In a perturbation treatment these terms must be small for a valid calculation to be made. Normally this is not the case and exact calculations must be carried out.

By the stochastic Liouville approach various diffusional motions[20,22] have been detected from analysis of ESR spectral lineshapes of peroxylamine disulfonate (PADS) radical dissolved in 85% glycerol solution and in frozen H_2O and D_2O. Such motions are isotropic Brownian rotation,[23,8] anisotropic rotational reorientation,[24] free diffusion,[9,8,20,25,26] and jump diffusion.[9,20,25,26] Isotropic Brownian rotation is obtained from a simple model of a spherical molecule of radius a embedded in a fluid of viscosity η. As the sphere rotates it experiences a viscous torque. Equating this to the Stokes–Einstein relation for rotational diffusion results in an equation for the rotational correlation time $\tau_c = 4\pi \eta a^3/3kT$ as we have used before.

Anisotropic rotational reorientation[24] assumes that the radical undergoes an anisotropic motion instead of the isotropic motion of isotropic Brownian motion.[20] Jump diffusion occurs when a molecule has a fixed orientation for a time τ_c and then jumps instantaneously to a new orientation.[20,25] Free diffusion occurs when the molecule reorients freely for a time τ_c (inertia motion) and then jumps instantaneously to a new orientation. However even Kubo's stochastic Liouville method for calculating ESR lineshapes has its limitations because the unsaturated lineshapes of ESR spectra are sensitive to rotational correlation times ranging only from 10^{-11} sec to $>10^{-6}$ sec. In fact, the rigid limit in glasses is considered to be $>10^{-6}$ sec. Because various biological molecules exhibit rotational motion on the order of 10^{-3} to 10^{-7} sec,[8] various nonlinear electron spin resonance techniques have been used to try to measure these times.[8,27,28] The term *nonlinear* refers to ESR or double resonance experiments where the form of the signal observed depends on the relaxation processes. By studying saturated ESR lineshapes, Goldman, Bruno, and Freed[27] were able to extend the range over which τ_c could be measured to slower motions than possible with unsaturated lineshapes. Hyde and Dalton[28] have shown that the modulation frequency dependence of adiabatic rapid passage signals appears to be an effective technique to estimate very long $\tau_c (10^{-7} < \tau_c < 10^{-3}$ sec). Another study[8,9] showed that ELDOR spectra are sensitive to molecular motion characterized by correlation times in the range of 10^{-3} to 10^{-7} sec. Only this last technique will be described here.

It has been shown that the response of spin systems to an intense microwave field is critically dependent on the efficiency with which spins transfer energy to the lattice in addition to the efficiency with which energy is transferred between resonant and nonresonant portions of the spin system.[29] This effect is known as *spectral diffusion*. If the radical concentration is of the order of $10^{-3} M$ or greater, a transfer of spin energy (spectral diffusion) can occur by a Heisenberg exchange mechanism (an intermolecular relaxation between neighboring electron spins). However, it was shown[29] that spectral diffusion at low concentration can also occur by modulation of the anisotropic magnetic interaction by the

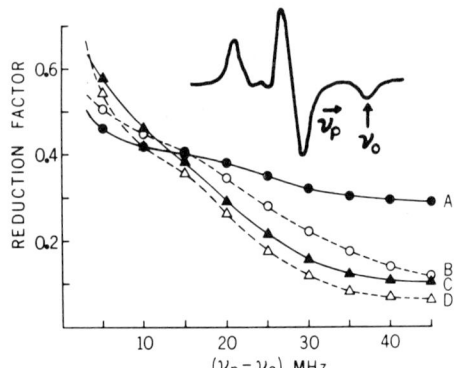

Figure 5-8. The ELDOR reduction factor as a function of the frequency difference $(\nu_p - \nu_0)$ between 5 to 45 MHz for 10^{-3} M tanol (2,2,6,6-tetramethyl-4-pyrolidinol-1-oxyl) in sec-butylbenzene at temperatures of (A) 166.5 K, (B) 159 K, (C) 153 K, and (D) 143 K. Correlation times estimated from the microscopic viscosities for these temperatures are (A) $\eta = 110P$, $\tau_c = 2 \times 10^{-6}$ sec; (B) $\eta = 1100P$, $\tau_c = 2 \times 10^{-5}$ sec; (C) $\eta = 11,000P$, $\tau_c = 2 \times 10^{-4}$ sec; (D) $\eta = 3 \times 10^6 P$, $\tau_c = 5 \times 10^{-2}$ sec. Field modulation of 14 G peak to peak amplitude at a frequency of 270 Hz, a pump microwave field of 0.32 G, and an observer microwave field of 0.063 G were used. From M. D. Smigel et al., *Proc. Nat. Acad. Sci. U.S.*, **71**, 1925 (1974).

molecular motion. This occurs in the following manner. In viscous media paramagnetic molecules with different orientations contribute to different portions of the ESR spectrum. If the energy levels belonging to one group of orientations are saturated, upon molecular reorientation the saturation will be transferred to that portion of the spectrum belonging to a second orientation. In this way a transfer of saturation to another part of the spectrum has occurred.

To measure saturation transfer by ELDOR,[8] the observing microwave field is positioned at the high field turning point (the point labeled ν_o on the ESR spectrum in Fig. 5-8) of an ESR spectrum of a nitroxide radical, tanol (Fig. 5-8), or HDA (Fig. 5-9) in sec-butylbenzene.[30] Then the frequency of the primary microwave field is applied at +45 MHz from the observing field and a field swept ELDOR spectrum is obtained. This gives a value for R at 45 MHz on line A in Fig. 5-8 or Fig. 5-9. Additional experiments are run at other frequency differences, resulting in line A (Fig. 5-8). Results are obtained from 166.5 K (line A, Fig. 5-8) to 143 K (line D, Fig. 5-8). As the temperature decreases with a consequent increase in viscosity, there is a decrease in the reduction factor at $\Delta \nu = 45$ MHz. This is a consequence of the rotational correlation time decreasing from 2×10^{-6} to 5×10^{-2} sec. Magnetic field modulation effects on R are eliminated by using 270 Hz modulation.

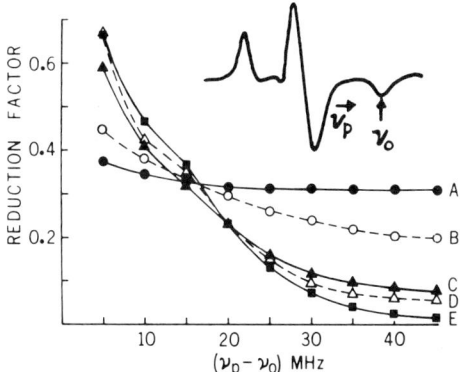

Figure 5-9. The ELDOR reduction factors for $10^{-3}\,M$ HDA (17β-hydroxy-4',4'-dimethylspiro[5α-androstane-3,2'-oxazolidin]-3'-oxyl) in sec-butylbenzene at temperatures of (A) 175.5 K, (B) 166.5 K, (C) 159 K, (D) 153 K, and (E) 143 K. The spectra were obtained for the same instrument settings as used in Fig. 5-8. From M. D. Smigel, *Proc. Nat. Acad. Sci. U.S.*, **71**, 1925 (1974).

A calculation of the reduction factors based on the stochastic Liouville method shows good agreement at intermediate temperatures (A, B, and C) with the experimental results of a jump diffusion model when a diffusive step size of approximately 0.15 rad is used. A diffusive step is defined as the net angular movement in time τ. Considerable deviation is found between the calculated and experimental curves D and E (Fig. 5-9) suggesting that the spin labels continue to rotate after appreciable ordering of the solvent exists. Preliminary studies on larger biological molecules indicate that their random motions are better described by Brownian diffusion.

5.2.4 Application to Magnetic Relaxation

We now turn our attention to using ELDOR reduction factors to test the theoretical model that is used to describe a given relaxation mechanism. A number of ELDOR active relaxation mechanisms are known to occur in solution; included among these are Heisenberg exchange (HE), chemical exchange, spectral diffusion (both rotational and translational diffusion), and nuclear relaxation. In Section 5.2.3 it was shown that a rotational correlation time could be calculated from the experimental reduction factors if an assumption were made concerning the predominant contributions to the relaxation. However, in this section we show that the reduction factors can also be used to test the model employed to describe a relaxation mechanism (in this particular instance, Heisenberg exchange) and to determine the relaxation rates for multiequivalent nuclei.

At concentrations of radicals above 10^{-3} M, Heisenberg exchange can be a significant relaxation mechanism.[15,10] Qualitatively this relaxation mechanism occurs because an electron-electron dipolar interaction between electron spins on neighboring radicals occurs that significantly contributes to the spin-lattice relaxation of all hyperfine lines of a given radical. Chemical exchange is a related relaxation mechanism in which a collision between a radical and a parent molecule with a different nuclear spin configuration transfers the electron spin to a different environment.[15] In other words, in chemical exchange it appears that the unpaired electron is being transferred to a different nuclear site. Since the behavior of these two intermolecular mechanisms is similar they will be considered together.

Based on the preceding model of Heisenberg and chemical exchange,[1] the theoretical reduction factors for all entries in Table 5-1 have been found to be equal to $b''/1+2b''$ where b'' is equal to $W_{ex}/6W_e$ (assuming Heisenberg or chemical exchange dominates). W_{ex} is the exchange frequency and equal to $W_{HE}+W_{CE}$ where W_{HE} and W_{CE} are the Heisenberg and chemical exchange frequencies, respectively. The effect of W_{ex} is to equalize the population differences between all pairs of hyperfine levels. Since most Heisenberg exchange studies appear to be consistent with a strong exchange,[31,18] $W_{HE} = 16\pi Da[R]$ where D is the translational diffusion coefficient defined in a Stokes–Einstein model by $D = kT/6\pi a\eta$ and $[R]$ is the radical concentration in molecules per cubic centimeter. By substituting D into $W_{HE} = 16\pi Da[R]$ we can define $W_{HE} = 6C[R]T/\eta$ so that if W_{HE} predominates, then $b'' = W_{HE}/6W_e = (C/A)[R]$. Chemical exchange is usually not diffusion controlled so that its temperature dependence is generally different from that of D, yet its rate increases with temperature.[32]

If this model is correct, then one would observe the ELDOR intensity to be independent of the hyperfine frequency interval in addition to being independent of temperature since b'' is independent of temperature. In fact, this has been verified quantitatively[6] by a study of the reduction factors (R) measured for aqueous solutions of peroxylamine disulfonate dianion radicals (PADS). From such a study it is also possible to show that the spin-lattice relaxation time (T_{1e}^λ) for the λth (degenerate) hyperfine line equals

$$T_{1e}^\lambda = T_{1e}(0)\left(\frac{1+D_\lambda b''}{1+\frac{1}{2}Nb''}\right) \qquad (5.12)$$

$$T_{1e}(0) = (2W_e)^{-1} \qquad (5.13)$$

where $T_{1e}(0)$ is the concentration independent value of T_{1e}, D_λ is the degeneracy of the λth transition, $b'' = W_{HE}/NW_e$ where W_{HE} is the exchange frequency, N is equal to the number of spin eigenstates, and W_e is the electron spin-flip transition probability. For instance, in the case of a nitroxide radical, $D_\lambda = 1$ and $N = 6$.

In addition, b'' is related to the experimental reduction factor extrapolated to infinite power R_∞ by the following equation:

$$R_\infty^{-1} - 1 = (D_p b'')^{-1} \qquad (5.14)$$

where D_p is the degeneracy of the pumped line and R_∞ is the experimental reduction factor extrapolated to infinite pump power. A value of R_∞ for each concentration permits a measurement of b'' from eq. 5.14. From a progressive saturation measurement under slow passage conditions[33] of each line, a value of T_{1e}^λ can be obtained if the linewidth is only a function of T_{2e}. A value of $T_{1e}(0)$ can then be determined from eq. 5.12 and used to obtain a value of W_e from eq. 5.13. Since $b'' = W_{HE}/NW_e$, a value of W_{HE} can be calculated for each concentration. One can then determine the contributions of these terms to the linewidth. From this a residual linewidth presumably due to g-tensor and spin-rotational terms can be found. Experimentally when Heisenberg exchange dominates, b'' has been found to be greater for Coppinger's radical than for a nitroxide radical because of the differences in $T_{1e}(0)$ for the two radicals.

Experiments of this type have also been used in a study of the relaxation in orbitally degenerate free radicals[5] to determine the contributions of the Heisenberg exchange mechanism to the linewidth. This permits an independent check on the anomalous residual linewidth, which suggests that the residual linewidth is indeed due to some anomalous spin-orbit-type process. The dominant ELDOR mechanism for the benzene radical anion is electron exchange with unreduced benzene.

Although the general relaxation theory for ELDOR spectroscopy in terms of the magnitude of the lattice-induced spin relaxation rates such as W_e (electron spin-flips), W_n (nuclear spin-flips), and W_{ex} (Heisenberg and/or chemical exchange frequencies) is fully applicable to complicated magnetic resonance spectra involving many magnetic nuclei, calculations have been reported for only a few simple radicals with a small number of magnetic nuclei. Such a calculation[1] for the nitroxide radical was given in Section 5.2.3. In more complicated cases a separate computer solution is required for each situation. However as the number of nuclei increases, even the computer solution becomes unwieldy.[4] For instance, an exact computer calculation of the magnetic relaxations for three or more equivalent methyl groups is nearly impossible.

In order to study those cases where many nuclei interact, approximate expressions have been derived[4] and are given in Table 5-2 for the

Table 5-2. Average ELDOR Reduction Factors[a]

Number of Completely Equivalent Nuclei		R[b]
	1	$\dfrac{\frac{1}{2}b(1 \pm 2M_o)}{2-b}$
	2	$\dfrac{\frac{1}{2}b(1 \pm M_o)}{1-b}$
(1 methyl group)	3	$\dfrac{\frac{1}{2}b(3 \pm 2M_o)}{2-3b}$
	4	$\dfrac{\frac{1}{2}b(2 \pm M_o)}{1-2b}$
	5	$\dfrac{\frac{1}{2}b(5 \pm 2M_o)}{2-5b}$
(2 methyl groups)	6	$\dfrac{\frac{1}{2}b(3 \pm M_o)}{1-3b}$
(3 methyl groups)	9	$\dfrac{b}{2}\dfrac{(9 \pm 2M_o)}{2-9b}$
(4 methyl groups)	12	$\dfrac{\frac{1}{2}b(6 \pm M_o)}{1-6b}$

[a] $b'' = 0$ (no Heisenberg exchange), END mechanism dominates. If Heisenberg exchange predominates, replace all R values by $D_p b''$ (D_p = degeneracy of the pumped line).

[b] The R factors have been calculated assuming that the separation between the pump and observing microwave frequencies equals one hyperfine interval. The plus (+) sign is used if $M_p = M_o - 1$ (the nuclear spin quantum number for the pumped line is one less than the observed line) and the negative (−) sign if $M_p = M_o + 1$. See eq. 4.8 of ref. 4 for reduction factors involving larger numbers of equivalent nuclei. If one includes the effects of cross transitions (i.e., combined electron-nuclear spin-flips) b is replaced by $(b^2 - c_1 c_2)/[b + \frac{1}{2}(c_1 + c_2)]$ where c_1 and c_2 are proportional to the cross-relaxation rates W_{x1} and W_{x2}, respectively, and are defined in eqs. B9a and B9b of ref. 4.

expected field swept ELDOR reduction factors for dilute concentrations of free radicals in liquids where $b \ll 1$, $b \equiv W_n/W_e$, the END relaxation mechanism predominates, and Heisenberg exchange has been neglected. This situation can arise when W_n results from rotational modulation of the electron-nuclear dipolar (END) interactions. In this situation W_n is usually much smaller than W_e, providing W_e results from spin-rotational or g-tensor interactions. This seemingly does occur for methyl protons because their internal rotational motion averages the END terms more than, say, for a ring proton. The approximate equations given for R in Table 5-2 are referred to as *average* ELDOR reductions.[4] These expressions take the simple form of an average ELDOR lineshape and will reproduce the exact expressions of b when $b \ll 1$. The equations are only valid for $b'' = 0$ (negligible Heisenberg exchange).

These equations have been derived for completely equivalent nuclei. However in many cases equivalent nuclei are observed that are not completely equivalent. This occurs when nuclei possess identical average hyperfine splittings but their relaxation properties are not identical. This may be a result of an out-of-phase correlation of the fluctuation in the isotropic hyperfine interaction or it may be due to the relative orientational position of their respective END interactions. Despite the assumption of complete equivalence it has been found that satisfactory results may be obtained by treating each equivalent group of nuclei as being a completely equivalent group whether it is or not. Thus Table 5-2 can be used to predict the magnitude of b for a number of chemically interesting systems.

If chemical or Heisenberg exchange dominates, then the asymptotic reductions (reduction factors extrapolated to infinite pump power) observed for very large pump powers and small observing power will depend on the degeneracy of the pump line D_p times b'' for each line where $b'' = W_{ex}/6W_e$.

In general, when both END and exchange terms contribute to the ELDOR signal, the two contributions may be separated by measuring the ELDOR reductions for low enough concentration ($10^{-4} M$) so as to remove exchange effects or by cooling samples of moderate concentrations to enhance the END contribution. These reduction factors can then be extrapolated to infinite pump powers and used to calculate the parameters of the relaxation mechanism under study.

5.2.5 Modulation Frequency Influence on *R* Factors

In Section 1.5.4 qualitative reasons were given why ELDOR reduction factors are dependent on the modulation frequency whenever the cycle time of the modulation frequency is competitive with the spin-lattice relaxation time (T_{1e}) or with the rotational correlation time of the radical. Quantitatively this modulation frequency dependence has been evaluated both theoretically and experimentally[10] as a function of $\omega_J T_{1e}$ where ω_J is the molecular energy transfer rate (ω_J can be the jump rate between two or more sites caused by molecular tumbling, Heisenberg spin exchange between two electron spins, W_{ex}, or intramolecular nuclear spin relaxation W_n). The frequency dependence also has been determined as a function of the ratio of the pump to the observing microwave power at different degrees of saturation of the observed ESR signal; as a function of the ratio T_{1e}/T_{2e} where T_{2e} is the spin-spin relaxation time; and as a function of different modes of ESR detection.

In order to appreciate the marked frequency dependence that can be found, one must first be aware of the field swept ELDOR lineshapes that result for different modes of ESR detection when a reduction in the ESR signal is observed. These are given in Fig. 5-10 for the first derivative presentation of (a) the absorption ESR signal in phase with the applied modulation and (b) the dispersion signal in phase with the modulation. In addition, the field swept ELDOR lineshape is given in Fig. 5-10 for the second derivative presentation of (c) the absorption ESR signal in phase with the applied modulation, and (d) the dispersion signal in phase with

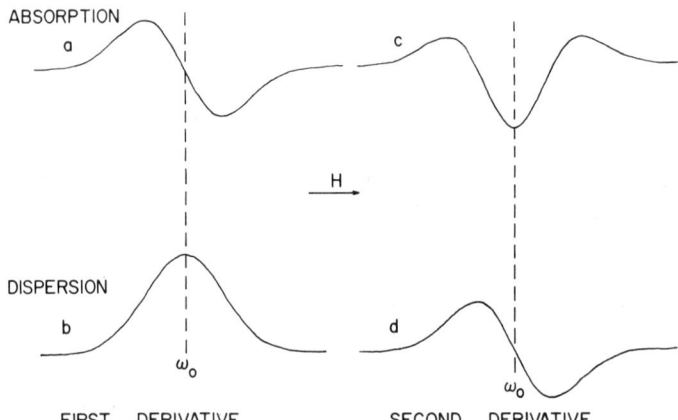

Figure 5-10. The lineshape of the first derivative presentation (first harmonic of the modulation) of the (a) adsorption and (b) dispersion ESR signal in phase with the modulation and the lineshape of the second derivative presentation (second harmonic of the modulation) of the (c) adsorption and (d) dispersion ESR signal in phase with the modulation. The magnetic field increases to the right. All out-of-phase ESR signals have similar lineshapes with increasing magnetic field. Adapted from B. H. Robinson et al., *Chem. Phys. Lett.*, **28**, 169 (1974).

the modulation. Note that as the magnetic field increases to the right, the first derivative presentation of the absorption (a) appears as a positive lobe and then a negative lobe with increasing magnetic field, similar in appearance to the second derivative presentation of the dispersion mode (d). On the other hand, the second derivative presentation of the absorption has a peak below the base line with increasing field and is opposite in phase to the first derivative presentation of the dispersion mode. Equivalent terms often used to describe the first and second derivative presentation are the first and second harmonic of the modulation, respectively. It is also possible under certain conditions to detect reduced ESR signals of each of these modes when the detector is set out of phase with the applied field modulation. Examples of this phenomena will be given later in this section but first we consider the in-phase frequency dependence.

As defined in Section 5.2 all field swept R factors are calculated according to the definition in Section 5.2 as $R = 1 - I/I_o$ where I is usually taken experimentally as the ESR signal height with the pump on and I_o as the ESR signal height with the pump off.

Using this definition the field swept reduction factor (R) for the first derivative absorption mode can be calculated from the heights of the ESR lines derived theoretically from a modified stochastic Liouville equation using the spin density matrix representation of the spin system.[10] Similar results are also obtained from an analysis of the Bloch equation.[11] As an example of the type of modulation frequency dependence that might appear, a plot of the reduction factors calculated for a nitroxide radical as a function of $\omega_J T_{1e}$ is given in Fig. 5-11 for no modulation (open circles, $\omega_m T_{1e} = 0$) and for an applied modulation (solid circles, $\omega_m T_{1e} = 3$), assuming homogeneously broadened ESR lines. The reduction factors in the absence of field modulation are larger than those in the presence of field modulation over the entire range of $\omega_J T_{1e}$ values plotted. Specifically if the modulation frequency ν_m (where $\omega_m = 2\pi\nu_m$) equals 100 kHz, the lower curve (solid circles) corresponds to the situation where $T_{1e} = 4.8 \times 10^{-6}$ sec. If T_{1e} is longer, for example 1.6×10^{-6} sec, then $\omega_m T_{1e} = 1$, a value corresponding to a curve intermediate between the two shown in Fig. 5-11. Furthermore if $T_{1e} = 1.6 \times 10^{-6}$ sec and lower modulation frequencies (270 Hz or 1 kHz) are employed, the reduction factors are approximately independent of modulation frequency and vary with $\omega_J T_{1e}$ according to the top curve in Fig. 5-11. However if T_{1e} is longer, such as typically found for nitroxide spin labels[9] where $T_{1e} = 10^{-5}$ sec, then $\omega_m T_{1e} = 6.28$ at 100 kHz field modulation and equals 0.017 at 270 Hz. In this situation modulation frequency effects are predicted to be observed at most modulation frequencies above 270 Hz.

The absolute magnitude of the difference in R factors with and without

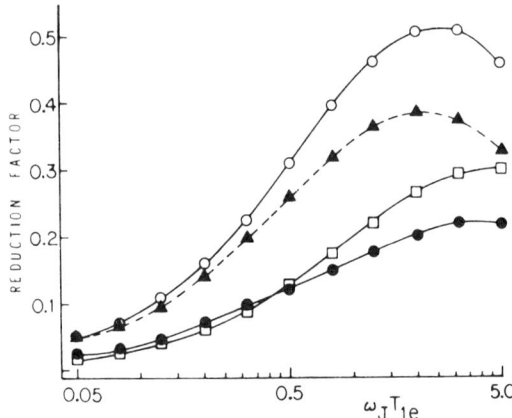

Figure 5-11. A plot of the calculated reduction factors as a function of the product of the molecular energy transfer rate ω_J and T_{1e} for the in-phase first derivative field swept absorption ^{14}N ELDOR signal for a value of $\omega_m T_{1e} = 0$ (open circles) and a value of $\omega_m T_{1e} = 3$ (solid circles) where $\omega_m = 2\pi\nu_m$ and ν_m equals the modulation frequency. The dashed line (solid triangles) represents the calculated first derivative in-phase field swept dispersion ^{14}N ELDOR for the same values of $\omega_m T_{1e}$. For comparison, the open squares represent the calculated first derivative frequency swept absorption in-phase ELDOR signal (discussed in Section 5.3) with $\omega_m T_{1e} = 0$. The calculations were carried out for the field swept ELDOR spectra with a frequency separation between the pumping and the observing microwave frequencies equal to $2f$, the exact frequency separation between the two ESR lines. For the frequency swept spectra $(\nu_p - \nu_o)$ equals the hyperfine splitting. Other parameters utilized in the calculation include the ratio of the pump to observer power (d_p/d_o) equal to 5, $T_{1e} = 10T_{2e}$, $f/2d_o = 1000$, $4d_o^2 T_{1e} T_{2e} = 0.07$, and the assumption of no interacting nuclei except for one ^{14}N. From B. H. Robinson et al., *Chem. Phys. Lett.*, **28**, 169 (1974).

modulation is also a function of the molecular energy transfer rate (ω_J) and increases with increasing values of $\omega_J T_{1e}$. For instance, at a value of $\omega_J T_{1e} = 0.05$, the difference in the expected R values equals approximately 0.02, whereas at a value of $\omega_J T_{1e} = 5$, the difference equals approximately 0.25. The decrease in reduction factors at large $\omega_J T_{1e}$ arises from spectral diffusion processes shortening T_{1e} and T_{2e}, making it more difficult to saturate the observed transition. These calculations are computed using $T_{1e} = 10T_{2e}$ with the ratio of the pump power to the observing power equal to 8. In addition, one may recall that average ELDOR reduction factors for field swept spectra were given in Table 5-2 for $b \ll 1$ where $b = W_n/W_e$. In terms of Freed's notation,[1] which was used in Section 5.2.3, $\omega_J T_{1e}$ equals $2\omega_J/\omega_e = 2b$ when $\omega_J = W_n$. From the graph in Fig. 5-11 a small modulation frequency effect is predicted for $b < 1$; however it would be insignificantly small at low modulation frequencies.

On the other hand, calculations show that the reduction factors for the dispersion mode ESR signal are independent of modulation frequency. For instance, in Fig. 5-11 the dashed line represents the calculated first derivative field swept dispersion ELDOR signal for $\omega_m T_{1e} = 0$ as well as for $\omega_m T_{1e} = 3$. In addition, we can observe that the frequency swept reduction factors (open squares, Fig. 5-11) are smaller than the field swept factors. A more detailed description of frequency swept ELDOR spectra will be given in Section 5.3.1.

Calculations have also been carried out for the second derivative presentation of the in-phase absorption signal that show a modulation dependence similar to the first derivative spectra.

In a calculation of the field swept reduction factor versus the ratio of the pumped (P_p) to the observing (P_o) microwave power, there is an interesting dependence on the degree of saturation of the observed transition. In Fig. 5-12 are plotted four graphs of reduction factor versus

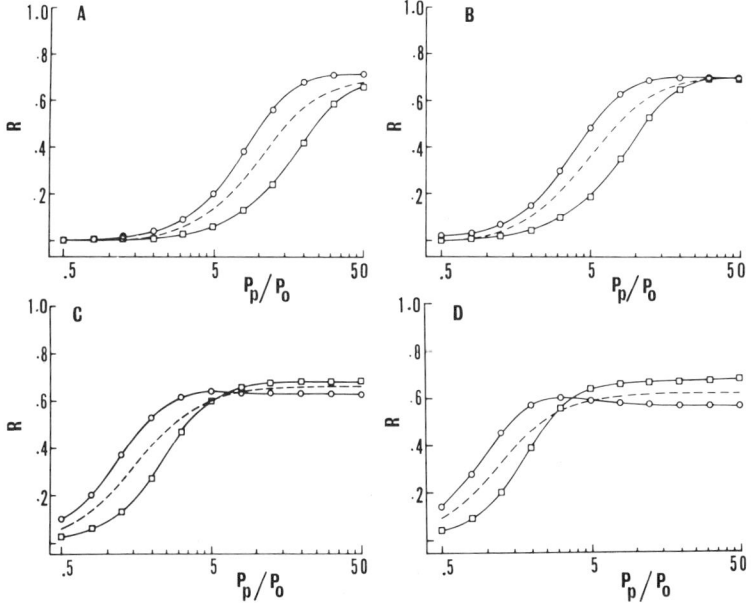

Figure 5-12. Calculated plots A, B, C, and D of the field swept ELDOR reduction factors for the first derivative in-phase absorption ESR signals for $\omega_m T_{1e} = 0$ (circles) and for $\omega_m T_{1e} = 3$ (squares) as a function of the ratio of the pump to the observer power (P_p/P_o). The observer powers used in plots A, B, C, and D correspond to values A, B, C, and D on the observer transition saturation curve given in Fig. 5-13. The dashed line represents the dispersion signal spectra, which are approximately independent of $\omega_m T_{1e}$. Other parameters used are $T_{1e} = T_{2e}$, $\omega_1 T_{1e} = 2.5$, and $f/2d_o = 1000$. From B. H. Robinson et al., *Chem. Phys. Lett.*, **28**, 169 (1974).

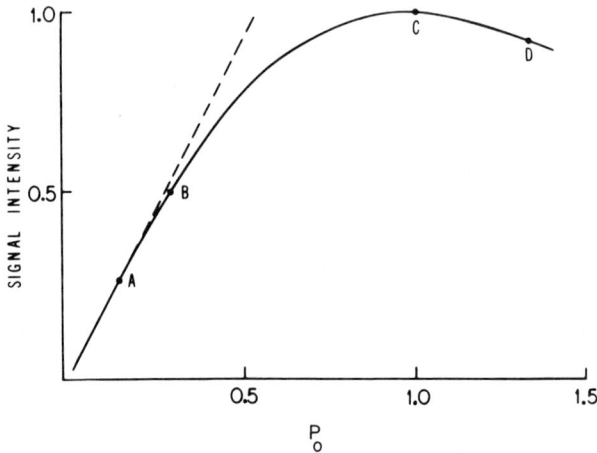

Figure 5-13. A calculation of signal intensity versus observer power (i.e., a power saturation curve) for a homogeneously broadened ESR line. Calculations for Fig. 5-12 were carried out at points A, B, C, and D where A and B lie on the linear response region of the saturation curve.

P_p/P_o for two $\omega_m T_{1e}$ values. The calculated points of the field swept ELDOR reduction factors for the first derivative in-phase absorption ESR signals for no modulation ($\omega_m T_{1e} = 0$) are denoted by circles, whereas those using modulation ($\omega_m T_{1e} = 3$) are denoted by squares. The dashed lines represent calculated reduction factors for the first derivative of the dispersion signal, which is independent of modulation frequency. Graphs A, B, C, and D correspond to the values of P_o denoted on the power saturation curve in Fig. 5-13. The general shape of the reduction factor curve is independent of P_o, merely being displaced along the axis. However most ELDOR measurements are recorded in the linear region of the saturation curve as denoted by the dashed line in Fig. 5-13. It is for these measurements (points A and B) that the greatest modulation frequency effect occurs for the first derivative in-phase absorption ESR signals, providing the P_p/P_o ratio is between a value of 2 and 20. A much smaller difference in reduction factors as a function of modulation frequency dependence is observed when $P_p/P_o > 5$ and the observing power is set at C. The reduction factors were also found to be insensitive to modulation amplitude as long as the modulation amplitude was much less than the spin packet linewidth. However measurable effects do occur when the amplitude approaches the linewidth.

In Fig. 5-14 a plot is given of the calculated field swept reduction factor versus modulation frequency (more specifically, $\omega_m T_{1e}$) when the ratio of T_{1e}/T_{2e} is varied from 1 (circles) to 10 (diamonds). A minimum in the

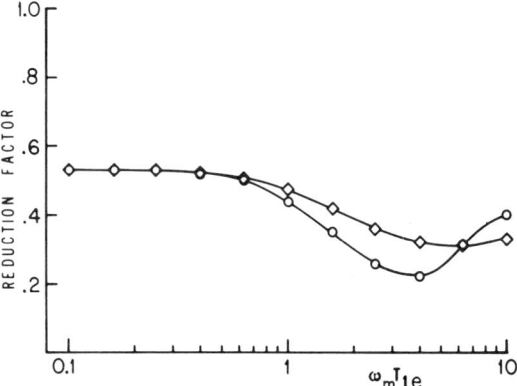

Figure 5-14. Calculated plots of the field swept ELDOR reduction factor for the first derivative in-phase absorption ESR signals as a function of $\omega_m T_{1e}$ for $T_{1e}/T_{2e} = 1$ (○) and $T_{1e}/T_{2e} = 10$ (◇). Other parameters used are $\omega_J T_{1e} = 2.5$, $P_P/P_o = 12$, and $f/2d_o = 1000$; P_o corresponds to point A in Fig. 5-13. From L. R. Dalton, unpublished results.

reduction factor is observed when $\omega_m T_{1e} = 3$ with the largest decrease in R found when $T_{1e} = T_{2e}$. Again insignificant effects are found if $\omega_m = 1.7 \times 10^3$ rad Hz (270 Hz) and $T_{1e} < 10^{-5}$ sec; however, measurable effects can be observed for nitroxide spin labels[11] if $\omega_m = 100$ kHz (6.3×10^5 rad Hz) since typically $T_{1e} = 10^{-5}$ sec for such radicals.

The decrease in the calculated value of the field swept absorption ELDOR reduction factors with increasing modulation frequency has been verified experimentally for the spin label perdeuterio-2,2,6,6-tetramethyl-4-piperidone-1-oxyl (perdeuterio-tanone) in viscous sec-butylbenzene at 204 K.[11] Furthermore for this system the field swept dispersion ELDOR reduction factors were found to be relatively insensitive to changes in modulaation frequency, a feature found to be characteristic of homogeneously or pseudohomogeneously broadened hyperfine lines.[11] On the other hand, when the ELDOR reduction factors were determined for a 1×10^{-3} M solution of 2,2,6,6-tetramethyl-4-piperidinol-1-oxyl in sec-butylbenzene at 204 K, the dispersion reduction factors decreased with decreasing modulation frequency although the frequency dependence of the absorption reduction factors remained the same.[11]

This difference is a direct consequence of the presence of proton hyperfine interactions that cause an inhomogeneous broadening of the hyperfine lines. In Fig. 5-15 a plot is given of the field swept dispersion ELDOR reduction factors computed from a stochastic Liouville equation treatment for the first derivative presentation in phase with the modulation as a function of P_o/P_p (the ratio of the observing power to pump

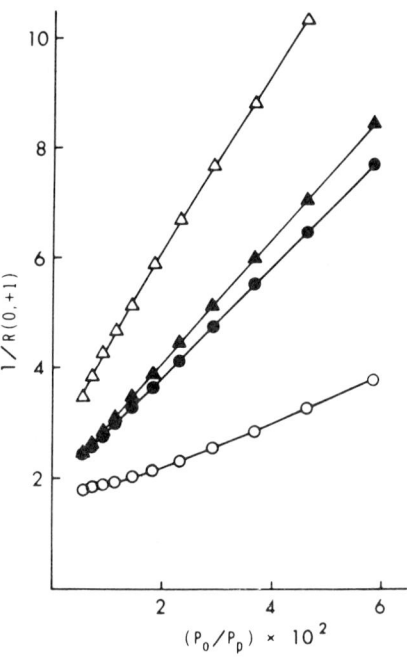

Figure 5-15. A plot of $1/R(0, +1)$ [where $R(0, +1)$ is the ELDOR reduction measured when the pumping microwave field pumps the $M_I(^{14}N) = 0$ ESR line while the observing microwave field monitors the $M_I(^{14}N) = +1$ ESR line] as a function of the ratio of the observing to pumping power (P_o/P_p) for the computed in-phase first derivative field swept dispersion ELDOR signals when the modulation frequency equals 10^5 Hz (○) and 10^4 Hz (△). The open circles and triangles are for calculations that include proton hyperfine interactions but assume proton nuclear spin relaxation rates are zero, and the solid triangles and circles correspond to calculations where proton hyperfine interactions are neglected. In these calculations $2H_m = 0.24$ G (the modulation field), $H_{obs} = 0.017$ G (observing microwave field), $\Omega_I = 9.1 \times 10^5$ sec^{-1}, $T_{1e} = 1.3 \times 10^{-6}$, and $T_{2e} = 2.76 \times 10^{-6}$ sec. From L. A. Dalton et al., *Chem. Phys.*, **6**, 166 (1974).

power) when proton superhyperfine interactions are included (open circles and triangles) and when they are not (solid circles and triangles). These results are in good agreement with experiment. Note that there exists relatively little difference between the calculated solid triangles (10 kHz modulation) and the solid circles (100 kHz modulation), indicating little frequency dependence for homogenously broadened lines. However the large difference in magnitude between the calculated first derivative dispersion reduction factors indicated by the open triangles and open circles demonstrates a very clear frequency dependence in which the reduction factors decrease with decreasing modulation frequency. It is also to be noted that a plot of R^{-1} versus P_o/P_p for the dispersion ELDOR R yields a straight line except at high pump power. This was predicted in Section 5.2.2.

Another experimental parameter that should be mentioned is the observation that an ESR signal can be observed with the modulation 90° out of phase with the applied modulation. A variation of the reduction factors with phase angle can also be obtained and will be given in more detail in the next section concerning frequency swept ELDOR studies.

In summary, these calculations and experimental measurements point out that modulation frequency effects are present to some degree in all

ELDOR measurements. However it should be pointed out that generally the modulation frequency dependence is neglible if modulation frequencies of 270 Hz or lower are employed.

Modulation frequency effects as a function of ω_J, T_{1e}, and T_{2e} can also be minimized if the modulation amplitude is much less than the spin packet linewidth, if an observing power is selected that results in the largest ESR signal height, if the ratio of the pump power to the observing power is greater than 5, and, in cases of homogeneous line broadening, if the ELDOR spectra are recorded in the dispersion mode.

In cases where the magnitude of the relaxation parameters or other quantitative values are to be deduced from the reduction factors, it is necessary to carry out an exact calculation of reduction factors using a time dependent spin Hamiltonian (solving the stochastic Liouville equation) that includes modulation effects. Such a calculation is nontrivial but necessary for deduction of quantitative values from the ELDOR data.

5.3 FREQUENCY SWEPT ELDOR SPECTRA: HYPERFINE LINES AND COMBINATION LINES

Although a great deal of information can be obtained from a field swept ELDOR experiment, it does require knowledge of the hyperfine splitting constants. Such information can be obtained from a field swept experiment by a tedious trial and error procedure. A spectroscopically more satisfactory method is to use the frequency swept ELDOR technique described in Chapter 2.

5.3.1 Conditions for Setting the Observing Field

As in the field swept experiment, an ELDOR line can appear when the difference frequency between the pumping and observing microwave frequencies equals a hyperfine interval. This is apparent if one considers the energy diagram in Fig. 5-1A. In a frequency swept ELDOR experiment, the magnetic field is set at the resonance position of one of the ESR lines. In the example here this magnetic field is that of the high field line (K) of Fig. 5-1A. The observing microwave frequency is set to a constant frequency ν_o, and the pump microwave frequency is swept to higher frequencies. As the pump frequency approaches the value ν_p (where $\nu_p - \nu_o$ = hyperfine splitting interval) depicted in 5-1A, there will be a transfer of saturation to the low field portion of the observed ESR line (K) followed by a transfer to the high field portion of the observed

ESR line. Because of this the lineshape of a frequency swept ELDOR line can vary markedly depending on the observing field position. Note from Fig. 5-1A that when $\nu_p > \nu_o$, the pump microwave frequency will sweep through energy levels that give rise to ESR lines at lower magnetic fields than the observed ESR line, whereas when $\nu_p < \nu_o$ (Fig. 5-18), the pump frequency sweeps through energy levels that give rise to ESR lines at higher magnetic fields than the observed ESR line.

Since the frequency swept ELDOR lineshape does vary with field position, Hyde et al.[3] have derived equations for the ELDOR lineshapes and frequency positions as a function of the observing magnetic field for both homogeneously and inhomogeneously broadened lines in the absence of modulation frequency effects. If the observing field is set at the crossover (zero slope of the absorption curve) of a first derivative homogeneous or inhomogeneous absorption ESR line, a first derivative, frequency swept ELDOR line will be observed. Figure 5-16 explains this schematically for the situation where $\nu_p > \nu_o$. The field modulation causes the experimental detection system to see a portion of the ESR of width equal to the modulation amplitude H_m centered at ω_o (Fig. 5-16a). If H_m equals the ESR derivative linewidth, when the observing ELDOR frequency reaches the low field peak of the derivative ESR line an ELDOR response will be observed (Fig. 5-16b). This response may be a reduction or an enhancement as shown in the two columns in Fig. 5-16. As the observing ELDOR frequency moves across the ESR line, the ELDOR

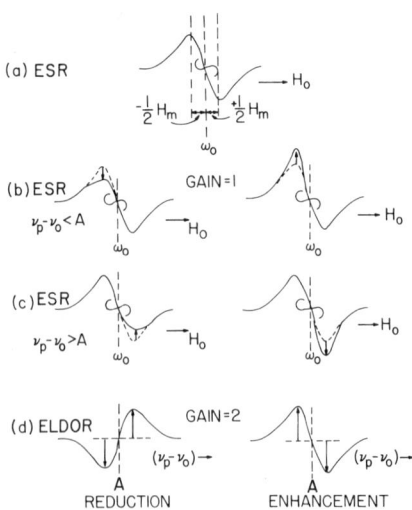

Figure 5-16. (a) A first derivative presentation of the absorption ESR line with a superimposed field modulation of amplitude equal to H_m (greatly exaggerated for clarity) centered at the crossover point of the ESR line (ω_o). The magnetic field increases to the right. (b) As the frequency difference between the pump (ν_p) and the observing (ν_o) microwave frequency approaches the value of the hyperfine splitting A, the intensity of the low field side of the ESR line is altered in the direction indicated by the arrow for either a reduction or an enhancement situation. (c) The intensity of the high field side is altered in the direction indicated by the arrow when $\nu_p - \nu_o > A$. (d) A plot of the resulting change in the ESR line of (c) and (d) as a function of $\nu_p - \nu_o$ for either reduction or enhancement.

response changes accordingly (Fig. 5-16c) and traces out a derivative ELDOR response as shown in Fig. 5-16d. For the conditions shown, an ELDOR reduction produces an ELDOR line of opposite phase to the ESR line and an ELDOR enhancement produces an ELDOR line of the same phase as the ESR line. This simple explanation only applies when the magnetization follows the effective magnetic field (Section 1.5.4). Deviations from this idealized behavior are often observed under practical experimental conditions in liquids. For example, in our experience the ELDOR spectra of nitroxides show the opposite phase from that predicted. This is presumably related to the fact that the magnetization does not follow the effective magnetic field for the 100 kHz modulation frequency typically employed.

If the observing position is set to the top of a first derivative homogeneous absorption ESR line (most ESR lines with no detectable fine structure will qualify) and a reduction in the ESR intensity is detected with $\nu_p > \nu_o$, the resulting ELDOR lineshape will appear as an inverted absorption curve centered at $\omega_o - \Delta\omega$ where ω_o is the ELDOR frequency obtained with the observing position at the crossover position and $\Delta\omega$ is one-half of the peak to peak ESR linewidth. If one positions the observing field at the bottom of the ESR first derivative absorption curve, an absorptionlike line will occur, positioned at $\omega_o + \Delta\omega$. If $\nu_p < \nu_o$, then the absorptionlike line will occur at $\omega_o + \Delta\omega$ and $\omega_o - \Delta\omega$ for the observing position centered at the top and bottom, respectively, of the first derivative absorption ESR line. To find ω_o one must average the two ELDOR line positions for observing the ESR derivative extrema.

In the case of inhomogeneous lineshapes, if the inhomogeneous linewidth becomes large with respect to the spin packet (sp) linewidth ($\Delta H_{obs} \gg \Delta H_{sp}$; see Fig. 1-16), ELDOR lines resembling derivatives will be obtained regardless of the setting of the resonant condition. Physically this occurs because the presence of a modulation field will sample both the positive and negative lobes of the first derivative absorption spin packet lineshapes irrespective of the observing position. Since it is difficult to know the ratio of the ESR linewidth to spin packet linewidth, ELDOR lines obtained at the top or bottom of most experimental first derivative ESR lines will tend to have distorted lineshapes from a mixture of first derivative and absorption shapes whose center frequency positions are difficult to estimate. Thus it is necessary to position the observing resonant condition at the true center of the observed ESR line in order to determine hyperfine splittings accurately.

In some cases the true center of an observed ESR line is difficult to determine as a result of overlap with neighboring ESR lines. In these cases if a distorted line is observed, one should experimentally shift the

Table 5-3. Summary of ELDOR Lineshapes Observed from ESR First Derivative Absorption Spectra for Different Experimental Conditions

ESR Line Type	Observing Field Position	ELDOR Lineshape	ELDOR Line Position
Homogeneous	derivative max/min	absorption or inverted absorption[a]	$\omega_o \pm \frac{1}{2}\Delta H_p$
Homogeneous	crossover	first derivative	ω_o
Inhomogeneous	derivative max/min	first derivative	ω_o
$\Delta H_{obs} \gg \Delta H_{sp}$	crossover	first derivative	ω_o
Inhomogeneous	derivative max/min	distorted	$\omega_o \pm \delta$
$\Delta H_{obs} \sim \Delta H_{sp}$	crossover	first derivative	ω_o

[a] Shape and position depend on phase of ESR spectrum and $\omega_p > \omega_o$ or $\omega_p < \omega_o$.

observing resonant conditions until the ELDOR line becomes symmetrical. Table 5-3 summarizes the ELDOR lineshapes seen for different experimental conditions when detecting first derivative ESR absorption spectra.

As in Section 5.2.5, the frequency swept ELDOR spectra can be obtained by detecting not only the first derivative ESR absorption curves in phase with the field modulation, but also the first and second derivative of the dispersion ESR signal, and the second derivative of the absorption ESR signal all in phase with the field modulation. The lineshapes will appear similar to those in Fig. 5-10 except the variable magnetic field base will be replaced by a variable frequency base. ELDOR signals may also be detected 90° out-of-phase with respect to the modulation with the observing field set on an ESR derivative extremum. However they often have an intensity that is dependent on the correlation times of the motion and the modulation frequency relative to T_{1e}. As an example, an interesting variation in the ELDOR lineshape and intensity of the first derivative dispersion or absorption ESR curve with phase angle at a modulation frequency of 10^5 Hz for the nitroxide spin label tanol is given in Figs. 5-17 and 5-18. As the phase angle changes from 0° toward 90° for the frequency swept dispersion ELDOR signal (Fig. 5-17), there is actually a minimum in the intensity near a phase angle of 60°, instead of 90° as would be expected for any spin system that can relax quickly between each modulation cycle so that the detected spins possess the same modulation phase relationship as excited spins. Because they do not, due to the jump rate ω_J and magnitude of T_{1e} competing with the modulation frequency (10^5 Hz), the minimum and maximum ELDOR

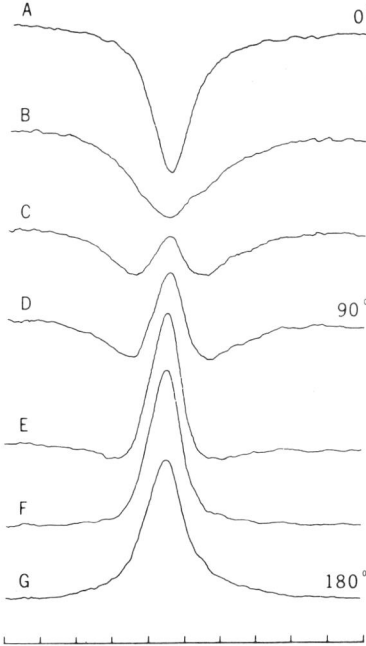

Figure 5-17. The experimental variation with phase angle of the first derivative frequency swept dispersion ELDOR signal for 1×10^{-3} M tanol in *sec*-butylbenzene at 210 K using a modulation frequency of 10^5 Hz and an amplitude of 0.24 G. The reference phase angle settings are (A) 0°, (B) 30°, (C) 60°, (D) 90°, (E) 120°, (F) 150°, (G) 180°, with the pump and observer power settings equal to 860 mW and 5 mW, respectively. The observing ESR position is at the top of the dispersion curve given in Fig. 5-10b. From L. A. Dalton et al., *Chem. Phys.*, **6,** 166 (1974).

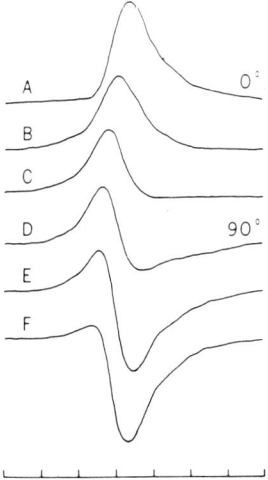

Figure 5-18. The experimental variation with phase angle of the first derivative frequency swept absorption ELDOR signal for 1×10^{-3} M tanol in *sec*-butylbenzene at 210 K using a modulation frequency of 10^5 Hz and an amplitude of 0.24 G. The reference phase angle settings are (A) 0°, (B) 30°, (C) 60°, (D) 90°, (E) 120°, (F) 150°, with the same settings as used in Fig. 5-17 except that the observing position is set at the bottom of the absorption ESR signal in Fig. 5-10a.

intensities actually depend on the reference phase angle. Note that the maximum dispersion mode ELDOR signal occurs at 150° in Fig. 5-17 and not at 180° as might be expected. This same sort of dependence is observed for the first derivative absorption presentation in Fig. 5-18 where the intensity at a phase angle of 90° is larger than at 60°. Although it is not possible to give a qualitative meaning at this time to this shift from 0° maximum and 90° minimum for the specific case of the nitroxide spin label tanol, it is important to realize in those cases of poor signal-to-noise ratio that an increase in ELDOR signal might result if the reference phase is changed. This is also true of the ESR signal in some cases.

5.3.2 Hyperfine Lines and Combination Lines

Examples of frequency swept ELDOR spectra of $5 \times 10^{-4}\,M$ α,α-diphenyl-β-picrylhydrazyl (DPPH) in toluene at 293 K are given in Fig. 5-19. Two intense lines in addition to several weaker lines are observed (Fig. 5-19d) when the magnetic field is set to the low field ESR line $M_{N_\alpha} = +1$ and $M_{N_\beta} = +1$ (+1, +1) of DPPH (Fig. 5-19d) and the pump frequency is swept over frequencies lower than the observing frequency. The ESR spectrum of DPPH is characterized by five partially resolved broad lines due to two large splittings from two nonequivalent nitrogens of approximately 22 MHz (A_α) and 27 MHz (A_β). These broad lines are made up of small splittings from the different aromatic ring protons. A number of attempts,[3] previous to ELDOR investigations of DPPH,

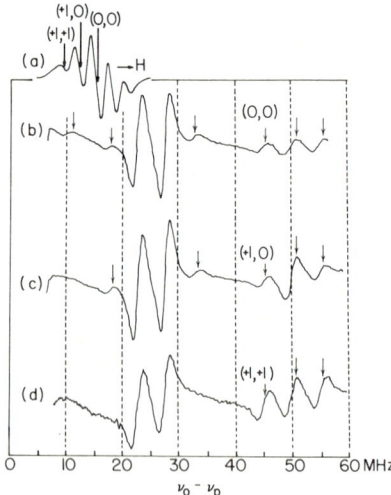

Figure 5-19. (a) An ESR spectrum for $5 \times 10^{-4}\,M$ DPPH in toluene at 293 K. The arrows denote various observing positions for ELDOR spectra where each position is coded by the nuclear quantum numbers of the α and β nitrogens. The observed frequency swept ELDOR spectra for unlabeled DPPH in toluene is shown when the observing ESR position is set at (b) $M_{N_\alpha} = 0$ and $M_{N_\beta} = 0$ (0, 0); (c) $M_{N_\alpha} = +1$, and $M_{N_\beta} = 0$ (+1, 0), and (d) $M_{N_\alpha} = +1$ and $M_{N_\beta} = +1$ (+1, +1). Weak combination lines are denoted by small arrows in the ELDOR spectra. The (0, 0) and (+1, 0) traces are at identical instrumental gain and the gain is 2.5 times higher for the (+1, +1) trace. From J. S. Hyde et al., J. Chem. Phys., **51**, 1404 (1969).

resulted in several different reported nitrogen hyperfine splittings as a result of the poorly resolved ESR spectrum. Even the best ESR spectrum obtainable for a ^{15}N-enriched sample of DPPH at the β position still results in an overlapped ESR spectrum. However the ELDOR spectrum of the unlabeled DPPH is well resolved and the two intense ELDOR lines are assigned to the hyperfine splittings $A_\alpha = 22.22$ MHz and $A_\beta = 27.27$ MHz. This assignment is verified by the ELDOR investigation of the ^{15}N$_\beta$ substituted compound in which case intense lines at 22.22 and 38.30 MHz are observed (Fig. 5-20). The difference in the nuclear

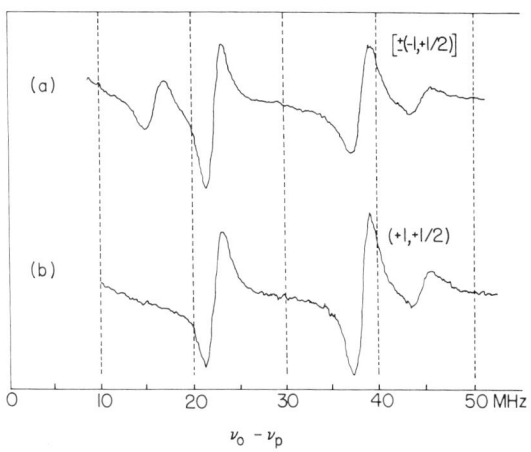

Figure 5-20. The frequency-swept ELDOR spectra of the ^{15}N$_\beta$ substituted DPPH in toluene at 293 K when the observing ESR position is located at (*a*) the crossover of the center ESR line $[\pm(-1, +\frac{1}{2})]$ and (*b*) the crossover of the low field ESR line $(+1, +\frac{1}{2})$. The lower trace is recorded at twice the instrument gain as the upper trace. From J. S. Hyde et al., *J. Chem. Phys.*, **51,** 1404 (1969).

moments and nuclear spins of ^{15}N and ^{14}N ($A_\alpha^{14}/A_\beta^{15} = 0.71294$) converts the larger ^{15}N splitting of 38.30 MHz to a ^{14}N splitting of 27.31 MHz. The difference between 27.27 and 27.31 is primarily due to second order hyperfine differences of 0.04 MHz.

Also notable are the weaker lines which vary in intensity as the observing magnetic field is set at different ESR lines (Fig. 5-19). Various intermolecular and intramolecular relaxation mechanisms are, in general, possible and thus numerous lines might be expected.

However in the ELDOR experiments given here, low radical concentrations are used (5×10^{-4} M) so that only intramolecular relaxations are likely. From other investigations nuclear relaxations are expected to be the most important. In this case modulation of the electron-nuclear dipolar (END) interaction as the molecule tumbles in solution is the dominant nuclear relaxation mechanism.

From Section 5.2.3 we know that for a dominant END relaxation mechanism, the ELDOR signal that appears at the hyperfine frequency depends on b, the ratio of the electron to nuclear longitudinal relaxation times. It has been observed that nuclei that have large hyperfine splittings usually have shorter nuclear relaxation times (larger b) than nuclei associated with the small hyperfine splittings. Because of this, ELDOR lines are observed at the α- and β-nitrogen hyperfine splitting whereas no lines are observed for nuclei with smaller hyperfine splittings. Thus the weaker lines are not due to proton splittings. Instead the weaker lines in Fig. 5-19 are found to appear at a multiple of the nitrogen hyperfine coupling or at a sum or difference of the two nitrogen hyperfine couplings. Such lines are called *combination lines*.[3] Combination lines are found to be strongly dependent on the observing and pumping microwave powers as well as on temperature. Combination lines (in megahertz) are observed from natural (^{14}N substituted) DPPH at $A_\beta - A_\alpha$ (5.05), $2(A_\beta - A_\alpha)$ (10.0), $2A_\alpha - A_\beta$ (17.2), $2A_\beta - A_\alpha$ (32.3), $2A_\alpha$ (44.5), $A_\alpha + A_\beta$ (49.5), and $2A_\beta$ (54.6). All but the 5.05 MHz lines are observed in Fig. 5-19b and are denoted by arrows. Note that the line at 10.1 MHz is not observed in Fig. 5-19c, whereas lines at 10.1, 17.2, and 32.3 observed in Fig. 5-19b are missing in Fig. 5-19d.

As a model for understanding the origin of these combination lines a stick ESR spectrum arising from the interaction of two nonequivalent nitrogens coupled to an electron is given in Fig. 5-21a. To determine the frequency position of each possible ELDOR line, a calculation could be carried out to determine the value of each energy level and derive the ELDOR line position from this. However since only $\Delta M_I = 0$ ESR lines are observed, we can carry out a more convenient calculation.

Each ESR line is labeled using the notation $(M_{I_1}, M_{I_2}, M_{I_3} \cdots)$ where M_{I_i} is the component of the nuclear spin quantum number of the ith nucleus for the particular line. The position of each line in frequency units relative to the center of the spectrum is then given to first order by $-A_1 M_{I_1} - A_2 M_{I_2} - A_3 M_{I_3} \cdots - A_i M_{I_i}$ where A_i is the hyperfine splitting constant of the ith nucleus. If the hyperfine splitting constants are positive, then the low field lines are denoted by positive M_I components. An ELDOR line position can now be predicted to occur at a frequency corresponding to the difference in the line positions of the observed and the pumped ESR lines.

To see just why this is so let us defer the discussion of the two nonequivalent nitrogen spectrum for a moment and consider only the ESR spectrum of a H atom. The low and high field ESR lines for a

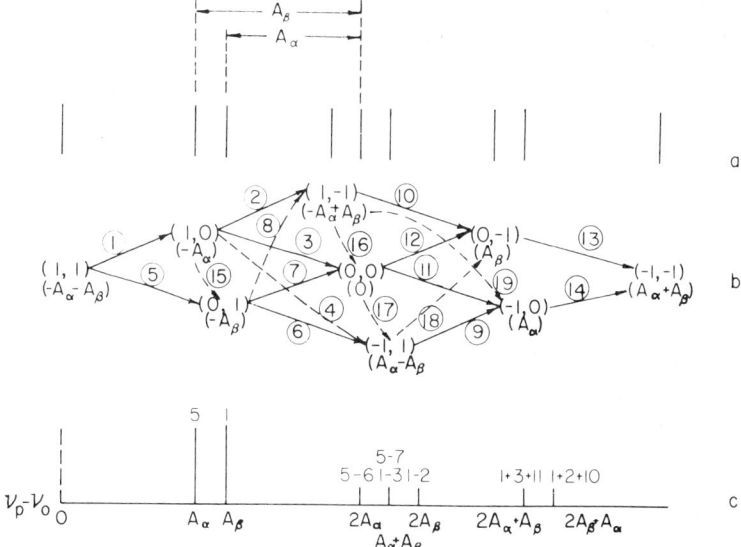

Figure 5-21. (a) A stick spectrum for a free radical containing two nonequivalent nitrogens with hyperfine splittings equal to A_α and A_β. (b) The possible allowed relaxation paths utilizing the selection rules $\Delta M_{N_\alpha} = \pm 1$; $\Delta M_{N_\beta} = 0$ or $\Delta M_{N_\alpha} = 0$; $\Delta M_{N_\beta} = \pm 1$ at each step of the pathway (solid lines) for an ELDOR spectrum (c) obtained with the observer field position set at the ($M_{N_\alpha} = +1$, $M_{N_\beta} = +1$) low field ESR line. The dashed lines indicate forbidden relaxation pathways that utilize other selection rules (see Table 5-4). The relaxation pathways responsible for each ELDOR line are assigned in (c). Adapted from J. S. Hyde et al., *J. Chem. Phys.*, **51**, 1404 (1969).

hydrogen atom ($M_I = \frac{1}{2}$) have line positions of $-A/2$ and $+A/2$, respectively. Observing the low field line and pumping the high field line results in an ELDOR line at a frequency according to the preceding recipe equal to the difference in the value of the pumped and observed lines: $(A_H/2) - (-A_H/2) = A_H$. This is in agreement with the predicted spectrum consisting of a line at A_H given in Fig. 1-27.

We now return to the discussion of two nonequivalent nitrogens. If each of the ESR lines is assigned according to this scheme, a detailed explanation can be given of the ELDOR transitions shown in Fig. 5-21. The ESR lines are labeled in the form M_{N_α}, M_{N_β} where α and β denote the two nonequivalent nitrogen nuclei. The position of each line relative to the center of the spectrum is also given in terms of A_α and A_β, the hyperfine splittings of the α and β nitrogen nuclei. The observed ESR position was set at the low field ESR line labeled (1, 1) in Fig. 5-21b and the pumped frequency was swept throughout the spectrum. Assuming that the selection rules $\Delta M_{N_\beta} = \pm 1$, $\Delta M_{N_\alpha} = 0$ or $\Delta M_{N_\alpha} = \pm 1$, $\Delta M_{N_\beta} = 0$ hold for each relaxation pathway consisting of a one step, one nuclear spin-flip process, then relaxation via pathway 1 gives rise to a line at $-A_\alpha - (-A_\alpha - A_\beta) = A_\beta$. Similarly, relaxation via pathway 5, where the selection rules $\Delta M_{N_\alpha} = \pm 1$ and $\Delta M_{N_\beta} = 0$ apply, gives rise to a line at A_α (Fig. 5-21c). Combination lines arise when these selection rules also hold for each step of a multiple step pathway. For example, by application of the selection rule $\Delta M_{N_\beta} = -1$, $\Delta M_{N_\alpha} = 0$ twice, path $1+2$ gives rise to a line at $2A_\beta$. Applying the selection rule $\Delta M_{N_\beta} = -1$, $\Delta M_{N_\alpha} = 0$ followed by $\Delta M_{N_\alpha} = -1$, $\Delta M_{N_\beta} = 0$ path $1+3$ gives rise to a line at $A_\alpha + A_\beta$, but path $1+4$ is forbidden according to the preceding selection rules. Note that these particular combination lines result from a two step process resulting in two nuclear spin-flips and are significantly weaker than those for a one step, one flip process. Similarly combination lines are also observed at $2A_\alpha$ for path $5+6$ and at $A_\alpha + A_\beta$ for path $5+7$ but are forbidden for path $5+8$. Note that the intensity ratio of the combination lines should be in the ratio of $1:2:1$ at $2A_\alpha$, $A_\alpha + A_\beta$, and $2A_\beta$, respectively, assuming that each pathway yields the same ELDOR intensity (Fig. 5-21c). Experimentally, the line at 49.5 MHz ($A_\alpha + A_\beta$) is more intense than those at 49.5 ($2A_\alpha$) and 54.6 MHz ($2A_\beta$) in Fig. 5-19d, although not exactly in the ratio of $1:2:1$. In addition, notice that it is not possible to observe lines at $2A_\beta - A_\alpha$ (32.3 MHz), $2A_\alpha - A_\beta$ (17.2 MHz), $2A_\beta - 2A_\alpha$ (10.1 MHz), and $A_\beta - A_\alpha$ (5.05 MHz) when the observing position is set at the low field position (1, 1) as all one step and two step pathways have been accounted for, leaving no combination of relaxation paths connecting ESR lines with a difference in frequency units of these values. This agrees with experiment. As a further instructive example, ELDOR combination lines can be calculated for a three step process where the selection rules $\Delta M_{N_\alpha} = \pm 1$ and $\Delta M_{N_\beta} = 0$ or $\Delta M_{N_\alpha} = 0$ and $\Delta M_{N_\beta} = \pm 1$ hold at each step. For instance, path $1+3+11$, path $5+6+9$ or path $5+7+11$ are allowed three-step processes according to these selection rules giving rise to ELDOR lines at $2A_\alpha + A_\beta$. Similarly, path $1+2+10$, path $5+7+12$, or path $1+3+12$ gives rise to ELDOR lines at $A_\alpha + 2A_\beta$ (Fig. 5-21c). These lines are expected to be very weak and the expected frequency range for these lines was not scanned in Fig. 5-19d.

On the other hand, when the observing magnetic field is set on the overlapping (+1, 0) and (0, +1) ESR lines in Fig. 5-21, a somewhat different set of combination lines will be allowed as summarized in Table 5-4. As was the case when the observing field was set at (1, 1), intense ELDOR lines occur at A_β via a one flip process along path 2 or 7 and at A_α via a one flip process along path 3 or 6. Two flip processes give rise to combination lines at $2A_\alpha$ via path $3+11$, at $A_\alpha + A_\beta$ via paths $7+11$, $6+9$, $2+10$, and $3+12$, and at $2A_\beta$ via path $7+12$. Note that the intensity ratio of 1:4:1 is in agreement with that observed in Fig. 5-19c. Further one and two spin-flip processes are also possible if the selection rules for the observation of combination lines are expanded to include $\Delta M_{N_\alpha} + \Delta M_{N_\beta} = 0$, in which case pathway 15 gives rise to a combination line at $A_\beta - A_\alpha$ (5.05 MHz). Incorporating the selection rule $\Delta M_{N_\alpha} + \Delta M_{N_\beta} = -1$ (reverse sign when $\nu_p > \nu_o$) give rise to combination lines at $2A_\beta - A_\alpha$ (32.3 MHz) and $2A_\alpha - A_\beta$ (17.2 MHz) via pathways 8 and 4, respectively. Previously these pathways were not accessible when the observing magnetic field was sitting at the low field line. Note that the combination lines that occur in Fig. 5-19c for the selection rules $\Delta M_{N_\alpha} + \Delta M_{N_\beta} = -1$ ($2A_\beta - A_\alpha$) are weaker than those where $\Delta M_{N_\alpha} + \Delta M_{N_\beta} = -2$ (i.e., $\Delta M_{N_\alpha} = -1$, $\Delta M_{N_\beta} = 0$ for a two step process) ($2A_\alpha$, $2A_\beta$, etc.).

When the observing position is set to the overlapping (1, 1), (0, 0), and (−1, 1) ESR lines in Fig. 5-21, the possible one and two spin-flip processes as summarized in Table 5-4 give rise to lines at A_α and A_β by a one spin-flip process, combination lines at $2A_\alpha$, $A_\alpha + A_\beta$, and $2A_\beta$ by a two spin-flip process, and at $A_\beta - A_\alpha$, $2A_\alpha - A_\beta$, and $2A_\beta - A_\alpha$. In addition, a new ELDOR combination line occurs at $2A_\beta - 2A_\alpha$ by the application of the selection rule $\Delta M_{N_\alpha} + \Delta M_{N_\beta} = 0$ to a two step process involving pathways 16 + 17. This is in agreement with the experimentally observed ELDOR spectrum given in Fig. 5-19b. Lastly, when the observing field is set to the overlapped (0, −1) and (−1, 0) lines, only lines at A_α and A_β are observed, as it is not possible to have relaxation pathways that give rise to combination lines at $2A_\alpha$, $2A_\beta$, and $A_\alpha + A_\beta$ when the variable pump frequency is less than the observing frequency.

The ELDOR spectrum of DPPH will be identical to that just described for two nonequivalent nitrogens as the long proton relaxation in DPPH prevents the coupling of the two nonequivalent nitrogen relaxation pathways to those of the proton. Thus when proton splittings are added, we need only to add the requirement that $\Delta M_{H_i} = 0$ to the selection rules we have already used. The effect of this selection rule is given in Fig. 5-22 where a proton with a splitting equal to $A_\beta - A_\alpha$ has been added. Note that when the observing position is set to the overlapping $(\overline{1, 0})$ and (0, 1) lines belonging to the $M_H = -\frac{1}{2}$ and $M_H = +\frac{1}{2}$ proton quantum numbers, respectively, that two equivalent relaxation pathways result (one denoted by the solid line, identical to that given in Fig. 5-22, and one denoted by a dashed line). Thus all lines that appeared without the addition of the proton will be observed.

Combination lines are always weaker in intensity and are usually wider than the principal line at A_α and A_β. This is because[1] the intensity of the primary ELDOR lines at A_N goes approximately as $b = T_{1e}/T_{1n}$ when $b \ll 1$ while combination lines go as b^2 (for two spin-flips). In addition,

Table 5-4. The ELDOR Line Positions for Two Nonequivalent ^{14}Nitrogen ($I = 1$) Nuclei as a Function of Observing Magnetic Field Position

Observing[a] Position	Selection Rules for Each Step	One Step	Path[b]	Two Steps	Path[b]	Three Steps	Path[b]
(1, 1)	$\Delta M_{N_\alpha} = \pm 1; \Delta M_{N_\beta} = 0$	A_α	5	$2A_\alpha$	$1+2$		
	$\Delta M_{N_\alpha} = 0; \Delta M_{N_\beta} = \pm 1$	A_β	1	$2A_\beta$	$5+6$	$2A_\alpha + A_\beta$	$\begin{cases} 5+6+9 \\ 5+7+11 \\ 1+3+11 \end{cases}$
				$A_\alpha + A_\beta$	$\begin{cases} 5+7 \\ 1+3 \end{cases}$	$2A_\beta + A_\alpha$	$\begin{cases} 1+2+10 \\ 1+3+12 \\ 5+7+12 \end{cases}$
(1, 0) and (0, 1)	$\Delta M_{N_\alpha} = \pm 1, \Delta M_{N_\beta} = 0$	A_α	$\begin{cases} 6 \\ 3 \end{cases}$	$2A_\alpha$	$3+11$		
	$\Delta M_{N_\alpha} = 0; \Delta M_{N_\beta} = \pm 1$	A_β	$\begin{cases} 2 \\ 7 \end{cases}$	$2A_\beta$	$7+12$	$2A_\alpha + A_\beta$	$\begin{cases} 3+11+14 \\ 2+10+13 \\ 3+12+13 \end{cases}$
				$A_\alpha + A_\beta$	$\begin{cases} 6+9 \\ 2+10 \\ 7+11 \\ 3+12 \end{cases}$	$2A_\beta + A_\alpha$	$\begin{cases} 6+9+14 \\ 7+11+14 \\ 7+12+13 \end{cases}$
	$\Delta M_{N_\alpha} + \Delta M_{N_\beta} = 0$	$A_\alpha - A_\beta$	15				

	$\Delta M_{N_\alpha} + \Delta M_{N_\beta} = -1^c$	$2A_\beta - A_\alpha$	8		
		$2A_\alpha - A_\beta$	4		
(1, 1)	$\Delta M_{N_\alpha} = \pm 1, \Delta M_{N_\beta} = 0$	A_α	$\begin{cases} 10 \\ 11 \end{cases}$	$2A_\alpha$	$10 + 13$
(0, 0)					
(−1, 1)	$\Delta M_{N_\alpha} = 0; \Delta M_{N_\beta} = \pm 1$	A_β	$\begin{cases} 12 \\ 9 \end{cases}$	$2A_\beta$	$9 + 14$
				$A_\alpha + A_\beta$	$\begin{cases} 11 + 14 \\ 12 + 13 \end{cases}$
	$\Delta M_{N_\alpha} + \Delta M_{N_\beta} = 0$	$A_\beta - A_\alpha$	$\begin{cases} 17 \\ 16 \end{cases}$		
	$\Delta M_{N_\alpha} + \Delta M_{N_\beta} = -1^c$	$2A_\alpha - A_\beta$	19	$2A_\alpha - 2A_\beta$	$16 + 17$
		$2A_\beta - A_\alpha$	18		
(0, −1)	$\Delta M_{N_\alpha} = \pm 1; \Delta M_{N_\beta} = 0$	A_α	13		
(−1, 0)	$\Delta M_{N_\alpha} = 0; \Delta M_{N_\beta} = \pm 1$	A_β	14		

[a] The observing position is defined as the position of the overlapped lines indicated.
[b] Path number defined in Fig. 5-21.
[c] The opposite sign occurs when $\nu_p > \nu_o$.

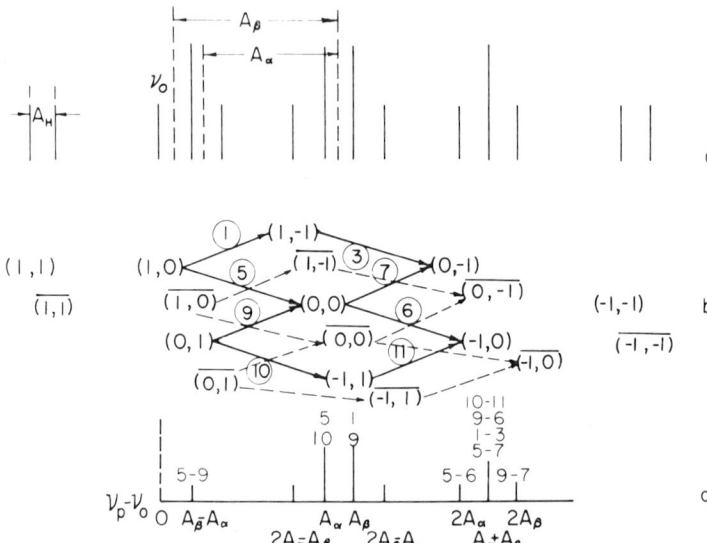

Figure 5-22. (a) The ESR spectrum for two nonequivalent nitrogens with splittings $A_\alpha \neq A_\beta$ interacting with a proton with a splitting equal to $A_\beta - A_\alpha$ and with an electron (b) The allowed ELDOR relaxation pathways utilizing the selection rules $\Delta M_{N_\alpha} = \pm 1$; $\Delta M_{N_\beta} = 0$ or $\Delta M_{N_\alpha} = 0$; $\Delta M_{N_\beta} = \pm 1$ at each step of the pathway when the observing field position is set on the overlapped $(+1, 0)$ and $(0, +1)$ ESR lines for $M_H = +\frac{1}{2}$ (solid lines) and $M_H = -\frac{1}{2}$ (dashed lines). (c) The resulting ELDOR spectrum is the same as that found when the observing ESR position is set at the overlapped $(+1,0)$ and $(0, +1)$ ESR lines in Fig. 5-21. Adapted from J. S. Hyde et al., *J. Chem. Phys.*, **51**, 1404 (1969).

these combination lines are wider because of second order shifts that will broaden the line $A_\alpha + A_\beta$ since these couplings correspond to the relaxation path where the β nitrogen nuclear spin is first flipped followed by the flip of the α nitrogen nuclear spin. These two relaxation paths will not be the same and will have slightly different shifts. The second order shifts for $2A_\beta$ and $2A_\alpha$ will cancel since the same nuclear spin-flip occurs twice for each case. Fortunately from a spectroscopic viewpoint, the difference in the width and intensity of the combination lines relative to the main lines at A_α and A_β make it possible to identify the main lines. In addition, splittings can be measured nearly an order of magnitude more accurately than by ESR methods.

5.4 SEPARATION OF OVERLAPPING SPECTRA

If intramolecular relaxation is the dominant ELDOR mechanism, then the spectral components that make up a multiradical system can be separated. As an example let us consider a mixture of 10^{-4} M DPPH and 10^{-4} M nitroxide for which the spectral components are each assignable by carrying out various field swept ELDOR spectra (Fig. 5-23). The five line ESR spectrum of DPPH with a nitrogen hyperfine separation of 25 MHz is given in Fig. 5-23a, whereas the three line spectrum of the 4-N-maleimido-2,2,6,6-tetramethylpiperidine nitroxide radical with a hyperfine splitting of 44 MHz is given in Fig. 5-23b. The ESR spectrum from a mixture of DPPH and the nitroxide radical is given in Fig. 5-23c. If the separation between the pumping and observing frequency $\Delta \nu = \nu_p - \nu_o = +88$ MHz (i.e., twice the nitroxide nitrogen hyperfine splitting) and the magnetic field is swept, only the low field ESR line corresponding to the low field nitroxide radical line will decrease in intensity. Likewise if $\Delta \nu = -88$ MHz only the high field line of the ESR pattern will decrease. In a number of cases these changes in the ESR signal intensity are difficult to detect so an electronic subtraction system is utilized. Typically this can be done by modulating the pumping microwave klystron with a known frequency, and detecting not only the field modulation that is employed, but also the superimposed klystron modulation frequency. In this

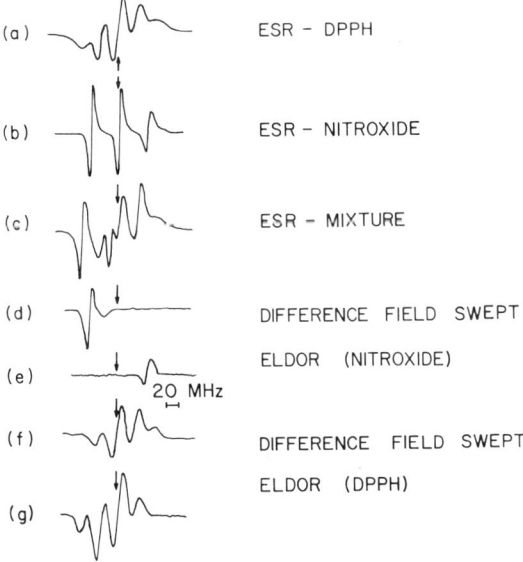

Figure 5-23. ESR spectra of (a) a 10^{-4} M solution of DPPH, (b) a 10^{-4} M solution of a nitroxide radical, and (c) a mixture of samples (a) and (b) at 193 K. Field swept difference ELDOR spectra of the mixture in (c) with (d) $\nu_p - \nu_o = -88$ MHz (the nitroxide spectrum) (e) $\nu_p - \nu_o = 88$ MHz, (f) $\nu_p - \nu_o = -25$ MHz (the DPPH spectrum) and (g) $\nu_p - \nu_o = 25$ MHz. See text for interpretation. Adapted from J. S. Hyde, unpublished work.

300 LIQUID PHASE ELDOR

manner the difference field swept ELDOR spectra are obtained as given in Figs. 5-23d and e, showing the high and low field lines of the nitroxide radical. On the other hand, if the difference frequency $\Delta \nu = \nu_p - \nu_o$ is set to +25 MHz (the average nitrogen splitting in DPPH), a difference field swept ELDOR spectrum shows the four higher field lines of the resolved DPPH spectrum (Fig. 5-23f). The four lower field ELDOR lines are observed (Fig. 5-23g) when $\Delta \nu = -25$ MHz. By frequency swept ELDOR, spectra similar to Fig. 5-23g are recorded by positioning the observing field at the high field ESR line and by sweeping the frequency difference $\nu_p - \nu_o$ where $\nu_p > \nu_o$.

5.5 COMPARISON OF ELDOR AND ENDOR MEASUREMENTS IN SOLUTION

The relaxation conditions under which ELDOR spectra are observed are quite different from the conditions required for ENDOR. An excellent example of these differences is found in the ELDOR[3] and ENDOR[34] investigations of DPPH in solution.

Optimum ELDOR intensity can occur for large magnitudes of W_n^{END} or equivalently for $b = W_n/W_e$. Such is the case for nuclei with large anisotropic hyperfine splittings because W_n^{END} increases with dipolar anisotropy. For DPPH the nitrogen nuclei possess a larger W_n^{END} magnitude than protons as a result of the ^{14}N nucleus interacting with its own $2p\pi$ unpaired electron density, and thus the magnitude of the dipolar term, which varies as r^{-6}, is much larger than that for the ring protons where the electron spin density is on an adjacent carbon atom. Since $W_n \propto T_{1n}^{-1}$, a short nitrogen relaxation time will be observed and will give rise to nitrogen ELDOR lines. Because of the long proton nuclear relaxation time, the large number of weakly coupled protons will contribute only to the ESR spectrum and not to the ELDOR spectrum.

In contrast, ENDOR investigations[34] of DPPH in mineral oil at room temperature show only proton ENDOR signals. A primary condition for observing ENDOR, as given in Chapter 1, is the requirement that the nuclear transition be saturated. The failure to observe nitrogen ENDOR lines suggests that the tumbling conditions in mineral oil are such that it is difficult to saturate the nitrogen nuclear transition with the available rf power. It is also necessary for the ESR line to be as strong as possible and still be saturable by the microwave power. The observation of the proton ENDOR lines suggests that sufficient rf power is available to saturate the proton nuclear transitions.

An important point to notice from the study of DPPH in solution is the way in which ENDOR and ELDOR complement each other. From ELDOR measurements accurate nitrogen hyperfine splittings are obtained for the α and β nitrogens and it is deduced that one of the proton splittings can be equal to the difference between the two nitrogen splittings. The ENDOR measurements show that the difference between the hyperfine splittings of the two equivalent ortho and the two equivalent meta protons of each phenyl ring is approximately equal to the difference between the two nitrogen splittings. Thus the ENDOR measurements substantiate the solution ELDOR interpretation.

In summary, ENDOR studies enable the measurement of small hyperfine splittings, the identification of nuclides, the determination of quadrupole couplings, and the observation of higher resolution than ELDOR measurements. ELDOR studies enable accurate measurements of large hyperfine splittings and are probably better for studying relaxation processes.

REFERENCES

1. J. S. Hyde, J. C. W. Chien, and J. H. Freed, *J. Chem. Phys.*, **48,** 4211 (1968).
2. V. A. Benderskii, P. A. Stunkas, and A. I. Rakoed, *Mol. Phys.*, **24,** 449 (1972).
3. J. S. Hyde, R. C. Sneed, Jr., and G. H. Rist, *J. Chem. Phys.*, **51,** 1404 (1969).
4. J. H. Freed, D. S. Leniart, and H. D. Connor, *J. Chem. Phys.*, **58,** 3089 (1973).
5. M. R. Das, S. B. Wagner, and J. H. Freed, *J. Chem. Phys.*, **52,** 5404 (1970).
6. M. P. Eastman, G. V. Bruno, J. H. Freed, *J. Chem. Phys.*, **52,** 321 (1970).
7. V. A. Benderskii, V. I. Gol'danskii, A. I. Rakoed, P. A. Stunzhas, E. A. Sokolov, *Dokl. Akad. Nauk. SSSR*, **204,** 1143 (1972) [English transl.: *Dokl. Phys. Chem.*, **204,** 478 (1972)].
8. M. D. Smigel, L. R. Dalton, J. S. Hyde, and L. A. Dalton, *Proc. Nat. Acad. Sci. U.S.*, **71,** 1925 (1974).
9. J. S. Hyde, M. D. Smigel, L. R. Dalton, and L. A. Dalton, *J. Chem. Phys.*, **62,** 1655 (1975).
10. B. H. Robinson, J. L. Monge, L. A. Dalton, L. R. Dalton, and A. L. Kwiram, *Chem. Phys. Lett.*, **28,** 169 (1974).
11. L. A. Dalton, J. L. Monge, L. R. Dalton, and A. L. Kwiram, *Chem. Phys.*, **6,** 166 (1974); P. W. Percival, J. S. Hyde, L. A. Dalton, and L. R. Dalton, *J. Chem. Phys.*, **62,** 4332 (1975).
12. H. Yoshida, D. F. Feng, and L. Kevan, *J. Chem. Phys.*, **58,** 4924 (1973).
13. J. H. Freed, *J. Chem. Phys.*, **43,** 2312 (1965).
14. J. H. Freed and G. K. Fraenkel, *J. Chem. Phys.*, **39,** 326 (1963).
15. J. H. Freed, *J. Phys. Chem.*, **71,** 38 (1967).
16. P. W. Atkins and D. Kivelson, *J. Chem. Phys.*, **44,** 169 (1966) and references cited therein.

17. O. H. Griffith, D. W. Cornell, and H. M. McConnell, *J. Chem. Phys.*, **43**, 2909 (1965); T. J. Stone, T. Buckman, P. L. Nordio, and H. M. McConnell, *Proc. Nat. Acad. Sci. U.S.*, **54**, 1010 (1965).
18. D. Kivelson, *J. Chem. Phys.*, **27**, 1087 (1960).
19. J. H. Freed, G. V. Bruno, and C. F. Polnaszek, *J. Phys. Chem.*, **75**, 3385 (1971).
20. S. A. Goldman, G. V. Bruno, C. F. Polnaszek, and J. H. Freed, *J. Chem. Phys.*, **56**, 716 (1972).
21. R. Kubo, *Adv. Chem. Phys.*, **15**, 101 (1969).
22. R. Kubo, *J. Phys. Soc. Japan Suppl.*, **26**, 1 (1969).
23. A. Abragam, *Principles of Nuclear Magnetism*, Oxford University Press, New York, 1961, p. 301.
24. J. H. Freed, *J. Chem. Phys.*, **41**, 2077 (1964).
25. P. A. Egelstaff, *J. Chem. Phys.*, **53**, 2590 (1970).
26. M. O. Smigel, L. A. Dalton, L. R. Dalton, and A. L. Kwiram, *Chem. Phys.*, **6**, 183 (1974).
27. S. A. Goldman, G. V. Bruno, and J. H. Freed, *J. Chem. Phys.*, **59**, 3071 (1973).
28. J. S. Hyde and L. A. Dalton, *Magn. Resonance Rev.*, **2**, 361 (1973).
29. L. R. Dalton, A. L. Kwiram, and J. A. Cowen, *Chem. Phys. Lett.*, **17**, 495 (1972); L. R. Dalton, A. L. Kwiram, and J. A. Cowen, *Chem. Phys. Lett.*, **14**, 77 (1972); L. R. Dalton and A. L. Kwiram, *J. Chem. Phys.*, **57**, 1132 (1972).
30. Tanol = 2,2,6,6-tetramethyl-4-piperidinol-1-oxyl; HDA = 17β-hydroxy-4',4',dimethyl-spiro-[5α-androstane-3,2'-oxazolidin]-3'-oxyl.
31. G. E. Pake and T. R. Tuttle, Jr., *Phys. Rev. Lett.*, **3**, 423 (1959); J. D. Currin, *Phys. Rev.*, **126**, 1995 (1962); C. S. Johnson, Jr., *Mol. Phys.*, **12**, 25 (1967).
32. R. L. Ward and S. I. Weissman, *J. Amer. Chem. Soc.*, **79**, 2086 (1957); C. S. Johnson Jr., *Adv. Magn. Resonance*, **1**, 89 (1965).
33. C. P. Poole, Jr., *Electron Spin Resonance*, Wiley-Interscience, New York, 1967, p. 705.
34. N. S. Dalal, D. E. Kennedy, and C. A. McDowell, *J. Chem. Phys.*, **59**, 3403 (1973).

6. Single Crystal and Powder ELDOR

6.1 Introduction
6.2 Interpretation of Organic Single Crystal ELDOR Spectra ($S = \frac{1}{2}$)
    6.2.1 Intramolecular Motion—Methyl Groups
    6.2.2 α Protons—No Intramolecular Motion
    6.2.3 Hyperfine Splitting Anisotropy
    6.2.4 Intramolecular Proton Spin Exchange
    6.2.5 Intramolecular Admixture of Nuclear Spin States (Forbidden Lines)
    6.2.6 Quadrupole Interaction
    6.2.7 Deuterium Hyperfine Splittings
    6.2.8 Resolution of Small Hyperfine Splittings
    6.2.9 Spin-Flip Transitions
    6.2.10 Modulation Frequency Dependence
    6.2.11 Intermolecular Spin Diffusion
        6.2.11.1 Radical Distribution
        6.2.11.2 Overlapped Lines
    6.2.12 Pulsed ELDOR
6.3 Applications—Oriented Radicals ($S = \frac{1}{2}$) in Single Crystals
    6.3.1 Separation of Overlapping Spectra
        6.3.1.1 Intramolecular Motion
        6.3.1.2 Temperature Dependence of R
        6.3.1.3 Fluorine Anisotropy and Motion
        6.3.1.4 Quadrupole Interaction and Motion
    6.3.2 Hydrogen-Deuterium Exchange
    6.3.3 Tunneling Methyl Groups
6.4 Powder ELDOR
    6.4.1 Determination of Hyperfine Splittings
    6.4.2 Spin Diffusion

6.5 Triplet State ($S = 1$)
  6.5.1 Excitons in Crystals
  6.5.2 Optical Detection in Polycrystalline Matrices
  References

6.1 INTRODUCTION

ELDOR investigations of radicals in solids differ in several respects from those in solutions. First the magnitude of the hyperfine splittings in single crystals depends on crystal orientation and thus the interactions are more complex, as already pointed out in Chapter 4. Second near neighbor nuclear dipole-dipole interactions result in ESR linewidths on the order of 3 G instead of less than 1 G, as found in solution spectra. In powders or glasses the composite ESR spectrum resulting from the averaging of many radical orientations is composed of broad lines centered about the three principal g values and separated by the principal hyperfine splittings. Because the relaxation parameters can depend on the hyperfine splitting magnitude, the ELDOR spectral line intensity varies with crystal angle; in addition, the broader ESR line in crystals results in ELDOR linewidths of the order of 5 to 6 MHz, which limits the inherent ELDOR resolution. In powders the ELDOR line intensity varies with the observing field position and depends largely on the averaging process that produces the composite ESR lineshape.

Although these major differences are found between the ELDOR spectra of liquids and solids, similarities do exist. In Chapter 5 the magnitudes of the ELDOR reduction factors for dilute solutions of radicals are shown to be dependent on the Brownian rotational diffusion correlation time of the radicals. Although it may not be possible for a radical trapped in a solid to possess the mobility to rotate freely and thus undergo Brownian rotational diffusion, radical substituents in single crystals such as CH_3 in $(CH_3)_2\dot{C}OOH$ (ref. 1), $(CH_3)_2\dot{C}OOD$ (ref. 1), and $CH_3\dot{C}OOD$ (ref. 1), NH_3^+ in $NH_3^+\dot{C}HCOO^-$ (ref. 2), CF_2 in $\dot{C}F_2CONH_2$ (ref. 2), $\dot{C}H_2$ in $\dot{C}H_2COO^-$ (ref. 3), and CD_2 in $\dot{C}D_2COOD$ (ref. 4) can undergo intramolecular rotational or torsional oscillatory motion and cyclical structures such as the cyclopentane ring can undergo pseudorotation due to two puckered conformations.[5] This intramolecular rotational motion gives rise to enhanced or reduced R factors that vary predictably with temperature, in some cases even more spectacularly than in solution.

Of course, intramolecular motion is not the only factor that leads to an ELDOR active relaxation mechanism for radicals in solids. Other factors, some of which are similar to those discussed in Chapter 5 for radicals in solution, also give rise to characteristic ELDOR spectra. These are quadrupole relaxation of α-chloro substituents attached to groups in radicals that do not exhibit motion on an ESR time scale ($\dot{\text{C}}$ClFCONH$_2$) (ref. 6) and those that do ($\dot{\text{C}}$Cl$_3$) (ref. 7); relaxation induced by the fluorine hyperfine splitting anisotropy[2] in radicals that do not undergo motion ($\dot{\text{C}}$FHCONH$_2$) as well as those that undergo torsional rotation ($\dot{\text{C}}$F$_2$CONH$_2$); relaxation induced by spin exchange of two nonequivalent nuclei[3] ($\dot{\text{C}}$H$_2$COO$^-$); relaxation induced by the admixture of nuclear spin states[8] (occurs when strong forbidden ESR lines are observed as a result of $h\nu_n \simeq A/2$); spectral diffusion in powders and glasses;[9,10] and Heisenberg and chemical spin exchange. In addition to these factors, the spectral dependence is also dependent on the field modulation frequency.[11,12] Most published spectra have not been corrected for field modulation frequency dependence and most of the spectra in this chapter have similarly not been corrected.

In the first part of this chapter we present the spectral analysis of specific oriented radicals in single crystals in order to demonstrate the factors that produce an ELDOR spectrum characteristic of a particular radical substituent. From these studies we derive empirical relationships that can be used to assign the spectral lines of complex overlapping ESR spectra. Particular attention is given to the identification of hydrogen-deuterium exchange reactions in irradiated amino acids,[13] the separation of overlapping spectra in the presence of significant intermolecular relaxation,[11] and the separation of overlapped ESR spectra from radicals containing substituents that each undergo internal rotation at a different rate.[14] An example is also given in which a methyl group undergoes tunneling rotation.

The next part of the chapter is devoted to the ELDOR study of radicals in powders and frozen glasses. Considerable information can be obtained from these studies because there exists a turning point in the ESR spectrum that corresponds predominantly to radicals in a unique orientation to the magnetic field. The anisotropic hyperfine coupling for this orientation can be determined by selecting the observing resonant condition that corresponds to one of these turning points while the pumped microwave source is swept. This effect was demonstrated in an ELDOR study of frozen solutions of DPPH.[15] ELDOR studies of frozen solutions have also shown that spectral diffusion[9,10] and the transfer of saturation[9] between unlike radicals can be measured.

The final part of the chapter is devoted to the ELDOR study of triplet excitons. From studies by Benderskii and his colleagues,[16-19] it is possible to measure an activation energy for the spin exchange process involved, to determine that the onset of exchange can be detected at a much lower temperature from ELDOR than from ESR measurements, and to show that the diffusion process between excitons and local paramagnetic centers is temperature independent.

6.2 INTERPRETATION OF ORGANIC SINGLE CRYSTAL ELDOR SPECTRA ($S = \frac{1}{2}$)

As discussed in Chapter 4 it has been shown that a characteristic hyperfine splitting anisotropy exists for different nuclei in an oriented radical.[20,21] For instance, alpha protons exhibit a hyperfine anisotropy varying from -90 to -30 MHz. Beta protons exhibit a nearly isotropic component that can vary from 0 to 140 MHz, depending on the orientation of the C_β—H_β bond to the p orbital for a given radical conformation. Chlorine hyperfine splittings can vary from 0 to 58 MHz, nitrogen hyperfine splittings from 0 to 110 MHz, and fluorine splittings from 0 to 600 MHz and in a few cases even more. In Chapter 2 it was noted that the frequency sweep range of the commercial Varian ELDOR spectrometer pump mode can cover the frequency range (with variable temperature dewars) from 340 MHz above the observer to approximately 100 MHz below; therefore with this spectrometer it is not possible to observe anisotropic hyperfine splittings that exceed 340 MHz. This is not a severe limitation, as the frequency swept ELDOR intensity of lines at large fluorine hyperfine splittings is shown later in this chapter to be quite weak and therefore ELDOR lines would probably not be seen even if a larger frequency range were available. Only in the case where multiple hyperfine transitions are observed (such as with six equivalent protons) or in triplet state studies might it be advantageous to have a wider frequency range such as is possible with a helical cavity structure (see Section 2.4.3).

To a first order approximation the experimental procedure for obtaining the principal hyperfine splitting tensor components for each nucleus from an ELDOR spectrum of an oriented radical (where $S = \frac{1}{2}$ and $I = \frac{1}{2}$) is identical to that given in Section 4.2.2 for ENDOR. In brief, one plots the allowed-allowed ELDOR line position at the apparent hyperfine splitting for each nucleus as a function of angle in each ij plane and the resulting curve is equated to eq. 4.7 where $R(\theta) = (\sin^2 \theta\, T_{ii} + \cos^2 \theta\, T_{jj} + 2 \sin \theta \cos \theta\, T_{ij})^{1/2}$. The T_{ij} components form a matrix that is subsequently diagonalized and the diagonal components obtained are the squares of the principal hyperfine splittings. The matrix required to diagonalize the T matrix contains the direction cosines between the applied magnetic field and the axes of the principal hyperfine splittings.

However in addition to the allowed-allowed transitions, one may recall from Chapter 1 that forbidden-allowed lines (or combination lines from

Chapter 5) often appear for radicals in single crystals. In order to predict the positions of these lines and thus account for all observable ELDOR lines, it is necessary to examine further the equations for the energy levels that result from eq. 4.1. Also, we will later describe the ELDOR spectra of two or more nuclei interacting with the electron, and anticipating this we will expand eq. 4.1 to include multiple nuclei.

Under these conditions and assuming small g anisotropy the first order equation for the energy levels of multiple interacting nuclei at constant magnetic field equals[8]

$$E(M_s, M_I^1, M_I^2, \ldots, M_I^n) = g_{hh}\beta H M_s + \sum_{i=1}^{n} A_i(M_s) M_I^i \qquad (6.1)$$

where $g_{hh} = (\mathbf{hgh})^{1/2}$, $\mathbf{h}$ is the unit vector along the applied magnetic field whose components equal l_x, l_y, and l_z, the direction cosine given in Section 4.2.2, and i is the subscript which varies from 1 to n where n is the total number of interacting nuclei. The hyperfine splitting $A_i(M_s)$ in eq. 6.1 is an effective hyperfine splitting at a given orientation of the crystal with respect to the applied magnetic field. This effective hyperfine splitting can be expressed[8] in terms of the NMR frequency of the nucleus in question (ν_n) and the principal hyperfine splitting tensor $A_i(M_s)$ by eqs. 6.2 and 6.3.

$$A_i(M_s) = \{\mathbf{h}[\mathbf{A}_i(M_s)]^2 \mathbf{h}\}^{1/2} \qquad (6.2)$$

and

$$\mathbf{A}_i(M_s) = M_s \mathbf{A}_i - \nu_n \mathbf{E} \qquad (6.3)$$

where $\mathbf{E}$ is the unit tensor and $\mathbf{h}\mathbf{A}_i(M_s)$ is the effective hyperfine field felt by a proton. To calculate the energy correctly to the first order requires the value of ν_n and the components of the hyperfine splitting tensor obtainable from procedures outlined in Section 4.2.2.

As an instructive example utilizing eqs. 6.1 through 6.3 let us consider the idealized situation in which the magnetic field lies in the XY plane where X and Y are the principal axis of the hyperfine tensor. In this situation the hyperfine tensor contains only diagonal elements A_{XX}, A_{YY}, and A_{ZZ} and no off-diagonal elements such as the A_{ij} components given in eq. 4.5. For the moment we will consider only one interacting nucleus and later will generalize to multiple nuclei. Since we are in the XY plane, the direction cosine, l_Z, given in eq. 4.5, equals $\cos 90° = 0$ and thus $\mathbf{h} = (l_X, l_Y, 0)$. Also in this case

$$\mathbf{A}_i(M_s) = \begin{pmatrix} (M_s A_{XX} - \nu_n) & 0 & 0 \\ 0 & (M_s A_{YY} - \nu_n) & 0 \\ 0 & 0 & (M_s A_{ZZ} - \nu_n) \end{pmatrix}$$

Substituting h and $A_i(M_s)$ into eqs. 6.1, 6.2, and 6.3 gives

$$E = M_s \nu_e \pm \tfrac{1}{2}[l_X^2(M_s A_{XX} - \nu_n)^2 + l_Y^2(M_s A_{YY} - \nu_n)^2]^{1/2} \tag{6.4}$$

where $g\beta H/h = \nu_e$, $g_N \beta_N H/h = \nu_n$; $M_s = \pm\tfrac{1}{2}$, and A_{XX} and A_{YY} are the principal hyperfine tensor components along the X and Y principal axes. For simplicity let us define

$$A_+ \equiv A_i(M_s = +\tfrac{1}{2}) \tag{6.5}$$
$$A_- \equiv A_i(M_s = -\tfrac{1}{2}) \tag{6.6}$$

where $A_i(M_s)$ was defined in eq. 6.2 so that,

$$A_+ = [l_X^2(\tfrac{1}{2}A_{XX} - \nu_n)^2 + l_Y^2(\tfrac{1}{2}A_{YY} - \nu_n)^2]^{1/2} \tag{6.7}$$

and

$$A_- = [l_X^2(\tfrac{1}{2}A_{XX} + \nu_n)^2 + l_Y^2(\tfrac{1}{2}A_{YY} + \nu_n)^2]^{1/2} \tag{6.8}$$

From eq. 6.4 the two energy levels 3 and 4 of Fig. 1-28 for $M_s = +\tfrac{1}{2}$ are equal to $E_{4,3} = \tfrac{1}{2}\nu_e \pm \tfrac{1}{2}A_+$ whereas the two levels 2 and 1 for $M_s = -\tfrac{1}{2}$ equal $E_{2,1} = -\tfrac{1}{2}\nu_e \pm \tfrac{1}{2}A_-$. Thus if we consider that transition 2–3 of Fig. 1-28 is observed ($\Delta E = \nu_e - \tfrac{1}{2}(A_+ + A_-)$) and transition 1–4 is pumped [$\Delta E = \nu_e + \tfrac{1}{2}(A_+ + A_-)$], then an ELDOR line will occur at $(E_4 - E_1) - (E_3 - E_2) = A_+ + A_-$. To simplify further, consider that the magnetic field lies along the X principal axis so that $l_X = 1$, $l_Y = 0$. In this case

$$A_+ + A_- = \tfrac{1}{2}A_{XX} - \nu_n + \tfrac{1}{2}A_{XX} + \nu_n = A_{XX}$$

exactly as would be expected. On the other hand, if the magnetic field lies along neither the X nor the Y principal axis but in the XY plane, a weighted average of the two splittings A_{XX} and A_{YY} will be measured. Note also that ν_n gives rise to a positive contribution from the A_- term but a negative contribution from the A_+ term. Because of this it turns out that when $A_{ii} > 2\nu_n$, ν_n gives a neglible contribution to the observed splitting when the magnetic field scans the XY plane. Thus the ELDOR spectra will appear anisotropic and dependent only on the principal hyperfine splittings.

This is not the case when a forbidden line is pumped. For instance, if transition 2–3 is observed and transition 2–4 is pumped in Fig. 1-28 with the magnetic field positioned along the X axis, a forbidden-allowed ELDOR line at $A_+ = \tfrac{1}{2}A_{XX} - \nu_n$ is observed. In this case the ELDOR line is dependent on ν_n.

Normally when $A > \nu_n$ the NMR term is dropped in the original spin Hamiltonian because the allowed ESR lines are not dependent on ν_n. However in view of the fact that forbidden-allowed ELDOR lines do depend on ν_n from the example given above, one will find it practical to

Table 6-1. The First Order ELDOR Transitions for Two Unequal Couplings (CFH-R)[a]

Forbidden-Allowed	Allowed-Allowed	
$\frac{1}{2}A_H \pm \nu_H$	$\frac{1}{2}A_F \pm \nu_F$	A_H
$\frac{1}{4}A_H + \frac{1}{2}A_F \pm \nu_H \mp \nu_F$	$A_H + \frac{1}{2}A_F \mp \nu_F$	$A_H + A_F$
$\frac{1}{2}A_H + \frac{1}{2}A_F \pm \nu_H \pm \nu_F$		A_F
$A_F + \frac{1}{2}A_H \pm \nu_H$		

From L. Kispert and K. Chang, *J. Magn. Resonance*, **10**, 162 (1973). This table was constructed assuming the observing position is set at the high field line and $\nu_p > \nu_o$. If $\nu_p < \nu_o$ then the observing position is set at the low field position. In the case of more than two unequal nuclei, a table of ELDOR transitions must be calculated for each observing position from eq. 6.9.

[a] Assuming at a given crystal orientation,

$$E(M_I^F, M_I^H) = g\beta H M_s + A_H M_s M_I^H + A_F M_s M_I^F - \nu_F M_I^F - \nu_H M_I^H.$$

approximate the energy levels for a radical in a crystal by the following expression:

$$E(M_s, M_I^1, M_I^2, \ldots, M_I^n) = \nu_e M_s + \sum_{i=1}^{n} A_i(\text{eff}) M_s M_I^i - \sum_{i=1}^{n} \nu_n^i M_I^i \quad (6.9)$$

where $\nu_e = g\beta H/h$ and $\nu_n^i = g_n\beta_n H/h$ as before and $A_i(\text{eff})$ is the hyperfine splitting observed at any given angle. Making this assumption, Table 6-1 has been constructed for two nonequivalent nuclei, namely, a fluorine and a proton. Note that all forbidden-allowed lines are dependent on ν_n^i. This table is of practical importance when assigning forbidden-allowed ELDOR lines without resorting to extensive calculations. But when $A \sim 2\nu_n$ eq. 6.1 and 6.2 must be used. This case is covered in Section 6.2.5.

So far in determining hyperfine splittings from ELDOR spectra we have ignored the second order corrections to the ELDOR line positions. Generally when a line position fit is made to eq. 4.7, it is assumed for all practical purposes that such corrections are small. Indeed in most cases of protonated radicals, a first order perturbation treatment is adequate to interpret the frequency swept ELDOR spectra since the ELDOR linewidths are from 4 to 6 MHz and the second order shift is of the order of 0.3 MHz. In these cases the allowed-allowed ELDOR transitions at a given angle will be observed at $\sum A_i(M_i^p - M_i^o)$ where M_i^p is the ith quantum number for the pumped line and M_i^o is the ith quantum number for the observed line at a position A_i. Then the use of eq. 4.7 is appropriate. However in some cases second order theory will be needed. For example, the hyperfine splitting constant for the six methyl protons of $(CH_3)_2\dot{C}COOH$ in irradiated α-aminoisobutyric acid is nearly isotropic and equal to 64 MHz. To a good approximation the second order downfield shift for each ESR line from that of a first order spectrum is $(A^2/2H_o)[I(I+1)-M_1]$ where M_1 is the nuclear quantum number for each line and I is the total quantum number. Thus an ELDOR line will occur at $A+5A^2/2H_o$ when the observing field is set on the resonance position of the high field $M_I^o = -3$ ESR line and the $M_I^p = -2$ line is pumped. For $A = 64$ MHz, this shift from the first order splitting A equals 1.3 MHz, a small but measurable quantity. As noted in Table 6-2, this correction varies depending on the observed and pumped lines.

If a large hyperfine anisotropy is observed such as for the fluorine nucleus in $\dot{C}FHCONH_2$, the second order equation is also angularly dependent.[20] For example, if the principal hyperfine splittings $A_X = A_Y = B$ and $A_Z = A$ where $A \gg B$ are observed for a particular radical, then an ELDOR line will be observed along the Z direction at $A(M_I^p - M_I^o) + (B^2/2H_o)[(M_I^o)^2 - (M_I^p)^2]$ for $\nu_p > \nu_o$ where M_I^p and M_I^o are the nuclear quantum numbers for the pumped and observed lines, respectively, ν_p is the pumping frequency, and ν_o is the observing frequency. It is to be noted that the second order shift along the Z principal axis direction is dependent on the magnitude of the hyperfine splitting in the X or Y direction. On the other hand, the ELDOR line along the X principal axis direction

Table 6-2. Second Order Shift for Six Equivalent β Protons[a]

Observing Position[b] (on Resonance) M_I^o	Pumping Position[b] M_I^p	Second Order Corrections,[c] Units of $A^2/2H_o$
-3	-2	-5
-2	-1	-3
-1	0	-1
0	1	1
1	2	3
2	3	5

[a] An allowed-allowed ELDOR line is possible at an experimental frequency of $-A_H[M_I^o - M_I^p] + (A^2/2H_o)[(M_I^o)^2 - (M_I^p)^2]$.
[b] M_I^o is the total quantum number for the observed line. M_I^p is the total quantum number for the pumped line.
[c] To be added to the experimentally observed ELDOR line to obtain the A value to first order when $\nu_p > \nu_o$; when $\nu_p < \nu_o$, the M_I^o and M_I^p labels are interchanged and the sign of the correction is reversed.

is observed at $B(M_I^p - M_I^o) + [(A^2 + B^2)/4H_o][(M_I^o)^2 - (M_I^p)^2]$. Note that the second order shift in the X direction is dependent largely on the magnitude of the largest splitting in the Z direction. An additional difficulty is that single crystal spectra are usually measured in a nonprincipal axis system, in which case the second order terms also include significant cross terms that are functions of angle. However to a good approximation the second order ELDOR shift in a direction near the largest principal splitting will depend on the smallest hyperfine splitting. Such a shift may be difficult to detect for $B < 20$ MHz, whereas in a direction near the observed smallest hyperfine splitting, a measurable second order shift will be observed for $A \geq 100$ MHz.

Nevertheless eq. 4.7 can still be used to determine principal hyperfine splittings in those cases where second order effects are measurable, if the ELDOR line positions are first shifted to a first order position. An example of this has been given in Table 6-2 for six equivalent β protons. Generally when $\nu_p > \nu_o$, the observing ELDOR frequency must be decreased when sitting on the high field ESR lines and increased when sitting on the low field ESR lines.

6.2.1 Intramolecular Motion—Methyl Groups

The rate at which intramolecular motion occurs greatly affects the relaxation times T_{1e}, T_{1n}, T_{x1}, and T_{x2}.[1-5] Therefore the ELDOR spectral intensity can vary significantly as the rotational correlation times of substituents change with temperature. The quantitative manner in which molecular motion affects T_{1n} and T_x processes in solids has not been studied. Nevertheless considerable insight into the influence of motion on T_{1n} and T_x can be deduced by examining the definitions of W_n, W_{x1}, and W_{x2} derived for the tumbling motion of a radical in solution. If the isotropic dipolar contribution is neglected,[1] then the ratio of

$$\frac{W_n}{W_{x2}} = \frac{1}{4}(1 + \omega_n^2 \tau_c^2) \quad (6.10)$$

where ω_n is the nuclear magnetic resonance frequency and τ_c is the rotational correlation time of the substituent. For X-band ESR, ω_n^{-1} is about 1.1×10^{-8} sec so that if the motion has a correlation time (τ_c) much longer than 1.9×10^{-8} sec, W_n will be larger than W_{x2}.

A calculation of the reduction factors in terms of a four level energy diagram including the transition probabilities W_n, W_e, W_{x1}, W_{x2} for the situation where the pumping frequency is at resonance and the observing mode is not saturated was shown in Section 1.5.2.2 to equal

$$R = \frac{W_n^2 - W_{x1}W_{x2}}{W_e(2W_n + W_{x1} + W_{x2}) + (W_n + W_{x1})(W_n + W_{x2})} \quad (6.11)$$

where $W_n = 1/T_{1n}$, $W_e = 1/T_{1e}$, $W_{x1} = 1/T_{x1}$, $W_{x2} = 1/T_{x2}$. Thus if

$$W_{x1}W_{x2} > W_n^2 \quad (6.12)$$

R will be negative and an enhanced ESR signal will be predicted. On the other hand, if

$$W_n^2 > W_{x1}W_{x2} \quad (6.13)$$

a reduction is predicted. Substituting eq. 6.10 into the condition for observing enhanced spectra $W_{x1}W_{x2} > W_n^2$ and setting $W_{x2} = 6W_{x1}$ yields $\tau_c = 7 \times 10^{-9}$ sec (W_{x2} is expected to be larger than W_{x1}, because of the presence of hyperfine anisotropy). Thus by analogy to molecular reorientation rates in solution, enhanced spectra would be predicted whenever τ_c, the intramolecular reorientation rate of a substituent group, is less than 7×10^{-9} sec. Slower rotational times than this would yield reduced ELDOR spectra. Of course remember this is a calculation based on a radical in solution. The exact τ_c would require a calculation based on an oriented radical; nevertheless, this calculation will form the basis for the qualitative explanation given when one or more substituents of a radical undergoes internal motion.

As an example let us consider the frequency swept ELDOR spectra observed for the high temperature conformation of the $(CH_3)_2\dot{C}COOH$ radical formed when a 77 K irradiated crystal of α-aminoisobutyric acid is warmed to room temperature. From ESR[22] and ENDOR[23] measurements, the methyl groups freely rotate about their own axis at or near room temperature resulting in equivalence of the methyl protons for each methyl group. Above 375 K the methyl groups become equivalent as a result of each methyl group oscillating between two or more conformations. Upon cooling to 77 K or lower, the simple seven line pattern with a binomial intensity ratio of 1:6:15:20:15:6:1 at 375 K changes reversibly to a complex pattern because of the freezing out of a conformation in which the one methyl group is stationary while the other freely rotates.[23]

The frequency swept ELDOR spectra obtained by setting the observing field position at the bottom of the first derivative $M_I = -2$ ESR absorption line are given as a function of temperature in Fig. 6-1 over a frequency range of 12 to 300 MHz. A reduction in the ESR intensity is observed at 323 K, resulting in intense ELDOR lines at 66, 131, 195, and 260 MHz flanked on each side by ELDOR lines occurring at ±14 MHz of the observed ELDOR line. Near 283 K the ESR lines remain unchanged

ORGANIC SINGLE CRYSTAL ELDOR SPECTRA 313

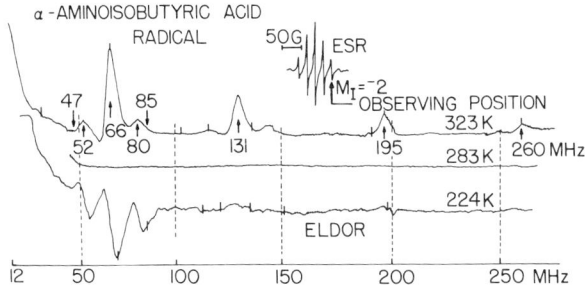

Figure 6-1. Typical ELDOR spectra obtained as a function of temperature for an oriented π radical with rotating methyl groups attached to the carbon atom containing the unpaired electron. The observing position is located at the bottom of the $M_I = -2$ first derivative ESR line of the $(CH_3)_2\dot{C}COOH$ radical in irradiated α-aminoisobutyric acid crystals. At 323 K a reduction (as indicated by an absorptionlike peak) in the ESR line is observed at $A_H = 66$ MHz, $2A_H$, $3A_H$, and $4A_H$. No change in ESR intensity is observed near 283 K while at 224 K an enhancement in the ESR intensity is observed at A_H, a reduction at $2A_H$, and a near zero enhancement at $3A_H$. The forbidden lines at 47.0 MHz and 85 MHz are barely observable, being partially obscured by the spin-flip lines at 52.0 and 80.0 MHz. 100 kHz field modulation was used. From L. D. Kispert et al., *J. Chem. Phys.*, **58**, 2164 (1973).

and no ELDOR lines are observed. Below 283 K an enhancement of the ESR lines occurs for the ELDOR line at 66 MHz; however a reduction in the ESR line is observed for the ELDOR line at 131 MHz with a very weak ELDOR line at 195 MHz. This same enhancement and reduction dependence is also observed for the $(CH_3)_2\dot{C}COOH$ radical in irradiated α-aminoisobutyric acid and in N,N-dideutero-α-aminoisobutyric acid.[1]

The transition responsible for the ELDOR line at 66 MHz (Fig. 6-1) while observing the $M_I = -2$ ESR line at 323 K is given in Fig. 6-2. Since the proton hyperfine splitting constants for β protons are nearly isotropic and are significantly larger than $2\nu_H$ (where ν_H is the NMR frequency of a free proton), the energy level diagram is given to the first order by eq. 6.9. However if the energy is expressed in terms of M_I, the component of the total nuclear quantum number for six equivalent protons, then

$$E(M_s, M_I) = g\beta H M_s + A_H M_I - \nu_H M_I \qquad (6.14)$$

where M_I is the component of the total nuclear quantum number for six equivalent protons. Using this description, allowed-allowed ELDOR lines are predicted at A_H, $2A_H$, $3A_H$, $4A_H$, and $5A_H$. All except the line at $5A_H$ (which occurred outside the spectrometer sweep range) were experimentally observed.

Utilizing eq. 6.14, forbidden-allowed ELDOR lines are calculated to occur at $f_{p_1} = A_H/2 + \nu_H = 47$ MHz and $f_{p_3} = 3/2 A_H - \nu_H = 85$ MHz where

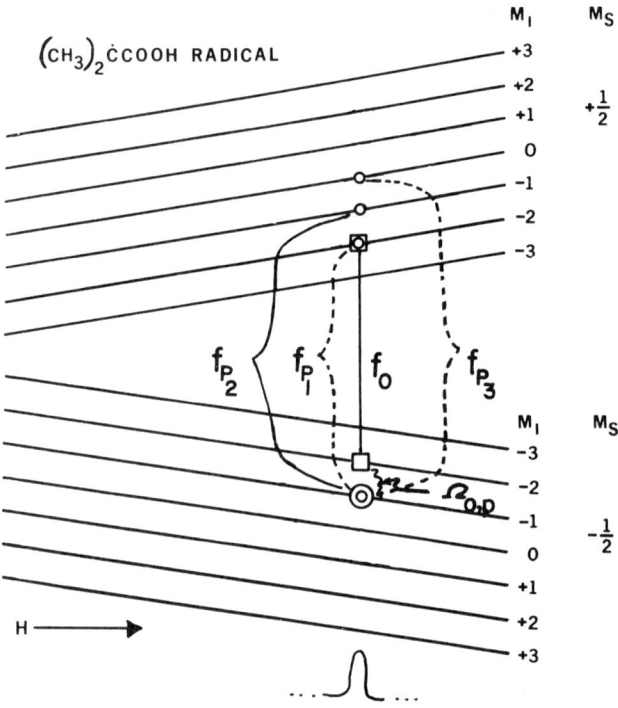

Figure 6-2. The energy level diagram indicating the transitions f_{P_1} and f_{P_3} (dotted lines) responsible for the forbidden-allowed ELDOR lines at 47.0 and 85.0 MHz and the allowed-allowed ELDOR line (f_{P_2}) at $A_H = 66.0$ MHz in Fig. 6-1. When the observing position is corrected to the center of the first derivative line, a shift to 45.9, 82.1, and 64.0 MHz, respectively, occurs. From L. D. Kispert et al., *J. Chem. Phys.*, **58**, 2164 (1973).

A_H is the effective hyperfine separation at a given angle and is not one of the principal values of the hyperfine tensor. Experimentally these lines are not observed in Fig. 6-1.

Instead the lines that are observed on either side of the ELDOR line at 66 MHz occur at $A_H \pm \nu_H$ and are referred to as ELDOR spin-flip transitions. For the moment we will ignore these lines, as they will be treated in more detail in Section 6.2.9. If only allowed-allowed ELDOR lines occur, the ELDOR spectrum will contain lines at the same positions from the observed line as the ESR spectrum. As one may recall from Table 5-3 the difference between the experimentally observed hyperfine splitting, $A_H = 64$ MHz, and the center of the ELDOR peak, 66 MHz, is due to the observing position.[15] For instance, when the observing position

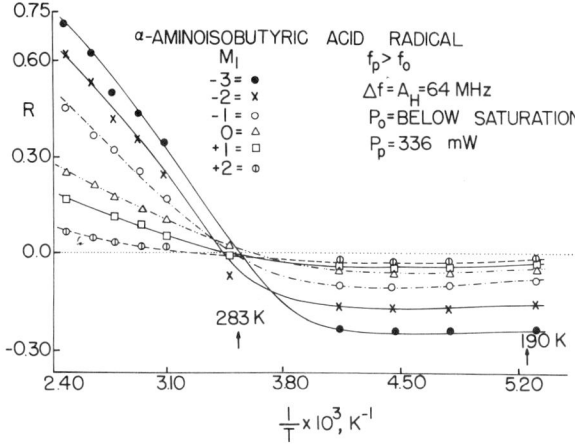

Figure 6-3. Typical temperature dependence for the reduction factor R of the ELDOR line at A_H as a function of M_I when each methyl group of the $(CH_3)_2\dot{C}COOH$ radical in irradiated α-aminoisobutyric acid crystals undergoes rapid rotation below 283 K and the pseudo-exchange of the two methyl groups above 300 K. An M_I dependence is observed over the entire temperature range with a reduction in the ESR intensity above 283 K and an enhancement in the ESR intensity below 283 K. From L. D. Kispert et al., *J. Chem. Phys.* **58**, 2164 (1973).

is situated at the bottom of a first derivative homogeneously (or approximately so) broadened ESR line, the center of the ELDOR absorptionlike peak occurs at $A_H + \frac{1}{2}\Delta H$, where ΔH is the peak to peak ESR linewidth.

The frequency swept ELDOR spectral intensity for $(CH_3)_2\dot{C}COOH$ at A_H varies with temperature and with M_I, the quantum number of the observed line. The spectral intensity variation is given in Fig. 6-3 for a temperature change from 187 to 403 K for the α-aminoisoburyric acid crystals. Above 283 K the reduction factor is dependent both on temperature and M_I, suggesting that W_n (the lattice-induced spin-flip probability) is the primary contributor to the ELDOR spectrum observed. (See Section 1.5.2.2.) Below 283 K an M_I dependent enhancement of the ESR line at A_H is observed. Particular note should be given to the weak temperature dependence observed below 243 K in contrast to the nearly linear temperature dependence observed for the ELDOR intensity above 283 K.

To further understand the observed ELDOR temperature dependence given in Fig. 6-3 a calculation can be carried out to determine the contribution of each relaxation pathway to the ELDOR spectrum. To simplify matters it is assumed that the six protons are completely equivalent, that the probability of a double quantum jump is zero, and that the relaxation can be described in terms of W_e, W_n, W_{x1}, and W_{x2} probabilities. The results of such calculations[1] indicate that above room temperature, the spectral dependence arises from a competition between W_n/W_e, W_{x1}/W_e, and W_{x2}/W_e. It is the increase in the W_{x2} and W_{x1} probabilities relative to W_n that causes the observed change from a reduced ELDOR line at A_H above 283 K to an enhanced ELDOR line at 224 K. This same change in W_n/W_e and W_{x1}/W_e also predicts the M_I dependence of the ELDOR lines at $2A_H$, $3A_H$, etc., at 323 K and the very weak reduced lines at $2A_H$ and $3A_H$ (see Fig. 6-1) at 224 K.

In summary, it appears then that a group undergoing internal motion should give rise to an ELDOR spectrum of lines at multiples of A_H when the correlation time is longer than 10^{-8} sec, that is, if the electron-nuclear dipolar relaxation mechanism predominates as is observed for the $(CH_3)_2\dot{C}COOH$ radical above room temperature. As the rotational correlation time becomes shorter than 10^{-8} sec and $W_{x1} \simeq W_n$, an enhanced spectrum is expected at A_H, with very weak reduced peaks being observed at $2A_H$ and $3A_H$. For all practical purposes only an enhanced peak at A_H is observed.

6.2.2 α Protons—No Intramolecular Motion

In a large number of cases the free radicals that contain rotating groups also contain α protons. Although rapid reorientation of the methyl protons usually occurs at room temperature and is easily detected from the ESR spectrum, large amplitude torsional motion by the α protons in many cases is not observed at room temperature. However such motion can occur above room temperature. Since the presence of intramolecular motion gives rise to ELDOR active transitions, one might ask what the ELDOR intensity variation is for the α protons in the presence of rotating groups. Two examples will demonstrate this point. The first one is the frequency swept ELDOR investigation of $CH_3\dot{C}HCOOD$ in irradiated deuterated *l*-alanine crystals.[1] This example will also demonstrate the observed frequency swept ELDOR line shape as a function of temperature that results from the overlap of ESR lines from both the methyl and the α protons. In a second example, that of $NH_3^+\dot{C}HCOO^-$ in irradiated glycine, the effect of rotating groups other than methyl will be shown.[2]

The ESR spectrum of the $CH_3\dot{C}HCOOD$ radical in deuterated *l*-alanine is, in general, complex[24,25] because of the anisotropy of the α proton and the presence of two magnetically nonequivalent radical sites. However along the c axis, all four protons appear to be equivalent,

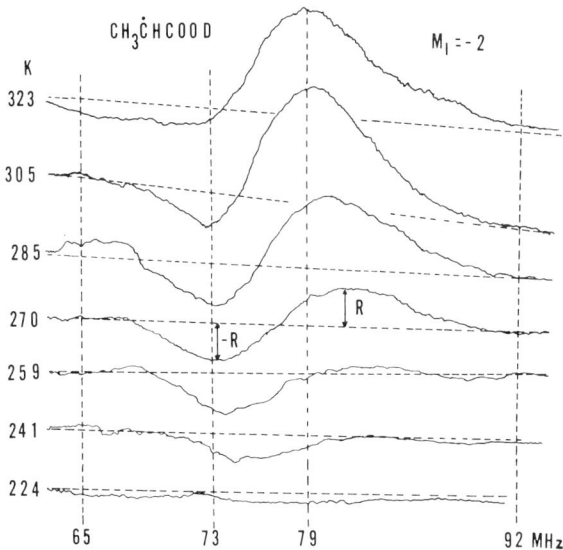

Figure 6-4. The ELDOR spectrum of CH₃ĊHCOOD in irradiated *l*-alanine single crystals obtained along the *c* crystal axis as a function of temperature where the hyperfine splitting for the methyl protons is almost equal to that of the α protons. The observing ESR field is positioned at the bottom of the first derivative $M_I = -2$ ESR line in order to demonstrate that the ELDOR line is composed of an enhanced ELDOR line at 75 MHz due to the rotating $10^{-11} < \tau_c < 10^{-9}$ methyl group and a reduced ELDOR line at 78 MHz due to the α proton which decreases with decreasing temperature. From L. D. Kispert et al., *J. Chem. Phys.*, **58**, 2164 (1973).

resulting in a five line ESR spectrum with intensities near the expected 1:4:6:4:1. Analysis of the ELDOR spectrum shows that the β proton splitting ($A_H^{CH_3} = 73$ MHz) differs from the α proton splitting ($A_H^\alpha = 75$ MHz) by approximately 2 to 3 MHz.

The temperature dependence of the frequency swept ELDOR spectrum of the CH₃ĊHCOOD radical in irradiated *l*-alanine single crystals (along the *c* axis) is shown in Fig. 6-4. Only the portion of the ELDOR spectrum near the $A_H^{CH_3} = A_H^\alpha$ frequency is shown. The observing ESR field is positioned at the bottom of the first derivative $M_I = -2$ absorption ESR line in order to dramatize the complex change in the ELDOR lineshape with temperature. For this observing position an ELDOR peak will occur at the hyperfine splitting frequency plus one-half of the linewidth (ΔH). Note that at 323 K, an ELDOR peak is observed at 78 MHz ($A_H^{CH_3} + \Delta H$) that results from a 17% reduction in the ESR line. As the temperature is lowered to 285 K there appears an increase in the intensity of a peak below the baseline (denoted by the dotted line) and a decrease in the peak observed above the baseline at 323 K. At 270 K the contributions from both positive and negative reductions are approximately equal, giving rise to an apparent first derivative-like lineshape. At 241 K only a 4% enhancement in the ESR line is observed at 75 MHz ($A_H^\alpha + \Delta H$); note the change in frequency from the ELDOR line at higher temperature. It should also be pointed out that if the observing ESR field is moved to the center of the ESR line below 305 K, the ELDOR intensity is barely detectable. In fact, the lineshape is quite dependent on the precise observing field position as a result of the contributions from both reduced and enhanced lines. This is in contrast to the first derivative ELDOR signal for which a maximum ELDOR intensity is observed for $(CH_3)_2\dot{C}COOH$ when the observing field is set at the center of the ESR line.[11] (See Fig. 5-16 and the associated text for an explanation of the lineshape.)

Qualitatively the complex ELDOR lineshape appears to result from a competition between the reduction in the α proton ESR line intensity at 78 MHz, which decreases with decreasing temperature,[26] and the enhancement of the methyl proton ESR line at 76 MHz, which increases with decreasing temperature. Quantitatively Miyagawa and Itoh[24] report that the methyl group in $CH_3\dot{C}HCOOH$ has a rotational correlation time τ_c equal to 3×10^{-10} sec at 224 K and 2.6×10^{-11} sec at 323 K. Based on eqs. 6.1 and 6.2 an enhanced ESR spectrum would be predicted at 224 K as is observed. At higher temperature the longer correlation time of the C—H torsional motion results in a significant ESR reduction that dominates the ELDOR spectrum.

The observation that enhanced and reduced ELDOR lines can be observed in the same spectra, depending on the rotational correlation time of the substituents to which each hyperfine splitting belongs, is further noted in irradiated glycine. The ELDOR spectrum observed[2] for $NH_3^+\dot{C}HCOO^-$ at 313 K is given in Fig. 6-5 for the crystal orientation where the c crystal axis is nearly parallel to the magnetic field. Setting the observing position at the ESR line position indicated by the arrow results in an ELDOR spectrum with enhanced lines at the NH_3^+ proton hyperfine splittings (53 and 107 MHz) and reduced lines at 79 MHz, the hyperfine splitting of C_α—H protons. The appearance of enhanced lines above room temperature is a consequence of the larger barrier to rotation exhibited by the NH_3^+ group than that for the methyl protons. In other words, short rotational correlation times are possible only above room temperature. This dependence on rotational correlation time results in an ELDOR spectral intensity that varies with temperature in a manner depicted for $NH_3^+\dot{C}HCOO$ in Fig. 6-6. The intensity for α protons decreases below detectability below 270 K.

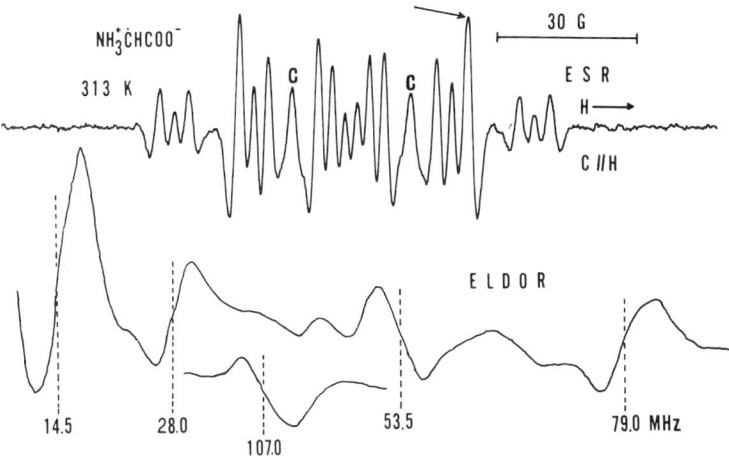

Figure 6-5. (a) The second derivative ESR spectrum of $NH_3^+\dot{C}HCOO^-$ and $\dot{C}H_2COO^-$ (the low and high field line denoted by the letter C), obtained with the magnetic field along the c crystal axis at 313 K. (b) The ELDOR spectrum was obtained by placing the observing field at the position of the arrow in the $NH_3^+\dot{C}HCOO^-$ spectrum. Particularly noteworthy is observance of an enhanced ELDOR line at the hyperfine splitting of the rotating amine protons (53.5 MHz) and a reduced line at 79.0 MHz, the hyperfine splitting of the α proton. The ELDOR line at approximately 28 MHz occurs at the difference between the amine and α proton splitting as predicted, utilizing eq. 6.9 to calculate the ELDOR transitions.

Once again note that when the α proton splitting is approximately equal to the amine protons, distorted ELDOR lines will result at some temperatures from the imperfect addition of an enhanced and a reduced line.

6.2.3 Hyperfine Splitting Anisotropy

The hyperfine splitting anisotropy present for each radical can cause a large variation in ELDOR intensity with angle, providing no intramolecular motion on an ESR time scale is present to average out the hyperfine

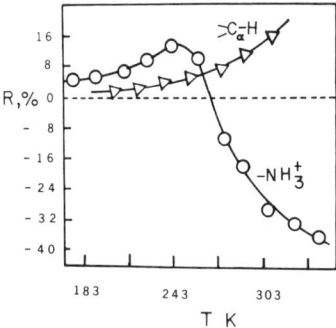

Figure 6-6. Temperature dependence of the allowed-allowed ELDOR line intensity at 53.5 MHz (O) and 79.0 MHz (▷) for the $NH_3^+\dot{C}HCOO^-$ radical given in Fig. 6-5. Note the near zero intensity for the α proton ELDOR line below 273 K and the nonzero intensity for the amine protons, which varies from a reduced line below to an enhanced line above 273 K. The observing position was set at the high field ESR line of the $NH_3^+\dot{C}HCOO^-$ radical.

anisotropy. An example of this effect is observed in the ELDOR investigations of ĊFHCONH$_2$, where a large fluorine anisotropy occurs.[2]

The ESR spectrum consists of four first derivative absorption lines with principal fluorine hyperfine splittings equal to 530 (perpendicular to the radical plane), −11, and −45 MHz (parallel to the C—F bond), whereas the proton hyperfine splittings equal −63 (perpendicular to the radical plane), −96 (perpendicular to the C—H bond), and −31 MHz (parallel to the C—H bond). Therefore an assessment of the effect of a large hyperfine anisotropy on a proton hyperfine splitting is possible by varying the fluorine hyperfine splitting from 530 to 40 MHz, which causes the proton splitting to vary from 63 to 82 MHz. In this way a large fluorine anisotropy can be observed while maintaining a small proton anisotropy. Any variation observed in the ELDOR intensity as a function of fluorine hyperfine splitting is assumed to be a result of the fluorine hyperfine anisotropy since no motion on an ESR timescale is observed for this radical.

The relative intensities of the ĊFHCONH$_2$ ELDOR lines observed as a function of angle are given in Table 6-3 for the allowed-allowed and allowed-forbidden ELDOR transitions given in Table 6-1. It is immediately noted from Fig. 6-7b and Table 6-3 that a complex ELDOR spectrum is observed when the observing magnetic field is set at the high

Table 6-3 Fluorine Hyperfine Splittings MH$_z$ versus Selected ELDOR Frequencies for the ĊFHCONH$_2$ Radical at 233 K in CFH$_2$CONH$_2$

Experimental		Reduction Factors[a]			
$A_F(\theta)$	$A_H(\theta)$	$\frac{1}{2}A_H - \nu_H$	$\frac{1}{2}A_H + \nu_H$	A_H	$\frac{1}{2}A_F \mp \nu_F \pm \nu_H^{NH_2}$
39.9	82.2	0.09	0.05	0.05	(0.49)
79.2	79.2	0.05	0.10	0.05	0.27
108.6	81.8	0.09	(0.09)	0.02	0.22
152.9	81.8	0.07	0.07	0.02	0.19
211.1	80.1	0.08	0.07	0.02	0.04
252.8	79.8	0.09	0.08	0.02	
330.0	77.8	0.06	0.09	<0.01	
399.3	73.5	0.06	0.17	<0.01	
498.0	67.5	0.20	0.19	<0.01	
530.0	63.2	0.23	0.04	<0.01	

From L. Kispert and K. Chang, *J. Magn. Resonance*, **10**, 162 (1973).

[a] R is approximated as ELDOR lineheight/ESR lineheight; no corrections are made for the differences between the inhomogeneous ESR linewidth of approximately 7 to 9 Gauss and the ELDOR linewidth of 4 to 5 MHz. For the allowed lines at $A_F = 79.2$, 152.9, and 211.1 MHz, R equals 2 to 3%.

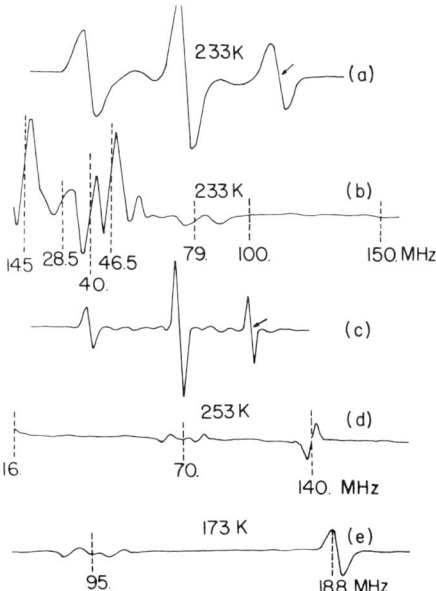

Figure 6-7. The typical complex ELDOR spectrum (*b*) obtained for the ĊFHCONH$_2$ radical at 233 K when $A^F = A^H = 84$ MHz and the observing magnetic field is set at the high field ESR line (*a*). This is to be contrasted with the simpler ELDOR spectrum composed of a forbidden-allowed transitions at 61 and 79 MHz and an allowed-allowed transition at 140 MHz observed for ĊF$_2$CONH$_2$ (*d*) when the observing field is set at the high field ESR (*c*) and $A_F = 140$ MHz. The allowed-allowed ELDOR lines from ĊF$_2$CONH$_2$ are observed to change from a reduced ($R = 10\%$) to an enhanced ($R = 19\%$) spectrum over the temperature range 253 to 173 K while the forbidden-allowed lines remain as reduced ELDOR lines. Adapted from L. Kispert and K. Chang, *J. Magn. Resonance*, **10**, 162 (1973).

field ESR line (Fig. 6-7*a*) with rather intense forbidden-allowed lines observed at $A_H/2 \pm \nu_H$ and $A_F/2 \pm \nu_F$. Particular attention should be given to certain features. When the observing field position is perpendicular to the radical plane (a direction for which $A_F(\theta) = 530$ MHz), a rather intense line occurs at $A_H/2 - \nu_H$; however none is observed at A_H. As the fluorine splitting is decreased, an increase in the intensity of the $A_H/2 + \nu_H$ line is observed; however still no detectable line is observed at A_H. Upon decreasing the fluorine hyperfine splitting below 253 MHz, the $A_H/2 \pm \nu_H$ lines remain constant in intensity with a weak but detectable line at A_H being observed. The predominance of forbidden-allowed lines at large A_F values is assumed to be due to the influence of the hyperfine anisotropy on the relaxation involved. ELDOR spectra taken of crystals that contain smaller hyperfine anisotropy exhibit this effect to a much smaller degree. It is also noted that the intensity of the ELDOR lines for ĊFHCONH$_2$ slowly increases with decreasing temperature when the observing power is kept at a constant value. It appears that the slow increase in the ELDOR intensity may be a reflection of an increase in saturation at lower temperatures.

A somewhat simpler ELDOR spectrum arises for fluorinated radicals such as ĊF$_2$CONH$_2$ that contain equivalent nuclei, which are known to undergo a torsional oscillation about the C—C bond.[2] In Fig. 6-7*d* the ELDOR spectrum obtained by setting the observing position at the crossover of the high field absorption ESR line at 153 K (Fig. 6-7c) consists of an allowed-allowed reduced ELDOR line at 140 MHz and a weaker forbidden-allowed reduced ELDOR lines at 61 and 79 MHz. Upon decreasing the temperature, (Fig. 6-7e) the A_F value increases and an allowed-allowed enhanced ELDOR line is observed. Even though the relative intensity of the allowed-allowed and forbidden-allowed lines do change with hyperfine splitting, the forbidden-allowed lines never approach the intensity observed for $\dot{C}HFCONH_2$. The change in the allowed-allowed ELDOR intensities from a reduced to enhanced line at 173 K is attributed to the competition between the slower but dominant torsional oscillatory motion near room temperature and the rapid out-of-plane in-phase wag of the CF_2 group, which appears to be the dominant motion at 173 K.[2] The appearance of reduced forbidden-allowed lines at all temperatures is in keeping with the prediction given in Section 1.5.2.2 that forbidden-allowed ELDOR lines always appear as reduced lines.

6.2.4 Intramolecular Proton Spin Exchange

One may recall from Section 6.2.1 that the presence of intramolecular motion results in an ELDOR spectrum composed of allowed-allowed transitions that vary from enhanced to reduced as the correlation time increases. However the forbidden-allowed transitions are weak or not observed. On the other hand, when analysis of the ESR spectrum shows the absence of motion on an ESR time scale in addition to the presence of a large hyperfine anisotropy, intense forbidden-allowed ELDOR lines appear with weak allowed-allowed ELDOR lines. We now present an interesting combination of these two effects when two protons undergo spin exchange or jump processes between a finite number of configurations.[3]

For example, such jump processes appear to occur for the $\dot{C}H_2COO^-$ or $\dot{C}H_2COOH$ radicals found in irradiated crystals of malonic acid,[27] glycine,[28,29] sodium acetate trihydrate,[30,31] and zinc acetate dihydrate.[32,33] The four line ESR spectrum of $\dot{C}H_2COO^-$ observed at low temperatures is that of two nonequivalent protons. At higher temperatures the four line spectrum collapses to a three line pattern attributable to two equivalent protons and the outer lines shift toward the center of the spectrum. Despite these changes with temperature, the g values remain constant[30] and the direction of the carbon p oribtal remains quenched in space.[30] Several models have been suggested; however none have proved adequate for the description of the motion.[30,32-34] Recently Hayes et al.[34] proposed that a nonadiabatic spin exchange is responsible for the observed temperature dependence of $\dot{C}H_2COO^-$ and they were able to

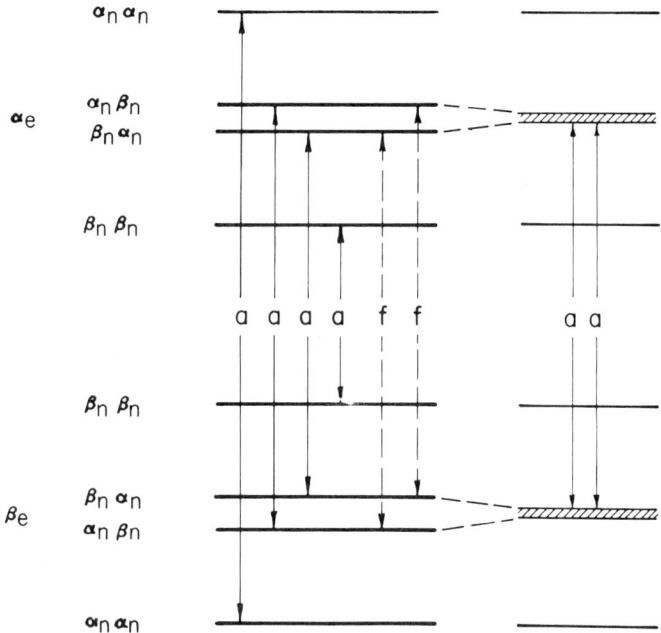

Figure 6-8. The energy level diagram for the two nonequivalent protons of $\dot{C}H_2COO^-$ showing the allowed (a) ESR transitions and the forbidden (f) transitions which mix together to give a doubly degenerate allowed transition for two equivalent protons when the spins states $\alpha_e\alpha_n\beta_n$ and $\alpha_e\beta_n\alpha_n$ become degenerate as well as levels $\beta_e\beta_n\alpha_n$ and $\beta_e\alpha_n\beta_n$.

reproduce many of the features of the spectrum. In their model the exchange of the two protons in a crystal results in the effective exchange of the $\alpha_N\beta_N$ proton nuclear spin states for the $\beta_N\alpha_N$ spin states and the appearance of a shift of the high and low field ESR lines to smaller hyperfine values. The four line ESR spectrum arises at low temperatures from the allowed transitions indicated in Fig. 6-8. The indicated forbidden transitions are not observed as long as the correlation time for the motionally averaged spectra is $>10^{-6}$ sec. The forbidden lines are observed in the ESR spectrum when the correlation time is between 10^{-7} to 10^{-9} sec, as the levels $\alpha_e\alpha_n\beta_n$ and $\alpha_e\beta_n\alpha_n$ become degenerate as well as levels $\beta_e\beta_n\alpha_n$ and $\beta_e\alpha_n\beta_n$.

The typical behavior for the ELDOR spectrum as a function of temperature for either $\dot{C}H_2COO^-$ in irradiated zinc acetate or $\cdot CH_2COOH$ in irradiated malonic acid when the observing position is set at D and $\nu_p > \nu_o$ is given in Fig. 6-9. Noteworthy is the decrease in the intensity of the allowed-allowed ELDOR lines at 45 and 67 MHz for two

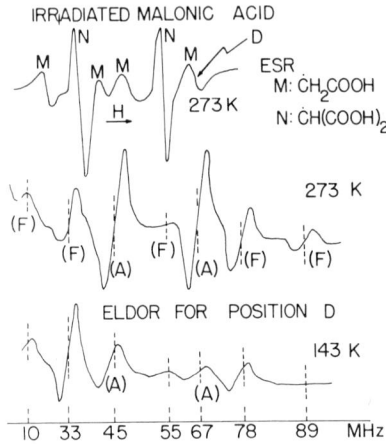

Figure 6-9. Typical intensity variation with temperature of the ELDOR spectrum for two nonequivalent protons in the $\dot{C}H_2COOH$ radical in irradiated malonic acid crystals. Note the decrease in intensity of the allowed-allowed (A) lines at 45 and 67 MHz with decreasing temperature and the increase in intensity of the forbidden-allowed (F) line at 33 MHz.

nonequivalent protons with decreasing temperature (273 to 143 K) and the increase in the forbidden-allowed line at 33 MHz. Similar behavior is found in a crystal direction where only three ESR lines occur.

The temperature dependence of the frequency swept ELDOR spectrum obtained from the first derivative absorption ESR of the $\dot{C}H_2COO^-$ radical in single crystals of zinc acetate at 100 kHz modulation is given in Fig. 6-10. The observing field is positioned at the crossover of the high field ESR line of a three line pattern with an intensity ratio of 1:2:1 at 300 K. The three line ESR spectrum was observed over the entire temperature range investigated. The ELDOR reduction factors (R) for the allowed-allowed lines A and B show a maximum from 200 to 220 K with the maximum intensity of line A occurring at a different temperature than that of line B. Upon lowering the temperature the R values of lines D and C increase, whereas R values of the allowed lines A and B decrease. The maximum R value of the allowed line A occurs at 200 K where the spin exchange time equals 0.2×10^{-6} sec.

A similar temperature dependence for the ELDOR spectral intensity is observed for the $\dot{C}H_2COOH$ radical in irradiated malonic acid over a temperature range where the four line ESR pattern at low temperature changes to a three line pattern at higher temperature. The observed reduction factors R are plotted as a function of temperature in Fig. 6-11. The allowed-allowed ELDOR lines occur at 64.9 and 48 MHz whereas the forbidden-allowed lines occur at 36.5 and 19.0 MHz. The maximum R value for both allowed-allowed lines occurs at approximately 273 K whereas the maximum R values for the forbidden-allowed lines occur from 220 to 240 K. At 323 K the central two lines of the four line ESR pattern begin to collapse noticeably to a single line as evidenced by a

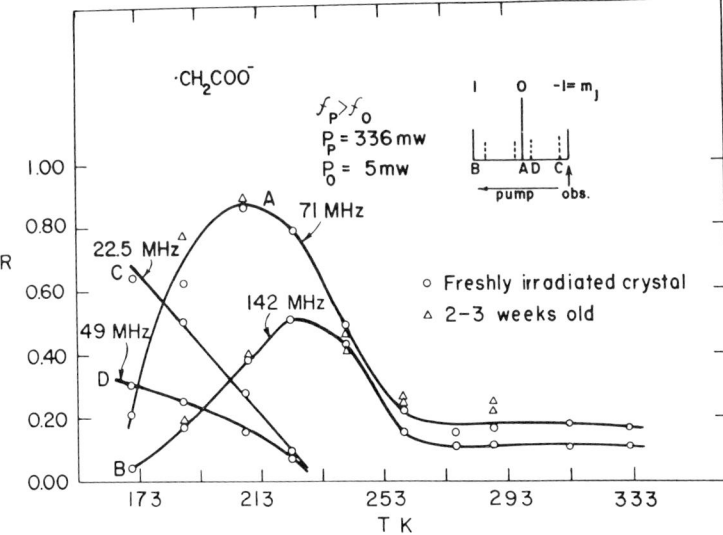

Figure 6-10. ELDOR reduction factors for $\dot{C}H_2COO^-$ (in zinc acetate) versus temperature. A and B are the allowed-allowed ELDOR lines, and C and D are the forbidden-allowed ELDOR lines. For all curves the $M_I = -1$ ESR line is the observing ESR line. Below 223 K the intensity of the allowed-allowed ELDOR lines decreases and that of the forbidden-allowed lines increases. From L. D. Kispert et al., *J. Chem.*, **77**, 629 (1973).

change in separation of the two central lines from 5.5 G at 273 K to 2.5 G at 323 K. In fact, the change in the ESR hyperfine pattern from 273 to 323 K appears to be similar to the change in the four line pattern shown for $\cdot CH_2COO^-$ in Fig. 1a (203 K) and 1b (242 K) of ref. 34 where the correlation time is calculated to change from 0.2×10^{-6} to 0.3×10^{-7} sec. The only difference between Figs. 6-10 and 6-11 appears to be the temperature at which the maximum is observed.

An exact calculation[3] using a density matrix approach and a four level scheme failed to predict any condition of W_{x1}, W_{x2}, W_e, or W_n that results in the ELDOR spectral dependence observed in Figs. 6-10 and 6-11. However the ELDOR spectral dependence observed was predicted by a density matrix calculation of an eight level energy diagram changing to a six level energy diagram. In this calculation a significant pseudo electron spin-flip transition probability between nearly degenerate energy levels is the main contributor to the appearance of the ELDOR spectra in Figs. 6-10 and 6-11. In somewhat simplified terms these results can be interpreted in the following way. Near the temperature at which the four line ESR pattern begins to change to a three line ESR pattern, the transition probability of the forbidden lines increases as an indirect result of the onset of motion.

326 SINGLE CRYSTAL AND POWDER ELDOR

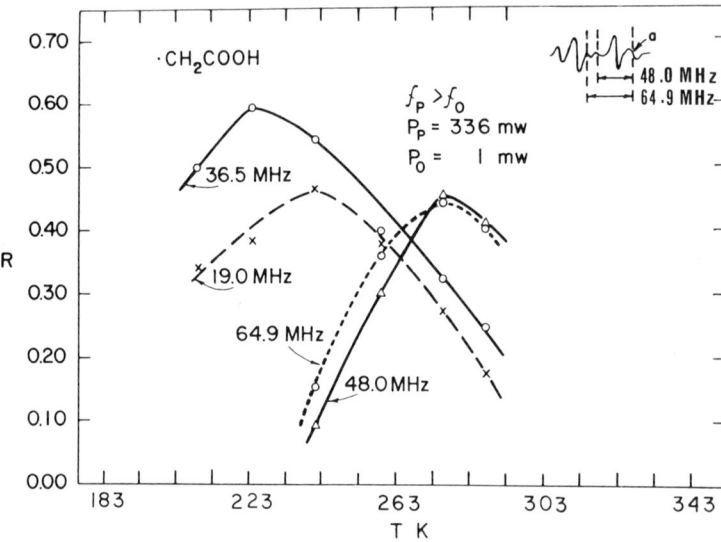

Figure 6-11. ELDOR reduction factors for ĊH$_2$COOH (in malonic acid) versus temperature. Only the allowed-allowed ELDOR lines observed at 64.9 (○) and 48.0 MHz (△) and the forbidden-allowed ELDOR lines observed at 36.5 (○) and 19.0 MHz (×) were plotted. A maximum occurs at approximately 273 K for the allowed ELDOR lines and from 223 to 243 K for the forbidden ELDOR lines. The observing field is set at position a. From L. D. Kispert et al., *J. Phys. Chem.*, **77**, 629 (1973).

As this forbidden transition is pumped, a spin population is transferred to the observed allowed-allowed lines, resulting in the appearance of forbidden-allowed lines at low temperatures. As the temperature is raised, the forbidden lines became equivalent to the allowed central lines. At this point the motion produces significant W_n processes, which give rise to intense allowed ELDOR lines. This ELDOR spectral pattern as a function of temperature is very typical whenever there exist two exchanging protons and is used to identify such phenomena.

6.2.5 Intramolecular Admixture of Nuclear Spin States (Forbidden Lines)

In the previous section we found that so-called forbidden transitions ($\Delta m_s = \pm 1$, $\Delta m_I = \pm 1$) can provide an important relaxation pathway for ELDOR whenever a perturbation such as intramolecular motion results in mixing of the nuclear spin states. A similar phenomenon can also occur[8] whenever a rotation of the crystal changes the proton hyperfine splitting A from $A > 2\nu_p$, where ν_p is the proton NMR frequency at the applied field, to $A < 2\nu_p$. In this case not only do the allowed ESR line positions depend on both A and ν_p as eqs. 6.1 to 6.3 imply, but also the nuclear spin states are mixed, causing the forbidden ESR lines to become allowed. This in turn results in the intensity of the observed frequency swept ELDOR lines being directly dependent on the size of A relative to ν_p. Since most studies of radicals in single crystals involve angular rotation measurements, it is important that we understand why the ELDOR intensity varies with angle when $A \simeq 2\nu_p$. To demonstrate the principles involved we examine the ELDOR results of radical I trapped in irradiated single crystals of potassium hydrogen maleate (KHM):

H   H

O⋯C⋯C⊖⋯C⋯C⋯O

O⋯⋯⋯⋯⋯⋯⋯⋯O

(I)

The principal hyperfine splitting values of the two protons in radical I are identical, each equal to $A_1 = 5.9$, $A_2 = 19.6$, $A_3 = 28.4$ MHz, with the principal directions different for each proton because of the different C—H bond directions. The ESR spectrum and the energy level transition diagram that result for radical I when the magnetic field is along the vinylene C=C bond where the two protons have the same coupling is given in Fig. 6-12. The four transitions allowed for both protons are labeled aa, those four allowed for one proton and forbidden for the other are labeled af and fa, and those four forbidden for both protons ff. These transitions give rise to a nine line spectrum due to the coalescence of some lines. The notation $(--)$ next to each energy level denotes the nuclear spins $\beta_1\beta_2$, $(++)$ denotes α_1, α_2, etc.

One might wonder why so many ESR lines occur for two equivalent protons, especially since the selection rules that apply for the case $A > 2\nu_p$ (valid in Section 6.2) predict that only three ESR lines should appear. The answer lies in the transition probability expression that governs the ESR intensity for two equivalent protons when $A \simeq 2\nu_p$.

Previously it has been shown that for a single nucleus with $I = \frac{1}{2}$ interacting with an electron the transition probability for allowed and forbidden ESR lines is proportional to $\cos^2(\theta/2)$ and $\sin^2(\theta/2)$, where θ is the angle between the two vectors $hA_i(M_s = \frac{1}{2})$ and $hA_i(M_s = -\frac{1}{2})$. These vectors correspond to the directions of the nuclear spin before and after the transition. Evaluation of the direction cosine between these two

328 SINGLE CRYSTAL AND POWDER ELDOR

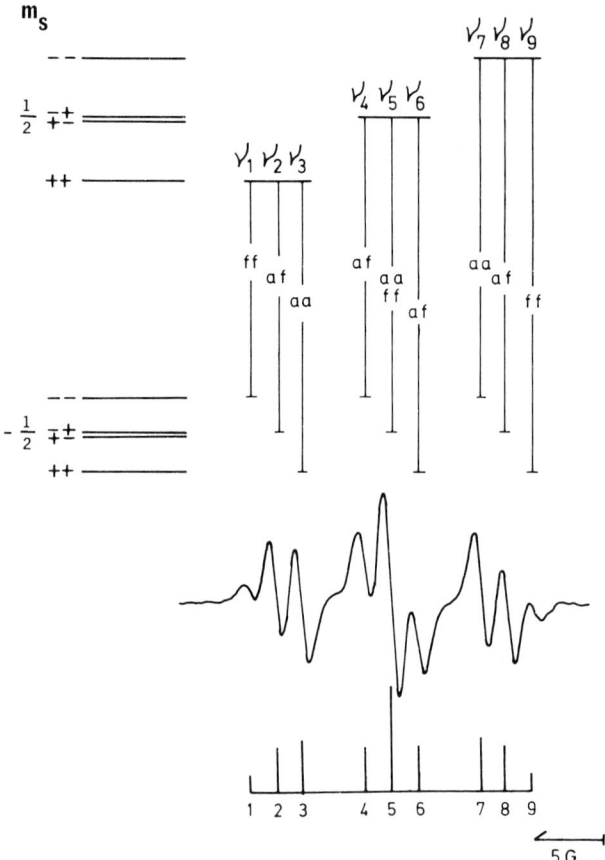

Figure 6-12. The ESR spectrum and the energy level transition diagram for OOCHĊHCOO⁻ (radical I) in an irradiated single crystal of potassium hydrogen maleate, with a stick diagram showing the calculated intensities. The notation $(--)$ denotes the nuclear spin state $\beta_1\beta_2$, $(++)$ denotes $\alpha_1\alpha_2$, etc. From M. Iwasaki et al., *J. Chem. Phys.*, **61**, 106 (1974).

vectors yields

$$\cos\theta = \frac{h\mathbf{A}(\tfrac{1}{2})\mathbf{A}(-\tfrac{1}{2})\mathbf{h}}{A_+ A_-}. \tag{6.15}$$

To understand the implications of eq. 6.15 refer to the instructive example given in Section 6.2 where the magnetic field lies in the XY plane, X and Y being the principal axes of the hyperfine tensor. Then

$$\cos\theta = \frac{[A_{XX}^2 - (2\nu_p)^2]l_X^2 + (A_{YY}^2 - (2\nu_p)^2)l_Y^2 + (A_{ZZ}^2 - (2\nu_p)^2)l_Z^2}{4A_+ A_-} \tag{6.16}$$

where $l_Z = 0$; l_X and l_Y are the direction cosines defined previously, and A_+ and A_- have been defined in eqs. 6.7 and 6.8. In this particular example $A_+ = A_1(\frac{1}{2}) = A_2(\frac{1}{2})$ and $A_- = A_1(-\frac{1}{2}) = A_2(-\frac{1}{2})$. We will let I_a be the intensity of the allowed line and I_f be the intensity of the forbidden line. Thus

$$I_a = \cos^2\frac{\theta}{2} \tag{6.17}$$

$$I_f = \sin^2\frac{\theta}{2} \tag{6.18}$$

where θ has been defined in eq. 6.15. In addition, the transition probabilities for two equivalent protons are products or cross products of I_a and I_f for each proton, so

$$I_{aa} = I_a I_a \tag{6.19}$$

$$I_{af} = I_a I_f = I_f I_a \tag{6.20}$$

$$I_{ff} = I_f I_f \tag{6.21}$$

for the aa, af, or fa and ff transitions. Note that if the ESR spectrum were recorded along the X axis for the example used to produce eq. 6.16, then $l_X = 1$, $l_Y = l_Z = 0$, and $\cos\theta = 1$ or $\theta = 0°$ when $A_{XX}^2 > (2\nu_p)^2$. Indeed in this case $I_{aa} = 1$ and $I_{ff} = 0$ for the transitions given in Fig. 6-12. Note that the selection rules, $\Delta m_I = 0$, $\Delta m_s = \pm 1$, used in Section 6.2 where $A > 2\nu_p$ would also label transition ν_3 as an allowed and ν_1 as a forbidden transition. However note what happens when $A_{xx}^2 = (2\nu_p)^2$, so $\cos\theta = 0$ or $\theta = 90°$. Then $I_{aa} = (\frac{1}{2})(\frac{1}{2})$ and $I_{ff} = (\frac{1}{2})(\frac{1}{2})$. Thus both transitions are equally likely and the terms allowed and forbidden take on a new meaning. The fact that the intensity of ν_1 and ν_3 are not experimentally equal for KHM reflects the fact that different direction cosines and hyperfine splittings actually exist.

Now that we have an expression for the transition probability, the field swept ELDOR reduction factor expression for the condition of no saturation in the observing mode and very strong saturation in the pumping mode given in Section 1.2.2.1 for a four level energy diagram can be used to calculate R. However in our example here we require an eight level energy diagram. Thus eq. 1.26 for the four level diagram must be modified to read

$$R = \frac{W_{n21}W_{n34} - W_{24}W_{31}}{W_{23}(W_{24} + W_{31} + W_{n21} + W_{n34}) + (W_{24} + W_{n21})(W_{31} + W_{n34})} \tag{6.22}$$

The W_{ij}'s denote either the electron spin transition or the cross-relaxation probabilities depending on which levels are stimulated. The W_{nij}'s denote

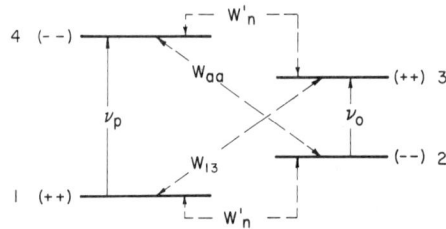

Figure 6-13. The four level energy equivalent diagram when ν_1 (ff) is observed (ν_o) and ν_9 (ff) is pumped (ν_p) in Fig. 6-12.

the pure nuclear spin transition probabilities. From this equation a prediction can be made as to whether a reduced or an enhanced field swept ELDOR line will be observed for each possible transition. For instance, if transition $\nu_1(ff)$ (Fig. 6-12) is observed and $\nu_9(ff)$ is pumped, we can write down a four level diagram as given in Fig. 6-13. Note that we have labeled each level with the same nuclear configuration as given in Fig. 6-12 for the levels connecting transitions ν_1 and ν_9. In order to apply eq. 6.21, we label the observing levels as 2 and 3 and the pumping levels by 1 and 4. Next it is noted that $W_{24} = W_{13}$ is actually W_{aa} or the probability of the lattice-induced aa transition.

In addition, $W_{n21} = W_{n34}$, which is nothing more than the nuclear spin-flip probability of both protons (W'_n). It is usually assumed that W'_n is much smaller than W_n, the nuclear spin-flip probability for one proton, since the simultaneous flip of both protons is less likely. Thus the numerator of eq. 6.21 becomes $(W'_n)^2 - W^2_{aa}$. In other situations W_{af} and W_{ff} will be needed and are defined as the probability of the lattice-induced af and ff transitions, respectively. To a first approximation, the terms W_{aa}, W_{af}, and W_{ff} are assumed to be proportional to the ESR transition probabilities I_{aa}, I_{af}, and I_{ff}. Thus for the experiment in Fig. 6-13 $(W'_n)^2 - W^2_{aa}$ will be negative since $W_{aa} \propto \cos^2(\theta/2)$ while W'_n is small, and evaluation of eq. 6.21 results in large enhancements.

On the other hand, when transition ν_1 is observed and the aa component of ν_5 or the ff component of ν_5 is pumped, we have the four level scheme to consider given in Fig. 6-14, where the labels are defined in the same manner as in Fig. 6-13. In Fig. 6-14 $W_{34} = W_{21} = W_n$ where W_n is the nuclear spin-flip probability of one proton. If we consider Fig. 6-14 we find that the same transition probabilities W_{af} and W_n are present. In this instance the sign of $W_n^2 - W_{af}^2$ depends on the magnitude of W_{af}, which is proportional to $\cos^2(\theta/2) \sin^2(\theta/2)$ and thus on the magnitude of $\sin^2(\theta/2)$. In the c crystal direction the forbidden line intensity of this radical is quite large [i.e., $\sin^2(\theta/2)$ is large], so we may expect W_{af}^2 to be large in this direction. On the other hand, an enhancement may not occur in the a crystal direction because the forbidden line is quite weak

ORGANIC SINGLE CRYSTAL ELDOR SPECTRA 331

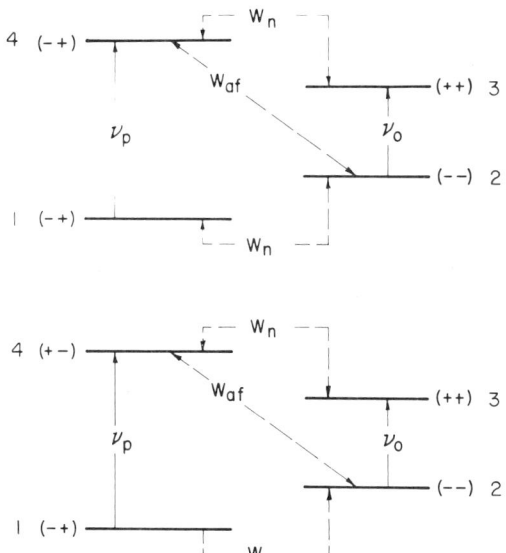

Figure 6-14. The four level equivalent energy diagram when ν_1 (*ff*) is observed (ν_o) and ν_5 (*aa*, upper diagram) or (*ff*, lower diagram) is pumped (ν_p) in Fig. 6-12.

$[\sin^2(\theta/2) \simeq 0]$, so W_{af}^2 may be small and a reduction in the ESR height may occur.

For those ELDOR experiments having a level in common, it has been shown rigorously by Freed[35] that only reductions will be observed. In order to predict the value of the reduction factor for any of the preceding situations detailed knowledge of all the relaxation contributions from all the possible paths is required. So far this is not possible although estimates can be given.

Experimentally, the preceding predictions of reduced and enhanced ELDOR lines were observed for a frequency swept ELDOR spectrum and are shown in Figs. 6-15a, b, c for the observed ELDOR frequencies ν_1, ν_2, and ν_3 given in the upper half of Table 6-4 for two equivalent protons with the magnetic field along the c axis using 100 kHz modulation. For any ELDOR frequency listed in Table 6-4 the corresponding observing ESR frequency is given by the label listed down the left column and the pump ESR frequency is denoted by the label read across the top of the table. The separation of the corresponding hyperfine lines is given in the lower half of Table 6-4. The symbols R and E in Fig. 6-15 denote reduction and enhancement, respectively. It should be noted that only enhanced lines are observed where no level is in common with another;

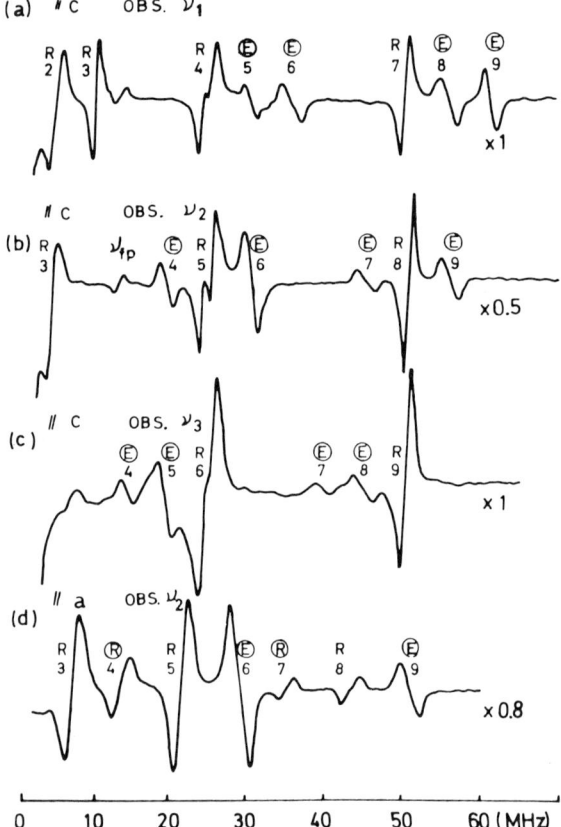

Figure 6-15. The ELDOR spectra for OOCHĊHCOO⁻ (radical *I*) in an irradiated single crystal of potassium hydrogen maleate. The magnetic field is applied along (*a*), (*b*), (*c*) the *c* axis, and (*d*) the *a* axis. The observing transition is (*a*) ν_1, (*b*), (*d*) ν_2, and (*c*) ν_3 as indicated in Fig. 6-12. The numbers indicate the pumped ESR lines. The symbols *R* and *E* denote reduction and enhancement, respectively. The circles indicate the ELDOR transitions involving no level in common. From M. Iwasaki et al., *J. Chem. Phys.*, **61**, 106 (1974).

these transitions are denoted by circles. Enhancement implies that W_{aa} and W_{af} are quite large. On the other hand, with the magnetic field along the crystallographic *a* axis (Fig. 6-15*d*) reduced lines are observed where no level is found in common (lines 4 and 7), indicating a significant decrease in W_{af}.

At room temperature the ELDOR reduction factors (defined as the ratio of the ELDOR to the ESR signal heights for a frequency swept experiment and as given in section 5.2 for a field swept experiment) can be calculated for those ELDOR transitions that do not involve a level in

Table 6-4. The Separations of the Successive Hyperfine Lines of the OOCCHCHOO⁻ Radical in Terms of $A_{\pm}$ for Two Equal Couplings (below the diagonal) and the Corresponding ELDOR Frequencies in Megahertz (above the diagonal) Obtained with the Magnetic Field Parallel to the c Axis at Room Temperature[a,b]

		ν_1	ν_2	ν_3	ν_4	ν_5	ν_6	ν_7	ν_8	ν_9
Observing Frequency	ν_1		5.3	10.4	25.3	30.3	35.8	50.5	56.0	61.4
	ν_2	A_-		5.3	19.7	25.3	30.5	45.0	50.5	56.0
	ν_3	$2A_-$	A_-		14.8	19.7	25.2	39.8	45.3	50.5
	ν_4	A_+	$A_+ - A_-$	$A_+ - 2A_-$		5.3	10.3	25.3	30.5	36.0
	ν_5	$A_+ + A_-$	A_+	$A_+ - A_-$	A_-		5.2	20.0	25.3	30.5
	ν_6	$A_+ + 2A_-$	$A_+ + A_-$	A_+	$2A_-$	A_-		14.7	19.7	25.0
	ν_7	$2A_+$	$2A_+ - A_-$	$2(A_+ - A_-)$	A_+	$A_+ - A_-$	$A_+ - 2A_-$		5.3	10.4
	ν_8	$2A_+ + A_-$	$2A_+$	$2A_+ - A_-$	$A_+ + A_-$	A_+	$A_+ - A_-$	A_-		5.3
	ν_9	$2(A_+ + A_-)$	$2A_+ + A_-$	$2A_+$	$A_+ + 2A_-$	$A_+ + A_-$	A_+	$2A_-$	A_-	

From M. Iwasaki et al., J. Chem. Phys., 61, 106 (1974).

[a] $A_- = [\mathbf{h}(\frac{1}{2}\mathbf{A} + \mathbf{E}\nu_p)^2 \mathbf{h}]^{1/2}$. See eq. 6.8 for a specific example.
[b] $A_+ = [\mathbf{h}(\frac{1}{2}\mathbf{A} - \mathbf{E}\nu_p)^2 \mathbf{h}]^{1/2}$. See eq. 6.7 for a specific example.

common from the assumed parameters $b = W_n/W_{aa} = 0.2$ and $b' = W'_n/W_{aa} = 0.04$ along the c crystal axis and $b = 0.3$ and $b' = 0.09$ along the a axis. In Table 6-5 the ELDOR effect and the observed and calculated reduction factor are given for the ELDOR lines denoted by $i-j$ where i is the observed and j is the pumped line. Notably good agreement is found between the observed and calculated reduction factors, further substantiating the fact that significant W_{aa} and W_{af} transition probabilities exist for all ELDOR transitions along the c axis where $A \sim 2\nu_H$ and where forbidden lines are the most intense. Note that 100 kHz field modulation was used in these experiments. Along the a axis the forbidden line intensities decrease and thus W_{aa} and W_{af} decrease, changing the enhanced ELDOR lines when $c \| H$ to reduced ELDOR lines in some cases. Along both axes there is also a marked variation in the reduction factor depending upon which levels are observed and pumped. This is not the case for the ELDOR transitions involving a level in common where reduced ELDOR lines with a considerably smaller variation are observed.

Competing with the relaxations induced by the admixture of nuclear spin states at room temperature is a temperature dependence of W_e and W_n. In general, the R factors change from a negative value (enhanced) to a positive value with a maximum reduction around 173 K and then decrease.

6.2.6 Quadrupole Interaction

Nuclei of spin $I > \frac{1}{2}$ that possess an electric quadrupole moment can relax via the interaction of the quadrupole moment with the electric field gradient at the nucleus. In fact, for molecules in solution the quadrupole relaxation can be orders of magnitude faster than the relaxation arising from the magnetic dipole-dipole interactions.[37] Quadrupolar nuclei have been incorporated into molecules to study anisotropic rotation in liquids by NMR quadrupolar relaxation[38] and have been used in radicals to examine anisotropic rotational diffusion by ESR.[39,40] Frequency swept ELDOR studies of the ·CClFCONH$_2$ radical in irradiated CCl$_2$FCONH$_2$ crystals[6] and the ĊCl$_3$ radical in irradiated CCl$_3$CONH$_2$ crystals[7] demonstrate that quadrupolar relaxation can dominate the relaxation induced by hyperfine splitting anisotropy and intramolecular rotational motion, respectively.

Proof that the quadrupole-induced relaxation is dominant over the relaxation induced by the hyperfine splitting is based on the observed absence of a large variation in the intensity of the allowed-allowed and forbidden-allowed ELDOR lines for ĊClFCONH$_2$ as a function of fluorine hyperfine splitting anisotropy. One may recall from Section 6.2.3

Table 6-5. Observed and Calculated R Factors for ELDOR Transitions Involving No Level in Common

ELDOR Lines	ELDOR Effect		Competition[a]	c axis		a axis	
	c Axis	a Axis		R_{obs}	R_{calc}[b]	R_{obs}	R_{calc}[c]
1–9	E	E	$W'_n - W_{aa}$	−0.36	−0.32	−0.36	−0.43
1–8	E	E	$W_n W'_n - W_{aa} W_{af}$	−0.25	−0.29	−0.45	−0.32
1–6	E	E	$W_n W'_n - W_{aa} W_{af}$	−0.22	−0.29	−0.53	−0.32
1–5	E	R	$W_n - W_{af}$	−0.18	−0.15	+0.22	+0.08
2–9	E	E	$W_n W'_n - W_{aa} W_{af}$	−0.19	−0.19	−0.36	−0.20
2–7	E	R	$W_n W'_n - W_{af} W_{ff}$	−0.06	−0.06	+0.08	+0.03
2–6	E	E	$W_n^2 - W_{aa}(W)$[d]	−0.46	−0.25	−0.95	−0.29
2–4	E	R	$W_n^2 - W_{ff}(W)$	−0.20	−0.02	+0.39	+0.07
3–8	E	R	$W_n W'_n - W_{af} W_{ff}$	−0.06	−0.07	+0.07	+0.03
3–7	E	E	$W'_n - W_{ff}$	−0.02	−0.04	−0.09	+0.02
3–5	E	R	$W_n - W_{af}$	−0.19	−0.15	+0.48	+0.08
3–4	E	R	$W_n W'_n - W_{aa} W_{af}$	−0.07	−0.06	+0.18	+0.03
4–9	E		$W_n W'_n - W_{aa} W_{af}$	−0.20	−0.19		
4–8	E		$W_n^2 - W_{aa}(W)$	−0.44	−0.25		
5–9	E		$W_n - W_{af}$	−0.03	−0.05		
5–7	E		$W_n - W_{af}$	−0.05	−0.07		
6–8	E		$W_n^2 - W_{ff}(W)$	−0.18	−0.02		
6–7	E		$W_n W'_n - W_{af} W_{ff}$	−0.06	−0.06		

From M. Iwasaki et al., *J. Chem. Phys.*, **61**, 106 (1974).
[a] Fourth column indicates the competition between the reduction and enhancement paths; see text.
[b] Parameters used, $b = 0.2$ and $b' = 0.04$.
[c] Parameters used, $b = 0.3$ and $b' = 0.09$.
[d] $(W) = \frac{1}{2}(W_{aa} + W_{ff})$.

that radicals (such as ĊFHCONH₂) for which the relaxation is dominated by hyperfine splitting anisotropy give rise to a large variation in the intensity of the spectral lines. Evidence for the dominance of the chlorine quadrupole relaxation over intramolecular rotational motion is currently based on the observed absence of any significant ELDOR spectral intensity for the ĊCl₃ radical in irradiated trichloroacetamide crystals.[7] Above room temperature the ESR spectrum of ĊCl₃ appears as a ten line pattern due to a rapidly time-averaged spectrum. However as the temperature is lowered to 224 K a broadening of the ESR lines occurs, obscuring the ESR spectral lines that distinguish the different isotopic species of ĊCl₃. This occurs because of an increase in the rotational correlation time for the motion exhibited by the ĊCl₃ radical. By analogy to the observed ELDOR spectral variations with molecular motion given in Sections 6.2.1 and 6.2.2, intense ELDOR spectra are expected if relaxation is dominated by molecular motion modulating the dipolar anisotropy. However this does not appear to be the case for ĊCl₃. The fact that the ELDOR intensity increases with decreasing temperature for both the ĊClFCONH₂ and ĊCl₂CONH₂ radicals (below 223 K) further suggests the predominance of chlorine quadrupole relaxation over other relaxation mechanisms and such a temperature dependence appears to be typical when quadrupole relaxation predominates. Furthermore since quadrupole relaxation exists between states that differ only in M_I ($\Delta M_I = \pm 1$ or ± 2), only reduced ELDOR spectra are observed as was explained in Chapter 1 (Section 1.5.2.2).

As an example of ELDOR dominated by quadrupole relaxation, let us consider the ĊClFCONH₂ radical in irradiated CCl₂FCONH₂ crystals. The first derivative ESR absorption spectrum using 100 kHz modulation is shown in Fig. 6-16a. The crystal is mounted so that the magnetic field lies in a direction perpendicular to the radical plane where the quadrupole coupling $Q_z = 37$ MHz, the chlorine hyperfine splitting $A_z(^{35}Cl) = 50$ MHz and $A_z(F) = 471$ MHz. The ESR spectrum is complex because of the breakdown of the first order selection rules as a result of the large quadrupole interaction relative to the chlorine splitting. This results in several $\Delta M_I = \pm 2$ ^{35}Cl transitions with intensities one-half that of the $\Delta M_I = 0$ transitions in addition to a similar spectrum one-third the intensity due to ^{37}Cl. Furthermore each of these lines is broadened by partially resolved fine structure due to small splittings from the amine nitrogen and protons.

The frequency swept ELDOR spectrum shown in Fig. 6-16b consists of two intense reduced ELDOR lines at approximately 50 and 74 MHz plus several weaker lines when the observing field is set at any one of the positions A, B, or C of the high field ^{35}Cl ESR line indicated in Fig.

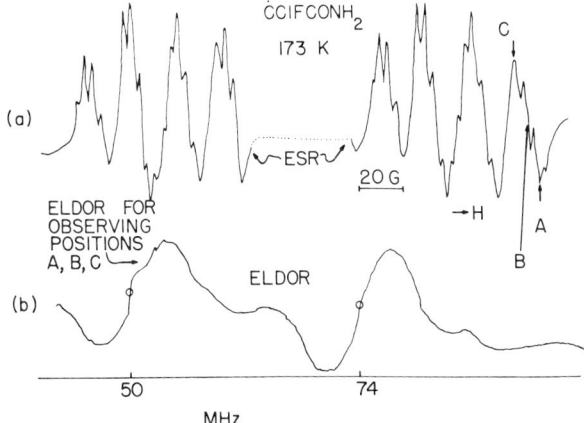

Figure 6-16. (a) The first derivative absorption ESR spectrum of ĊClFCONH$_2$. (b) The ELDOR spectrum of the ĊClFCONH$_2$ radical in irradiated dichlorofluoroacetamide single crystals at 173 K. A first derivative spectrum is obtained for all ESR observing positions A, B, and C because of the inhomogeneous broadening from the amide nitrogen and proton splittings. Very little or no ELDOR is observed at room temperature; however below 173 K a substantial reduction ($R > 30\%$) is observed. From L. D. Kispert et al., *Chem Phys. Lett.*, **17**, 529 (1972).

6-16a. No lines are observed above 100 MHz, nor are lines observed at the hyperfine splitting of nitrogen or hydrogen nuclei. The two intense peaks arise because the allowed ELDOR transitions in the presence of quadrupole relaxation are governed by the selection rule $\Delta M_I = \pm 1$ or ± 2. Therefore ELDOR active transitions will occur when the pump frequency is set at f_{p_2} or f_{p_1} in Fig. 6-17. Furthermore a first order calculation for the ĊFClR fragment that includes the chlorine quadrupole interaction shows (Table 6-6) that these ELDOR lines occur at $A(\text{Cl}) = 50.5$ MHz and $\tfrac{3}{2}A(\text{Cl}) - \nu(\text{Cl}) = 74.8$ MHz, respectively, and belong to a class of transitions that do not include the quadrupole term. Experimental ELDOR lines assignable to possible transitions that do contain a quadrupole term were either not observed or had an intensity less than 10% of the allowed line at $A(^{35}\text{Cl})$. As the observing position is changed to lines of different M_I values, a small M_I dependence is observed.

In summary, quadrupolar relaxation of the chlorine nucleus appears to be dominant over all other relaxation processes. The fact that no ELDOR lines are observed from F, H, or N gives rise to a large increase in spectral resolution and allows an immediate measurement of $A(\text{Cl})$. The lack of quadrupole interactions for the allowed ELDOR lines simplifies the analysis. The presence of quadrupolar relaxation is conceptually similar to the ELDOR experiment on DPPH where the nitrogen couplings can be

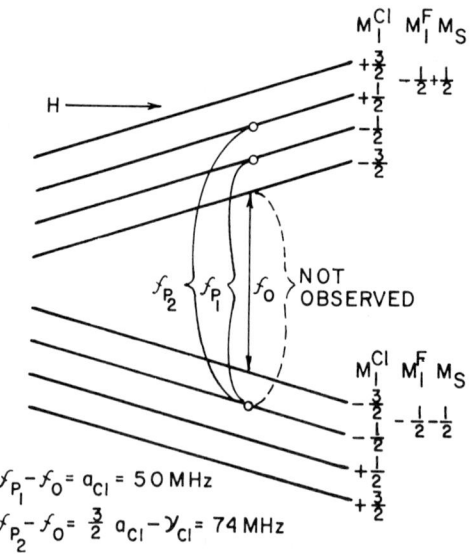

Figure 6-17. The energy diagram for the high field group of ESR lines of the ĊClFCONH$_2$ radical where $M_I^F = -\frac{1}{2}$ indicating the possible ELDOR transitions at 50 and 75 MHz while observing the $M_I(\text{Cl}) = -\frac{3}{2}$ line and sweeping the pump frequency. From L. D. Kispert et al., *Chem. Phys. Lett.*, **17**, 592 (1972).

Table 6-6. The First Order ELDOR Transitions for Chlorine in the ĊClFR Radical[a]

$\frac{1}{2}A\,(\text{Cl}) \pm \nu_{Cl} \pm \frac{1}{2}Q$	$A\,(\text{Cl})$	$= 50.5$ MHz
	$\frac{3}{2}A\,(\text{Cl}) \pm \nu_{Cl}$	$= 76.8$
		74.8
$A\,(\text{Cl}) \pm 2\nu_{Cl} \pm \frac{1}{2}Q$	$\frac{3}{2}A\,(\text{Cl}) \pm 3\nu_{Cl}$	$= 79.2$
		72
$2A\,(\text{Cl}) \pm 2\nu_{Cl} \pm \frac{1}{2}Q$		
$\frac{5}{2}A\,(\text{Cl}) \pm \nu_{Cl} \pm \frac{1}{2}Q$	$2A\,(\text{Cl})$	$= 101.0$
	$3A\,(\text{Cl})$	$= 151.5$

From L. D. Kispert et al., *Chem. Phys. Lett.* **17,** 592 (1972).
[a] Assuming $E_m = M_s g\beta H + A\,(\text{Cl})M_s M_I(\text{Cl}) - M_I(\text{Cl})\nu_{Cl} + (Q/12)[3(M_I(\text{Cl}))^2 - I(I+1)]$.

extracted from a complicated spectrum because of the presence of long proton nuclear relaxation times (see Section 5.3.2). The increasing ELDOR intensity with decreasing temperature is characteristic of chlorinated radicals and this feature may be useful in determining the presence of a chlorinated radical in a overlapped spectrum containing several radicals.

6.2.7 Deuterium Hyperfine Splittings

From Chapter 1 we saw that measurable ELDOR reductions occur when W_n processes are competitive with W_e processes for the END relaxation mechanism when other possible relaxation processes are negligible. Freed and co-workers have also shown that W_n processes in solution are proportional to γ_n^2 in addition to other parameters, where γ_n is the nuclear gyromagnetic ratio. Thus, all other factors being equal, the W_n probability decreases by a factor of $\gamma_H^2/\gamma_D^2 = 42$ when a deuteron is substituted for a proton. In this event little ELDOR intensity will be observed if the ELDOR intensity of the protonated radical has a signal-to-noise ratio of less than 42. This seems to be the explanation for the failure to observe deuterium combination lines with protons in $CD_2H^+\dot{C}DCOO^-$, $CH_2D\dot{C}HCOOD$, and $CH_3\dot{C}DCOOD$ in irradiated l-alanine crystals.[13] Note that this observation is somewhat similar to the frequency swept ELDOR study of DPPH where no ELDOR lines are observed from the smaller ESR splittings. In the case of DDPH the proton nuclei with the smaller splittings have longer nuclear relaxation times than the nitrogen nuclei with the larger splittings, which prevents the observation of ELDOR combination lines. Similarly when $W_n \propto \gamma_D^2/\gamma_H^2$, only weak deuterium ELDOR spectra will be seen. Furthermore it is expected that when a radical contains both protons and deuterons the ELDOR active transitions will occur via the fast W_H processes rather than the slow W_D process.

Nevertheless, intense frequency swept deuterium ELDOR lines are observed from the first derivative ESR absorption mode of $\dot{C}D_2COOD$ using 100 kHz modulation at room temperature.[4] This radical lacks α protons, methyl groups, chlorine quadrupoles, and nitrogens and thus a number of competitive relaxation mechanisms have been eliminated. A relaxation mechanism that does give rise to the observed ELDOR intensity of $\dot{C}D_2COOD$ is the onset of cross relaxation between the nearly degenerate energy level as the crystals are warmed to room temperature. A plot of the frequency swept ELDOR intensity in terms of R is given in Fig. 6-18 as a function of temperature when the observing position is set

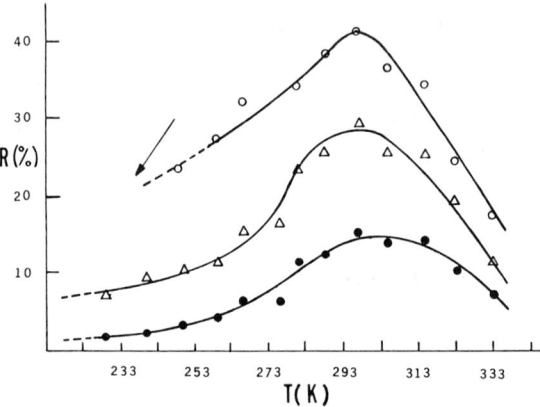

Figure 6-18. A plot of the temperature dependence of R with the observing ESR position set at the bottom of the $M_I = -1$ ESR line of $\dot{C}D_2COOD$. Frequency swept ELDOR spectra show three transitions corresponding to the hyperfine intervals, a_D (○), $2a_D$ (△), and $3a_D$ (●), using a freshly irradiated crystal. The ELDOR line at a_D becomes badly overlapped below 263 K because of a broad unresolved peak that occurs between 8 and 15 MHz. From L. D. Kispert and P. S. Wang, *J. Phys. Chem.*, **78**, 1839 (1974).

at the bottom of the $M_I = -1$ ESR line of $\dot{C}D_2COOD$ as indicated in Fig. 6-19 by the letter a. The temperature dependence of the intensity is similar to that observed for the allowed-allowed ELDOR lines of $\dot{C}H_2COOH$ radical in malonic acid shown in Fig. 6-11.

The ELDOR spectrum observed at 323 K is given in Fig. 6-19 where the observed field is set at the bottom of the first derivative high field line of $\dot{C}D_2COOD$. The ELDOR line intensity is close to the $2:3:2:1$ ratio expected from the ESR spectrum of $\dot{C}D_2COOD$, which consists of a five line pattern with an intensity of $1:2:3:2:1$. The ESR spectrum in Fig. 6-19 is the composite spectra of two radicals: a three line (central three lines) ESR pattern with a $1:1:1$ intensity ratio due to $\dot{C}D(COOD)_2$ overlapped by the five line $1:2:3:2:1$ pattern of $\dot{C}D_2COOD$.

The poor resolution obtained in the frequency swept ELDOR spectrum is discussed more fully in Section 6.2.10.2. If the observing field is set at the bottom of an overlapped line of the $\dot{C}D_2COOD$ and $\dot{C}D(COOD)_2$ radicals, the ELDOR intensity ratios are about the same and suggest little ELDOR contribution to the spectrum from the $\dot{C}D(COOD)_2$ radical. A complete analysis of this effect shows that the intramolecular motion of $\dot{C}D_2COOD$ causes a cross relaxation between levels and gives rise to the ELDOR active transitions in $\dot{C}D_2COOD$. No indication of motion is observed for $\dot{C}D(COOD)_2$, giving rise to longer nuclear relaxation and the absence of ELDOR spectral lines.

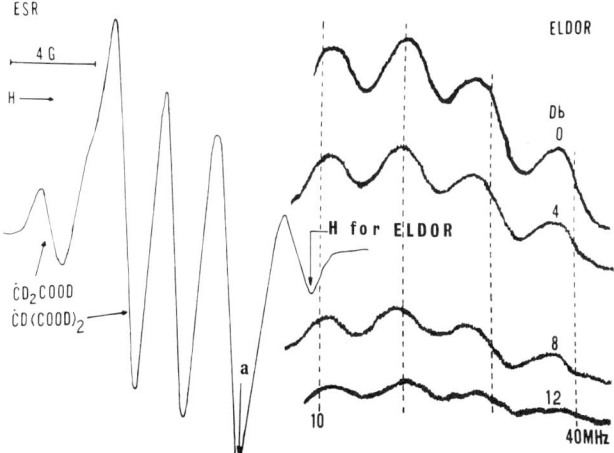

Figure 6-19. ELDOR spectra taken at 323 K as a function of pump power with H nearly parallel to the b crystal axis. The observing ESR position was placed at the bottom of the $M_I = -2$ line of $\dot{C}D_2COOD$ (as indicated by the arrow) when the concentration ratio of $\dot{C}D(COOD)_2/\dot{C}D_2COOD$ equaled $\frac{3}{2}$. Note the 2:3:2:1 ratio of the ELDOR heights as would be expected for a spectrum containing only the $\dot{C}D_2COOD$ radical, suggesting very little contribution from $\cdot CD(COOD)_2$. From L. D. Kispert and P. S. Wang, *J. Phys. Chem.*, **78,** 1839 (1974).

6.2.8 Resolution of Small Hyperfine Splittings

In the ELDOR study of DPPH given in Section 5.3 the small proton splittings (from 5.6 to 2 MHz) were not observed, whereas the larger nitrogen splittings (27.4 and 22.2 MHz) were detected. To observe an ELDOR spectrum generally requires short nuclear relaxation times more typical of nuclei that are strongly coupled to the electron (larger couplings), and thus only strongly coupled nuclei are observed. This would seem to explain the failure to observe frequency swept deuterium ELDOR splittings (11.7 MHz) in $CH_3\dot{C}DCOO^-$ (ref. 2) and the ^{14}N splittings (9.2 MHz) in $NH_3^+\dot{C}HCOO^-$ (ref. 13) while proton ELDOR splittings (50 to 90 MHz) are observed. From these few examples it can be concluded the splittings on the order of 12 MHz or less may not be observed in an ELDOR spectrum so that a considerable increase in spectral resolution over the ESR spectral resolution is possible.

Normally the ESR spectral resolution for radicals containing ^{14}N can be increased by substituting ^{15}N ($I = \frac{1}{2}$) for ^{14}N ($I = 1$) so that the triplet ^{14}N pattern complicated by the small quadrupole interaction of the ^{14}N is replaced by the ^{15}N doublet. So far it has been found that as the ESR

342 SINGLE CRYSTAL AND POWDER ELDOR

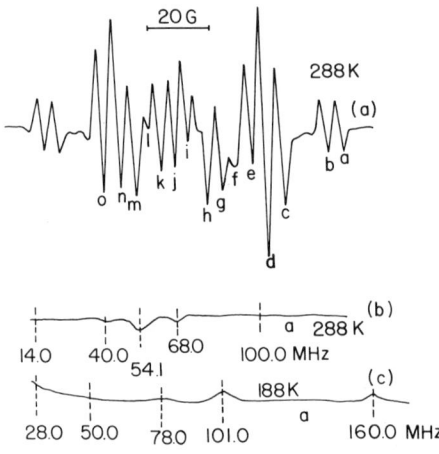

Figure 6-20. (a) The first derivative ESR spectrum of $^{15}NH_3^+\dot{C}HCOO^-$ and minor amounts of $\cdot CH_2COO^-$ at 288 K. (b) The ELDOR spectrum obtained by setting the observing position at the bottom of the high field ESR line of $^{15}NH_3^+\dot{C}HCOO^-$ in (a). Only the enhanced ELDOR line at the amine proton hyperfine splitting is observed. (c) The ELDOR spectrum obtained under the same conditions as (b) except at 188 K, which shows amine proton splittings at 101 and 160 MHz, and a weak line at 78 MHz. A third amine proton ELDOR line occurs at a frequency too small (1 MHz) to be observed. Results of K. Chang and L. Kispert.

resolution increases so does the frequency swept ELDOR resolution. However this is not the case for ^{15}N substitution. In Fig. 6-20a the first derivative absorption ESR spectrum of $^{15}NH_3^+\dot{C}HCOO^-$ in the bc plane with minor amounts of $\dot{C}H_2COO^-$ at 288 K is given. A frequency swept ELDOR spectrum obtained by setting the observing position at the bottom of the high field line (a) and then scanning the pumping frequency where $\nu_p > \nu_o$ results in the ELDOR spectrum given in Fig. 6-20b. Note that at 288 K only the enhanced ELDOR line of the amine proton (NH_3^+) and its associated spin-flip lines are observed. No combination lines between ^{15}N splittings and the amine protons nor the α-proton splitting are observed at 288 K. As one might recall from Fig. 6-6, the α-proton ELDOR line is nearly absent in the ^{14}N-substituted radical presumably because of the lack of intramolecular motion at this temperature for the C_α—H proton.

When the temperature is lowered to 188 K, the central portion of the ESR spectrum appears to sharpen as the rotational motion of the amine group slows and better resolution is observed (Fig. 6-21a). An ELDOR spectrum taken with the observing position set at the bottom of the high field ESR line a consists of a weak line at 78 MHz (α proton) and amine proton lines at 101 and 160 MHz (Fig. 6-20c). A third amine proton ELDOR line occurs at a frequency too small (1 MHz) to be observed on the frequency sweep covered. Note the absence of ^{15}N splittings. However, this is to be contrasted with the ELDOR spectrum obtained when the observing position is set to position d in Fig. 6-21a, which is given in Fig. 6-21b. It consists of a large number of lines at the hyperfine splittings of the amine protons, the α proton, and the ^{15}N. The reason for the

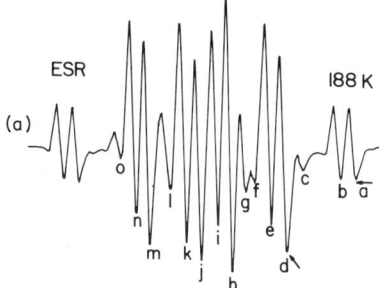

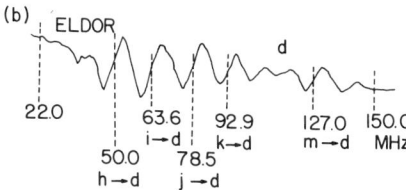

Figure 6-21. (a) The first derivative ESR spectrum of $^{15}NH_3^+\dot{C}HCOO^-$ at 188 K in the bc crystal plane. (b) The ELDOR spectrum at 188 K observed at position d. The ELDOR lines are denoted by the letters of the allowed pump lines h, i, j, k, and m from which they arose. Significant is the observance of the ^{15}N splitting (line h minus line i). Results of K. Chang and L. Kispert.

detection of the small ^{15}N splitting is not definitely known. However, the magnetic moment for ^{14}N (0.40358) is smaller than the magnetic moment of ^{15}N (−0.5660). Thus the ^{14}N splitting of 9.2 MHz is equivalent to 13 MHz for ^{15}N. At 188 K the relaxation time for ^{15}N may be just short enough for the $m_I^{NH_3} = \frac{1}{2}$ lines to give rise to an ELDOR line. It is interesting to note that if the temperature is raised to 223 K and the crystal is rotated in the bc plane to give poorer resolution, as shown in Fig. 6-22 (smaller α proton splitting), the ^{15}N splitting is no longer observed when the observing position is set at D. Thus poor ESR resolution may result in a well resolved ELDOR spectrum if a number of small splittings are observed. Of course this effect may not only be due to the magnitude of the ^{15}N splittings but also depend on the magnitude of the α proton and amine proton splittings. It was previously pointed out in Section 6.2.3 that significant intensity occurred for the forbidden-allowed lines in a crystal direction where a large hyperfine splitting occurred. In any event this example can serve as a warning that for a well resolved ESR spectrum, the ELDOR spectrum may contain an equal number of lines and thus an increase in resolution will not be observed.

6.2.9 Spin-Flip Transitions

In Sections 6.2.1 and 6.2.2 frequency swept ELDOR spectra of the first derivative absorption ESR mode were given in which satellite lines appeared at ±14 MHz from the main ELDOR line with an intensity equal

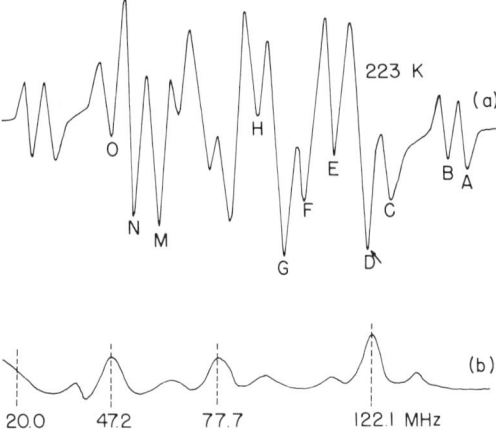

Figure 6-22. The first derivative ESR spectrum of irradiated ^{15}N-glycine observed at a different orientation in the bc^* plane at 223 K than Fig. 6-21. (b) Despite the lower ESR resolution than that in Fig. 6-20 and Fig. 6-21 ELDOR lines obtained with the observing positions set at d occur at the hyperfine splitting of the amine proton (47 MHz), the alpha proton (77), and at the sum of the two splittings (124 MHz). The ^{15}N splittings are not seen. Results of K. Chang and L. Kispert.

to 25 to 50% of that of the main line. These ELDOR lines are due to spin-flip lines observed in the ESR spectra of most irradiated organic single crystals.[41] A calculation based on eqs. 6.1 through 6.3 assuming $A < 2\nu_n$ (in particular, $A = 0$) shows the spin-flip separation from the main ESR line to be independent of angle and equal to ± 14 MHz at 3400 G. Physically, the spin-flip lines represent a weak magnetic dipole-dipole interaction coupling the electron spin of a radical to the nuclear spin of a nucleus that is bonded to a diamagnetic lattice molecule surrounding the radical. They occur when there is a change in the spin state of the nonbonded lattice protons concurrent with the change in the spin state of the electron on the paramagnetic fragment. The ratio of the intensity of either satellite line (S_1) to the main ESR line (M) is given by the following equation:

$$\frac{S_1}{M} = \frac{9}{4} \sum_i \frac{g_e^2 \beta_e^2}{H^2 r_i^6} \sin^2 \theta_i \cos^2 \theta_i \tag{6.23}$$

where θ_i is the angle between the r_i vector and H, H is the applied magnetic field, r_i is the vector distance between the ith nucleus and the unpaired electron, and g_e and β_e are the gyromagnetic ratio of the electron and the Bohr magneton, respectively. As can be seen from eq. 6.23 the satellite intensity is angularly dependent and reaches a maximum when $\theta = 45°$. The satellite also saturates at higher power than the main ESR line. Because of this saturation behavior, the intensity of the frequency swept ELDOR spin-flip lines decreases with decreasing pump power more rapidly than the main (allowed-allowed) frequency swept ELDOR line. The power dependence of these spin-flip lines is given in

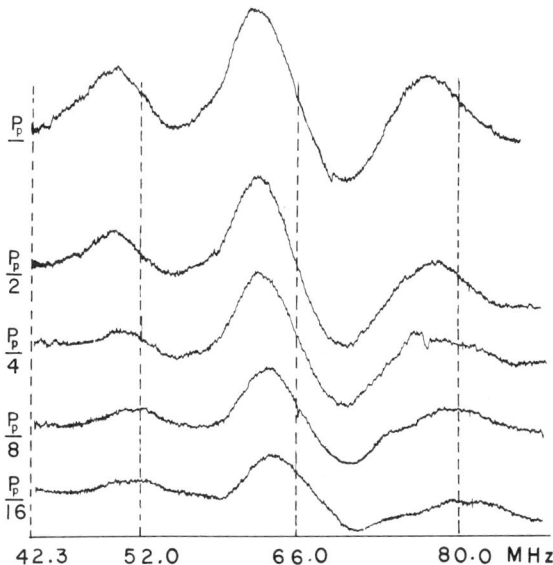

Figure 6-23. Typical dependence of ELDOR spin-flip line intensity as the pump power is varied from $P_p = 336$ mW to $P_p/16 = 21$ mW. A more rapid decrease in the spin-flip line intensity than the main ELDOR line is observed for irradiated α aminoisobutyric acid single crystals. From L. D. Kispert et al., *J. Chem. Phys.*, **58**, 2164 (1973).

Fig. 6-23 for the enhanced line occurring at 66 MHz for $(CH_3)_2\dot{C}COOH$ in irradiated α-aminoisobutyric acid single crystals at 274 K as the pump power is varied from $P_P = 336$ mW to $P_P/16 = 21$ mW. A first derivative ELDOR line is observed because the observing position is set at the resonance position ($\omega_o = 0$) of the ESR line. The lineshape phase of the spin-flip lines always follows that of the main line. In other words, if enhanced (reduced) main lines are observed, then enhanced (reduced) spin-flip lines are also observed. Because of the pump power dependence of these lines, the frequency swept ELDOR resolution can be increased by simply reducing the pump power until most of the spin-flip line intensity disappears. It is noted at 21 mW that the main line is still observable, as it decreases at a slower rate with pump power.

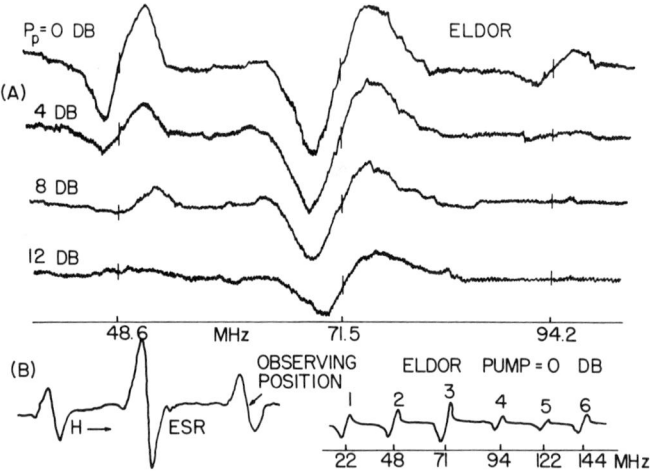

Figure 6-24. The intensity variation of the forbidden-allowed ELDOR lines at 48.6 and 94.2 MHz and the allowed-allowed ELDOR line at 71.5 MHz with pump power for the $\dot{C}H_2COO^-$ radical at 173 K in irradiated zinc acetate crystals. The ELDOR spectrum at 0 dB (336 mW) is recorded between 15 and 150 MHz while observing the high field ESR line and is given in the lower part of Fig. 6-24.

An example of the intensity variation with pump power of the forbidden-allowed lines discussed in Section 6.2.5 relative to the allowed-allowed lines is given in Fig. 6-24 for $\dot{C}H_2COOH$ at 173 K employing 100 kHz field modulation. The observing position is set at the crossover of the high field first derivative ESR absorption line and the pump frequency is swept to a frequency higher than the observing frequency. Forbidden-allowed ELDOR lines are observed at 23, 48, 94, and 122 MHz whereas allowed-allowed ELDOR lines are observed at 71.5 and 144 MHz. As the pump power (P_p) is decreased from 0 dB to 12 dB, the forbidden-allowed line at 94.2 MHz disappears first, followed by the line at 48.6 MHz. At 12 dB, the allowed-allowed line intensity has decreased; however it is still observable. Note that spin-flip lines at 57.5 and 85.5 are not observed in this example even at $P_p = 0$ dB. Although the intensity dependence with pump power for forbidden-allowed lines is similar to that of spin-flip lines, it is not possible to predict which set of lines will be more intense under a given set of conditions. For radicals that undergo little motion, intense forbidden-allowed lines can be expected (as was demonstrated in Section 6.2.3) that decrease in intensity with the onset of motion, yet it is possible to observe intense spin-flip lines when the radical is undergoing intramolecular motion as was evident for $(CH_3)_2\dot{C}COOH$ in Fig. 6-1 at 224 K.

Because of the similarity of the pump power dependence, the spin-flip lines can be mistaken for forbidden-allowed lines when the hyperfine splitting is about 60 MHz. For instance, frequency swept ELDOR spectra of $(CH_3)_2\dot{C}COOH$ were recorded along the crystal axes of irradiated dimethylmalonic acid where $A_H = 60$ MHz. In this case the forbidden-allowed lines at $\frac{1}{2}A_H + \nu_H = 44$ MHz and at $\frac{3}{2}A_H - \nu_H = 76$ MHz can be mistaken for the spin-flip lines at $A_H \pm \nu_H = 46.5$ and 76 MHz, respectively. Only by rotating the crystal to an orientation where the hyperfine splittings are larger or smaller than 60 MHz can the difference be discovered and an assignment made. Of course in some special cases, where enhanced forbidden-allowed lines and reduced allowed-allowed lines are observed, the spin-flip lines will be reduced and can be definitely distinguished from the forbidden-allowed lines.

6.2.10 Modulation Frequency Dependence

As discussed in Section 1.5.4 the frequency swept ELDOR spectral intensity obtained from the first derivative ESR absorption mode of radicals in various media exhibits a dependence on the modulation frequency that varies depending on the ability of the electrons to relax during each modulation cycle. Because the various relaxation times are not usually known over a given temperature range in irradiated crystals, the spectral variations are more difficult to predict than in solution and they can vary widely from radical to radical.

For example, when the observing frequency swept ELDOR position is set on the crossing point of the high field first derivative ESR absorption line of $\dot{C}H_2COO^-$ in zinc acetate crystals,[32,33] the ELDOR intensity of the line at $2A_H$ varies[14] according to the plot in Fig. 6-25. The modulation frequency was varied from 1 kHz (□) to 10 kHz (△) to 100 kHz (○) over a temperature range from 153 to 353 K. Over this range the correlation time of the motion that changes the ESR spectrum from a four line ESR spectrum at 153 K to a three line ESR spectrum above 275 K varies from 6×10^{-6} to 9×10^{-9} sec. Only at 153 K does the modulation frequency of 100 kHz ($\omega_s = 1.6 \times 10^{-6}$ sec) compete with the correlation time of 6×10^{-6} sec at 153 K. If such a competition controls the modulation frequency dependence, the largest effect should be observed at 153 K. Instead possibly the smallest dependence occurs at this temperature. It should be noted that the form of the frequency dependence is approximately the same at all modulation frequencies but is shifted along the temperature axis (at some orientations the 100 kHz ELDOR signal did vary from $+R$ to $-R$). At 1 kHz an enhanced ELDOR line is observed between 330 and 190 K whereas at 100 kHz a reduced ELDOR line is observed for this crystal orientation. The ELDOR spectrum at 10 kHz is enhanced above 240 K and reduced below 240 K.

A plot of the ELDOR intensity at A_H is complicated by the fact that the central ESR line broadens to near zero intensity at approximately 260 K and thus the reduction factors at A_H for all modulation frequencies also decrease to zero. Nevertheless a large modulation frequency dependence is also observed, as enhanced lines are observed above 260 K for 1 and 10 kHz whereas a reduced line is observed for 100 kHz modulation. Below 260 K, only the 1 kHz modulation gives rise to an enhanced ELDOR spectrum. Since this modulation frequency dependence is somewhat clearer in Fig. 6-25 (uncomplicated by the coalescence problem) for pumping the low field line while observing the high field line, only the dependence at $2A_H$ is shown.

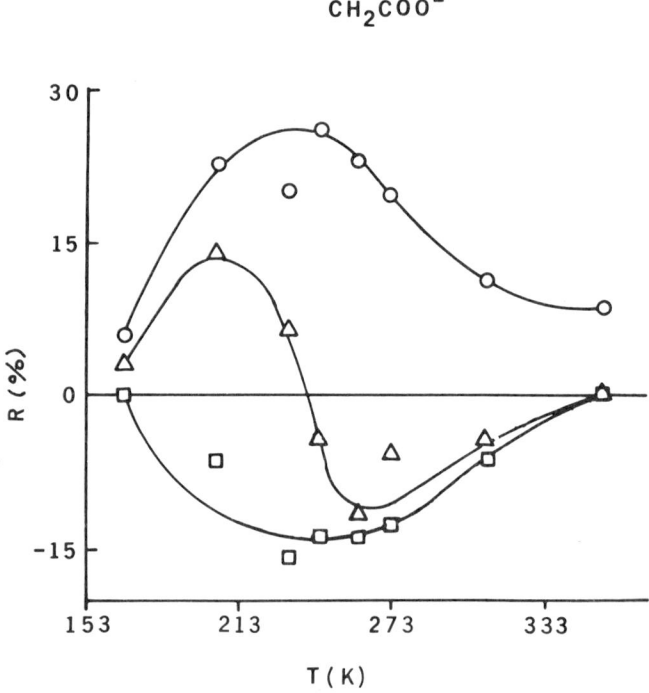

Figure 6-25. The temperature dependence of R at $2A_H$, as the modulation frequency is varied from (O) 100 kHz, to ($\triangle$) 10 kHz to ($\square$) 1 kHz, when the observing condition is set at the cross over of the high field first derivative absorption line of $\dot{C}H_2COO^-$ in irradiated zinc acetate crystals and the low field line is pumped. From C. Mottley, K. Chang, and L. Kispert, *J. Magn. Resonance,* **19,** 130 (1975).

This remarkable change is not always observed when a radical is known to undergo intramolecular motion. A modulation frequency dependence plot of the reduction factors for $(CH_3)_2\dot{C}COOH$, which is known to undergo intramolecular motion (see Section 6.2.1), shows only a 10 to 20% change in the frequency swept ELDOR intensity.[11] Above 285 K a reduced line is observed, whereas at 240 K an enhanced line is observed for all modulation frequencies.

The difference observed in these two examples may possibly arise from the fact that the correlation time for the dominant motion in $\dot{C}H_2COO^-$ varies from 6×10^{-6} to 9×10^{-9} sec over the investigated temperature range, whereas for $(CH_3)_2\dot{C}COOH$ the correlation time of the methyl group rotation is shorter than 10^{-9} sec between 240 and 315 K. If this is the case, one may even need to take into account the exchange of the two methyl groups, which have a correlation time varying from 10^{-6} to 10^{-9} over this temperature range.

A second, probably more important, difference may be the spin-lattice relaxation times as noted previously in Section 5.2.5. Some preliminary measurements of methyl radicals in various metal acetate salts have shown that the spin-lattice relaxation can vary over several orders of magnitude as the cation is varied. Thus if $T_{1e} \simeq 10^{-4} - 10^{-5}$ sec, large modulation effects would be observed whereas little would be observed if T_{1e} were shorter than 10^{-6} sec.

In view of these frequency variations, any attempt to deduce the correlation times of any intramolecular motion of radicals in crystals by ELDOR spectroscopy must be done by an exact calculation that includes the modulation frequency in the spin Hamiltonian.

6.2.11 Intermolecular Spin Diffusion

6.2.11.1 Radical Distribution

In Section 1.5.2.2 we noted that intermolecular diffusion of spins between the energy levels of different radicals causes an increase in the reduction factor for the radical being observed. Although any factor that increases the ELDOR spectral intensity is generally favorable, the presence of spin diffusion can be troublesome spectroscopically whenever the assignment of the spectral lines of a complex ESR spectrum is being attempted. In the presence of significant spin diffusion, all the lines are connected and no ELDOR spectral separation is possible. Spin diffusion effects are known to decrease with decreasing radical concentration, suggesting that all spectral assignments should be carried out at as low a concentration as possible.

However radicals formed in irradiated crystals at low temperatures (77 K) tend to form in clusters as a consequence of inhomogeneous radiation energy deposition. Thus even though the average concentration is low, the local concentration may be high enough to give significant spin diffusion effects. This has been found to be a particular problem in irradiated crystals that have not been annealed.[42] Once the irradiated crystals are annealed, spin diffusion tends to be less of a problem as is seen in the spectral separation of $NH_3^+\dot{C}HCOO^-$ from $\dot{C}H_2COO^-$ (denoted by the letter C) obtained in Fig. 6-5. This same spectral resolution is also possible at low temperatures.

Generally, poorer ESR spectral resolution occurs before annealing than after, so that it may not be surprising that spectral separation can be difficult. However even for a well resolved first derivative ESR absorption spectrum such as that given in Fig. 6-26 for irradiated glycine crystals, spectral separation using ELDOR techniques can be difficult. The resolved four line first derivative ESR spectrum of $\dot{C}H_2COO^-$ is denoted by the letters B, C, D, and E, whereas the remaining ESR lines are due to $NH_3^+\dot{C}HCOO^-$ (Fig. 6-26a). When the observing condition is set at the crossover of the high field first derivative absorption ESR line of the $NH_3^+\dot{C}HCOO^-$ radical (A), the frequency swept ELDOR spectrum consists of lines from both $NH_3^+\dot{C}HCOO^-$ and $\dot{C}H_2COO^-$ when a pump power of 330 mW is used (Fig. 6-26b). The intense lines at 44.0, 93.6,

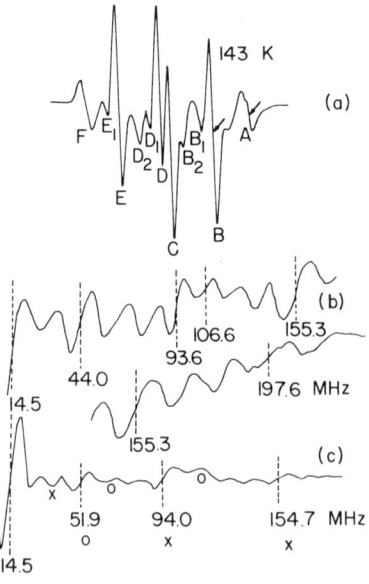

Figure 6-26. (a) The first derivative ESR spectrum at 143 K of glycine crystals irradiated at 77 K and warmed to 143 K. The $\dot{C}H_2COO^-$ radical is denoted by the letters E, D, C, and B and the remaining lines are due to the $NH_3^+\dot{C}HCOO^-$ radical where nonequivalent proton splittings are observed for the restricted amine group. (b). The complex ELDOR spectrum obtained by setting the observing condition at the crossover point of the high field line of $NH_3\dot{C}HCOO^-$ with the pump power equal to 330 mW. The intense signals at 44.0, 93.6, and 155.3 MHz are the intermolecular transitions between $\dot{C}H_2COO^-$ and $NH_3^+\dot{C}HCOO^-$. (c) The ELDOR spectrum observed at the crossover point of line B and the pump power equal to 41 mW. Both intra (denoted by 0) and intermolecular (denoted by ×) transitions are observed. Results of K. Chang and L. Kispert.

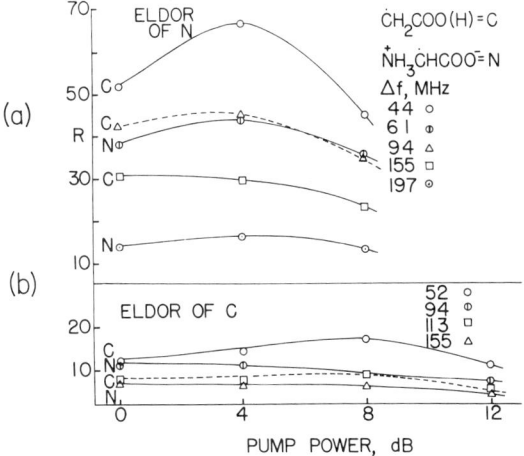

Figure 6-27. The variation in the frequency swept reduction factors (defined as ELDOR signal height divided ESR height) at 143 K as a function of pump power for (a) the ELDOR lines at 44 (○), 61 (◐), 94. (△), 155 (□), and 197 (◎) MHz in Fig. 6-26a when the observing condition is set at the crossover position of the high field line (A) of the $NH_3^+\dot{C}HCOO^-$ radical; (b) the ELDOR lines at 52 (○), 94 (◐). 113 (□), and 155 (△) MHz when the observing condition is set at the crossover position of the highfield line (B) of the $\dot{C}H_2COO^-$ radical in Fig. 6-26a. The notation C and N refers to the radical that is being pumped and that is therefore responsible for the observed ELDOR line. Small differences in the power dependences from one line to another are observed. Results of K. Chang and L. Kispert.

and 155.3 MHz are due to intermolecular transitions between CH_2COO^- and $NH_3^+\dot{C}HCOO^-$. The relative ELDOR signal height does vary as the pump power is reduced and for some lines an increase in resolution can be obtained by decreasing the pump power. This is observed in Fig. 6-26c where the pump power has been reduced to 41 mW when the observing condition is set at the crossover of line B. Notable is the intramolecular transition (○) at 51.9 MHz and intermolecular transitions (×) at 94 and 154.7 MHz. Other inter (×) and intra (○) molecular transitions are not as intense.

The variation in the frequency swept reduction factors as a function of pump power is given in Fig. 6-27a when the observing position is set at the crossover of the high field ESR line (A) of $NH_3^+\dot{C}HCOO^-$ in Fig. 6-26a and in Fig. 6-27b for the observing position set at the crossover of the high field line of $\dot{C}H_2COO^-$ (line B) of Fig. 6-26a. It is noted empirically that when the high field line of CH_2COO^- is observed (Fig. 6-27b). a maximum in the reduction factor occurs for the lines of CH_2COO^- at 8 dB, whereas such a maximum does not occur for the

352 SINGLE CRYSTAL AND POWDER ELDOR

intermolecular $NH_3^+\dot{C}HCOO^-$ lines. From this data it would appear that an assignment of the ELDOR lines could be made on the basis of the pump power dependence, since radicals C and N appear to saturate at considerably different power. Note, however, that in Fig. 6-27a, a maximum occurs at a pump power of 4 dB for both the intramolecular lines of N and the intermolecular lines of C, making it difficult to separate the two radicals when the observing field is set at the high field line of N. Nevertheless by noting the power dependence at different observing magnetic field settings, it should be possible to make a spectral assignment.

6.2.11.2 Overlapped Lines

Another difficulty that arises in the assignment of a complex spectrum is the doubling of peaks when crystals are misaligned and two magnetically nonequivalent sites are observed.[42] Generally the first derivative absorption ESR lines from the two radical sites are partially overlapped. When this occurs spin diffusion from one spin packet to another occurs

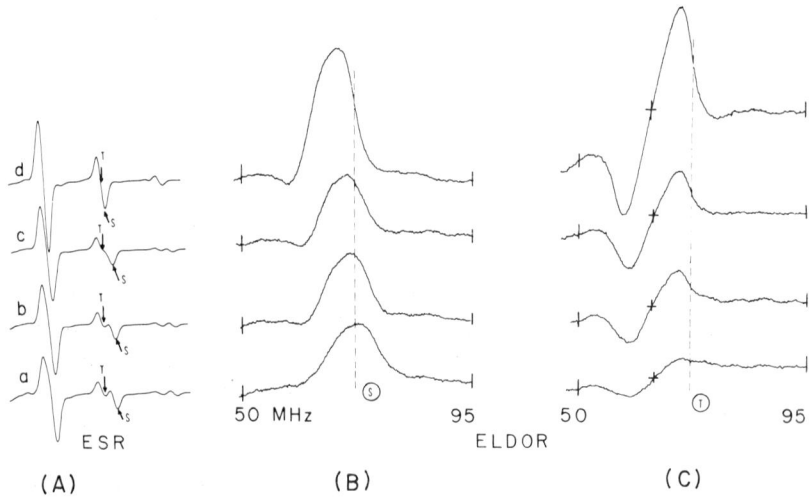

Figure 6-28. (A) the $M_I = -2$ ESR line of the $(CH_3)_2\dot{C}COOH$ radical in irradiated α-aminoisobutyric acid as a function of the separation in megahertz ($a = 13.7$, $b = 12.9$, $c = 10.6$, and $d = 0.0$) between the nonequivalent radical sites. (B) The frequency swept ELDOR spectrum at A_H when the observing position is set to the bottom of the $M_I = -2$ ESR line at position S and (C) between the nonequivalent sites at the crossover position T. Note that a consistent ELDOR lineshape and height is observed for position S for separations a, b, and c whereas a continued variation in shape and height is observed at position T due to the overlapped ESR lines.

and two ESR lines instead of one can be observed in the ELDOR spectrum, such as was observed for line 4 of Fig. 6-15a, where the observing field was set at the crossover of a first derivative ESR line. In Fig. 6-28 the first derivative ESR absorption spectra and the frequency swept ELDOR spectra are given as a function of the separation in megahertz between the two nonequivalent radical sites of $(CH_3)_2\dot{C}COOH$. If one sits at position S, an absorptionlike ELDOR line is observed that exhibits a consistent intensity over separations a to c. In contrast, the ELDOR spectrum observed at T gives rise to an asymmetric derivativelike spectrum that varies in intensity with separation, increasing as the separation between radical sites is decreased. The consistent ELDOR intensity observed for position S over separation a to c is due largely to the fact that one is far off resonance of the other radical site and only one line is contributing to the ELDOR. However, by sitting at position T, two lines are contributing to the ELDOR line in unpredictable amounts. Because of this it is helpful to remember that by sitting at crossover positions of overlapped lines, it is possible in unfortunate situations even to observe little or no ELDOR; yet positioning the observing field to the top or bottom of an overlapped line generally gives rise to an ELDOR signal largely due to one ESR line.

6.2.12 Pulsed ELDOR

In a few ELDOR experiments the pumping microwave power is pulsed on and off. In this mode it is possible to observe transient ELDOR as discussed in Section 1.5.2.1. The primary reason for doing this is to permit the measurement of the individual relaxation rates rather than the measurement of some averaged relaxation rate as is normally obtained with the Varian ELDOR spectrometer. Experimentally the pump microwave power is usually pulsed by using a microwave diode switch with the observing cavity mode connected to a wide-band receiver sensitive to the transient change of the absorption ESR signal. The transient signal obtained can be stored in a boxcar integrator or in a multichannel analyzer and later fed to a recorder.

In this way the spin-lattice relaxation time of a V_1 center in electron-irradiated MgO crystals has been measured[43] to be 1.1 sec at 4.2 K, the spin-lattice and cross-relaxation times of a CH fragment in crystals of irradiated malonic acid were found to equal 40 μsec and 300 μsec, respectively, at ambient temperature,[44] the cross-relaxation time of nitrogen centers in diamond varied between 7 and 135 msec at 1.6 K, depending on the orientation of the nitrogen center,[45] a number of different relaxation rates were measured at 1.6 K for Co^{2+} ions (eight allowed transitions) in a crystal of $La_2Zn_3(NO_3)_{12} \cdot 24H_2O$ (ref. 46) and were found to be strongly dependent on the direction of the applied magnetic field, and spin-lattice relaxation rates were measured for $NiSiF_6 \cdot 6H_2O$ diluted in diamagnetic $ZnSiF_6 \cdot 6H_2O$ between 2.2 and 4.2 K, which enabled a relaxation mechanism to be deduced.[47] Although the measurement of the relaxation times is necessary if the details of a relaxation mechanism is to be verified, the emphasis of this chapter is on pointing out the uses of ELDOR spectroscopy in assigning the spectral lines of a complex pattern. Thus a complete discussion of the relaxation times will not be given. However two studies do bear mentioning in detail because their application could be helpful in certain spectral analyses.

The temperature dependence of the ESR spectrum of radicals in single crystals can often be difficult to understand in terms of the motion of a substituent of the radical. However in some cases at very low temperature, small fragments such as the hole trapped at an isolated cation vacancy can jump from one orientation to another.[43] Although this may appear as a change in the ESR spectrum over an appropriate temperature range, such a mechanism would not be observed by ESR at low temperature.

In Fig. 6-29A the first derivative dispersion ESR spectrum of the V_1 center at 4.2 K with the magnetic field applied to the [110] crystal direction of MgO[43] is given. The low field line is due to a radical site of O^-, denoted by V_1 (90°), that lies 90° from the direction [110] and the central line is due to another radical site of O^-, denoted by V_1 (45°) that lies 45° from the [110] direction. If the difference between the pumping and observing frequencies equals the difference (in hertz) between the $V_1(90°)$ and $V_1(45°)$, then it is possible to monitor the $V_1(90°)$ line at very low power (1 mW) while simultaneously saturating the line at $V_1(45°)$ with 10 mW power when the magnetic field is swept. The field swept ELDOR spectrum that results is given in Fig. 6-29B and a large reduction in the intensity of the $V_1(90°)$ site is observed. It has been found from uniaxial stress experiments that the V_1 centers are not frozen and that they tend to orient parallel to the stress axis. From the ELDOR measurements the transfer of saturation between different configurations of the V_1 center could be interpreted as reorientational motion of the hole around the vacancy. It also could be intermolecular cross-relaxation between different sites of the V_1 center.

To differentiate between these two mechanisms, one can make use of the fact that the cross-relaxation time between radicals decreases with increasing concentration whereas the jump time between sites lengthens with increasing concentration. To measure this time a pump pulse is

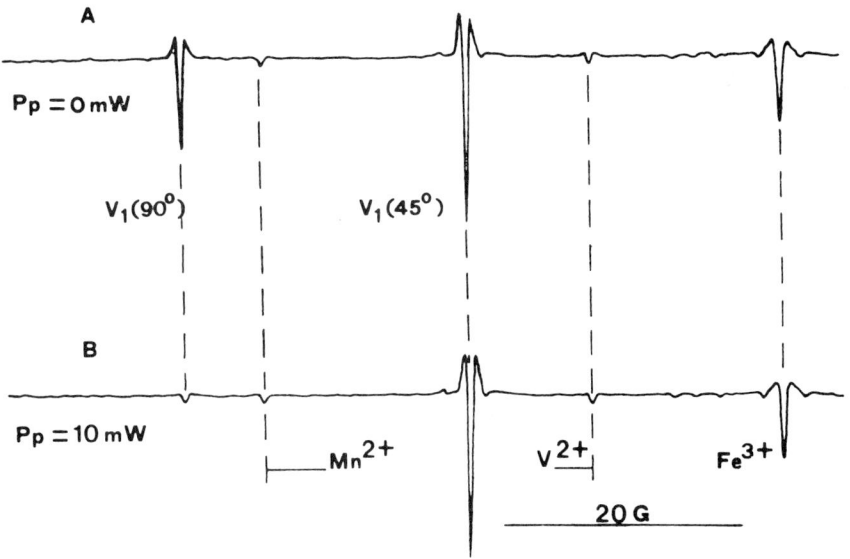

Figure 6-29. (A) The dispersion mode ESR spectrum of the V_1 center at 4.2 K and 9 GHz with $H_o \| [110]$. (B) A field swept ELDOR spectrum obtained with 10 mW of pump power and $\nu_p > \nu_o$ with the microwave frequency difference between the observing and pumping modes set so that at a given H_o field the $V_1(90°)$ site is observed and the $V_1(45°)$ site is pumped. From G. Ruis and A. Herve, *Solid State Commun.*, **15**, 421 (1974).

applied and the transient response of the observed signal is noted. This appears as an exponential increase in the time (τ_s) required for onset of saturation of the observed ESR signal as seen in Fig. 6-30b. The exponential decrease in the observed transient response after the pumping pulse has been removed (Fig. 6-30a) is the spin-lattice relaxation time (T_{1e}). A measurement of τ_s as a function of concentration showed an increase in time with concentration; therefore τ_s is the jump time of the hole vacancy from one orientation to another.

Another pulse experiment gave some evidence that very narrow ELDOR lines may be observed if the transient ELDOR signal intensity from a pulsed frequency swept experiment where the pumping pulse duration equals 10 μsec is recorded as a function of the difference frequency. In Fig. 6-31 the narrow ELDOR line (width at half height $\simeq$ 100 kHz) superimposed on a wider one arises when an observing resonant condition is positioned on the high field allowed line of the >CH fragment in irradiated malonic acid crystals and the pump frequency is swept through the transition corresponding to a forbidden line.[44] The width of the narrow line increases with decreasing observing power,

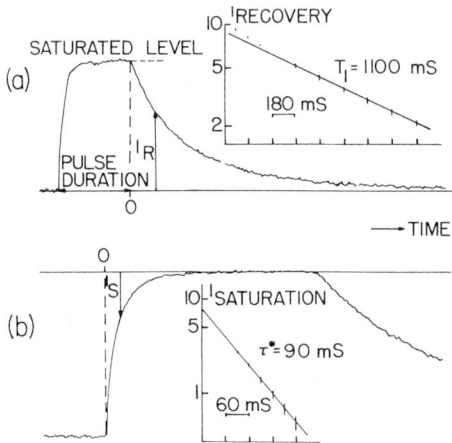

Figure 6-30. The pulsed ELDOR response of the V_1 center at 4.2 K with $H_o \| [110]$. (a) The variation of the ELDOR intensity of the $V_1(90°)$ ESR line during a 1-sec pumping pulse of the $V_1(45°)$ line at 10 mW of power. (b) Expansion of the trace in (a), showing the time dependence of the pumping rate during the pulse. From G. Ruis and A. Herve, *Solid State Commun.*, **15**, 421 (1974).

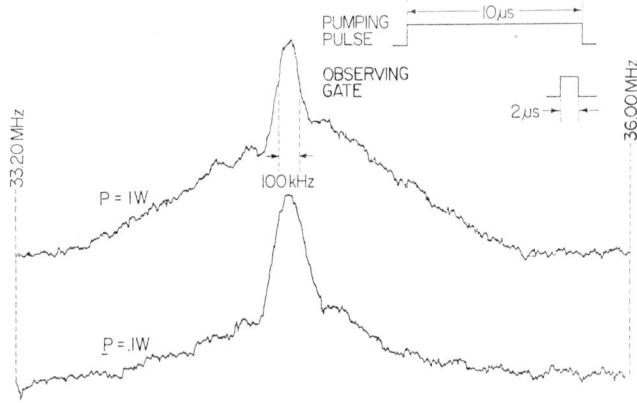

Figure 6-31. The frequency swept transient ELDOR intensity recorded as a function of the difference between the observing and pumping microwave frequencies for the $\dot{C}H(COOH)_2$ radical while the pumping pulse was on and a forbidden line was being pumped. From M. Nechtschein and J. S. Hyde, *Phys. Rev. Lett.*, **24**, 672 (1970).

whereas the width of the broad line is proportional to the pumping power. The origin of the narrow line is not known, however better resolution occurs at low pump powers and low observing microwave power.

6.3 Applications—Oriented Radicals ($S=\frac{1}{2}$) in Single Crystals

One of the major contributors to ELDOR active relaxation mechanisms in single crystals is intramolecular motion. Fortunately almost all radicals, especially those in irradiated crystals, undergo some sort of intramolecular motion, and therefore most organic radicals give an ELDOR response. Characteristic ELDOR responses from each of the different radicals given in Sections 6.2.1 through 6.2.12 can be used to assign spectral lines of a complex ESR spectrum, study hydrogen-deuterium exchange reactions, and assign forbidden lines when methyl groups undergo tunneling rotation. A few applications are explored in detail in the following section to emphasize the spectroscopic use that can be made of the preceding empirical observations from ELDOR studies.

6.3.1. Separation of Overlapping Spectra

6.3.1.1 Intramolecular Motion

Whenever a radical substituent undergoes intramolecular motion, nuclei that were nonequivalent at low temperature can become equivalent at higher temperatures. When this occurs, some of the rigid lattice ESR lines broaden and disappear, eventually giving rise to the high temperature ESR spectrum.

For instance, when the $\dot{C}H_2COO^-$ radical in irradiated zinc acetate undergoes a torsional oscillation,[14] the four line ESR spectrum at 155 K given in Fig. 6-32 changes to a three line spectrum at 275 K. The Arrhenius rate equation for the correlation time of the rotation calculated from a time dependent Hamiltonian[34] is found to equal

$$\tau_c^{-1} = 5.62 \times 10^{11} \exp\left(-4.63 \text{ kcal } (RT)^{-1}\right) \quad (6.24)$$

Over this temperature range the central two lines at low temperature broaden and collapse into a single narrow line above 275 K. The frequency swept ELDOR spectrum obtained by setting the observing condition at the crossover point of the high field first derivative absorption ESR line at 248 K using 100 kHz modulation consists of allowed-allowed

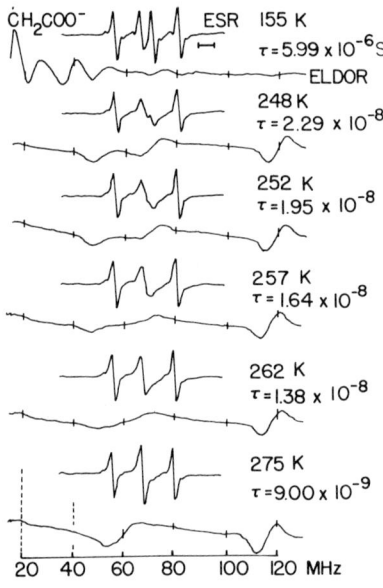

Figure 6-32. The ESR (upper) and ELDOR (lower) lineshapes at 100 kHz modulation of the $\dot{C}H_2COO^-$ radical in zinc acetate as a function of temperature. At 155 K the splitting between the central first derivative absorption ESR lines is 21.8 MHz. The bar below the ESR spectrum at 155 K represents 30 MHz for the ESR spectra and the scale at the bottom is for the ELDOR spectra. The ELDOR spectra were run with the observing position set at the crossing point of the high field ESR line. The correlation times were calculated using eq. 6.24. From C. Mottley, K. Chang, and L. Kispert, *J. Magn. Resonance*, **19**, 130 (1975).

lines at 51.0, 69.5, and 120.0 MHz. Because the central ESR lines are beginning to broaden, the linewidths of the ELDOR lines at 51.0 and 69.5 MHz have increased from a peak to peak linewidth of 6 MHz at 155 K to 9 MHz at 248 K. As the temperature is raised to 252 K, the ELDOR spectrum changes to a broad doublet (peak to peak linewidth = 26.5 MHz) centered at about 60 MHz and a line at 118.5 MHz. It is to be noted that the linewidth of the central corresponding "doublet" ESR line (23.2 MHz) at 252 K is slightly narrower than the ELDOR line. At 262 K the center ESR lines have coalesced into a single broadened line with a peak to peak width of 11.5 MHz and the outer lines have a peak to peak width of 8.5 MHz. This is reflected in the ELDOR spectrum, which consists of a single line at 60 MHz (peak to peak width of 21.5 MHz) and a line at 117.5 MHz with a peak to peak width of 7.0 MHz. The shift in the position of the 118.5 MHz peak is the direct result of the reorientation of a radical in a crystal. At 271 K the ESR lineshape approaches the 1:2:1 triplet expected for two equivalent protons and the ELDOR pattern consists of two lines at 60 and 116.4 MHz where the 60 MHz line has narrowed to 11.5 MHz. The temperature at which the two coalescing ELDOR or ESR lines are the broadest[14] is given by the requirement that

$$\Delta\omega\tau_c \simeq 2 \qquad (6.25)$$

where τ_c is the correlation time of the motion in seconds and $\Delta\omega$ is the frequency difference between the central lines of the rigid lattice in rad-

Hz.[32-33] The correlation time τ_c can be estimated experimentally in the slow exchange limit (two center ESR lines) from the relationship[48]

$$2\pi\Delta\nu = \frac{1-P_i}{\tau_c} \quad (6.26)$$

where $\Delta\nu$ is the increase in the peak to peak ELDOR linewidth at 60 MHz due to the exchange process and P_i is the probability for being in a given orientation ($\frac{1}{2}$ for the twofold rotor in zinc acetate).

In the fast exchange limit (one central ESR line) τ_c can be estimated from eq. 6.27 where ν_a and ν_b are the low temperature line positions of the coalescing lines relative to the center of the spectrum and $\Delta\nu$ is the increase in ELDOR linewidth over that of the central ELDOR line in

$$\Delta\nu = \frac{2\pi\tau_c}{4}(\nu_a - \nu_b)^2 \quad (6.27)$$

the rapidly rotating limit.

To find the temperature at which the largest ELDOR linewidth occurs, the value of τ_c obtained from eq. 6.25 is compared to that obtained from a plot of ln $(1/\tau_c)$ versus $1/T$ calculated from eqs. 6.26 and 6.27.

For example, the separation between the central two ESR peaks $(\Delta\omega)$ in Fig. 6-33 at 155 K (rigid lattice) is 36.1 MHz. For this orientation the largest linewidth of the central lines will occur when $\Delta\omega\tau = 2$ or $\tau_c = 5.5 \times 10^{-8}$ sec. From the plot of ln $(1/\tau_c)$ versus $1/T$, this value τ_c occurs at $T = 263$ K. This is a somewhat approximate method; however in all cases so far attempted,[14] the predicted temperature is within ± 5 K of the experimental temperature. Note that in Fig. 6-33 the ELDOR line at approximately 60 MHz is so broad that it is barely detectable.

This suggests an interesting spectroscopic application. If an ESR spectrum consists of several overlapping peaks from different radicals, a separation of these peaks is possible, providing that the correlation times of the motion in each radical are not the same. Normally, significant spin diffusion effects occur for badly overlapped lines (see Section 6.2.11.2) preventing ELDOR spectral separation. However by carefully selecting an orientation (and thus a $\Delta\omega$) and a temperature T where $\Delta\omega\tau_c = 2$ the central spectral lines from one radical broaden below detectability, allowing spectral separation from the spectrum of other radicals. It has also been noted experimentally that no ELDOR lines are recorded when the observing condition is set at the crossover of the high field inner line of the four line ESR spectrum over a temperature range where the inner lines begin to broaden (248 to 257 K, Fig. 6-32). This failure to observe ELDOR spectra can be attributed to the increase in linewidth of the observed line. At 155 K, where sharp line rigid lattice-type ESR spectra are observed, the ELDOR spectrum consists of a strong line from

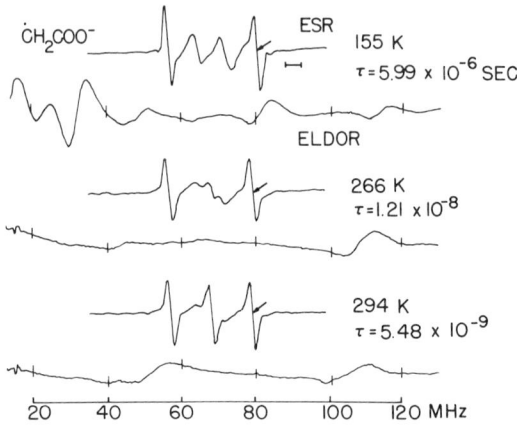

Figure 6-33. The first derivative ESR absorption (upper) and ELDOR (lower) lineshapes as a function of temperature of the $\dot{C}H_2COO^-$ radical in zinc acetate using 100 kHz modulation at a different orientation than in Fig. 6-32. The scales are the same as in Fig. 6-32. The splitting between the inner ESR lines is 36.1 MHz at 155 K. The observing point for the ELDOR spectra is the crossing point of the high field line as indicated. The correlation times were calculated using eq. 6.24. From C. Mottley, K. Chang, and L. Kispert, *J. Magn. Resonance*, **19**, 130 (1975).

pumping the low field inner line and a weak line corresponding to pumping the extreme low field line.

As an example of how these observations might be used, let us consider the spectral separation of the ESR spectrum of $NH_3^+\dot{C}HCOO^-$ from that of $\dot{C}H_2COO^-$ in irradiated glycine. At 77 K the amine protons in $NH_3^+\dot{C}HCOO^-$ are distinguishable whereas at 300 K rapid rotation about the C—N bond causes the three protons to appear equivalent.[50] On the other hand, the ESR spectrum of $\dot{C}H_2COO^-$ changes from a four line spectrum (77 K) to a three line pattern near room temperature.

The ELDOR spectrum obtained by setting the observing condition at the crossover of the first derivative high field ESR line of glycine crystals irradiated at 195 K is given in Fig. 6-34 for $b \parallel H_o$. Because spin diffusion effects are minimal in this particular case (the crystal had been annealed at 300 K) only the ELDOR spectrum of $NH_3^+\dot{C}HCOO^-$ is observed at 139 K with lines at 14.0 MHz (the proton frequency), 56.8 MHz (A_{NH_1}), 86.8 MHz (A_{NH_2}), and 144.0 MHz ($A_{NH_1}+A_{NH_2}$) plus the associated spin-flip lines (Section 6.2.9) and possible forbidden lines. The line at A_{NH_3} cannot be observed because it occurs at 1 MHz. The α proton splitting of 61 MHz is also absent. Just as expected, when the temperature is raised, rotation about the C—N bond increases and the ELDOR lines at A_{NH_1} and A_{NH_2} decrease in amplitude and broaden out until effectively disappearing at 175 K. There is little change in the $A_{NH_1}+A_{NH_2}$ line. At 221 K

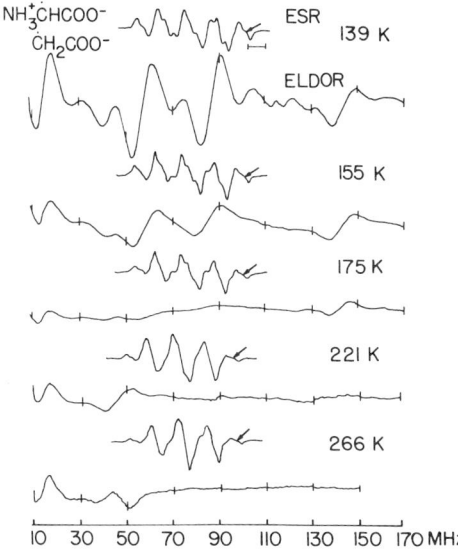

Figure 6-34. Temperature dependent first derivative ESR absorption (upper) and ELDOR (lower) spectra using 100 kHz modulation for glycine irradiated at 195 K. The crystal is mounted so that $b \parallel H_o$ in the bc^* plane. The observing position for ELDOR was the crossing point of the high field ESR line. The observed ELDOR lines are due to the $NH_3^+\dot{C}HCOO^-$ radical. The ESR and ELDOR scales are defined in Fig. 6-32. From C. Mottley, K. Chang, and L. Kispert, *J. Magn. Resonance*, **19**, 130 (1975).

the amine protons are nonequivalent and a reduced ELDOR line appears at 47.5 MHz $(A_{NH_1} + A_{NH_2} + A_{NH_3})/3$. At 266 K this line becomes enhanced.

In this particular setting of the observing ESR condition, the appearance of just the $NH_3^+\dot{C}HCOO^-$ ELDOR spectrum is due to the absence of spin diffusion and the absence of spectral overlap from other radicals. Thus τ_c can be determined experimentally by using the definition of τ_c in the slow exchange region (such as at 155 K) given by eq. 6.26 where $P_i = \frac{1}{3}$ for the threefold rotor of NH_3 (ref. 33). In the fast exchange limit (one average line, 221 K) τ_c is determined from the equation

$$\Delta\nu = \frac{2\pi\tau_c}{27}[(\nu_a - \nu_b)^2 + (\nu_b - \nu_c)^2 + (\nu_a - \nu_c)^2] \qquad (6.28)$$

where ν_a, ν_b, and ν_c are line positions in frequency units for the three protons relative to the $M_I = \pm\frac{1}{2}$ line positions of the rotating amine group and $\Delta\nu$ is the increase in ELDOR linewidth over that of the rapidly rotating amine protons. As before eq. 6.25 determines the value of the τ_c for which the A_{NH_1} and A_{NH_2} ELDOR lines coalesce and disappear for a given $\Delta\omega$. The temperature that corresponds to this τ_c can be obtained from a plot of $\ln(1/\tau_c)$ versus $1/T$. Along the b axis where $\Delta\omega \simeq$ 168.6 MHz, a temperature of 173 K is obtained that agrees favorably with the 175 K observed experimentally.

However an example of spectral separation can be demonstrated by setting the observing position at the crossing point of line 2 (denoted by the arrow) in Fig. 6-35. ELDOR lines from both radicals are observed at 139 K since the observing line is a superposition of lines from both radicals. We have, in addition to the proton line at 15.3 MHz, reduced lines at 30.0, 86.7, and 144.0 MHz due to the nonequivalent amine protons in the $NH_3^+\dot{C}HCOO^-$ radical and a reduced line at approximately 57.5 MHz probably due to the α proton line, which overlaps the lines from the $\dot{C}H_2COO^-$ radical. The lines at 44.0 and 73.0 MHz are spin-flip lines. To separate these lines the temperature must be raised to a point where one of the overlapping ESR lines increases in linewidth. Such a condition occurs at 175 K for the ESR line from $NH_3^+\dot{C}HCOO^-$ and, as a result, the ELDOR spectrum at 175 K is due only to the $\dot{C}H_2COO^-$ radical. In Fig. 6-35 the two nonequivalent protons of $\dot{C}H_2COO^-$ give rise to the ELDOR lines at 52.5 (A_{CH_1}) and 68.0 (A_{CH_2}) MHz. The proton line at 13.5 MHz and spin-flip lines at 38.3, 82.5, 107.0, and 136.0 MHz are also observed. As the temperature is raised and rotation occurs about the C—C bond in $\dot{C}H_2COO^-$, the A_{CH_1}, A_{CH_2}, and $A_{CH_1} + A_{CH_2}$ lines

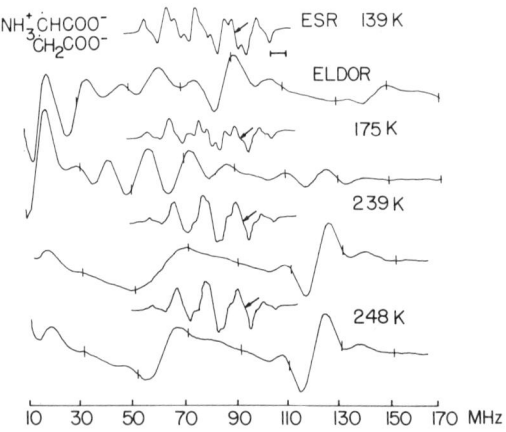

Figure 6-35. Temperature dependent first derivative ESR absorption (upper) and ELDOR (lower) spectra for glycine irradiated at 195 K so that $b \| H_o$ in the bc^* plane. The observing position is set at the crossing point of the high field inner line as indicated by the arrow. At 139 K ELDOR lines due to both the $NH_3^+\dot{C}HOO^-$ and the $\dot{C}H_2COO^-$ radicals are observed. The scales are defined in Fig. 6-32. From C. Mottley, K. Chang, and L. Kispert, *J. Magn. Resonance*, **19**, 130 (1975).

behave in a manner analogous to the zinc acetate system. At 239 K the protons are approximately equivalent and a single broad line at 61.0 MHz and a sharp line at 120.0 MHz are observed. On further warming the line at 61.0 MHz continues to sharpen.

From these observations it should be possible to solve more complex spectra, providing that two conditions are satisfied. If the rigid lattice hyperfine splittings for the radicals in a given orientation are approximately the same, then (1) the activation energies for rotation must be different enough to allow the condition $\Delta\omega\tau_c \simeq 2$ to be met at temperatures separated by at least 10 degrees for each species present or (2) the anisotropy in the hyperfine splittings must be such that even though the τ_c's may be similar at a given temperature the condition $\Delta\omega\tau_c \simeq 2$ is satisfied at a different orientation of the crystal for each radical species. That is, the condition $\Delta\omega\tau_c \simeq 2$ must not be satisfied for more than one radical species at a time.

6.3.1.2 *Temperature Dependence of R*

Even though a large number of complex spectra can be assigned by simply considering the correlation times of the motion for each radical, the temperature dependence of the reduction factor for each substituent can be used for the same purposes as well.

In Fig. 6-36 a plot of the temperature dependence of the reduction factor at 100 kHz modulation is shown for $CFH-$ (□) groups; chlorine substituents (◐), rotating methyl groups (●); exchanging protons ($\dot{C}H_2COOH$) (○), and $\dot{C}H_3CHR$ (△).

Generally the rotating methyl groups result in an ELDOR spectrum that varies between a reduced and enhanced ELDOR line, depending on the rotational correlation times in the radical. In addition, ELDOR spectra are observed over a large temperature range, from a temperature greater than 400 K to a temperature less than 77 K where tunneling rotation (refer to Section 6.3.3.) occurs. In contrast this type of temperature dependence is not observed for radicals containing chlorine where a zero ELDOR intensity is observed at room temperature, a sharp increase below 220 K, and a gradual increase below 160 K. This can be further compared to the near temperature independence of the fluorine ELDOR spectral intensity, providing that motion on an ESR time scale is absent.

Exchangeable protons ($\dot{C}H_2COO^-$) give a still different temperature dependence; the R factor shows a maximum as a function of temperature. Thus in any complex spectrum containing radicals with F, Cl, methyl groups, or exchangeable protons, the spectral peaks can be identified just by studying the temperature dependence of the reduction factors for each line.

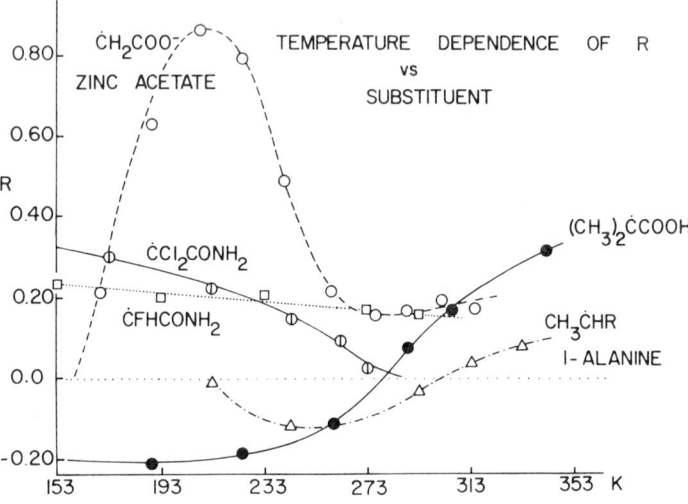

Figure 6-36. The temperature dependence of R versus substituent for the frequency swept absorption ELDOR spectra obtained with 100 kHz modulation for (○) the $M_I = -1$ observing line when $\Delta f = 71$ MHz for $\dot{C}H_2COO^-$; (●) the $M_I = -3$ observing line when $\Delta f = 62$ MHz of $(CH_3)_2\dot{C}COOH$; (⌀) the field line of $\dot{C}Cl_2CONH_2$ and $\dot{C}ClFR$ and $\Delta f = 74$ MHz; (□) the high field of $\dot{C}FHCONH_2$ and $\Delta f = 35$ MHz; and (△) the $M_I = -2$ line of $CH_3\dot{C}HR$ and $\Delta f = 73$ to 79 MHz. $\Delta f = \nu_p - \nu_o$. From L. Kispert and K. Chang, *J. Magn. Resonance*, **10**, 162 (1973).

6.3.1.3 Fluorine Anisotropy and Motion

The effects of fluorine hyperfine anisotropy given in Section 6.2.3 demonstrated that intense forbidden-allowed transitions are possible for radicals that contain nonequivalent nuclei and exhibit little apparent motion on an ESR time scale (e.g., $\dot{C}FHCONH_2$). Yet for those fluorinated radicals that contain equivalent fluorines (such as $\dot{C}F_2CONH_2$) and do exhibit torsional motion on an ESR time scale, relatively intense allowed-allowed ELDOR lines (relative to the forbidden lines) are observed. Thus several empirical rules of thumb for certain spectroscopic applications might be suggested.

In a complex ESR spectrum made up of the overlapping spectra of several fluorinated radicals and insignificant spin diffusion, the ELDOR spectra associated with radicals containing CF_2 will be composed of lines at the fluorine hyperfine splitting, which can change from enhanced to reduced lines as the temperature is varied. Intense forbidden-allowed lines and weak or unobservable allowed-allowed ESR lines will result from the radicals containing nonequivalent nuclei. Thus the spectrum of a radical containing a CF_2 group can be identified and separated from other fluorinated radicals. However care must be taken since at large hyperfine splittings ($A_F > 200$ MHz) the allowed-allowed lines decrease in intensity even for $\dot{C}F_2CONH_2$, as a result of the hyperfine anisotropy.[2] This is no major limitation since good spectral resolution usually exists for large hyperfine splittings.

The forbidden-allowed ELDOR intensity also appears to be dependent on the degree of symmetry. Thus a differentiation of radicals containing nonequivalent fluorine nuclei can be determined by an analysis of the forbidden-allowed ELDOR intensities.

6.3.1.4 Quadrupole Interaction and Motion

As pointed out in Section 6.2.6 chlorine quadrupolar relaxation can be orders of magnitude faster than the relaxation arising from the magnetic dipole-dipole interactions.[37] Because of this the quadrupolar relaxation is usually the dominant relaxation and thus determines the active ELDOR transitions. Typically whenever α chlorines are substituents of the radicals under study, the ELDOR spectral intensity increases with decreasing temperature, with little intensity observed above 223 K, giving rise to a simple pattern comprised primarily of intense lines at $A(Cl)$ and $\frac{3}{2}A(Cl) - \nu(Cl)$ for a completely chlorinated radical. Although intramolecular motion has been such a dominant factor in all other ELDOR active mechanisms, it apparently has little effect on the presence of quadrupole relaxation. For example, no ELDOR spectra are obtained from the freely rotating or inverting $\dot{C}Cl_3$ radicals at room temperature where the intramolecular rotation should provide a substantial influence.[7]

Likewise the influence of hyperfine anisotropy on the ELDOR spectral intensity appears to be neutralized in the presence of quadrupolar relaxation. The ELDOR spectral intensity and number of lines of $\dot{C}ClFCONH_2$ did not change in a manner like that reported in Table 6-4 for $\dot{C}FHCONH_2$ when the fluorine hyperfine splitting was changed from 467 to 150 MHz.

The ELDOR spectral resolution obtainable for radicals containing α chlorine should enable a number of investigations to be carried out that were not previously possible.

6.3.2 Hydrogen-Deuterium Exchange

Hydrogen-deuterium exchange reactions in irradiated crystals[24,25] have important implications for biological applications because they are stereo-specific and the rate constant for exchange (3×10^{-4} sec^{-1}) is similar to that for enzymatic exchange $2 \times 10^{-4} \text{ sec}^{-1}$). Itoh and Miyagawa[24] first reported in 1964 an example of hydrogen-deuterium exchange reactions in irradiated l-alanine (CH_3CHND_2COOD) and subsequently showed the importance of the crystal field for such reactions. When l-alanine is irradiated at 300 K, $CH_3\dot{C}HR$ is formed, which can easily be identified by the appearance of a five line spectrum with an intensity ratio of $1:4:6:4:1$ along the c crystal axis (Fig. 6-37a). However if the crystal is left at room temperature for two years or if it is heated for 2 hours at 373 K a new spectrum appears at the expense of the $CH_3\dot{C}HCOOD$ spectrum with an intensity ratio of $1:1:1:3:3:3:3:3:3:1:1:1$ [Fig. 6-37b]. This pattern is due to a mixture of $CH_3\dot{C}DR$ and $CH_2D\dot{C}HR$. If the crystals are heated for 10 hours at 423 K, the spectrum consists primarily of $CD_3\dot{C}DR$ (Fig. 6-37d). Less drastic heating conditions produce intermediate radicals such as $CHD_2\dot{C}HR$, $CH_2D\dot{C}DR$, $CD_3\dot{C}HR$, and $CD_2H\dot{C}DR$ as shown in Fig. 6-37c. Itoh and Miyagawa[24] found that the exchange process occurs by two processes: direct exchange between the protons of $CH_3\dot{C}HCOOD$ and the lattice deuterons and exchange between α and β protons (deuterons).

Hydrogen-deuterium exchange is also observed[25] in irradiated crystals of $CH_3CDND_3^+CO_2^-$ and $CH_3CDNH_3^+CO_2^-$ where $CH_3\dot{C}DR$, $CH_3\dot{C}HR$, $CH_2D\dot{C}HR$, or $CH_3\dot{C}DR$ result, depending on the length of the heating

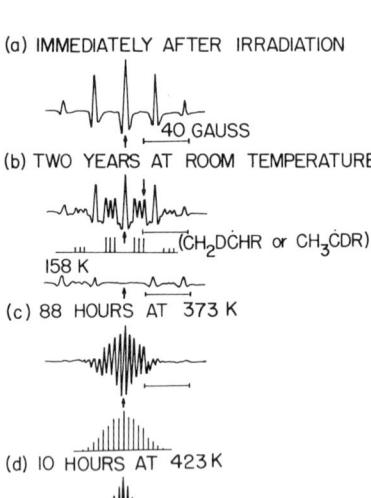

Figure 6-37. Second derivative ESR absorption spectra at room temperature of irradiated crystals of CH_3CHND_3COOD taken with the magnetic field parallel to the [001] axis. The crystals were heated at the temperature and for the period of time given above each spectrum. The spectra are for (a) $CH_3\dot{C}HR$ (b) a mixture of $CH_3\dot{C}HR$ and $CH_2D\dot{C}HR/CH_3\dot{C}DR$, ($c$) 25% $CH_2D\dot{C}DR$ and $CHD_2\dot{C}HR$, 50% $CD_3\dot{C}HR$ and $CHD_2\dot{C}DR$, and 25% $CD_3\dot{C}DR$, (d) $CD_3\dot{C}DR$. From K. Itoh and I. Miyagawa. J. Chem. Phys., **40**, 3328 (1964).

period. Three different hydrogen-deuterium exchange processes are detected. First, the appearance of CH$_3$ĊHR in equilibrium with CH$_3$ĊDR occurs by exchange between the α deuteron in the radical and the methyl hydrogen in an adjacent molecule. Second, the appearance of CH$_2$DĊHR occurs by an exchange of the methyl proton from CH$_3$ĊHR with an α deuteron of an adjacent molecule. Third, the appearance of CD$_3$ĊDR occurs by exchange of the amine deuterons from a large number of surrounding molecules with the radical protons. The large number of different exchange processes that can occur simultaneously also result in complex ESR spectra. In irradiated l-alanine, the ESR spectrum was fortunately quite easy to analyze along the c crystal axis and the various partially deuterated radicals were identified. However in general the ESR spectra are complex. The failure to observe deuterium ELDOR lines although proton lines are observed in radicals that contain both protons and deuteriums, as discussed in Section 6.2.7, suggests that ELDOR spectroscopy is ideally suited to study H/D exchange. Furthermore ENDOR investigations of the H/D exchange processes have failed so far to detect any signal.[51]

The increase in resolution obtainable by ELDOR for H/D exchange studies enables two types of problems to be solved. First in irradiated l-alanine CH$_3$ĊHR is initially formed, and upon heating either CH$_2$DĊHR or CH$_3$ĊDR or a mixture of these two radicals is formed (Fig. 6-37b). Since all four protons are equivalent along the c axis it is not possible to identify which of these radical assignments is correct without carrying out an angular ESR study. However ELDOR studies can determine the identity of the partially deuterated radicals without requiring an orientational study.[52] To accomplish this the observing ESR position is set at the bottom of the high field first derivative absorption ESR spectrum of CH$_2$DĊHR/CH$_3$ĊDR in Fig. 6-37b and a frequency swept ELDOR spectrum is obtained using 100 kHz modulation. We can anticipate from the data given in Fig. 6-36 and Section 6.2.7 that a frequency swept ELDOR spectrum for CH$_3$ĊDCOOD at room temperature would consist of an enhanced line (with a shape as in Fig. 6-1) at 76 MHz because of the rapidly rotating methyl group with no lines being observed from deuterium. On the other hand, if the extra ESR lines were due to CH$_2$DĊHCOOD, the ELDOR spectrum would consist of only a reduced line as the rotational correlation time of the CH$_2$D group has changed sufficiently so that a reduced ELDOR line at the CH$_2$D proton frequency would be observed. However neither of these were observed experimentally. Instead the ELDOR line for the deuterated radical appears to be a combination of an overlapped enhanced and a reduced line not so different from that given in Fig. 6-4 for the fully protonated

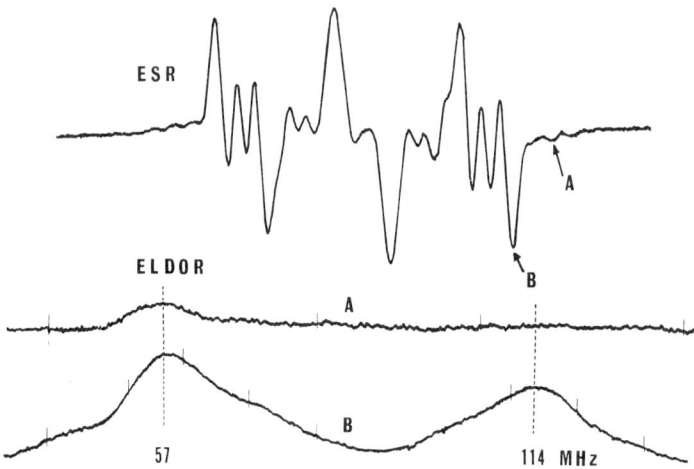

Figure 6-38. The first derivative absorption ESR spectrum (upper) of partially deuterated glycine-d_3 crystal irradiated at 77 K and measured at 193 K. The magnetic field is along the c crystal axis. The frequency swept ELDOR spectrum (lower) taken with the observing condition set at A (bottom of the first derivative curve) consists of a peak at 55 MHz that is assigned to the amine proton in $ND_2H^+\dot{C}HCOO^-$ whereas that at B consists of two peaks at 57 and 144 MHz from $\dot{C}H_2COO^-$. From L. Kispert and K. Chang, unpublished work.

$CH_3\dot{C}HCOOD$ radical. Thus the conclusions reached by the previously reported ESR studies[24] that the ESR lines are due to a mixture of $CH_2D\dot{C}HCOOD$ and $CH_3\dot{C}DCOOD$ radicals have been verified.

A further application is the identification of the products of hydrogen-deuterium exchange when the crystal is a mixture of partially (45% $NHD_2^+CH_2COOD$, 45% $ND_3^+CH_2COOD$, and 10% others) deuterated molecules. When the magnetic field is along the c crystal axis of a partially deuterated glycine crystal, the ESR spectrum given in Fig. 6-38 is observed when the crystal is irradiated at 77 K and warmed to 193 K. The frequency swept ELDOR spectrum given in Fig. 6-38 results when the observing ELDOR position is set at A (the bottom of the first derivative ESR line). Note the presence of a reduced ELDOR line at 55 MHz that corresponds to the amine proton splitting, but the absence of any line around 80 MHz, the hyperfine splitting of the α proton. The reason for this is clear if we refer back to Fig. 6-6, where it is found that the α proton ELDOR intensity is extremely weak at 193 K and would probably not be observed. Combining this ELDOR data with calculations of all possible ESR spectra that can result for partially deuterated radicals containing at least one amine proton shows the radical to be $NHD_2^+\dot{C}HCOO^-$. It is also important to realize that by obtaining the

ELDOR spectrum along the c crystal axis, the amine and α proton splitting magnitudes differ enough to make unique assignments of the ELDOR splitting possible. The ELDOR spectrum obtained from observing position B is that of $\dot{C}H_2COO^-$, as identified by two peaks, one at A_H (57 MHz) and one at $2A_H$ (114 MHz). When the crystal temperature is raised, the ELDOR spectra at A and B still show the presence of $\dot{C}H_2COO^-$ and $NHD_2^+\dot{C}HCOO^-$; however the absolute ESR intensity shows a decrease in these two radicals. With this ELDOR information the ESR spectrum can be calculated and compared to the experimental ESR spectrum. From this it is concluded that the following exchange reactions occur in partially deuterated glycine

$$NHD_2\dot{C}HCOO^- \rightarrow NHD_2^+\dot{C}DCOO^-$$
$$\cdot CH_2COO^- \rightarrow \dot{C}D_2COO^- \text{ (or } \dot{C}DHCOO^-)$$

Further identification of the H/D exchange processes can be carried out by obtaining the frequency positions of the protons in the new radicals. Following this the new radical structure can be calculated by using deuterium hyperfine splittings based on proton splittings deduced by ESR or ENDOR measurements at low temperature.

6.3.4 Tunneling Methyl Groups

The ELDOR applications presented so far have considered only the spectral identification of the allowed ESR lines in a complex overlapped spectrum. It is also possible to use the ELDOR technique to resolve forbidden ESR lines with an ESR intensity of 0.1 to 0.01 that of the allowed ESR lines from an overlapped spectrum. The conditions under which this might be possible are shown in an ELDOR investigation of the methyl group undergoing tunneling rotation in irradiated methylmalonic acid.

The ESR spectrum at low gain of a methyl group in methylmalonic acid undergoing tunneling rotation consists of a seven line pattern with an intensity ratio of $1:1:1:2:1:1:1$ below 40 K as given in the lower part of Fig. 6-39. The weak lines denoted by the arrows are due to radical impurities. At high gains (upper portion of Fig. 6-39) there appear forbidden lines (denoted by a, b, c, and d) associated with the seven line pattern at 8 K that are partially overlapped at a by one of the impurity lines. Numerous articles have been written about methyl groups that undergo tunneling rotation,[53] the essence of which was previously summarized in Section 4.4.4. Thus we will not discuss tunneling rotation in detail again but simply review a few aspects

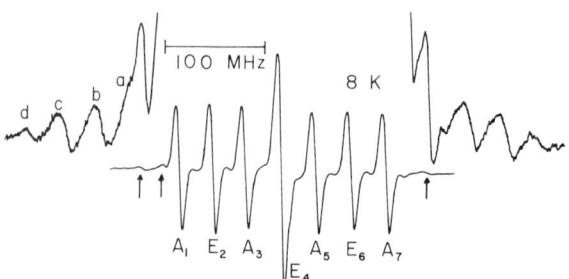

Figure 6-39. The first derivative ESR absorption spectrum at 8 K of irradiated methylmalonic acid crystal with the observing power at ~0.5 μW. The crystal was oriented to give a sharp seven line spectrum. The lines are labeled according to symmetry and line position. The weak sidebands a, b, c, and d are forbidden transitions resulting from tunneling rotation. From C. Mottley, L. Kispert, and S. Clough. *J. Chem. Phys.*, **63**, 4405 (1975).

relevant to the ESR spectrum obtained from $CH_3\dot{C}(COOH)_2$ in methylmalonic acid. At 4 to 30 K a seven line ESR spectrum instead of a four line ESR spectrum arises because the ground vibrational state is split into three levels due to the threefold rotational barrier of the methyl group. One level is a singlet and is described by a spin wavefunction that rotates symmetrically about the C_3 axis of the methyl group. Following group theory conventions this symmetrical level is designated A. The other two levels are degenerate and are described by spin wavefunctions that are unsymmetrical with respect to rotation and are thus designated as E levels. The splitting between the A and E levels in the lowest ground state is referred to as the tunneling splitting (energy units) or the tunneling frequency (frequency units). The lines in Fig. 6-39 labeled A_1, A_3, A_5, and A_7 arise from ESR transitions between energy levels with A symmetry as indicated in Fig. 6-40. Likewise the lines E_2, E_4, and E_6 in Fig. 6-39 arise from ESR transitions between energy levels with E symmetry as shown in Fig. 6-40. If the tunneling splitting is of the order of the hyperfine splitting, then second order terms become important and the forbidden transitions labeled a, b, c, and d in Fig. 6-40 become partially allowed, giving rise to the weak sidebands in Fig. 6-39. These sidebands are symmetrically placed about the center of the main ESR spectrum, and the distance from the center of the ESR spectrum to the center of one of the groups of sidebands corresponds to the tunneling frequency. Experimentally at 10 K the tunneling sideband a (Fig. 6-40) is obscured by a temperature independent impurity peak. The other lines are observed in Fig. 6-39 at 8 K with the gain increased by 100. If the impurity lines had not existed, then the ESR spectrum at high gain on the low field side would appear somewhat like the absorption spectrum

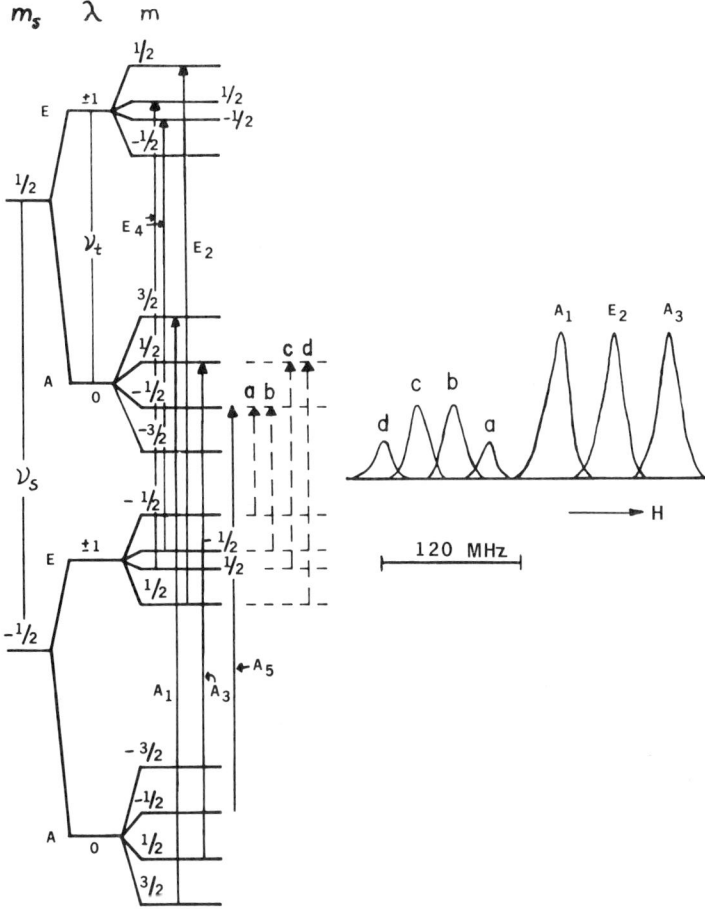

Figure 6-40. The energy level diagram and the low field half of the absorption ESR spectrum for $CH_3\dot{C}(COOH)_2$ in methylmalonic acid at 8 K. The main ESR transitions are labeled A_1, E_2, E_4, A_3 and A_5, giving their symmetry and line position. The sidebands are labeled a, b, c, and d with ν_τ being the tunneling frequency. The intensity of the sidebands in the ESR spectrum is greatly enhanced relative to the main lines for clarity.

shown in Fig. 6-40. At 35 K the sidebands shift toward the center of the ESR spectrum and only d and c are observed because the impurity peaks obscure a and b.

Two features of the tunneling spectrum can be examined by ELDOR techniques:[54] first the assignment of the forbidden lines a, b, c, and d to the transitions given in Fig. 6-40, and second the separation of the tunneling sideband from the impurity line despite the low observing temperature where spin diffusion may predominate.

From the energy level diagram in Fig. 6-40 it can be seen that transition E_2 has a level in common with sideband d and transition A_3 has a level in common with sidebands c and d. Analysis of a three level energy diagram similar to that done in Section 1.5.3.3 shows that ELDOR signals are observed for forbidden-allowed transitions only if W_n processes are nonzero. To verify the assignment of the transitions given in Fig. 6-40 the main ESR lines A_3 and E_2 are both observed while the sideband region is pumped. At low temperatures (<8 K) the A and E energy levels are not mixed as they are when classical rotation is present and only very weak ELDOR signals are observed, indicating that W_n must be small. At 12 K ELDOR reductions in E_2 and A_3 are observed when pumping the sidebands with an energy level in common with the observed transition. This is seen in Fig. 6-41 A and B. At 24 K intense ELDOR spectra are observed for all four sidebands when pumping A_3

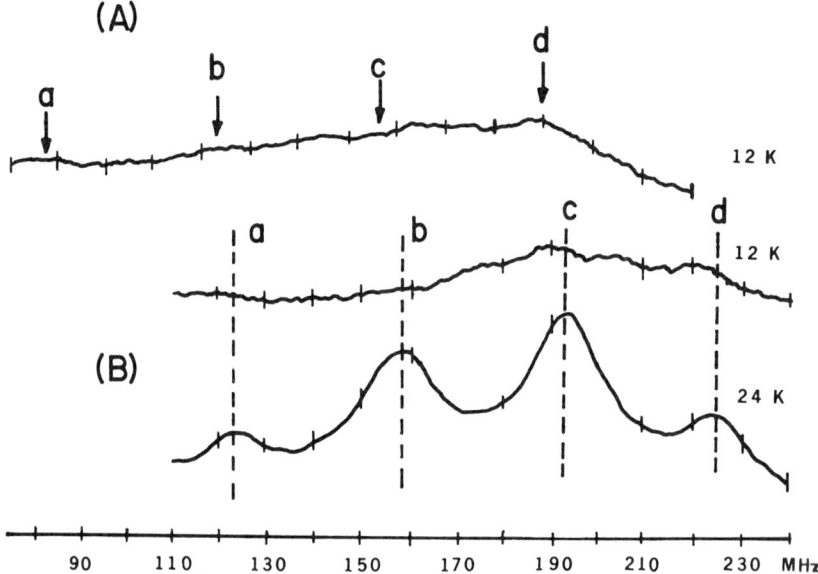

Figure 6-41. The frequency swept ELDOR spectra obtained by setting the observing condition at the bottom of the first derivative absorption ESR peak (A) E_2 and (B) A_3 at 12 K and at 24 K while pumping the low field sideband area. The observing power was 0.5 μW while the pump power was attenuated 5 dB from a 150 mW maximum. The dashed vertical lines represent the sideband positions a, b, c, and d at 17 K. At 12 K the line at 190 MHz (sideband d) in plot A is the most intense of the four lines a, b, c, and d since this line has a level in common with the observed line E_2 whereas lines at 192 and 223 MHz (sidebands c and d) are most intense for (B) because they have a level in common with the A_3 line. Adapted from C. Mottley, L. D. Kispert, and S. Clough, *J. Chem. Phys.*, **63**, 4405 (1975).

(Fig. 6-41B), suggesting that W_n has increased and that there is mixing of the A and E energy levels. It should also be noted that not only have the sidebands been definitely assigned to the given transitions by ELDOR spectra, but also all four sidebands are observed and they have thus been separated from the impurity lines. Therefore to observe forbidden ESR lines overlapped by impurity lines (at least in the case of tunneling methyl groups) a nonzero W_n process and little spin diffusion are required. At temperatures below 15 K, the relaxation processes also result in forbidden-allowed ELDOR lines being observed when the observing condition is set at the allowed ESR lines and the pump frequency scans the remaining allowed ESR lines. However at 24 K where W_n processes are more significant, only allowed-allowed ELDOR transitions are observed as predicted in Section 1.5.2.2. It thus appears possible to resolve weak forbidden ESR lines for other organic radicals, providing that the requirements of a nonzero W_n process and little spin diffusion are met.

6.4 POWDER ELDOR

6.4.1 Determination of Hyperfine Splittings

In Section 4.6 we learned that the ESR intensity I for radicals in powders or frozen glasses at a constant value of the microwave frequency ν and magnetic field H arises from the sum of the resonant ESR patterns of a large number of randomly oriented radicals. In addition, for certain magnetic fields one orientation of the g or hyperfine tensor dominates sufficiently to cause the appearance of a turning point in the ESR spectrum. It is indeed fortunate that certain orientations of the g or hyperfine tensor are dominant, for if the ESR lines were spread uniformly over the magnetic field range determined by the principal g and hyperfine components, it would be difficult to detect any absorption.

Computationally[15] the ESR intensity I can be calculated as a function of magnetic field for the randomly oriented radicals by using eq. 6.29:

$$I(H) = \sum C_{M_1 \cdots M_k \cdots M_n}(H) \qquad (6.29)$$

where

$$C_{M_1 \cdots M_k \cdots M_n}(H) = \int_\theta \int_\phi f_{M_1 \cdots M_k \cdots M_n}(H, \theta, \phi) \sin\theta \, d\theta \, d\phi \qquad (6.30)$$

In eq. 6.29, $C_{M_1 \cdots M_k \cdots M_n}(H)$ is the contribution to the ESR intensity at a magnetic field H from a nuclear spin configuration where there are n nuclei with nuclear quantum numbers $M_1 \cdots M_k \cdots M_n$. Quantitatively $C_{M_1 \cdots M_k \cdots M_n}(H)$ is expressed in eq. 6.30 as an integral of a function f

times the surface element $\sin\theta\, d\theta\, d\phi$. The function f depends on the nuclear quantum numbers, the magnetic field H, and the angles θ and ϕ, which define the orientation of the radicals to the field. The function f is actually a measure of whether a spin configuration with nuclear quantum number $M_1 \cdots M_k \cdots M_n$ has a resonance at a magnetic field H over the surface element $\sin\theta\, d\theta\, d\phi$. For instance, if the field H is set at the high field turning point of Fig. 4-18, f is nonzero only for those nitrogen spin configurations with $M_I = -1$ oriented with the p-orbital parallel to the magnetic field. At other magnetic field settings the ESR intensity results from the sum of spin configurations with different values of θ and ϕ and nuclear quantum numbers. Thus at an observing frequency ν_o, the ESR intensity $I(H)$ will be a function of $M_1 \cdots M_k \cdots M_n$, θ, and ϕ. If a pumping frequency ν_p that is smaller than the observing frequency is set at a portion of the powder spectrum described by the same θ and ϕ and by a set of nuclear quantum numbers $M_1 \cdots (M-1)_k \cdots M_n$, where the kth quantum number has been decreased by one unit, then a change in the ESR intensity will occur at H, giving rise to an ELDOR response.

Quantitatively[15] the component at $I(H)$ will give rise to an ELDOR signal whose intensity is proportional to

$$\int_\theta \int_\phi [f_{M_1 \cdots M_k \cdots M_n}(\nu_o, \theta, \phi)][f_{M_1 \cdots (M-1)_k \cdots M_n}(\nu_p, \theta, \phi)] \sin\theta\, d\theta\, d\phi, \quad (6.31)$$

that is, to the product of the observed and pumped components. This expression assumes that the relaxation processes are angularly independent.

The principles involved in these equations can best be explained by giving an example of an ELDOR study of a frozen solution of DPPH in toluene.[15] In Fig. 6-42 ESR spectra are given for a frozen solution of natural (upper curve) and ^{15}N substituted (lower curve) DPPH. The five line pattern arises from the interaction of an electron with two nearly equivalent nitrogens. The low and high field lines (a) and (e) (generally referred to as turning points; see Section 4.6.1) in the upper curve of Fig. 6-42 arise from configurations denoted by $[(+1, +1)\|]$ and $[(-1, -1)\|]$ where the numbers refer to the nuclear quantum number of the α and β nitrogen in DPPH (see Fig. 5-16 for formula) and the $\|$ sign indicates that the magnetic field is parallel to the p orbital of the two nitrogens and perpendicular to the molecular plane (the two p orbitals are assumed parallel). Alternatively the sign $\perp$ is used to indicate that the field is perpendicular to the p orbitals of the nitrogen. As we indicated in Section 4.6.1 a large nitrogen splitting is associated with the $\|$ direction, whereas a near zero splitting was observed in the $\perp$ direction. The intense central line[6] arises from several configurations, the largest contributor being $[(0, 0)\perp, \|]$ with some contribution arising from $[(\pm 1, 0)\perp]$, $[(0, \pm 1)\perp]$,

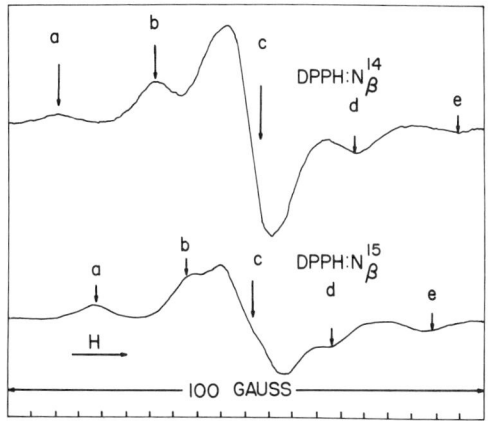

Figure 6-42. The first derivative absorption ESR spectrum of a solid solution of 5×10^{-4} M DPPH in toluene. The upper curve is for natural abundant ^{14}N and the lower is for ^{15}N substituted DPPH. The letters a, b, c, d and e indicate the turning points of the ESR spectrum. From J. S. Hyde, R. C. Sneed, Jr., and G. H. Rist, *J. Chem. Phys.*, **51**, 1404 (1969).

and $[(\pm 1, +1) \perp, \|]$. Turning point d arises from configurations $[(0, -1)\|]$ and $[(-1, 0)\|]$ and turning point b arises from configurations $[(0, +1)\|]$ and $[(+1, 0)\|]$. A similar notation is used for the ^{15}N substituted sample $[(+1, +\frac{1}{2})\|]$, $[(-1, -\frac{1}{2})\|]$ for the low and high field lines a and e; $[\pm(+1, +\frac{1}{2}) \perp]$, $[\pm(0, +\frac{1}{2}) \perp]$, and $[\pm(+1, -\frac{1}{2}) \perp, \|]$ for the center line c; and $[(0, -\frac{1}{2})\|]$ and $[(0, +\frac{1}{2})\|]$ for lines b and d on the high and low field side of the central line.

According to eqs. 6.29 and 6.30 the ELDOR response in a powder is dependent on the molecular orientation angles θ and ϕ. This means that a different ELDOR response will in general be observed for each setting of the observing field. However some settings are worth noting. For instance, since the largest contribution to the center of the spectrum arises from the nuclear spin configuration $[(0, 0)\|, \perp]$ where $M_I = 0$, the function f in eq. 6.30 is independent of θ and ϕ. Thus all radicals in the configuration $(0, 0)$ for all orientations contribute to the central line intensity with equal probability. Therefore it is impossible to select a preferred molecular orientation when the center of this powder spectrum is observed. On the other hand, when a high or low field line is observed, a unique molecular orientation can be studied, in this case a direction parallel to the nitrogen p orbital (a symmetry axis). For the ^{15}N substituted sample the center of the spectrum depends on angle; however the shoulders at $[(0, \pm\frac{1}{2})\|]$ correspond to those radicals where the p-orbital of the β nitrogen is oriented parallel to the field.

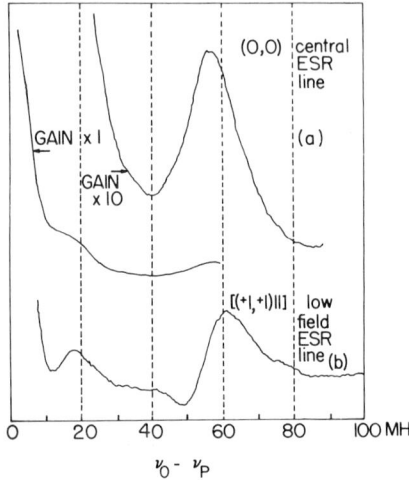

Figure 6-43. The frequency swept ELDOR spectra of DPPH in solid solutions of toluene for $\nu_p < \nu_o$. Spectrum (a) is obtained at 153 K with the observing resonant condition set on the crossover of the center $(0, 0)$ (position c in Fig. 6-42) line while spectrum (b) was obtained at 123 K while observing the peak of the low field turning point. (position a in Fig. 6-42). From J. S. Hyde, R. C. Sneed, Jr., and G. H. Rist, J. Chem. Phys., **51**, 1404 (1969).

When the observing field is set at the central line $(0, 0)$ of a frozen solution of natural DPPH and the pumping frequency is swept, then according to eq. 6.31, a buildup of ELDOR intensity occurs at those frequencies where $\nu_p - \nu_o$ corresponds to the principal frequency of the hyperfine tensor components of the α or β nitrogens. An example of such a situation is given in Fig. 6-43 where a single broad ELDOR line at 56.5 MHz occurs as a result of contributions from both $[(-1, 0) \|\,]$ and $[(0, -1) \|\,]$. Since the central line of a frozen solution of natural DPPH is not dependent on selected orientations, it is concluded that 56.5 MHz is the average of the anisotropic α and β nitrogen hyperfine tensors for the parallel direction, that is, $\frac{1}{2}(|A+2B|_\alpha + |A+2B|_\beta) = 56.5$. When the observing field is set on the low field ESR line a, $[(+1, +1) \|\,]$, the ELDOR intensity is given by eq. 6.31 to be proportional to

$$f_{(+1,\,+1)}(\nu_o, H \parallel \text{symmetry axis}) \times [f_{(0,\,+1)}(\nu_p, H \parallel \text{symmetry axis})$$
$$+ f_{(+1,\,0)}(\nu_p, H \parallel \text{symmetry axis})]. \quad (6.32)$$

The contributions from other spin configurations are neglected.

An ELDOR spectrum obtained under these conditions is given in Fig. 6-43b where a buildup of intensity at 56 MHz is also observed. This can only occur at the same frequency as observed in Fig. 6-43a if the symmetry axes (the direction of the p orbitals) for both the α and β nitrogens are parallel as had been assumed. If indeed the two axes were not parallel the low field line would have corresponded to an intermediate angle between the two axes and the ELDOR line would have depended on θ and ϕ.

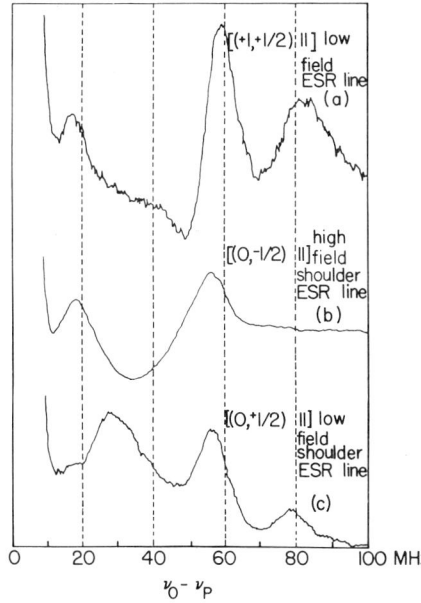

Figure 6-44. The frequency swept ELDOR spectra of ^{15}N substituted DPPH in solid solutions of toluene at 153 K with the bracketed notation indicating the observing points in the ESR spectrum. From J. S. Hyde, R. C. Sneed, Jr., and G. H. Rist, *J. Chem. Phys.*, **51**, 1404 (1969).

Because the ELDOR lines are quite broad, the different α and β nitrogen hyperfine splittings are not resolvable by ELDOR in a frozen natural sample of DPPH. However they are resolved in a $^{15}N_\beta$ substituted sample of DPPH. By setting the observing position on line b $[0, +\frac{1}{2}\|]$ in Fig. 6-42b and scanning the pump frequency to smaller frequencies, the ELDOR spectrum given in the lower part of Fig. 6-44 is observed. It results from separate nuclear spin-flips by the α and β nitrogens. The intensity of the ELDOR lines is given as

$$f_{(0, +\frac{1}{2})}(\nu_o, H \| \beta \text{ axis})[f_{(0, -\frac{1}{2})}(\nu_p, H \| \beta \text{ axis}) + f_{(-1, +\frac{1}{2})}$$

$$(\nu_p, H \text{ projected on } \beta \text{ axis})]. \quad (6.33)$$

The spectrum in Fig. 6-44 shows a peak at 79 MHz, which is assigned to the anisotropic coupling $|A+2B|$ of the $^{15}N_\beta$ nuclei in the parallel direction, and a peak at 56.6 MHz, which is assigned to the α nitrogen. This assignment can be made by noting that the ELDOR spectrum observed at $[(0, -\frac{1}{2})\|]$ contains a peak at 56 MHz but none at 79 MHz because only a transition from the $M_I = -1$ component of an α nitrogen is possible (there being no M_I component of the β nitrogen at high field transitions scanned by the pump transitions). On the other hand, both the ELDOR peaks at 56 and 79 MHz appear when the observing position is set at $[(+1, +\frac{1}{2})\|]$. The 79 MHz value for the ^{15}N nuclei translates into a value of 56.4 MHz for the ^{14}N nuclei at the β position. Thus it appears that the nitrogen splittings are equal to within the resolution here.

The shape of the lines is changed by small changes in the observing resonant condition. Theoretically the angle between the symmetry axes can be determined by this type of experiment. However experiments have so far only been performed by selecting an observing position that gives the most symmetrical lines. Certain features of the ELDOR spectra given in Figs. 6-43 and 6-44 are not understood. For instance, the ^{15}N ELDOR lines are always weaker than the ^{14}N lines. This could be due to the quadrupole moment of ^{14}N, which contributes to the nuclear relaxation, or to both the pump and the observing sources being on the resonance lines of ^{15}N, whereas for ^{14}N either the pump or the observing source will be on the angularly independent $M = 0$ lines. Some additional lines are observed. One occurs at 14 MHz that appears to be a forbidden-allowed transition from the protons on the DPPH radical. This is not due to the solvent (see Section 1.5.2.2), but possibly occurs at transitions equal to $\nu_H \pm A/2$ where A is quite small. Another transition appears at 28 MHz (Fig. 6-44c) that possibly is due to a $(+1, +1)$ configuration at intermediate angles.

Comparison of the ELDOR spectra to the frozen solution ESR spectra shows that the single splitting obtained from ELDOR is the same as that obtained from ESR; hence there is no improvement in resolution. However the origins of some forbidden lines and the asymmetry of the ELDOR lines suggest that an exact computer analysis of the powder spectra will enable a determination to be made of the principal direction of the hyperfine tensors of each nitrogen.

6.4.2 Spin Diffusion

When more than one radical exists in an organic glass or a powder, the ESR spectra of the two or more radicals overlap, resulting in magnetic energy transfer between the two radicals. The spin diffusion time and an estimate of the spatial distribution of the two radicals can be deduced according to the procedures outlined in an ELDOR study at 77 K of a trapped electron and a MTHF radical in γ-irradiated 2-methyl-tetrahydrofuran (MTHF) glass.[9] These same procedures are also applicable to single crystals.

The experiment is to pump a MTHF radical line not overlapping with the electron line and to observe the effect on the electron line. Saturation of the electron line is observed. The cross saturation or spin diffusion mechanism between two paramagnetic centers is consistent with dipolar

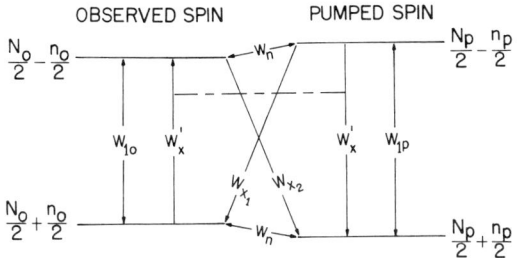

Figure 6-45. Energy levels of two two-level spin systems showing the relaxation probabilities W_n, W_{x1}, W_{x2}, W'_x, W_{1o}, and W_{1p} and the level populations in terms of N, the total number of spins in one system, and n, the excess number of spins in the lower Zeeman level. W'_x is a cross-relaxation probability in which a p electron spin is flipped down and an o electron spin is flipped up. Adapted from H. Yoshida, D. F. Feng, and L. Kevan, *J. Chem. Phys.*, **58**, 4924 (1973).

cross relaxation in which a MTHF radical spin flips down and a trapped electron spin flips up. The relaxation mechanisms for the transfer of spins from the MTHF radical that is pumped to the trapped electron that is observed are given in Fig. 6-45. The observed spin of the trapped electron is represented by a two level energy diagram with populations in terms of N, the total number of trapped electron spins, and n, the excess number of spins in the lower level. Likewise the spins pumped in the MTHF radical are represented by another two level energy diagram. The two two-level spin systems are connected by a cross-relaxation probability W'_x in which a pumped electron spin is flipped down and an observed electron spin is flipped up. Note that this same effect could be considered within a single spin system describable by a four level energy diagram consisting of W_n (nuclear spin relaxation) W_{x1} and W_{x2} (cross relaxation) relaxation probabilities.

Analysis of the relaxation processes shows[9] that the field swept ELDOR reduction factors are related to the relaxation times T_{po} (the spin diffusion time between the pumped (p) and the observed (o) spins), T_{1o} and T_{1p} (the spin-lattice relaxation times of the observed spins and the pumped spins, respectively), and W_{sp} the pump power by eq. 6.34:

$$R^{-1} = 1 + \frac{2T_{po}}{T_{1o}} + (2W_{sp}T_{1p})^{-1}\left(1 + \frac{2T_{po}}{T_{1o}} + \frac{T_{po}T_{1p}}{T_{1o}T_{op}}\right) \quad (6.34)$$

Thus a plot of R^{-1} for the observed spin versus (pump power)$^{-1}$ is predicted to be linear with an intercept of $1 + (2T_{po}/T_{1o})$. Such a plot is given in Fig. 6-46 for the trapped electron and radical in MTHF glass irradiated at 77 K when the difference between the pumped and observed microwave frequencies equals 58 MHz (◐) and 109 MHz (○) at 73.1 K

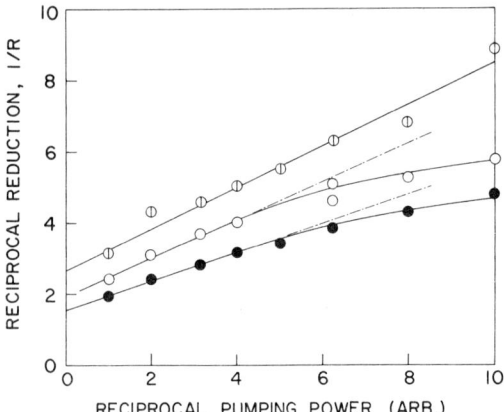

Figure 6-46. The field swept ELDOR saturation curves of the trapped electron in MTHF glass irradiated to 2.6 Mrad at 77 K and measured at 73.1 ± 0.5 K for (◐) $\Delta f = 58$ MHz and (○) $\Delta f = 109$ MHz, and at 58 K for (●) $\Delta f = 58$ MHz. From H. Yoshida, D. F. Feng, and L. Kevan, *J. Chem. Phys.*, **58**, 4924 (1973).

and 58 MHz at 58 K (●). The ratio of the cross-relaxation time to the spin-lattice time for the detected spins equals 0.5 at 73 K ($\Delta f = 58$ MHz), 0.8 at 73 K ($\Delta f = 109$ MHz), 0.3 at 58 K ($\Delta f = 58$ MHz). If the spin-lattice relaxation time for the observed spins is known independently, then numerical values of the cross-relaxation times can be obtained. Since the T_{po}/T_{1o} ratios are of the order of 1, the cross relaxation is significant for trapped electrons and radicals in MTHF. Because the energy transfer is efficient, it is assumed that the spatial distributions of the two spin systems are correlated.

6.5 Triplet States ($S = 1$)

So far all discussions of ELDOR studies have been confined to systems that contain only one unpaired electron. A free radical system that contains two unpaired electrons has $S = 1$ and is a triplet state. Assuming that the system contains only weakly coupled nuclei, one possible energy level diagram is given in Fig. 6-47. It is possible to measure a collision frequency of triplet-triplet collisions in crystals by analyzing the ESR line broadening with increasing temperature.[16,17] ELDOR studies of the same system yield the spin exchange frequency resulting from the triplet-triplet collisions.[16-19] An advantage of the ELDOR measurement is that lower frequency processes can be detected by ELDOR than by ESR methods. This is because the exchange frequency measured by ELDOR must be

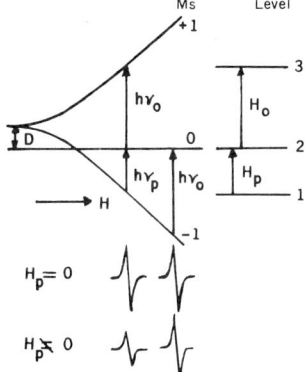

Figure 6-47. The triplet state energy diagram as a function of magnetic field with the $-1 \rightarrow 0$ transition being pumped while the $0 \rightarrow 1$ transition is observed. Adapted from V. A. Benderskii, L. A. Blumenfeld, P. A. Stunzas, and E. A. Sojolov, *Nature*, **220**, 365 (1968).

compared with $1/T_{1e}$ and not with $1/T_{2e}$ as for ESR. In solids T_{1e} is generally larger than T_{2e}. A brief summary of the work by Benderskii and his colleagues[16,19] is given below as an example of the chemical information that can be obtained from triplet state ELDOR studies.

6.5.1 Excitons in Crystals

Below 250 K the ESR spectrum of triplet excitons in crystals of tetracyanquinodimethane salt (TCNQ) containing a benzthiocarbocyanine dye contains two lines between 3000 and 3500 G. The splitting (A) between the two lines varies from 0 to 140 G for different crystal orientations.[16] These two lines arise from microwave transitions between levels 0 and 1 and levels -1 and 0 shown in Fig. 6-47.

An interesting dependence on temperature occurs for the ESR intensity when the $0 \rightarrow 1$ transition is observed and the $-1 \rightarrow 0$ transition is pumped in an ELDOR experiment. An enhancement of the observed ESR line $0 \rightarrow 1$ intensity is seen below 160 K, and a reduction is seen above 160 K that increases with temperature until a maximum is observed dependent on the hyperfine splitting A.

If a reduction factor is determined for the three level diagram in Fig. 6-47 in which the $0 \rightarrow 1$ transition is observed and the $-1 \rightarrow 0$ transition is pumped, then

$$R = -\frac{T_{23}}{T_{13}}\left(\frac{T_{13} + T_{23}}{T_{13}}\right)^{-1} \qquad (6.35)$$

where the spin-lattice relaxation time T_{13} exists between levels -1 and $+1$ and T_{23} between levels 0 and $+1$.

However eq. 6.35 predicts enhanced ELDOR spectra (i.e., negative R) over the entire temperature range. Additional relaxations therefore must be included. Experimentally the ESR doublet components broaden with increasing temperature because of the spin exchange of the electrons that make up the triplet state. The spin exchange is characterized by a collision frequency ω_c that is dependent on the exchange integral J, the correlation time τ_e, the concentration of triplet excitons N_T, the diffusion constant D_T, and the collision diameter a_T through the relation[17]

$$\omega_c = 8\pi D_T N_T a_T \frac{4J^2\tau_e^2}{1+4J^2\tau_e^2}. \tag{6.36}$$

If the relaxation proceeds via the spin exchange

$$^3T_o + {}^3T_o \rightleftarrows {}^3T_{+1} + {}^3T_{-1} \tag{6.37}$$

(two electrons in the 0 state exchange to produce one electron in the $+1$ state and another in the -1 state) we can characterize this by ω_e, the frequency of double spin transitions from level 0 to the other two levels. This has the tendency to equalize the populations in all levels. In this case analysis of the three level diagram leads to

$$R_\infty = \frac{b''-b}{1+b''+b} \tag{6.38}$$

where $b'' = \omega_e T_{23}$ and $b = \dfrac{T_{23}}{T_{13}}$

Since experimentally the pump power can never be infinite yet the reduction factors should be measured at infinite pump power, the observed reduction R is defined as

$$R = R_\infty (1-Z) \tag{6.39}$$

where Z is the saturation factor for the pumped transition ($-1 \to 0$) and R_∞ is the reduction factor at infinite pump powers. Z can be calculated from eq. 6.39 by knowing the experimental values of R and R_∞. $Z=1$ and 0 when no pump power and infinite pump power is applied, respectively. Experimentally this can be determined by obtaining R from the relationship $R = (1 - I/I_o)$, where I and I_o have been defined in Section 5.2 at the maximum available power used, and by obtaining R_∞ according to the methods described in Section 5.2.2.

A plot of the resulting saturation factor Z and R_∞ as a function of temperature for the hyperfine splittings $A = 75$ and 140 G is given in Fig. 6-48. Theoretically the observed variation of R_∞ with temperature can be explained as follows. At temperatures below 160 K $b > b''$, so R_∞ is negative, and thus enhanced ELDOR spectra are observed. Qualitatively

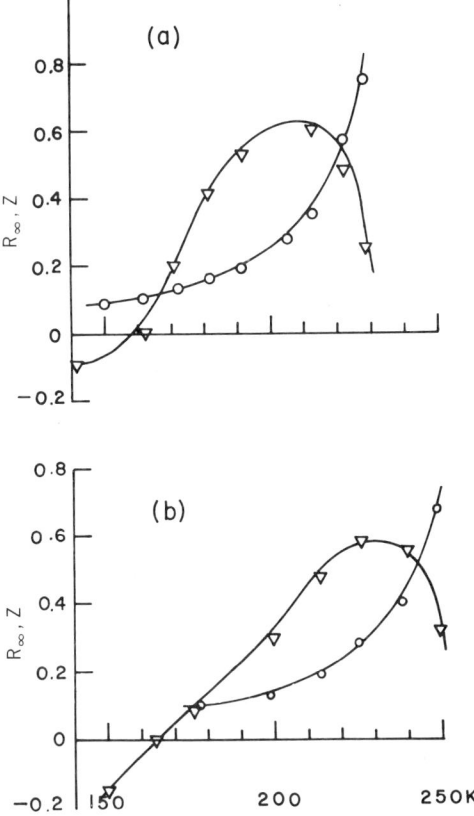

Figure 6-48. The temperature dependence of the ELDOR intensity $R(\triangledown)$ and the saturation factor $Z(0)$ for a splitting of (a) 75 G and (b) 140 G for the triplet excitons in crystals of tetracyanquinodimethane salt (TCNQ) containing a benzthiocarbocyanine dye. Adapted from V. A. Benderskii, L. A. Blumenfeld, P. A. Stunzas, and E. A. Sojolov, *Nature*, **220**, 365 (1968).

this means that saturation of the pumped transition $-1 \to 0$ increases the population of level 0 and thus the population difference between levels 0 and 1 is also increased. This is exactly what eq. 6.38 predicts in the absence of exchange (i.e., $b'' = 0$). However as the temperature is raised, ω_e increases, so that $b'' = \omega_e T_{23} > b = T_{23}/T_{13}$; then R becomes positive and an ELDOR reduction is observed. Physically the increase in $\omega_e T_{23}$ with temperature tends to equalize the populations of all levels. As the temperature is raised above 200 K, the R factor reaches a maximum and then decreases with further increase in temperature. This decrease is a direct consequence of the increasing saturation factor of the pumped transition ($-1\rightarrow 0$) at higher temperature. In other words, it becomes more and more difficult to saturate the pump transition (shorter spin-lattice relaxation time).

Note that Fig. 6-48 shows that the spin-lattice relaxation time of the pump transition is dependent on the hyperfine splitting. At a given temperature the larger A is associated with a longer relaxation time. It is assumed that this behavior is due to the occurrence of cross-relaxation processes between triplet excitons and local paramagnetic centers and that this process is more efficient than spin-lattice relaxation. The collision frequencies ω_c obtained from the analysis of the ESR lines broadening are found to be isotropic and larger by a factor of 10 than those (ω_e) obtained by ELDOR measurements. The exchange frequency ω_e obtained from ELDOR measurements is anisotropic and appears to be a measure of the efficiency with which collisional processes lead to double spin transitions. At small splittings almost all collisions lead to double spin transitions, whereas at larger splittings, the number of successful collisions decreases.

It is also possible to detect[17] the appearance of a line at $A/2$ by ELDOR in exciton systems. When $\omega_c \ll A$, the triplet state ESR spectrum consists of two lines separated by A centered about a weak absorption of relative intensity $4(\omega_c/A)^2$. This feature is clearly seen in the ELDOR spectrum as a small asymmetry in the ELDOR line. The line at $A/2$ is difficult to see in the ESR spectrum because the lifetime of the intermediate state which results in a line at $A/2$ is small compared to T_{1e}. Typically the ratio of the ELDOR to the ESR intensity of the line at $A/2$ is equal to or greater than 10. This ratio increases with increasing pump power as $1/Z$. Therefore these results imply that the triplet-triplet collisions can be detected at lower frequencies and thus lower temperatures by ELDOR than by ESR.

6.5.2 Optical Detection in Polycrystalline Matrices

The ability to detect triplet state ELDOR spectra is not limited to an ELDOR spectrometer that makes use of a bimodal microwave cavity such as that described in Chapter 2. It is also possible to carry out triplet state ELDOR experiments by using two concentric microwave helices.[55,56] Such an experimental setup has been used to optically detect triplet state ELDOR of phosphorescent molecules such as pyrimidine[55] and tetrachlorobenzene[56] at zero field. Optical detection of ELDOR can be used where optical detection of ESR fails for observing transitions at zero magnetic field that have equal populations or are nonradiative at low temperature.

At very low temperature where spin-lattice relaxation processes are very slow only two of the three zero field transitions ($-1 \to +1$ and $0 \to +1$) can be optically detected by monitoring the phosphorescence. The detection of the third transition depends on the average spin-lattice relaxation processes between the three levels. This third level can be detected if either the $-1 \to +1$ or the $0 \to +1$ transition in Fig. 6-47 is saturated by a resonant microwave radiation. If now a second microwave frequency is applied to the transition $-1 \to 0$, a change in population gives rise to change in the phosphorescence intensity. In this way the third transition is determined. ELDOR detection has also been useful[55] in detecting resonances in those cases where two zero field transitions have equal population and no resonance can normally be detected. This is accomplished by destroying the population equality of the two levels by saturating the appropriate transition. Further uses have also been found,[55] such as determining the rate constants of the spin-lattice relaxation processes between the zero field levels, determining population changes that cannot be detected or accomplished by use of conventional optical means, and eliminating inhomogeneous broadening in phosphorescent microwave double resonant spectroscopy.[56]

REFERENCES

1. L. D. Kispert, K. Chang, and C. M. Bogan, *J. Chem. Phys.*, **58,** 2164 (1973).
2. L. Kispert and K. Chang, *J. Magn. Resonance* **10,** 162 (1973).
3. L. D. Kispert, K. Chang, and C. M. Bogan, *J. Phys. Chem.*, **77,** 629 (1973).
4. L. D. Kispert and P. S. Wang, *J. Phys. Chem.*, **78,** 1839 (1974).
5. T. N. Margulis, L. R. Dalton, and A. L. Kwiram, *Nature* (Phy. Sci.), **242,** 82 (1973).
6. L. D. Kispert, K. Chang, and C. M. Bogan, *Chem. Phys. Lett.*, **17,** 592 (1972).
7. L. D. Kispert and M. T. Rogers, *J. Chem. Phys.*, **58,** 2065 (1973).
8. M. Iwasaki, K. Toriyama, and K. Nunome, *J. Chem. Phys.*, **61,** 106 (1974).
9. H. Yoshida, D. F. Feng, and L. Kevan, *J. Chem. Phys.*, **58,** 4924 (1973); *J. Amer. Chem. Soc.*, **94,** 8922 (1972).
10. H. Yoshida, D. F. Feng, and L. Kevan, *J. Chem. Phys.*, **58,** 3411 (1973).
11. L. D. Kispert and C. Mottley, unpublished results.
12. B. H. Robinson, J. L. Monge, L. A. Dalton, and L. R. Dalton, *Chem. Phys. Lett.*, **28,** 169 (1974); L. A. Dalton, J. L. Monge, and L. R. Dalton, *Chem. Phys.*, **6,** 166 (1974); P. W. Percival, J. S. Hyde, L. A. Dalton, and L. R. Dalton, *J. Chem. Phys.*, **62,** 4332 (1975).
13. L. D. Kispert, K. Chang, and P. S. Wang, *J. Magn. Resonance*, **14,** 339 (1974).

14. C. Mottley, K. Chang, and L. Kispert, *J. Magn. Resonance*, **19**, 130 (1975).
15. J. S. Hyde, R. C. Sneed, Jr., and G. H. Rist, *J. Chem. Phys.*, **51**, 1404 (1969).
16. V. A. Benderskii, L. A. Blumenfeld, P. A. Stunzas, and E. A. Sokolov, *Nature*, **220**, 365 (1968).
17. P. A. Stunzhas, V. A. Benderskii, L. A. Blumenfeld, and E. A. Sokolov, *Opt. Spektrosk.*, **28**, 278 (1970) [English Transl.: *Opt. Spectrosc.*, **28**, 150 (1970)].
18. P. A. Stunzhas, V. A. Benderskii, and E. A. Sokolov, *Opt. Spektrosk.*, **28**, 487 (1970) [English transl.: *Opt. Spectrosc.*, **28**, 261 (1970)].
19. P. A. Stunzhas, V. A. Benderskii, *Opt. Spektrosk.*, **30**, 1041 (1971) [English transl.: *Opt. Spectrosc.*, **30**, 559 (1971)].
20. J. E. Wertz and J. R. Bolton, *Electron Spin Resonance*, McGraw-Hill, New York, 1972.
21. A. Carrington and A. D. McLachlan, *Introduction to Magnetic Resonance*, Harper & Row, New York, 1967, p. 99.
22. H. C. Box and H. G. Freund, *J. Chem. Phys.*, **44**, 2345 (1966).
23. J. W. Wells and H. C. Box, *J. Chem. Phys.*, **46**, 2935 (1967).
24. K. Itoh and I. Miyagawa, *J. Chem. Phys.*, **40**, 3328 (1964).
25. K. Itoh, I. Miyagawa, and C. S. Chen, *J. Chem. Phys.*, **52**, 1822 (1970), and references cited therein.
26. J. S. Hyde, L. D. Kispert, R. C. Sneed, and J. C. W. Chien, *J. Chem. Phys.*, **48**, 3824 (1968).
27. A. Horsfield., J. R. Morton, and D. H. Whiffen, *Mol. Phys.*, **4**, 327 (1961).
28. J. R. Morton, *J. Amer. Chem. Soc.*, **86**, 2325 (1964).
29. R. F. Weiner and W. S. Koski, *J. Amer. Chem. Soc.*, **85**, 873 (1963); H. C. Box, H. G. Freund, and E. E. Budzinski, *J. Amer. Chem. Soc.*, **88**, 658 (1966).
30. M. Fujimoto and J. Janecka, *J. Chem. Phys.*, **55**, 5 (1971).
31. M. T. Rogers and L. D. Kispert, *Adv. Chem. Ser.*, **82**, 327 (1968).
32. W. M. Tolles, L. P. Crawford, and J. L. Valenti, *J. Chem. Phys.*, **49**, 4745 (1968).
33. H. Ohigashi and Y. Kurita, *Bull. Chem. Soc. Japan.*, **41**, 275 (1968).
34. R. G. Hayes, D. J. Steible, W. M. Tolles, and J. W. Hunt, *J. Chem. Phys.*, **53**, 4466 (1970).
35. J. H. Freed, *J. Chem. Phys.*, **43**, 2312 (1965).
36. J. S. Hyde, J. C. W. Chien, and J. H. Freed, *J. Chem. Phys.*, **48**, 4211 (1968).
37. W. T. Huntress Jr., in *Adv. in Magn. Resonance*, **4**, 1 (1965).
38. C. P. Poole Jr., and H. A. Farach, *Relaxation in Magnetic Resonance*, Academic Press, New York, 1971, p. 75.
39. J. H. Freed, *J. Chem. Phys.*, **41**, 2077 (1964), and references therein.
40. J. H. Freed, in *Electron Spin Relaxation in Liquids*, L. T. Muus and P. W. Atkins, eds., Plenum Press, New York, 1972, p. 165.
41. G. T. Trammell, H. Zeldes, and R. Livingston, *Phys. Rev.*, **110**, 630 (1958).
42. L. D. Kispert and K. Chang, unpublished results.
43. G. Rius and A. Herve, *Solid State Commun.*, **15**, 421 (1974).
44. M. Nechtschein and J. S. Hyde, *Phys. Rev. Lett.*, **24**, 672 (1970).
45. P. P. Sorokin, G. J. Lasher, and I. J. Gelles, *Phys. Rev.*, **118**, 939 (1960).

46. W. P. Unruh and J. W. Culvahouse, *Phys. Rev.*, **129,** 2441 (1963).
47. K. D. Bowers and W. B. Mims, *Phys. Rev.*, **115,** 285 (1959).
48. A. Horsfield, J. R. Morton, and D. H. Whiffen, *Mol. Phys.*, **5,** 115 (1962).
49. A. Carrington and A. D. McLachlan, *Introduction to Magnetic Resonance*, Harper & Row, New York 1967, Chapter 12. For more detail see C. S. Johnson, Jr., *Adv. Magn. Resonance*, **1,** 33 (1965).
50. M. A. Collins and D. H. Whiffen, *Mol. Phys.*, **10,** 317 (1966).
51. I. Miyagawa, personal communication.
52. K. Chang and L. D. Kispert, unpublished results.
53. For example, W. L. Gamble, I. Miyagawa, and R. L. Hartman, *Phys. Rev. Lett.*, **20,** 415 (1968); P. S. Allen and S. Clough, *Phys. Rev. Lett.*, **22,** 1351 (1969); S. Clough. *J. Phys. C.: Solid State Phys.*, **180,** (1971); F. Apaydin and S. Clough, *J. Phys. C.: Solid State Phys.*, **1,** 932 (1968); C. Mottley, T. B. Cobb, and C. S. Johnson, Jr., *J. Chem. Phys.*, **55,** 5823 (1971); R. Ikeda and C. A. McDowell, *Mol. Phys.*, **25,** 1217 (1973); S. Clough, M. Starr, and N. D. McMillan, *Phys. Rev. Lett.*, **25,** 839 (1974); P. S. Allen, *J. Phys. C.: Solid State Phys.*, **7,** L22 (1974); S. Clough and J. R. Hill, *J. Phys. C.: Solid State Phys.*, **7,** L20 (1974), and references cited therein.
54. C. Mottley, L. Kispert, and S. Clough, *J. Chem. Phys.*, **63,** 4405 (1975).
55. T. S. Kuan, D. S. Tinti, and M. A. El-Sayed, *Chem Phys. Lett.*, **4,** 507 (1970).
56. M. Leung and M. A. El-Sayed, *Chem Phys. Lett.*, **16,** 454 (1972).

7. Biochemical Applications

7.1 Biochemical Applications of ENDOR
    7.1.1 Flavoproteins
    7.1.2 Copper Proteins—Stellacyanin
    7.1.3 Metmyoglobin
    7.1.4 Bacteriochlorophyll
    7.1.5 Iron-Sulfur Proteins
    7.1.6 Vitamin Quinones
    7.1.7 Prognosis
7.2 Biochemical Applications of ELDOR
    7.2.1 Nitroxide Spin-Labeled Biomolecules
    7.2.2 Xanthine Oxidase
    References

7.1 BIOCHEMICAL APPLICATIONS OF ENDOR

ENDOR has found considerable applicability in the study of biochemical systems since 1968, but the significance of ENDOR in this area has only barely been tapped. In this chapter we define biochemical systems as those of direct biological significance with greatest emphasis on proteins. A number of single crystal studies of radicals produced in irradiated amino acids and related biochemical compounds have been carried out and were discussed in Chapter 4. As shown in Chapter 4 single crystal analysis certainly gives the most complete information about a radical, and two early ENDOR attempts dealt with single crystals of copper phthalocyanine[1] and metmyoglobin.[2] Although ENDOR signals were seen from both of these biochemical systems they were not analyzed in any detail and did not give significantly more information than was obtainable from the ESR spectrum. Indeed all the significant ENDOR studies of biochemical systems have been carried out on frozen solutions rather than on single crystals. In most cases it is simply not feasible to obtain single crystals of the proteins and other such biological systems of current importance. So the development of high power ENDOR instrumentation and the emergence of methods to look at disordered systems by ENDOR (see Section 4.6) were required to make the effective application of ENDOR to a number of biological problems feasible.

The several types of protein systems that have been successfully studied by ENDOR will be discussed in this chapter, but first we will indicate the types of information that might be available from incisive ENDOR studies. First, the matrix ENDOR line, generally from protons, will usually be observed in frozen solutions or in powders. This matrix line allows one to assess the role of water at the radical site. If the matrix line persists when the sample is exchanged with D_2O, then one may conclude that the radical site is a hydrophobic environment and probably embedded in the protein in some fashion. Of course in such an analysis one must also take into account the types of protons that might be exchangable in the particular system being studied.

Second, some hyperfine structure is often seen by ENDOR, even in disordered systems, which may give information about the identification of the radical site in the particular biological system being studied. In general, one expects to see both proton and nitrogen ENDOR in many protein systems. However, in practice, proton ENDOR is generally seen and nitrogen ENDOR is rather seldom seen. If both proton and nitrogen ENDOR lines are seen, they may be distinguished by recording the ENDOR spectra at two slightly different microwave frequencies by using different cavity modes. The proton ENDOR signals are generally found centered at the free proton frequency and split by their hyperfine coupling. If the resonant microwave frequency and consequently the magnetic field is changed by a slight amount, the proton ENDOR lines will shift accordingly. However nitrogen ENDOR lines typically occur at one-half the nitrogen hyperfine constant separated by twice the free nitrogen nuclear frequency because the free nitrogen nuclear frequency is typically less than the nitrogen hyperfine coupling. Thus a change in the magnetic field will not shift the nitrogen ENDOR lines. This distinction serves as a very useful way of distinguishing between proton and nitrogen ENDOR lines in protein systems.[3] Of the proton ENDOR lines the most prominent ones in disordered solids are usually those from rotating methyl groups because of the low anisotropy of the protons in these groups. Thus methyl group coupling constants can often be discerned and assigned to particular locations with respect to the radical site.[4] In the particular case of bacteriochlorophyll the ENDOR signals from rotating methyl groups demonstrated that the *in vivo* bacteriochlorophyll cation was a dimeric species with about half the coupling constants found from monomeric bacteriochlorophyll cation produced *in vitro*.[5]

In some cases it is also possible to determine a hyperfine tensor if the ESR spectrum shows considerable g anisotropy. In this case one can do ENDOR at the $g_\parallel$ position and look only at the molecules with their symmetry axes parallel to the magnetic field and consequently obtain the parallel component of hyperfine splittings. Similarly one can observe ENDOR at the $g_\perp$ position of the ESR spectrum and obtain the perpendicular component of the hyperfine interaction. Of course this assumes that the principal axes of the g and hyperfine tensors are the same, but in many cases this turns out to be true or nearly so.[6]

We now examine several different biological systems about which considerable information has been obtained by ENDOR.

7.1.1 Flavoproteins

Nicotinamide adenine dinucleotide phosphate (NADPH) dehydrogenase is a protein enzyme with a molecular weight of about 104,000 containing two flavin mononucleotides (FMN) per molecule of the dehydrogenase and containing no metal ions. In its biological action this flavoprotein undergoes reduction and it is thought that the site of the radical is the flavin mononucleotide in the flavoprotein. Thus this system is ideal for model system studies by looking at the ENDOR spectra of flavoproteins. A comprehensive study of this type was carried out by Eriksson et al.[4] that did allow assignment of the ENDOR lines of the reduced NADPH dehydrogenase. Some of the flavin molecules studied and the associated radical anions and cations formed are shown in Fig. 7-1. The radical anion is formed by electron addition to a neutral flavin and the radical cation is formed by effective H_2^+ addition to a neutral flavin so both the anion and cation are reduced forms of flavin molecules. However these two forms have a somewhat different spin density distribution. Under some conditions a neutral flavin radical is formed by hydrogen addition to N-1; this is similar to the cation radical and has a similar spin density distribution. In addition, radical chelates with zinc or cadmium coordinating between nitrogen 5 and the oxygen bonded to C-4 seem to have about the same spin density distribution as the flavin anion radical. The ENDOR spectrum of the lumiflavin radical zinc chelate in dimethylfor-

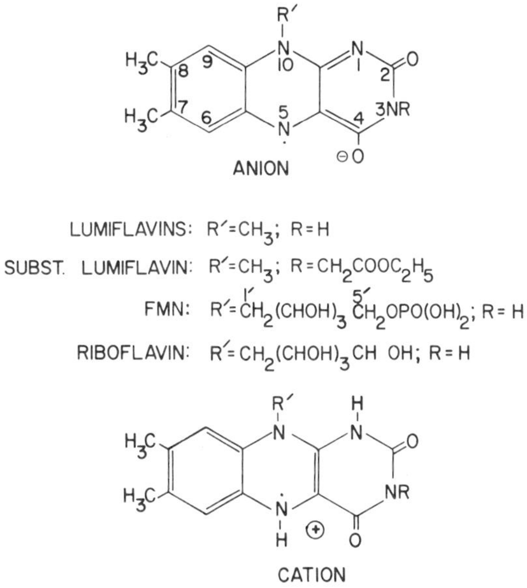

Figure 7-1. Structures of the anionic radical (semiquinoid) and cationic radical forms of various flavins. FMN means flavin mononucleotide. The numbers inside the rings and above the FMN formula denote the ring and side chain numbering system used.

LUMIFLAVINS: $R' = CH_3$; $R = H$
SUBST. LUMIFLAVIN: $R' = CH_3$; $R = CH_2COOC_2H_5$
FMN: $R' = CH_2(CHOH)_3 CH_2OPO(OH)_2$; $R = H$
RIBOFLAVIN: $R' = CH_2(CHOH)_3 CH OH$; $R = H$

mamide at 113 K is shown in Fig. 7-2. One might expect that the prominent ENDOR line between 19 and 20 MHz is due to rotating methyl groups. This is confirmed by substituting a CD_3 and/or Cl for the methyl groups at various positions in the flavin radical as shown in Fig. 7-3. Figure 7-3A compared to Fig. 7-3B shows that the C-8 CH_3 is responsible for the large ENDOR signal near 19 MHz and that the N-10 CH_3 is responsible for a weak ENDOR signal near 18 MHz. Figure 7-3C indicates a weak signal near 18.7 MHz that is assigned to the C-6 H based on calculated spin density distributions. Figure 7-3D is consistent with the preceding assignments. When riboflavin anion radicals are examined, it appears that the weak peak due to N-10 CH_3 near 18 MHz is replaced by a weak peak near 17.5 MHz, which is assigned to the methylene protons at N-10. In summary, it appears that flavin anion radicals are rather easily characterized by a strong ENDOR line corresponding to a 10 MHz coupling to the C-8 methyl.

When flavin radicals are looked at in an ice matrix there is a slight shift in the methyl coupling constants but the C-8 methyl coupling constant remains larger than that for the N-10 methyl. Furthermore when D_2O is

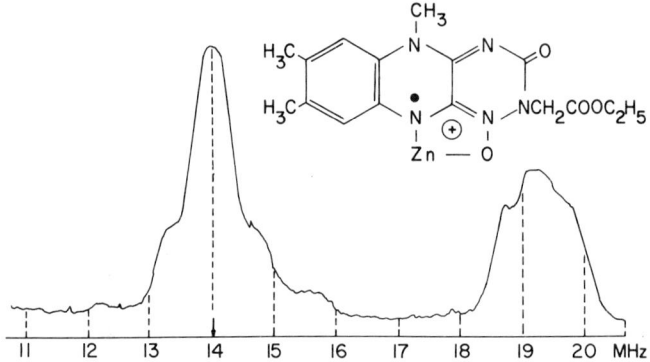

Figure 7-2. Proton ENDOR spectrum of lumiflavin radical chelate with zinc in dimethylformamide at about 113 K. The free proton frequency has been adjusted to 14.0 MHz for easy comparison with other figures. From L. E. G. Eriksson et al., *Biochim. Biophys. Acta*, **192**, 211 (1969).

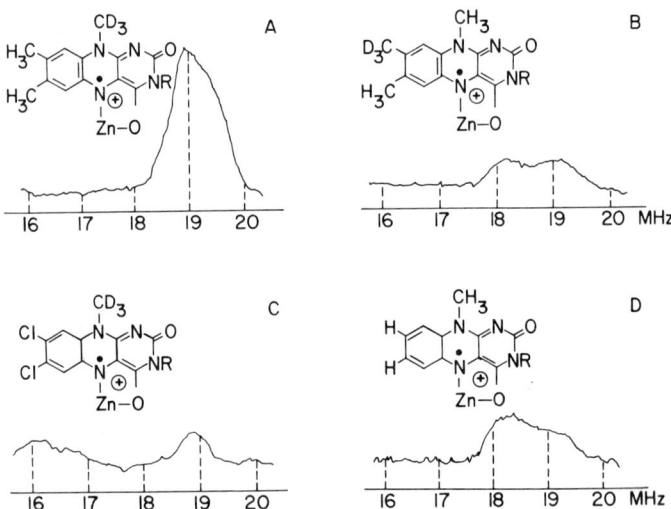

Figure 7-3. High frequency portion of proton ENDOR spectra for the indicated substituted lumiflavin radical chelates with zinc in dimethylformamide at about 113 K. The frequency range for the matrix ENDOR line is not shown but the free proton frequency has been adjusted to 14.0 MHz for easy comparison with other figures. The gain of (C) is four times that of the rest. From L. E. G. Eriksson et al., *Biochim. Biophys. Acta*, **192**, 211 (1969).

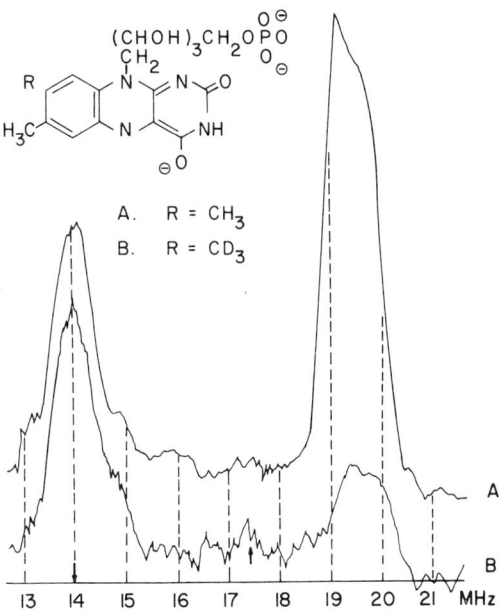

Figure 7-4. ENDOR spectra of photoreduced flavoproteins in 50 mM tris buffer and 10 mM EDTA at 153 K (A) 0.5 mM NADPH dehydrogenase natural flavoprotein with $R = CH_3$ and (B) 0.2 mM apoprotein of NADPH dehydrogenase combined with specifically deuterated flavin mononucleotide to reconstitute the flavoprotein. The free proton frequency has been adjusted to 14.0 MHz for easy comparison with other figures. The formula shown is for the flavin radical moiety of the flavoprotein. The gain of (B) is twice that of (A). The arrow denotes a weak peak that seems absent in Fig. 7-2. From L. E. G. Eriksson et al., *Eur. J. Biochem.*, **17,** 539 (1970).

substituted for H_2O, the matrix proton signal is almost completely removed indicating that it occurs largely from matrix protons as opposed to weakly coupled protons in the flavin radical.

One may compare these model system studies with the ENDOR spectrum of photoreduced NADPH dehydrogenase in frozen solution as shown in Fig. 7-4A. There is considerable similarity with the flavin anion radical spectrum in Fig. 7-2. This suggests that the radical site in the flavoprotein is in a flavin mononucleotide moiety. The prominent ENDOR line near 19 MHz can be confidently assigned to the methyl group in the C-8 position. In addition, a small peak appears at about 17.5 MHz in Fig. 7-4 that does not appear to be present in Fig. 7-2. By comparison with the appearance of a similar line in a riboflavin anion radical, this small line can be assigned to the methylene protons at the N-10 position in the flavin mononucleotide. To verify definitely the assignment of the prominent ENDOR signal near 19 MHz in Fig. 7-4 to the methyl protons at the C-8 position the following elegant experiment was performed. The FMN groups were separated from the NADPH dehydrogenase, followed by deuteration of the FMN at the methyl group in the C-8 position and reconstitution of the flavoprotein.[7] The resulting ENDOR spectrum is shown in Fig. 7-4B, which clearly shows a great drop in intensity in the 19 MHz region. The residual ENDOR line at this frequency can be assigned tentatively to the ring proton at C-6. Also, the ~10 MHz coupling constant of the methyl group at the C-8 position suggests that the FMN radical produced by photoreduction of the NADPH dehydrogenase is in the anionic form by comparison with the couplings found for model flavin anion radicals.

As indicated before, the matrix proton signals may be used to probe the accessibility or proximity of water molecules or matrix molecules to the radical site. When NADPH dehydrogenase is photoreduced in D_2O, the matrix proton line decreases by some 40%.[7] So one can conclude that the radical site in this flavoprotein is accessible to solvent water, but it is not as accessible as a free flavin anion radical, since for that case the matrix ENDOR line is almost completely eliminated in a D_2O matrix.

The model of the flavin radical produced when the NADPH dehydrogenase flavoprotein is reduced together with its characteristic signature of a methyl proton ENDOR line at ~19 MHz should be extendable to other flavoproteins. This has been confirmed for different flavoproteins isolated from *Azotobacter vinelandii*[7] and *Peptostreptococcus elsdenii*.[8] ENDOR spectra of photoreduced *P. elsdenii* are shown in Fig. 7-5. Figure 7-5A is similar to Fig. 7-4A except that the prominent ENDOR line has shifted from ~19.3 MHz to ~18.3 MHz. The assignment of the 18.3 MHz line to C-8 methyl protons was unambiguously shown by reconstituting the flavoprotein with FMN deuterated at the C-8 position (Fig. 7-5C). The 18.3 MHz line corresponds to a smaller coupling of about 8 MHz to the methyl protons in the C-8 position for the flavoprotein of *P. elsdenii* compared to the ~10 to 10.5 MHz coupling for the flavoprotein of NADPH dehydrogenase. From ESR work[7] this smaller coupling is consistent with the cationic form of the FMN radical as opposed to the anionic form. The change in spin density between anionic and cationic (or neutral) radicals of flavin model compounds indicates that the spin density is lower at both the C-8 and C-6 positions and higher in the N-10 position in the cation. Thus in the cation form of the FMN radical moiety in the *P. elsdenii* flavoprotein one expects a weak ENDOR line corresponding to the methylene group at the N-10 position appearing above ~17.5 MHz (see Fig. 7-4B). As shown in Fig. 7-5A a small

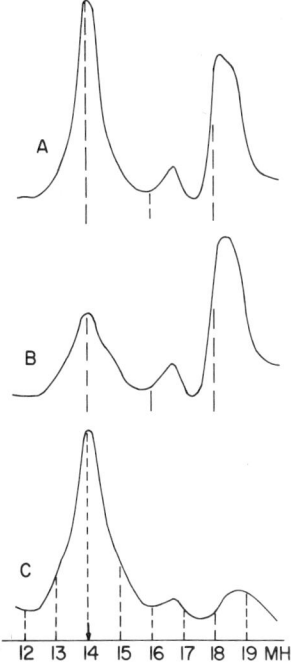

Figure 7-5. ENDOR spectra of photoreduced *Peptostreptococcus elsdenii* flavoprotein in 0.1 M potassium phosphate and 0.01 M EDTA at 118 K. (A) Native flavoprotein in H_2O, (B) native flavoprotein in D_2O, (C) flavoprotein reconstituted from C-8 CD_3-FMN in H_2O. The free proton frequency was adjusted to 14.0 MHz for easy comparison with other figures. From J. Fritz et al., *Helv. Chim. Acta*, **57**, 2250 (1973).

shoulder is observed at ~18.7 MHz that can be assigned to N-10 methylene protons. Also, the peak between 18 to 19 MHz in Fig. 7-5C seems shifted to ~18.7 MHz from ~18.3 MHz in Fig. 7-5A, B. The N-10 methylene protons should make a dominant contribution to this line in Fig. 7-5C if the deuteration is reasonably complete. The small, but prominent line at ~16.7 MHz in Fig. 7-5 has been shown to be due to the C-6 proton by selective deuteration of FMN and reconstitution of the flavoprotein.[8] This is consistent with the expected reduced spin density at C-6 in the cation radical. Thus the spectra in Fig. 7-5 appear consistently assignable to the cation radical. The photoreduced *A. vinelandii* flavoprotein also seems to be in the radical cation form.[7] It is noteworthy that the ENDOR results can apparently distinguish between anion and cation (neutral) forms of the radical site in flavoproteins; Table 7-1 summarizes this distinction.

When the photoreduced *A. vinelandii* flavoprotein is examined in a D_2O matrix, the matrix proton ENDOR line decreases by about 75%,[7] whereas the same experiment with the photoreduced *P. elsdenii* flavoprotein shows a decrease of only 55%.[8] Thus the FMN radical site in all the photoreduced flavoproteins studied seems rather accessible to solvent

Table 7-1. Characteristic Proton Hyperfine Couplings of Flavin Radical Sites in Photoreduced Flavoproteins Determined by ENDOR

Proton Position[a]	Anion Radical Site[b]	Cation (Neutral) Radical Site[c]
C-8 methyl	10.6 MHz[d]	8.4 MHz[d]
N-10 methylene	7.0	9.4
C-6	9.4	5.4

[a] See Fig. 7-1 for flavin ring numbering system.
[b] Found in NADPH dehydrogenase (ref. 7).
[c] Found in *Peptostreptococcus elsdenii* flavoprotein (ref. 8) and in *Azotobacter vinelandii* flavoprotein (ref. 7).
[d] Splittings are about ±0.2 MHz.

water, and the *A. vinelandii* flavoprotein shows the most accessible radical site. Table 7-2 summarizes these observations.

Since the ENDOR spectra of the flavin radicals seem to be relatively well understood and relatively well characterized, this information can be used to study the form in which flavin is bound in other biological systems. This has been utilized in a study of the binding of flavin to the active center of succinate dehydrogenase.[9] The spectrum of the reduced flavin cation radical in this system is shown in Fig. 7-6B. There is clearly no prominent ENDOR peak between 18 to 19 MHz from a methyl radical at the C-8 position. For comparison, the riboflavin radical cation in the same matrix clearly shows such a peak (Fig. 7-6A). This indicates

Table 7-2. Summary of Proton Matrix ENDOR Line Intensities in Different Biological Systems

System	Reduction in Matrix Proton ENDOR Line Intensity in D_2O	Ref.
Lumiflavin radical ions	≥95%	4
NADPH dehydrogenase[a]	~40%	7
A. vinelandii flavoprotein[a]	~75%	7
P. elsdenii flavoprotein[a]	~55%	8
Stellacyanin	~0%	3
Adrenodoxin	~0%	14

[a] Photoreduced.

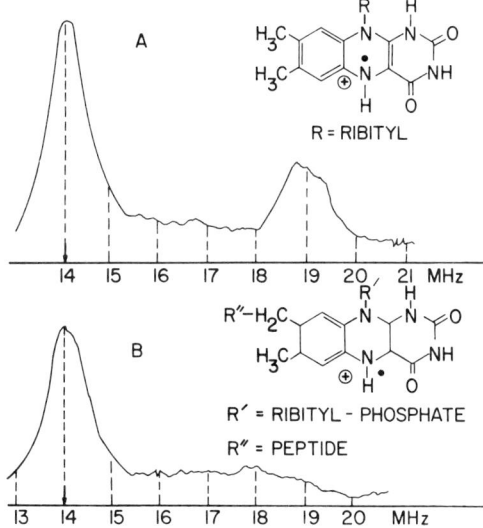

Figure 7-6. ENDOR spectra of (A) riboflavin radical cation and (B) succinate dehydrogenase flavin radical cation in 6 M HCl at 113 K. From W. H. Walker et al., *FEBS Lett.*, **5**, 237 (1969).

that the flavin is covalently bound to the succinate dehydrogenase through its C-8 position so that only methylene protons exist at that position. The broad weak signal between 17 and 18 MHz is probably due to coupling to the methylene protons in the C-8 position and to the proton at the C-6 position. It can be seen that a knowledge of the flavin radical ENDOR spectra can lead to a variety of useful and incisive information about the role of binding of flavins in various biological systems.

It should also be mentioned that nitrogen ENDOR was searched for in these various flavoprotein systems as well as in the model systems of flavin radicals.[4] Nitrogen ENDOR was never seen but this is perhaps because the temperature of the experiments was rather high, always being 113 K or above. As will be seen below, nitrogen ENDOR is observable in other protein systems but always at temperatures of the order 20 K or below.

7.1.2 Copper Proteins—Stellacyanin

Proteins containing copper play a significant role in respiration and metabolic processes. Two forms of paramagnetic copper can be identified in copper-containing proteins.[10] Type 1 copper is associated with a strong visible absorption near 600 nm that gives rise to a blue color. Type 2 copper is colorless. Both type 1 and 2 copper-containing proteins exhibit ESR spectra that are nearly axially symmetric. Type 1 copper has a unique narrow hyperfine splitting of $A_\| \sim 150$ MHz, while type 2 copper has ESR spectra quite similar to those from planar, low molecular weight copper complexes with typically $A_\| \sim 600$ MHz.

Stellacyanin is a blue copper protein containing type 1 copper. It has a molecular weight of about 20,000 and is obtained from the Japanese lacquer tree, *Rhus vernicifera*. The ESR spectrum shows considerable g anisotropy and gives little indication of the bonding of copper in this protein. However ENDOR has been used to demonstrate that the copper is bound to at least one and perhaps more nitrogens.[3]

Figure 7-7 shows ENDOR spectra at two different microwave frequencies at 15 to 20 K for an observation point at the low field extreme of the ESR spectrum. Observation at two different microwave frequencies can be used to distinguish between contributions from proton and nitrogen ENDOR in the same region. It can be seen that the line near 18 MHz is unshifted when the ENDOR spectra are run at the two different microwave frequencies, whereas the other ENDOR lines are shifted as would be expected for weak proton couplings. Thus the line at ~ 18 MHz is

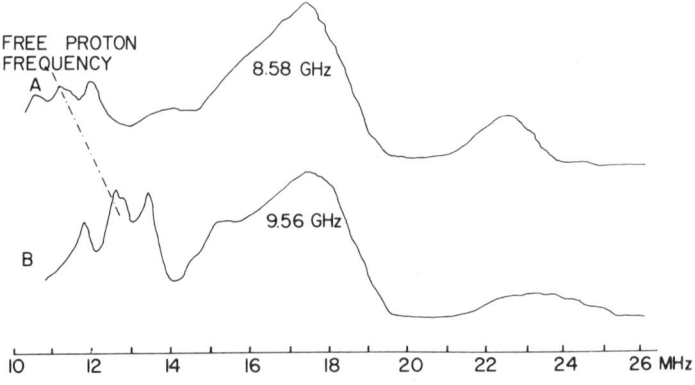

Figure 7-7. ENDOR spectra at 15 to 20 K of ~ 1.5 mM stellacyanin in H_2O at two microwave frequencies. The magnetic field is positioned at g_z, the low field peak of the ESR spectrum, which is dominated by g anisotropy. The absorption near 18 MHz is nearly independent of microwave frequency and is therefore assigned to ligand nitrogens ($A_\perp \sim$ 36 MHz). Part of the peak near 22 to 24 MHz also seems independent of frequency and may be assignable to ligand nitrogens ($A_\| \approx 48$ MHz). The other peaks that shift with frequency are assignable to protons. Adapted from G. H. Rist et al., *Proc. Nat. Acad. Sci. U.S.*, **67**, 79 (1970).

assigned to a nitrogen coupling. This is a broad line and one in general expects four lines due to hyperfine and quadrupole (Q) couplings from a set of equivalent nitrogens. These four lines occur in two pairs split by twice the free nitrogen nuclear frequency and are centered at $(A/2) \pm Q$ (see Section 4.3). At 3200 G twice the nuclear nitrogen frequency is 2 MHz, so in this spectrum no resolution of the nitrogen lines is observed. However one can assign a coupling of $A_\perp/2$ equal to ~18 MHz from the spectrum. Since this is observed at the low field (and high field) extreme of the ESR spectrum, it is argued that this is probably a perpendicular component of the nitrogen hyperfine splitting. Part of the peak at 22 to 24 MHz in Fig. 7-7 also seems independent of microwave frequency and may be attributable to a nitrogen coupling. This is presumably a parallel coupling. It seems apparent that the selection of molecules with their axes oriented only one way by sitting at g_z or g_y in the ESR spectrum is rather nonspecific in this case. Observation at other positions in the ESR spectrum corresponding to a parallel orientation also suggests that a nitrogen line may occur near 24 MHz, which corresponds to an $A_\parallel$ equal to 48 MHz. The couplings $A_\perp \sim 36$ MHz and $A_\parallel \sim 48$ MHz seem consistent with studies on model copper complexes.[11]

In Fig. 7-7A the line near 22 MHz shifts with frequency and is thus due to a strongly coupled proton that is possibly bonded to ligand nitrogen. The other resolved lines attributable to protons from 10 to 14 MHz can be assigned to protons on nearby amino acid residues, but they cannot be assigned in detail unless more information about the geometry of the copper ion is known.

The ENDOR line near the free proton frequency is essentially unaffected by preparing the sample in D_2O instead of H_2O. Thus the copper site does not seem to be accessible to solvent water, and there are apparently no exchangeable protons in this protein within a radius of several angstroms of the copper ion. This result is in considerable contrast to what is found for the flavoproteins (Table 7-2). The copper ion site is apparently embedded in the protein in such a way as to prevent access by water molecules.

7.1.3 Metmyoglobin

Metmyoglobin is a system in which ENDOR of the frozen solution allows resolution of the nitrogen ENDOR lines in sufficient detail to determine nitrogen hyperfine and quadrupole tensors. Metmyoglobin is an important heme protein in which the paramagnetic center is Fe^{3+} interacting with four nitrogens of a planar tetrapyrrole ring and with a fifth nitrogen

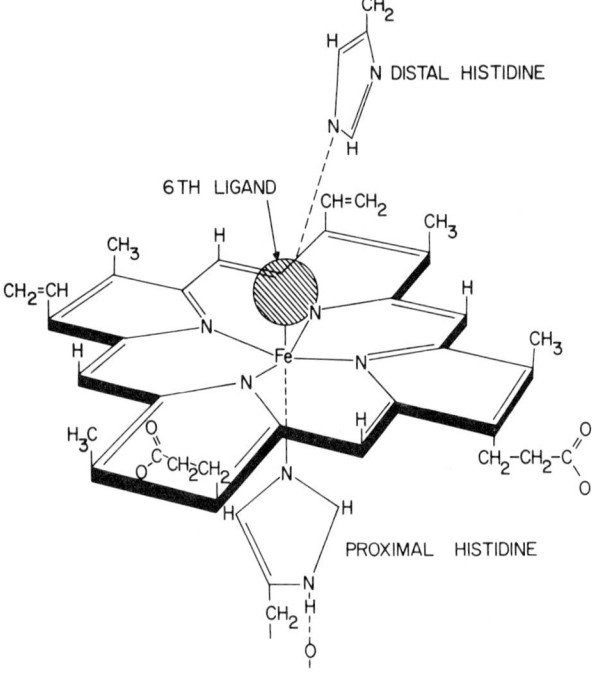

Figure 7-8. Structure of the heme group in myoglobin and hemoglobin.

in a proximal histidine residue located below the plane. This structure is shown in Fig. 7-8 in which the sixth ligand site is occupied by water in metmyoglobin.

The ESR spectrum is axially symmetric with $g_\| = g_z$ occurring near $g = 2$ and $g_\perp$ occurring near $g = 6$. Although the Fe^{3+} in metmyoglobin is in the high spin state, the ground state can be treated as having an effective electronic spin of $\frac{1}{2}$. By setting the magnetic field at the $g = 2$ portion of the ESR spectrum, one selects only those molecules that have their normals to the heme plane parallel to the magnetic field. In this case the ENDOR spectrum in Fig. 7-9 is obtained at 2.1 K in a glycerol-water mixture (1:1 by volume).[6] It is interesting that the normalized ENDOR signals are found to be much larger in the frozen solution than in single crystals of metmyoglobin. This is partly due to the fact that larger frozen solution samples can be used than the volumes obtainable as single crystals.

As described in Section 4.3 well resolved nitrogen ENDOR should give rise to four ENDOR lines for each set of equivalent nitrogens that occur as two pairs separated by twice the free nitrogen nuclear frequency and

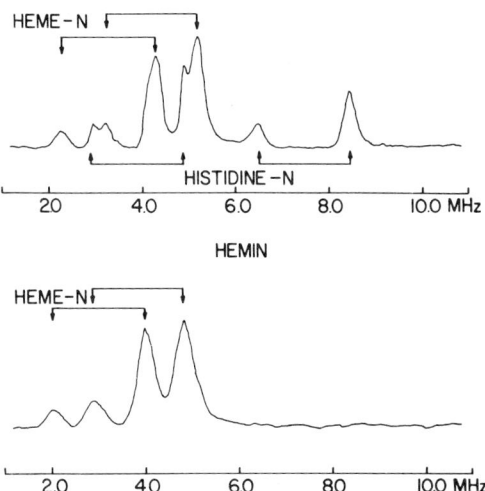

Figure 7-9. Low frequency part of the ENDOR spectrum of metmyoglobin and hemin showing the interaction of the Fe^{3+} spin with its ligand nitrogen nuclei. Metmyoglobin is 6 mM in glycerol-water (1:1 by volume), 0.1 M potassium phosphate buffer and pH = 6.0. Hemin is 3 mM hemin chloride in dimethylformamide-methanol (1:1 by volume) Spectra were obtained at 2.1 K, $H_o = 3.2$ kG, and $\nu_e = 8.9$ GHz. The ENDOR lines from a set of equivalent nitrogens appear as two pairs separated by twice the free nitrogen nuclear frequency and centered at one-half the hyperfine frequency ± the quadrupole coupling. Hemin does not contain a histidine nitrogen (see Fig. 7-8) and so shows only four ENDOR lines. The observing ESR position is near $g = 2$, which selects those molecules that have their normal to the heme plane parallel to H_o. Taken from C. P. Scholes et al., *Biochim. Biophys. Acta*, **263**, 448 (1972).

occurring at one-half the nitrogen hyperfine coupling constant plus or minus the quadrupole coupling constant. The four nitrogens in the heme plane are expected to be equivalent, and inequivalent to the histidine nitrogen. Thus eight ENDOR lines are expected, as observed. The lower frequency ones can be unambiguously assigned to heme nitrogens by comparison with the ENDOR spectrum from hemin, which contains no histidine nitrogen. There is a little bit of ambiguity in assigning the two lowest frequency transitions to the histidine nitrogen, and the assignment made is based on a consistent separation of the lines by twice the free nuclear frequency of nitrogen.

The assignment made of the ENDOR spectra in Fig. 7-9 leads to $A_{zz} = 7.60 \pm 0.02$ MHz and $Q_{zz} = 0.44 \pm 0.01$ MHz for the heme nitrogens and $A_{zz} = 11.46 \pm 0.03$ MHz and $Q_{zz} = 1.75 \pm 0.02$ MHz for the histidine nitrogen. To obtain the perpendicular components ENDOR must be done at the magnetic field corresponding to g = 6. ENDOR transitions have been seen in this case although they are much weaker because the ESR spectrum is much weaker, and no definite analysis has yet been given. In addition, proton ENDOR lines are seen near the free proton frequency and correspond to couplings with splitting constants of 0.80 MHz and 1.30 MHz. Preparation of the samples in D_2O matrices suggests that the 1.30 MHz protons are exchangeable. Further analysis of the proton ENDOR in this system seems warranted.

7.1.4 Bacteriochlorophyll

Chlorophylls contain magnesium coordinated to the four nitrogens in a tetrapyrrole ring as shown in the inset of Fig. 7-10. The primary act in photosynthesis has been postulated to involve electron transfer from chlorophyll to produce a chlorophyll cation. However, the exact nature of the chlorophyll cation as a dimeric cation has only been revealed by ENDOR studies.[5]

Bacteriochlorophyll from the photosynthetic bacteria *Rhodopseudomonos spheroides* and *Rhodopseudomonos rubrum* has been studied. Isolated bacteriochlorophyll in the monomeric form dissolved in 12% methanol in methylene chloride (v/v) was oxidized by elemental iodine to the cation and the ENDOR spectrum at 103 K is shown in Fig. 7-10a. Prominent ENDOR lines are observed at the free proton frequency at 13.7 MHz and at 16.1 and 18.3 MHz. These latter two strong lines are reasonably attributed to rotating methyl groups and have been so confirmed by looking at ENDOR spectra of specifically deuterated bacteriochlorophylls.[12] In contrast, the *in vivo* spectrum obtained by oxidation of intact cells or chromatophores prepared from the photosynthetic bacteria and oxidized with $K_3Fe(CN)_6$ produces the ENDOR spectrum shown in Fig. 7-10b. First, it is interesting that the matrix ENDOR signal is not very intense, which indicates that there are few protons near the unpaired electron site and that the active site is in a rather hydrophobic environment. Second, a prominent line occurs at 16 MHz that is reasonably associated with a rotating methyl group, but closer analysis shows it to correspond to the 18.3 MHz line in Fig. 7-10a. The other rotating methyl group with smaller coupling constant appears to absorb near 14.7 MHz. The absorption in the region of 17 to 19 MHz has been shown to be due to the β and δ methine protons in the bacteriochlorophyll by using suitably deuterated compounds.[12] Thus the interesting result is that the coupling constants to the same methyl groups appear to be smaller in the *in vivo* bacteriochlorophyll cation than in the *in vitro* bacteriochlorophyll

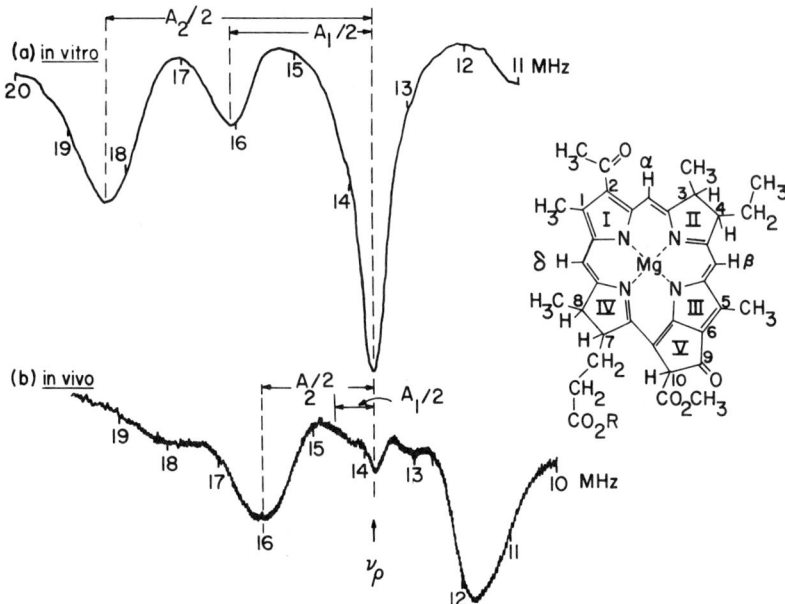

Figure 7-10. Proton ENDOR spectra from oxidized bacteriochlorophyll (BChl) in *vitro* and in *vivo* at 103 K. (*a*) Monomeric BChl in CH_2Cl_2-CH_3OH (88:12) by volume) oxidized to $BChl^+$ by I_2, (*b*) *Rhodopseudomonos rubrum* chromotophores in which the BChl has been oxidized by a minimal amount of $K_3Fe(CN)_6$. The insert shows the structure of BChl in which R stands for geranylgeraniol in the case of *R. rubrum*. In (*a*) the two prominent ENDOR lines near 16.1 and 18.3 MHz are assigned to two methyl groups and in (*b*) these two lines are shifted toward the free proton frequency ν_p at 13.7 MHz to correspond to coupling constants slightly less than one-half those in (*a*). Note that the frequency scale direction is reversed from the other figures. From J. R. Norris et al., *J. Amer. Chem. Soc.*, **95**, 1680 (1973).

cation. In fact, the difference in coupling constants is a little less than a factor of two. This indicates that the cation in the *in vivo* systems is dimeric with the spin density spread out over twice as many molecules with consequently half as much spin density at a given methyl proton site.

It will be noted that no nitrogen ENDOR is observed in the bacteriochlorophyll spectrum. This is at least partly due to the fact that observations were made at relatively high temperature. It seems possible that nitrogen ENDOR might be resolved at temperatures below 20 K by analogy to other proteins.

The ENDOR spectra of chlorophyll *a* and bacteriochlorophyll monomeric cations obtained by chemical oxidation have been characterized rather completely by a study of specific deuterated chlorophylls.[12]

Although chlorophyll contains some 15 protons as likely sites of significant unpaired electron interaction, the assignment of coupling constants to most of the sites by detailed ENDOR studies has been possible.

7.1.5 Iron-Sulfur Proteins

Proteins containing two irons and two labile sulfurs per molecule are called ferredoxins or adrenodoxins and have been found to serve as electron carriers in a variety of biochemical reactions. These proteins are known to be present in all photosynthetic organisms that utilize water as an electron donor and produce oxygen. These two-iron proteins, also called nonheme proteins, are found in plants (spinach and parsley ferredoxin), bacteria (putidaredoxin), and mammals (adrenodoxin). The amino acid sequence has been determined for a number of these iron-sulfur proteins and the number of amino acid residues varies between 97 and 112. The main information about the structure of the iron-sulfur protein active site has come from ENDOR studies.[13-15] The most likely structure is a binuclear tetrahedral configuration that consists of two iron atoms, two labile sulfur atoms, and four cysteine residues as shown schematically in Fig. 7-11. The reduced form consists of a high spin Fe(III) atom and a high spin Fe(II) atom antiferromagnetically coupled to form an $S = \frac{1}{2}$ system.

By using protein substituted with Fe^{57} ($I = \frac{1}{2}$) iron ENDOR signals have been studied in detail.[13] The ESR spectrum has a nearly axially symmetric g factor with principal values of $g_\| = 2.02$ and $g_\perp = 1.93$. The hyperfine tensor for the iron atoms can be determined by setting the magnetic field at $g_\|(H_z)$ to select only those molecules undergoing ESR that have their z axes aligned along the magnetic field. If we set the magnetic field at intermediate values, molecules of several orientations will contribute to the ESR spectrum and at some point those molecules whose y axes are

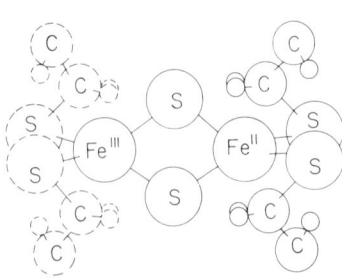

Figure 7-11. Schematic structure of the iron-sulfur complex in two-iron ferredoxins and adrenodoxin. The four sulfurs around each iron are arranged tetrahedrally. The two sulfurs bridging the two irons are labile. The small unidentified circles are hydrogens. The nonbridging sulfurs coordinated to iron are part of cysteinyl residues; the eight methylene protons of four cysteinyl residues are shown projecting above and below the irons. ENDOR is seen from these methylene protons and from the two iron atoms. Adapted from W. R. Dunham et al., *Biochim. Biophys. Acta,* **253,** 373 (1971).

along the magnetic field will dominate. By keeping track of which molecular orientations are contributing to the ESR and hence the ENDOR spectra it is possible to obtain the components of the hyperfine tensor. This is most simple for the case where the principal values of the g tensor and hyperfine tensor coincide. In general, these principal values will not coincide and small deviations from that situation can be determined by synthesizing ENDOR spectra and comparing with the experimental spectra.

Both iron and proton ENDOR lines are seen in the same region above the free proton frequency from 15 to 24 MHz. The iron ENDOR lines are identified by their presence or absence when ^{57}Fe is substituted into the protein or not and by the fact that the iron ENDOR signals do not change frequency when the resonant cavity frequency is changed slightly. This is the same technique that was used to distinguish proton and nitrogen ENDOR signals in stellacyanin. This works because the proton ENDOR signals have $A/2$ less than ν_p and are centered around ν_p while the iron ENDOR signals have $A/2$ greater than ν_{Fe} and are centered around $A/2$.

A summary of the iron ENDOR tensors for various ferredoxins and adrenodoxins is given in Table 7-3. It can be seen that the two irons are clearly nonequivalent and have different coupling constants; this corrects earlier interpretations from the ESR spectra alone in which ferredoxin substituted with ^{57}Fe exhibited a 1/2/1 triplet at the $g_\parallel$ position that was interpreted as indication of equivalent irons.[13] In this case the ESR spectral resolution is simply too low to show the true inequivalence of these two irons. From the ENDOR spectra it can also be concluded that the irons have a net spin of $S = \frac{1}{2}$ because the ENDOR lines occur at $A/2 \pm \nu_n$. Finally, some information about the relative orientations of the $g_\parallel$ and A tensors is deduced by computer simulations of the ENDOR spectra. This is indicated in Table 7-3. For spinach and parsley ferredoxins the x axes of the g and A tensors are nearly coincident whereas the y and z principal axes of the A tensor appear to be rotated about the x axis with respect to the g-tensor axis by an angle of about 30°. In adrenodoxin and putidaredoxin the g and A tensors are nearly coincident along the z axes, but there appears to be some difference between the g and A principal axes in the x and y directions.

Analysis of the proton ENDOR in adrenodoxin[14,15] shows that five proton couplings are observed at 20 K for ENDOR observation at the $g_\parallel$ position and at least three proton couplings are observed at the $g_\perp$ position (see Table 7-4). These proton ENDOR lines have been assigned to methylene protons from four cysteine residues bonded to the two irons (see Fig. 7-11). Thus there are eight β-CH$_2$ protons, which could all be

Table 7-3. Iron Hyperfine Constants in Iron-Sulfur Proteins Measured by ENDOR[a]

Protein (g_x, g_y, g_z)	Site 1 (Fe(III))			Site 2 (Fe(II))			
	A_x	A'_y	A'_z	A_x	A_y	A_z	
Spinach ferredoxin	51 ± 1	50^{+2}_{-7}	42 ± 1.5	?	?	35.5 ± 2	MHz
(1.89, 1.96, 2.05)	(19.3 ± 0.4)	$(18.2^{+0.7}_{-2.6})$	(14.6 ± 0.5)			(12.4 ± 0.7)	(G)
Parsley ferredoxin	51 ± 1	50^{+2}_{-7}	42 ± 2	?	?	34.5 ± 2.5	MHz
(1.90, 1.96, 2.05)	(19.2 ± 0.4)	$(18.2^{+0.7}_{-2.6})$	(14.6 ± 0.7)			(12.1 ± 0.9)	(G)
	$A_\perp$	$A'_\perp$	A_z	$A_\perp$	$A'_\perp$	A_z	
Adrenodoxin	50 ± 1.5	56^{+1}_{-3}	43^{-1}_{+2}	17 ± 4	24 ∓ 4	35 ± 1.5	MHz
(1.93, 1.935, 2.02)	(18.5 ± 0.5)	$(20.7^{+0.4}_{-1.1})$	$(15.2^{-0.4}_{+0.7})$	(6.3 ± 1.5)	(8.9 ∓ 1.5)	(12.4 ± 0.5)	(G)
Putidaredoxin	50 ± 1.5	56^{+1}_{-3}	43^{-1}_{+2}	17 ± 4	24 ∓ 4	35 ± 1.5	MHz
(1.93, 1.935, 2.02)	(18.5 ± 0.5)	$(20.7^{+0.4}_{-1.1})$	$(15.2^{-0.4}_{+0.7})$	(6.3 ± 1.5)	(8.9 ∓ 1.5)	(12.4 ± 0.5)	(G)

From J. Fritz et al., Biochim. Biophys. Acta, **253**, 110 (1971).

[a] For the upper two proteins the primed values A'_y and A'_z indicate that the g and A tensors are nearly coincident only for the x axis and that the y and z axes are apparently rotated about the x axis with respect to the g-tensor axes by 20° to 40°. For the lower two proteins the g and A tensors appear to be nearly coincident but the A tensor does not seem to be axially symmetric as is the g tensor; hence two $A_\perp$ values are given (primed and unprimed). The box indicates that these two components have the error flags correlated; i.e., if $A_\perp$ is in error by a positive increment, then $A'_\perp$ is in error by a negative increment or vice versa. All errors are intended to be the maximum possible values, inside which the actual value must lie.

Table 7-4. Proton and ^{57}Fe Hyperfine Coupling Constants of Native Adrenodoxin and Selena-adrenodoxin Determined by ENDOR

	A (MHz) at $g_\parallel$		A (MHz) at $g_\perp$	
Proton ENDOR:				
Native adrenodoxin	1.5, 2.7, 4.4, 7.2, 10.0 ± 0.2		1.8, 4.0, 5.2 ± 0.2	
Selena-adrenodoxin	1.0, 2.3, 4.3, 6.0, 9.8 ± 0.2		1.0, 2.6, 3.8 ± 0.2	
^{57}Fe ENDOR:	Fe(III) site	Fe(II) site	Fe(III) site	Fe(II) site
Native adrenodoxin	43.1 ± 2	35 ± 1.5	50 ± 1.5	24 ± 4
Selena-adrenodoxin	39.6 ± 0.5	33 ± 2	47.8 ± 0.7	26.6 ± 0.7

From M. Bowman et al., *Biochim. Biophys. Acta*, **328**, 244 (1973).

inequivalent. The five couplings observed indicate that at least five of these eight β-CH$_2$ protons are inequivalent.

It is also possible to substitute the labile sulfurs with selenium and still have a biologically active protein. Attempts to use ^{77}Se with $I = \frac{1}{2}$ have not revealed any selenium ENDOR,[15] but the effect of selenium on the proton and iron coupling constants can be studied in a very sensitive way by ENDOR. These results are summarized in Table 7-4. It is interesting that selenium does significantly affect the spin density in the active site but does not affect the biological activity. The results imply a slight shift of spin density from the Fe(III) to the bridging seleniums.

In this work[15] it was possible to resolve the iron and proton ENDOR signals by using temperature variation. At 20 K the proton signals were prominent in the spectrum, but at 10 K the proton signals were suppressed and the iron signals remained. In the previous detailed work on iron ENDOR at 20 K spectral subtraction techniques were used.[13]

The matrix proton ENDOR signal from adrenodoxin shows essentially no decrease when D$_2$O is substituted for H$_2$O.[14] This implies that the iron-sulfur site is embedded in the protein in a hydrophobic region and is not accessible to solvent water. This is similar to the copper site in stellacyanin but contrasts with the flavoprotein radicals (see Table 7-2).

7.1.6 Vitamin Quinones

Vitamins K, E, and ubiquinone are involved in biological electron transport and oxidative phosphorylation. So the role of such quinones in various biological reactions is of considerable importance. First, it is necessary to characterize the electronic structure of isolated biological quinones. The vitamin quinones are considerably simpler molecules than the protein systems discussed earlier. They can thus be studied in solution. By ENDOR a detailed assignment of the proton coupling constants with consequent spin density information has been obtained.[16]

The biological quinones studied include vitamin K_3 (menadione), vitamin K_1 (phytonodione), vitamin E (α-tocopherol quinone), and ubiquinone-10. For the most part, comparison with simpler substituted naphthosemiquinones indicates that replacement of methyl groups by the long side chains in the vitamins does not change the ring spin density distribution much. It is also possible to show that the preferred conformation of vitamin quinones in solution is not a static one. At lower temperatures ENDOR lines assigned to equivalent β-methylene protons split to show two inequivalent methylene proton splittings due to freezing out of internal free rotational motions. The analysis of such results has been treated in Section 3.3.

7.1.7 Prognosis

It has been seen that ENDOR had made significant contributions to the understanding of the paramagnetic centers in a variety of biological systems. As far as radical identification by ENDOR perhaps the most outstanding example is the identification of the cation in bacterial photosynthesis as a dimeric species.[5] The detailed work on the radical site in the flavoproteins is also of outstanding significance.[4] Other applications of this type to radical identification in biological systems by ENDOR should become increasingly significant.

It has been pointed out that although proton ENDOR is generally seen, the ENDOR from other nuclei is often not seen. This is primarily a matter of the relevant relaxation times being optimized for ENDOR detection. Thus temperature is a prime variable to use to try to search for ENDOR of nuclei that do not seem to be observable. It is noted that nitrogen ENDOR has only been observed in biological systems at temperatures of 20 K or below. Thus statements that it has not been observed at 110 K in flavoproteins, for example, only refer to that particular temperature. It is quite possible that nitrogen ENDOR might be observed at lower temperatures in these systems.

Finally the effect of deuteration on matrix proton ENDOR signals appears to be a very significant method for studying the involvement of water or the accessibility of water to the radical site. The full potential of this information has not yet been fully exploited. For example, if there exist protons in proteins that are exchangeable with D_2O only when the proteins are denatured, but are not exchangeable or are less completely exchanged with D_2O in the natural protein one can conceive a variety of denaturation, deuteration, reconstitution and subsequent protonation experiments in order to investigate the influence of the tertiary structure of the protein on proton exchangeability.[7] In addition, a detailed theory of the matrix ENDOR lineshape should yield structural information about the surrounding proton distribution. Certainly these and other significant applications of ENDOR to biological systems await future investigation.

7.2 BIOCHEMICAL APPLICATIONS OF ELDOR

Although the ENDOR studies in biochemical systems have been extended to a variety of topics, analogous ELDOR studies have been so far limited to spin-labeled biomolecules[17,18] and xanthine oxidase.[19] This has been due in part to the lack of available ELDOR instrumentation and in part to the lack of ELDOR signals from biological samples as a result of the absence of ELDOR active relaxation mechanisms.

Despite these problems it does appear that ELDOR studies of biochemical systems will be fruitful. This is because a large number of biochemical systems do undergo molecular motion of one form or another, which in turn generates ELDOR active transitions, a feature especially true of spin-labeled molecules (see Section 5.2.3). One might recall that in Section 1.5.2 and in Chapters 5 and 6, we discussed the relation between molecular motion and ELDOR active relaxation mechanisms and its importance for the observation of ELDOR spectra. In brief, the presence of intra- or intermolecular motion causes a modulation (a change with time) of the anisotropic magnetic interactions (such as the nitrogen anisotropic hyperfine splitting and g factors in nitroxide spin labels) that results in energy transfer occurring between the resonant and nonresonant portions of the spin system. This produces an ELDOR active relaxation mechanism and intense ELDOR spectra are observed.

As pointed out in Section 7.1, most biological systems of current interest are studied as disordered systems and thus exhibit powderlike ESR spectra. Energy transfer processes can be deduced by an ELDOR study of such a system whenever the paramagnetic fragments are undergoing molecular motion. In such a system, spins of a given orientation that have been saturated by the pump power will reorient, carrying the saturation to a different part of the spectrum. As one might recall from Section 5.2.3, this is referred to as spectral diffusion of saturation. By measuring the magnetic field range over which this diffusion of saturation occurs, and by knowing the anisotropy of the magnetic interaction and the memory time of the spin system (T_{1e}), one can estimate the rotational correlation time. From a theoretical analysis of the ELDOR spectrum, it is also possible to determine the diffusion relaxation mechanism (such as isotropic Brownian, anisotropic rotational free diffusion, or jump diffusion) that the spin label undergoes. Such a determination was previously described in Section 5.2.3 for the spin label tanol and is generally applicable to spin-labeled macromolecules. The results obtained for maleimido spin-labeled hemoglobin are given in Section 7.2.1.

It is also possible to obtain information such as dipolar anisotropy, reorientational rates, and an estimate of the environment surrounding the paramagnetic center from ELDOR studies of biological systems that have not been spin labeled. To stress the approach that is used and the extent of information obtainable, an ELDOR study of xanthine oxidase[19] is described in Section 7.2.2.

7.2.1 Nitroxide Spin-Labeled Biomolecules

As noted in Section 5.2.3 the correlation times for the molecular motion of spin labels attached to biological systems can vary from 10^{-3} to 10^{-10} sec. However, biological systems of general interest exhibit rotational correlation times longer than 10^{-7} sec, a correlation time range over which the ESR linewidth is insensitive. Fortunately, ELDOR studies of spin labels in highly viscous media such as maleimido-spin-labeled hemoglobin[18] have shown that correlation times can be measured on the order of 400 times longer than T_{1e}. Typically T_{1e} equals 10^{-5} sec for very slowly tumbling spin labels and does not vary with rotational correlation time. Thus it is presently possible to measure a correlation time as long as 4×10^{-3} sec. At some future date it may be possible to measure longer correlation times if spin labels can be synthesized that possess spin-lattice relaxation rates (T_{1e}) longer than 10^{-5} sec and lack substituents that undergo intramolecular motion. It has been noted that spin labels that undergo rapid intramolecular motion tend to mask the degree of mobility at the spin-labeled site and are thus inadequate for determining long rotational correlation times.

ELDOR of the maleimido-labeled hemoglobin molecule has also shown that the random motions of large molecules are best described by a Brownian diffusion model with small step sizes. This is in contrast to the jump diffusion model where a large step size of approximately 0.15 radians is required to describe slowly rotating, small, spin-labeled molecules.

It appears that molecular motion several orders of magnitude slower than previously detectable by ESR can be studied by ELDOR and that models can be deduced for the type of motion that occurs. Eventually such information should lead to a better structural model of macromolecules.

7.2.2 Xanthine Oxidase

The enzyme xanthine oxidase from bovine milk has been extensively studied to determine its enzymatic mechanism,[20,21] yet many questions remain. First among these is the role that the spin-spin interaction between molybdenum and one of the iron-sulfur systems of xanthine oxidase plays in the enzymatic mechanism.[21] From a magnetic resonance point of view there seems to be an inconsistency in the observed ESR results, as little dipolar coupling has been found between the Mo^V ion and the iron-sulfur system. Yet an isotropic coupling of 31 MHz to one of the iron systems is observed[19] below 45 K. Above 45 K this coupling is not detected and is thought to be due to an averaging process at high temperature caused by rapid spin-lattice relaxation of iron. An ELDOR study of this rather complex system has resulted in additional structural results.

The ESR spectrum of the low temperature form of the "slow" Mo^V signal from xanthine oxidase is given in Fig. 7-12. A frequency swept ELDOR spectrum is obtained by setting the observing resonant condition at point A and sweeping the pump frequency to lower frequencies. This gives rise to peaks at 14 MHz and at 35 MHz.[19]

The line at 14 MHz arises from the weak coupling to matrix protons.[22] Because of this it is possible to estimate whether or not the protons surrounding the immediate environment of the molybdenum in xanthine oxidase[20,21] are exchangeable with deuterium from D_2O by simply monitoring the change in the intensity of the 14 MHz line when a sample is prepared in a D_2O buffer. No decrease in intensity is observed, which implies that few of the protons in the neighborhood of the molybdenum are exchangeable.

Secondly, the line at 35 MHz corresponds to the low temperature splitting previously reported by Lowe et al.[21] to be 31 MHz. As the temperature is varied from 18 to 45 K no detectable shift occurs in this line. However, a shift does occur when the observing position is set to different points (A, B, C, and D) of the Mo spectrum as shown in Fig. 7-13. Note that the ELDOR peak observed between 35 to 45 MHz arises from an inhomogeneously broadened ESR line and thus is expected to be a composite of a derivative lineshape and a pure absorption lineshape.[22] If one assumes that the theoretical equations in the appendix by Hyde et

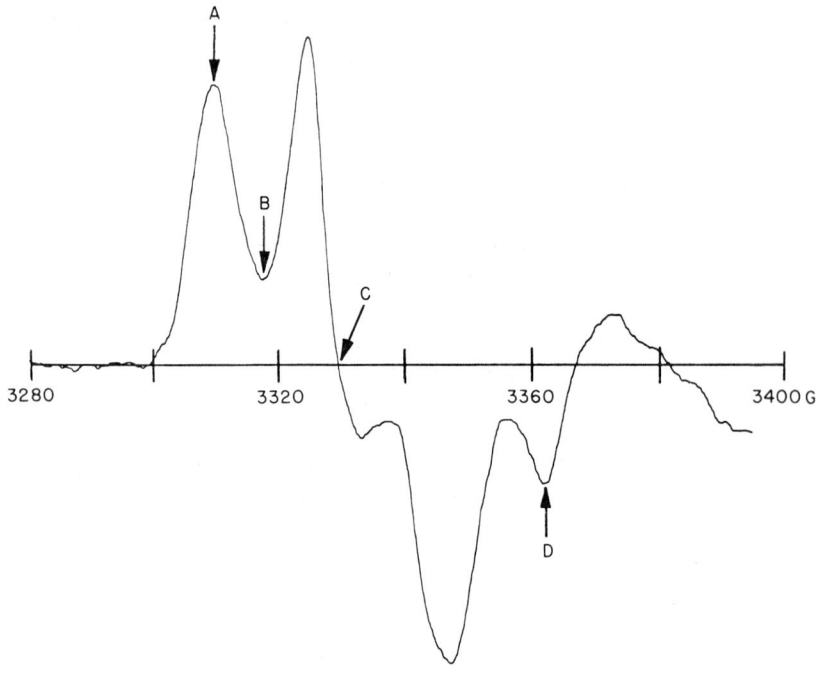

Figure 7-12. The 9.5 GHz ESR absorption spectrum for the "slow" Mo^V signal in xanthine oxisase at 30 K, 10 mW microwave power, and 2 G field modulation at 100 kHz. Frequency swept ELDOR spectra were obtained while observing points A to C with $\nu_p < \nu_o$ and D with $\nu_p > \nu_o$. From D. J. Lowe and J. S. Hyde, *Biochim. Biophys. Acta*, **377**, 205 (1975).

al.[22] are valid for the composite lineshape, the true line center of the 35 to 45 MHz peak in Fig. 7-13 is calculated to be that given by the position of the arrows. Note that the peak position varies from 35 MHz at the low field peak (A) to 44 MHz at the high field peak (D). This is an anisotropy of 9 MHz, which is somewhat greater than the 3 to 6 MHz dipolar anisotropy previously reported.[21] This suggests that the previously proposed separation of 40 Å between the iron-sulfur and the molybdenum[21] is improbably high.

One additional piece of structural information is obtained by noting that the intense ELDOR lines observed are approximately one-third of the ESR peak intensity. This can be understood by assuming that the observed low temperature ESR Mo spectrum arises from two Mo spectra

From saturation experiments the iron-sulfur spin-lattice relaxation time

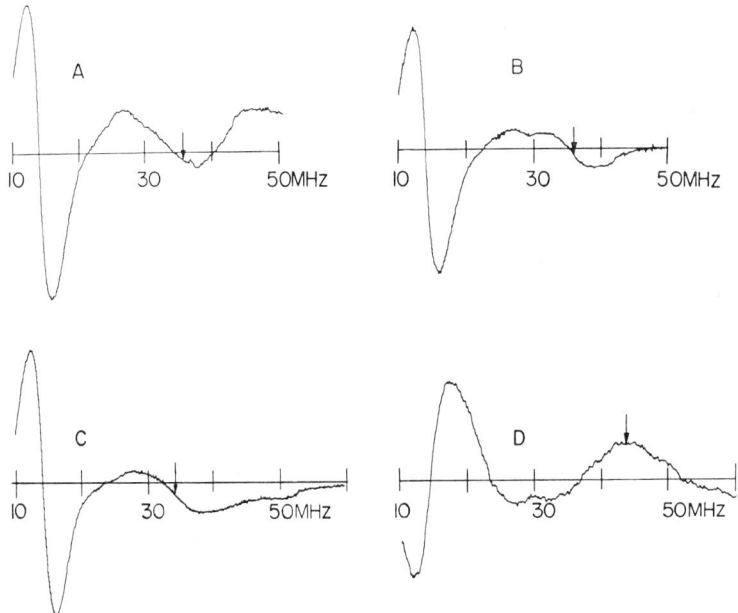

Figure 7-13. Frequency swept ELDOR spectra for xanthine oxidase obtained at the observing positions A, B, C, and D in Fig. 7-12 with a pump power attenuation of 800 mW except at C where it is 250 mW. The arrows indicate the true center of the 35 to 45 MHz peak obtained from a theoretical analysis of the lineshape. From D. J. Lowe and J. S. Hyde, *Biochim. Biophys. Acta*, **377**, 205 (1975).

has been found to be always less than that of Mo. This implies that the interconversion rate is more rapid than the Mo spin-lattice relaxation rate and thus according to Table 1-4 very strong ELDOR signals must arise. This model, which assumes that the low temperature Mo ESR spectrum arises from one radical interconverting between two spectral forms, is also consistent with the appearance of one ELDOR line at 35 MHz.

Although the question of why such a small Mo and iron-sulfur dipolar interaction is observed has been left unanswered by this ELDOR study, it is possible to demonstrate conclusively that only one site gives rise to the low temperature Mo spectrum. The fact that an exact time dependent calculation using density matrix techniques[18,23] has not been made yet also implies that further structural information can be deduced once the ELDOR lineshape, temperature dependence, and effect of rapid passage are properly analyzed.

REFERENCES

1. R. M. Deal, D. J. E. Ingram, and R. Srinivasan, in *Proceedings of Colloque Ampere XII*, R. Servant and A. Charrer, eds., North-Holland, Amsterdam, 1964, pp. 239–247.
2. P. Eisenberger and P. S. Pershan, *J. Chem. Phys.*, **47,** 3327 (1967).
3. G. H. Rist, J. S. Hyde, and T. Vänngard, *Proc. Nat. Acad. Sci. U.S.*, **67,** 79 (1970).
4. L. E. G. Eriksson, J. S. Hyde, and A. Ehrenberg, *Biochim. Biophys. Acta*, **192,** 211 (1969); **167,** 482 (1968).
5. J. R. Norris, M. E. Druyan, and J. J. Katz, *J. Amer. Chem. Soc.*, **95,** 1680 (1973).
6. C. P. Scholes, R. A. Isaacson, and G. Feher, *Biochim. Biophys. Acta*, **263,** 448 (1972).
7. L. E. G. Eriksson, A. Ehrenberg, and J. S. Hyde, *Eur. J. Biochem.*, **17,** 539 (1970).
8. J. Fritz, F. Müller, and S. G. Mayhew, *Helv. Chim. Acta*, **56,** 2250 (1973).
9. W. H. Walker, J. Salach, M. Gutman, T. P. Singer, J. S. Hyde, and A. Ehrenberg, *FEBS Lett.*, **5,** 237 (1969).
10. T. Vänngard, in *Magnetic Resonance in Biological Systems*, A. Ehrenberg, B. G. Malmstrom, and T. Vänngard, eds., Pergamon, Oxford, 1967, p. 213.
11. G. H. Rist and J. S. Hyde, *J. Chem. Phys.*, **52,** 4633 (1970); **50,** 4532 (1969).
12. J. R. Norris, H. Scheer, and J. J. Katz, *166th Amer. Chem. Soc. Nat. Meeting, Abstract Phys.* #25, (Fall, 1973).
13. J. Fritz, R. Anderson, J. Fee, G. Palmer, R. H. Sands, J. C. M. Tsibris, I. C. Gunsalus, W. H. Orme-Johnson, and H. Beinert, *Biochim. Biophys. Acta*, **253,** 110 (1971).
14. K. Mukai, T. Kimura, J. Helbert, and L. Kevan, *Biochim. Biophys. Acta*, **295,** 49 (1973).
15. M. Bowman, L. Kevan, K. Mukai, and T. Kimura, *Biochim. Biophys. Acta*, **328,** 244 (1973).
16. M. R. Das, H. D. Connor, D. S. Leniart, and J. H. Freed, *J. Amer. Chem. Soc.*, **92,** 2258 (1970).
17. M. D. Smigel, L. R. Dalton, J. S. Hyde, and L. A. Dalton, *Proc. Nat. Acad. Sci. U.S.* **71,** 1925 (1974).
18. J. S. Hyde, M. D. Smigel, L. R. Dalton, and L. A. Dalton, *J. Chem. Phys.*, **62,** 1655 (1975).
19. D. J. Lowe, and J. S. Hyde, *Biochim. Biophys. Acta*, **377,** 205 (1975).
20. R. C. Bray and J. C. Swann, *Struct. Bonding*, **11,** 107 (1972).
21. D. J. Lowe, R. M. Lynden-Bell, and R. C. Bray, *Biochem. J.*, **130,** 239 (1972).
22. J. S. Hyde, R. C. Sneed, and G. H. Rist, *J. Chem. Phys.*, **51,** 1404 (1969).
23. B. H. Robinson, J. L. Monge, L. A. Dalton, and L. R. Dalton, *Chem. Phys. Lett.*, **28,** 169 (1974).

Author Index

Numbers in parentheses are reference numbers. Numbers in *italics* indicate the pages on which the full reference appear.

Abragam, A., 14(6), 17(6), 28(6), *56;* 54(34), *57;* 166(1), 232(1), *252;* 271(23), *302*
Alger, R. S., 59(4), *93*
Allen, P. S., 369(53), *387*
Allendoerfer, R. D., 66(21), 74(21), 75(21), 76(21), 89(21), *93;* 100(9), *163;* 103(10), 105(10), 144(10), 148(10), 149(10), *163;* 105(7), *163;* 105(11), *163;* 105(12), 150 (12), *163;* 115(23), *163;* 123(30), *163;* 133(32), *163;* 135(7), *162;* 161(50), 162 (50), *164;* 235(60), *253*
Alexander, C., 178(7), *252*
Anderson, R., 404(13), 405(13), 407(13), *414*
Apaydin, F., 369(53), *387*
Aslop, L. E., 76(35), *94*
Astlind, T., 67(27), 75(27), *93*
Atherton, N. M., 30(19), *57;* 59(1), 62(1), *92;* 113(21), *163;* 135(5), *162;* 153(47), 154(47), 155(47), 157(47), *164;* 155(48), *164;* 159(49), 160(49), *164;* 166(3), *252*
Atkins, P. W., 41(26), *57;* 266(16), 267(16), *301;* 334(40), *386*

Baker, J. M., 74(33), *93;* 89(53), *94;* 178(8), 179(8), *252*
Bales, B. L., 74(30b), 88(30b), *93;* 244(67), *253;* 244(69), 246(69), *253;* 244(71), *253*
Bauer, G., 135(4), *162*
Bauld, N. L., 133(33), *163*
Beinert, H., 404(13), 405(13), 407(13), *414*
Benderskii, V. A., 76(37), 84(37), *94;* 254 (2), 255(2), 262(2), *301;* 254(7), 255(7), 265(7), 270(7), *301;* 305(16), 380(16), 381(16), *386;* 305(17), 380(17), 382(17), 384(17), *386;* 305(18), 380(18), *386;* 305 (19), 380(19), *386*
Bessent, R. G., 88(44)
Biehl, R., 66(23), 74(23), 75(23), 76(23), *93;* 111(20), 123(20), *163;* 123(31), *163;* 135(3), *162;* 135(6), 137(6), *162;* 138(37), 139(37), 140(37), *163;* 138(38), 139(38), 141(38), 143(38), *163*

Blackhurst, A. J., 30(19), *57;* 113(21), *163*
Blake, W. B. J., 89(53), *94;* 178(8), 179(8), *252*
Bleaney, B., 14(6), 17(6), 28(6), *56;* 166(1), 232(1), *252*
Blum, H., 66(10), *93;* 89(51), *94*
Blumberg, W. E., 89(50), *94;* 89(55), *94*
Blumenfeld, L. A., 305(16), 380(16), 381 (16), *386;* 305(17), 380(17), 382(17), 384(17), *386*
Bogan, C. M., 44(27), *57;* 47(30), *57;* 56(37), *57;* 92(62), *94;* 92(63), *94,* 304(1), 311(1), 316(1), *385;* 304(3), 305(3), 311(3), 322 (3), 325(3), *385;* 305(6), 334(6), *385*
Bohme, U. R., 209(33), *252*
Bolton, J. R., 59(1), 62(1), *92;* 306(20), 310 (20), *386*
Borcherts, R. H., 89(60), *94*
Bowers, K. D., 354(47), *387*
Bowman, M. K., 241(64), *253;* 244(70), 246(70), *253;* 249(75), *253;* 404(15), 405 (15), 407(15), *414*
Box, H. C., 66(18), *93;* 181(12), 182(12), *252;* 186(23), 201(23), *252;* 198(26), *252;* 199(27), 219(27), *252;* 199(28), 201(28), 204(28), 211(28), *252;* 201(29), *252;* 205(32), *252;* 210(34), 213(34), *252;* 212(35), *252;* 213(36), *252;* 233(57), *253;* 312(23), *386;* 322(29), *386*
Bray, R. C., 411(20), *414;* 411(21), 412(21), *414*
Breit, G., 12(5), *59*
Breslow, R., 105(13), *163;* 117(24), 119(24), *163*
Brunner, H., 76(39), 84(39), 86(39), *94*
Bruno, G. V., 76(38), *94;* 254(6), 255(6), 262(6), 265(6), 270(6), 274(6), *301;* 270 (19), *302;* 270(20), 271(20), *302;* 271(27), *302*
Buckman, T., 270(17), *302*
Budzinski, E. E., 181(12), 182(12), *252;* 199(28), 201(28), 204(28), 211(28), *252;* 201(29), *252;* 205(32), *252;* 210(34), 213 (34), *252;* 212(35), *252;* 213(36), *252;* 233(57), *253;* 322(29), *386*

SUBJECT INDEX

Carrington, A., 145(45), *164;* 306(21), *386*
Chadwick, J. R., 74(33), *93*
Chang, K., 44(27), *57;* 47(30), *57;* 56(36), *57;* 56(37), *57;* 90(61), *94;* 92(62), *94;* 92(62), *94;* 304(1), 311(1), 316(1), *385;* 304(2), 305(2), 311(2), 316(2), 318(2), 320(2), 321(2), 322(2), 341(2), 365(2), 384(2), *385;* 304(3), 305(3), 311(3), 322(3), 325(3), *385;* 305(6), 334(6), *385* 305(13), 339(13), 341(13), *385;* 305(14), 347(14), 357(14), 358(14), 359(14), *386;* 350(42), 352(42), *386;* 367(52), *387*
Chen, C. S., 316(25), 365(25), 366(25), *386*
Chien, J. C. W., 41(25), 43(25), 47(25), 55 (25), *57;* 76(36), 84(36), *94;* 254(1), 255 (1), 256(1), 259(1), 260(1), 262(1), 265(1), 267(1), 269(1), 270(1), 274(1), 275(1), 280(1), 295(1), *301;* 318(26), *386*
Clarke, R. H., 229(48), 230(48), 231(48), *253*
Clough, S., 219(41), 222(41), *253;* 219(42), 221(42), 222(42), *253;* 222(43), *253;* 369(53), *387;* 371(54), *387*
Cobb, T. B., 369(53), *387*
Cole, T., 89(48), *94;* 106(14), *163*
Collins, M. A., 360(50), *387*
Connor, H. D., 117(26), 121(26), *163;* 143 (42), *163;* 254(4), 255(4), 275(4), 277(4), *301;* 408(16), *414*
Cook, I. P., 30(19), *57*
Cook, R. J., 66(19), 73(19), *93;* 177(5), *252;* 178(6), *252;* 179(10), *252;* 184(18), 186 (18), *252;* 185(21), 186(21), *252;* 186(22), 201(22), *252*
Coope, J. A. R., 179(9), *252*
Copland, G. M., 89(53), *94*
Corbett, J. W., 66(15), *93*
Cornell, D. W., 270(17), *302*
Cowen, J. A., 271(29), *302*
Crawford, L. P., 322(32), 347(32), 359(32), *386*
Cross, L. G., 23(13), 30(13), *57*
Culvahouse, J. W., 76(35), *94;* 354(46), *387*
Currin, J. D., 274(31), *302*

Dalal, D. S., 66(22), 74(22), 75(22), *93;* 133 (34), 135(34), *163;* 179(9), *252;* 232(55), *253;* 300(34), *302*
Dalton, L. A., 54(33), *57;* 54(34), *57;* 254(8), 255(8), 270(8), 271(8), 272(8), *301;* 254 (9), 255(9), 271(9), *301;* 254(10), 255(10), 265(10), 274(10), 278(10), 279(10), *301;* 254(11), 255(11), 265(11), 279(11), 283 (11), *301;* 271(26), *302;* 271(28), *302;* 305(12), *302;* 305(12), *385;* 409(17), *414;* 409(18), 410(18), 413(18), *414*
Dalton, L. R., 54(34), *57;* 74(32), 88(32), *93;* 222(44), 223(44), *253;* 237(62), 238 (62), *253;* 254(8), 255(8), 270(8), 271(8), 272(8), *301;* 254(9), 255(9), 271(9), *301;* 254(10), 255(10), 265(10), 274(10), 278 (10), 279(10), *301;* 254(11), 255(11), 265(11), 279(11), 283(11), *301;* 271(26), *302,* 271(29), *302;* 304(5), 211(5), *385;* 305(12), *385;* 409(17), *414;* 409(18), 410 (18), 413(18), *414;* 413(23), *414*
Danner, J. C., 66(21a), 74(21a), 75(21a), 89(21a), *93;* 100(9), *163*
DAS, M. R., 117(26), 121(26), *163;* 254(5), 255(5), 275(5), *301;* 408(16), *414*
Davidson, R. B., 30(20), *57;* 66(24), 74(24), 75(24), 89(24), *93*
Davies, E. R., 75(34), *93*
Day, B., 135(5), *162;* 153(47), 154(47), 155(47), 157(47), *164*
Deal, R. M., 388(1), *414*
De Boer, C., 105(13), *163;* 117(24), 119(24), *163*
Decaillot, M., 234(58), *253*
Derouane, E. G., 248(74), *253;* 250(76), *253*
Dinse, K. P., 66(23), 74(23), 75(23), 76(23), *93;* 111(20), 123(20), *163;* 123(31), *163;* 135(3), *162;* 135(6), 137(6), *162;* 138(37), 139(37), 140(37), *163;* 138(38), 139(38), 141(38), 143(38), *163*
Doetschman, D. C., 231(53), *253*
Doyle, W. T., 66(11), *93*
Druyan, M. E., 390(5), 402(5), 408(5), *414*
Dyer, G. L., 89(59), *94*

Eastman, M. P., 76(38), *94;* 254(6), 255(6), 262(6), 265(6), 270(6), 274(6), *301*
Egelstaff, P. A., 271(25), *302*
Ehrenberg, B. G., 32(23), *57;* 67(27), 75(27), *93;* 390(4), 397(4), 408(4), *414;* 394(7), 395(7), 409(7), *414;* 396(9), *414;* 398(10), *414*

AUTHOR INDEX 417

Ehret, P., 66(17), *93;* 225(47), 230(47), 231(47), *253*
Eisenberger, P., 388(2), *414*
Eisinger, J., 89(55), *94*
El-Sayed, M. A., 384(55), 385(55), *387;* 384(56), 385(56), *387*
Engelmann, J. H., 105(11), *163*
Eriksson, L. E. G., 67(27), 75(27), *93;* 74 (29), 75(29), 88(29), 89(29), *93;* 107(16), *163;* 234(59), 239(59), *253;* 390(4), 397 (4), 408(4), *414;* 394(7), 395(7), 409(7), *414*
Eustace, E. J., 66(21b), 74(21b), 75(21b), 76(21b), 89(21b), *93;* 105(12), 150(12), *163*

Falle, H. R., 138(36), 140(36), 141(36), *163*
Farach, H. A., 334(38), *386*
Fee, J., 404(13), 405(13), 407(13), *414*
Feher, G., 12(1), *56;* 12(2), 19(2), *56;* 12(3), 21(3), 31(3), *56;* 15(8), *56;* 21(12), *57;* 26(17), *57;* 31(22), 34(22), *57;* 66(6), 89(6), *93;* 89(5), *94;* 390(6), 400(6), *414*
Feng, D. F., 49(31), 51(31), 52(31), *57;* 262(12), 263(12), *301;* 305(9), 378(9), 379(9), *385;* 305(10), *385*
Fessenden, R. W., 106(14), *163*
Fitzpatrick, J. D., 117(25), 120(25), *163*
Fraenkel, G. K., 136(35), *163;* 266(14), 267(14), 270(14), *301*
Freed, J. H., 19(11), *57;* 31(21), *57;* 41(25), 43(25), 47(25), 55(25), *57;* 41(26), *57;* 41(7), 43(7), *56;* 46(28), *57;* 76 (36a), 84(36a), *94;* 76(38), *94;* 110(19), 112(19), 143(19), 159(19), *163;* 117(26), 121(26), *163;* 122(28), 143(28), 144(28), 151(28), 153(28), *163;* 143(40), 144(40), 151(40), 153(40), *163;* 143(41), *163;* 143(42), 144(42), *163;* 254(1), 255(1), 256(1), 259(1), 260(1), 261(1), 265(1), 267(1), 269(1), 270(1), 274(1), 280(1), 295(1), *301;* 254(4), 255(4), 275(4), 277(4), *301;* 254(5), 255(5), 275(5), *301;* 254(6), 255(6), 262(6), 265(6), 270(6), 274(6), *301;* 266(13), 267(13), *301;* 266(14), 267(14), 270(14), *301;* 266(15), 274(15),*301;* 270(19),*302;* 270(20), 271(20), *302;* 271(24),*302;* 271(27),*302;* 331(35), *386;* 334(39),*386;* 334(40),*386;* 408(16),*414*

Freund, H. G., 66(18), *93;* 199(28), 201 (28), 211(28), *252;* 201(29), *252;* 210(34), 213(34), *252;* 233(57), *253;* 312(22), *386;* 322(29), *386*
Fritz, J., 394(8), 395(8), *414;* 404(13), 405 (13), 407(13), *414*
Fujimoto, M., 322(30), *386*
Fuller, C. S., 15(8), *56*

Gaillard, J., 232(56), *253*
Gallagher, P. E., 133(32), *163*
Gamble, W. L., 369(53), *387*
Garton, G., 74(33), *93*
Gazzinelli, R., 66(12), *93*
Gelles, I. J., 76(35), *93;* 353(45), *386*
Gere, E. A., 12(2), 19(2), *56;* 15(8), *56*
Geschwind, S., 89(55), *94;* 89(57), *94;* 89 (58), *94*
Giordmaine, J. A., 76(35), *94*
Gloux, P., 181(11), 183(11), 201(11), 207 (11), *252;* 181(13), 183(13), 217(13), *252;* 183(16), *252;* 232(56), *253*
Gol'danskii, V. I., 254(7), 255(7), 265(7), 270(7), *301*
Goldman, S. A., 270(20), 271(20), *302;* 271(27), *302*
Goncalves, A. L. Ponte, 231(52), *253*
Gordon, R. D., 133(33), *163*
Griffith, O. H., 270(17), *302*
Grimm, R., 135(4), *162*
Gunsalus, I. C., 404(13), 405(13), 407(13), *414*
Gunthard, H. H., 204(31), *252*
Gutman, M., 396(9), *414*
Gutowsky, H. S., 117(27), 119(27), *163*

Halford, D., 89(52), *94*
Hall, J. L., 66(13), *93*
Hampton, D. A., 178(7), *252*
Hartman, R. L., 369(53), *387*
Hase, H., 244(72), 246(72), *253*
Hausser, K. H., 76(39), 84(39), 86(39), *94*
Haustein, H., 138(37), 139(37), 140(37), *163;* 138(38), 139(38), 141(38), 143(38), *163*
Hayes, R. G., 322(34), 325(34), 357(34), *386*
Hayes, W., 88(44), *94*
Helbert, J. N., 74(30b), 88(30b), *93;* 240 (63), 244(63), 247(63), *253;* 244(67), *253;* 244(68), 249(68), 250(68), *253;*

404(14), 405(14), 407(14), *414*
Heller, C., 89(48), *94;* 106(14), *163*
Helms, H. A., Jr., 30(20), *57;* 66(24), 74(24), 75(24), 89(24), *93*
Herve, A., 353(43), 354(43), *386*
Hieke, S., 135(4), *162*
Hill, J. R., 219(42), 221(42), 222(42), *253;* 369(53), *387*
Holm, C. H., 117(27), 119(27), *113*
Holton, W. C., 89(51), *94;* 66(10), *93*
Hoogstraate, H., 25(15), 30(15), *57*
Horsfield, A., 106(15), *163;* 322(27), *386;* 359(58), *387*
Hudson, C. E., 133(33), *163*
Hunt, J. W., 322(34), 325(34), 357(34), *386*
Huntress, W. T., Jr., 334(37), 365(37); *386*
Hurrell, J. P., 74(33), *93;* 75(34), *93;* 89(54), *94*
Hutchison, C. A., Jr., 66(16), 89(16), *93;* 89(49), *94;* 229(48), 230(48), 231(48), *253;* 230(49), *253;* 230(50), 231(50), *253;* 230(51), *253;* 231(52), *253;* 231(53), *253*
Hyde, J. S., 19(10), *57;* 31(21), *57;* 32(23), *57;* 41(25), 43(25), 47(25), 55(25), *57;* 54(33), *57;* 54(34), *57;* 55(35), 56(35), *57;* 66(26), 67(26), 88(26), *93;* 67(27), 75(27); *93;* 74(29), 75(29), 88(29), 89(29), *93;* 74(30a), 88(30a), *93;* 74(31), 88(31), *93;* 76(36), 83(36), *94;* 88(40), *94;* 88(42), *94;* 88(45), 92(45), *94;* 96(1), *162;* 97(8), 115(8), 133(8), *162;* 105(13), *163;* 107(16), *163;* 108(18), *163;* 110(19), 112(19), 143(19), 159(19), *163;* 117(24), 119(24), *163;* 117(25), 120(25), *163;* 133(33), *163;* 135(2), 136(2), 137(2), *162;* 186(24), 201(24), *252;* 234(59), 239(59), *253;* 237(61), *253;* 237(61), 242(65), 243(65), *253;* 244(66), 248(66), 251(66), *253;* 251(77), *253;* 254(1), 255(1), 256 (1), 259(1), 260(1), 261(1), 265(1), 267 (1), 269(1), 270(1), 274(1), 275(1), 280 (1), 295(1), *301;* 254(3), 255(3), 286(3), 292(3), 300(3), *301;* 254(8), 255(8), 270(8), 271(8), 272(8), *301;* 254(9), 255(9), 271(9), *301;* 254(11), 255(11), 265(11), 279(11), 283(11), *301;* 271(28), *302;* 305(12), *385;* 305(15), 373(15), *386;* 318(26), *386;* 353 (44), 355(44), *386;* 389(3), 399(3), *414;* 390(4), 397(4), 408(4), *414;* 394(7), 395 (7), 409(7), *414;* 396(9), *414;* 409(17), *414;* 409(18), 410(18), 413(18), *414;* 409 (19), 410(19), 411(19), *414;* 411(22), 412 (22), *414*

Ikeda, R., 369(53), *387*
Imelik, B., 250(76), *253*
Ingram, D. J. E., 388(1), *414*
Isaacson, R. A., 26(17), *57;* 390(6), 400(6), *414*
Ishizu, K., 66(25), 74(25), *93*
Itoh, K., 316(24), 318(24), 365(24), 366(24), 368(24), *386;* 316(25), 365(25), 366(25), *386*
Iwasaki, M., 46(29), *57;* 184(20), 186(20), *252;* 215(37), *252;* 217(38), *252;* 217(39), *253;* 217(40), 218(40), *253;* 305(8), *385*

Janecka, J., 322(30), *386*
Jeffries, C. D., 66(8), *93*
Johnson, C. S., Jr., 274(31), *302;* 274(32), *302;* 369(53), *387*

Katz, J. J., 390(5), 402(5), 408(5), *414;* 402(12), 403(12), *414*
Kennedy, D. E., 66(22), 74(22), 75(22), *93,* 133(34), 135(34), *163;* 300(34), *302*
Kevan, L., 49(31), 51(31), 52(31), *57;* 74 (30b), 88(30b), *93;* 240(63), 244(63), 247(63), *253;* 241(64), *253;* 244(67), *253;* 244(68), 249(68), 250(68), *253;* 244(69), 246(69), *253;* 244(70), 246(70), *253;* 244(71), *253;* 244(72), 246(72), *253;* 249 (75), *253;* 262(12), 263(12), *301;* 305(9), 378(9), 379(9), *385;* 305(10), *385;* 404 (14), 405(14), 407(14), *414;* 404(15), 405 (15), 407(15), *414*
Keys, R. T., 66(21a), 74(21a), 75(21a), 89 (21a), *93;* 100(9), *163*
Kimura, T., 404(14), 405(14), 407(14), *414;* 404(15), 405(15), 407(15), *414*
Kispert, L. D., 44(27), *57;* 47(30), *57;* 56(36), *57;* 56(37), *57;* 76(36b), *94;* 90(61), *94;* 92(62), *94;* 92(63), *94;* 105(13), *163;* 117(25), 120(25), *163;* 304(1), 311(1), 316(1), *385;* 304(2), 305(2), 311(2), 316 (2), 318(2), 320(2), 321(2), 322(2), 341(2), 365(2), 384(2), *385;* 304(3), 311(3), 322(3), 325 (3), *385;* 304(4), 311(4), 339(4), *385;* 305(6), 334(6), *385;* 305(7), 334(7), 336 (7), 365(7), *385;* 305(11), 318(11), 349(11),

385; 305(13), 339(13), 341(13), *385;* 305(14), 347(14), 357(14), 358(14), 359(14), *386;* 318(26), *386;* 322(31), *386;* 350(42), 352(42), *386;* 367(52), *387;* 371(54), *387*

Kivelson, D., 266(16), 267(16), *301;* 270(18), 274(18), *302*

Kobayashi, M., 76(35), *94*

Kohler, B. E., 230(50), 231(50), *253*

Koma, A., 76(35), *94*

Kono, M., 66(25), 74(25), *93*

Koski, W. S., 322(29), *386*

Kotake, Y., 113(22), 115(22), *163;* 151(46), 153(46), 156(46), *164*

Kuan, T. S., 384(55), 385(55), *387*

Kubo, R., 270(21), *302;* 270(22), *302*

Kurita, Y., 322(33), 347(33), 359(33), 361(33), *386*

Kuwata, K., 113(22), 115(22), *163;* 151(46), 153(46), 156(46), *164*

Kwiram, A. L., 30(18), *57;* 54(34), *57;* 183(15), *252;* 222(44), 223(44), *253;* 223(45), *253;* 237(62), 238(62), *253;* 254(10), 255(10), 265(10), 274(10), 278(10), 279(10), *301;* 254(11), 255(11), 265(11), 279(11), 283(11), *301;* 271(26), *302;* 271(29), *302;* 304(5), 311(5), *385*

La Follette, D., 105(13), *163*

Lambe, J., 12(4), 19(4), *56;* 23(14), 25(14), 30(14), 31(14), *57;* 66(7), *93;* 89(48), *94;* 89(56), *94*

Lamotte, B., 181(11), 183(11), 201(11), 207(11), *252;* 181(13), 183(13), 217(13), *252;* 232(56), *253*

Lansbury, P. T., 133(32), *163*

Lasher, G. J., 76(35), *93;* 353(45), *386*

Laukien, G., 66(20), 67(20), 74(20), 89(20), *93*

Laurance, N., 12(4), 19(4), *56;* 23(14), 25(14), 30(14), 31(14), *57;* 66(7), *93;* 89(56), *94*

Leifson, O. S., 66(8), *93*

Lemart, D. S., 31(21), *57*

Leniart, D. S., 110(19), 112(19), 143(19), 159(19), *163;* 117(26), 121(26), *163;* 135(2), 136(2), 137(2), *162;* 143(42), 144(42), *163;* 242(65), 243(65), *253;* 244(66), 248(66), 251(66), *253;* 251(77), *258;* 254(4), 255(4), 275(4), 277(4), *301;* 408(16), *414*

Leung, M., 384(56), 385(56), *387*

Lilga, K. T., 66(18), *93;* 205(32), *252;* 212(35), *252;* 233(57), *253*

Livingston, R., 17(9), *56;* 344(41), *386*

Locher, P. R., 89(57), *94;* 89(58), *94*

Lohr, L. L., 89(60), *94*

Lowe, D. J., 409(19), 410(19), 411(19), *414;* 411(21), 412(21), *414*

Luckhurst, G. R., 138(36), 140(36), 141(36), *163*

Ludwig, G. W., 66(14), *93*

Lund, A., 184(19), 186(19), *252*

Lynden-Bell, R. M., 411(21), 412(21), *414*

Makhov, G., 23(13), 30(13), *57*

Maki, A. H., 66(21a), 74(21a), 75(21a), 89(21a), *93;* 96(1), *162;* 100(9), *163;* 103(10), 105(10), 144(10), 148(10), 149(10), *163;* 105(7), *163;* 107(17), 123(17), 132(17), *163;* 123(30), *163;* 135(7), *162*

Malmstrom, B. G., 32(23), *57;* 398(10), *414*

Margulis, T. N., 304(5), 311(5), *385*

Mayhew, S. G., 394(8), 395(8), *414*

Mc Calley, R. C., 30(18), *57;* 73(28), 89(28), *93;* 223(45), *253*

Mc Cann, V. H., 230(51), *253*

Mc Connell, H. M., 106(14), 201(14), *163;* 140(39), 151(39), *163;* 183(14), *252;* 270(17), *302*

Mc Dermed, J. D., 133(33), *163*

Mc Dowell, C. A., 66(22), 74(22), 75(22), *93;* 133(34), 135(34), *163;* 179(9), *252;* 232(55), *253;* 300(34), *302;* 369(53), *387*

Mc Irvine, E. C., 12(4), 19(4), *56;* 23(14), 25(14), 30(14), 31(14), *57;* 66(7), *93*

Mc Lachlan, A. D., 123(29), *163;* 145(45), *164;* 306(21), *386*

Mc Millan, N. D., 369(53), *387*

Mieher, R. L., 66(12), *93*

Mims, W. B., 354(47), *386*

Miyagawa, I., 30(20), *57;* 66(24), 74(24), 75(24), 89(24), *93;* 316(24), 318(24), 365(24), 366(24), 368(24), *386;* 316(25), 365(25), 366(25), *386;* 367(51), *387;* 369(53), *387*

Miyamae, T., 66(25), 74(25), *93*

Miyoshi, K., 89(46), *94*

Mobius, K., 66(23), 74(23), 75(23), 76(23), *93;* 107(17), 123(17), 132(17), *163;* 111(20), 123(20), *163;* 123(31), *163;* 135(3), *162;* 135(6), 137(6), *162;* 138(37), 139(37),

140(37), *163;* 138(38), 139(38), 141(38), 143(38), *163*
Monge, J. L., 54(24), *57;* 254(10), 255(10), 265(10), 274(10), 278(10), 279(10), *301;* 254(11), 255(11), 265(11), 279(11), 283(11), *301;* 305(12), *385;* 413(23), *414*
Moran, P. R., 53(32), *57;* 76(35), *94*
Mori, Y., 89(46), *94*
Morton, J. R., 106(15), *163;* 322(27), *386;* 322(28), *386;* 359(48), *387*
Mottley, C., 305(11), 318(11), 349(11), *385;* 305(14), 347(14), 357(14), 358(14), 359 (14), *386;* 369(53), *387;* 369(54), *387*
Mukai, K., 66(25), 74(25), *93;* 404(14), 405(14), 407(14), *414;* 404(15), 405(15), 407(15), *414*
Muller, F., 394(8), 395(8), *414*
Muus, L. T., 41(26), *57;* 334(40), *386*
Muto, H., 215(37), *252;* 217(38), *252;* 217 (39), *253;* 217(40), 218(40), *253*

Nash, F. R., 76(35), *94*
Nechtschein, M., 353(44), 355(44), *386*
Ngo, F. Q., 181(12), 182(12), *252;* 244(72), 246(72), *253*
Nordio, P. L., 270(17), *302*
Norris, J. R., 390(5), 402(5), 408(5), *414;* 402(12), 403(12), *414*
Nunome, K., 46(29), *57;* 217(38), *252;* 217 (39), *252;* 305(8), *385*

Ohigashi, H., 322(33), 347(33), 359(33), 361(33), *386*
Ohkura, H., 89(46), *94*
Orme-Johnson, W. H., 404(13), 405(13), 407(13), *414*

Pake, G. E., 274(31), *302*
Palmer, G., 404(13), 405(13), 407(13), *414*
Papez, R. J., 115(23), *163*
Pauling, L., 247(73), *253*
Pearson, G. A., 66(16), 89(16), *93;* 89(49), *94;* 230(49), *253*
Percival, P. W., 54(34), *57;* 254(11), 255 (11), 265(11), 279(11), 283(11), *301;* 305(12), *385*
Pershan, P. S., 388(2), *414*
Plato, M., 111(20), 123(20), *163;* 135(3), *162;* 135(6), 137(6), *162;* 138(38), 139 (38), 141(38), 143(38), *163*

Poindexter, E. H., 240(63), 244(63), 247(63), *253*
Poldy, F., 219(41), 222(41), *253;* 219(42), 221(42), 222(42), *253;* 222(43), *253*
Polnaszek, C. F., 270(19), *302;* 270(20), 271(20), *302*
Poole, C. P., Jr., 59(2), *92;* 61(2), *92;* 275 (33), *302;* 334(38), *386*
Poulis, N. J., 25(15), 30(15), *57*

Rabi, I. I., 12(5), *56*
Rakoed, A. I., 254(2), 255(2), 262(2), *301;* 254(7), 255(7), 265(7), 270(7), *301*
Ranon, U., 88(45), 92(45), *94*
Read, F. J., 183(17), 184(17), *252*
Rim, Y. S., 133(33), *163*
Rist, G. H., 46(28), *57;* 55(35), 56(35), *57;* 74(29), 75(29), 88(29), 89(29), *93;* 74 (30a), 88(30a), *93;* 74(31), 88(31), *93;* 88(40), *94;* 88(42), *94;* 107(16), *163;* 186(24), 201(24), *252;* 204(31), *252;* 234(59), 239(59), *253;* 237(61), *253;* 254(3), 255(3), 286(3), 292(3), 300(3), *301;* 305(15), 387(15), *386;* 389(3), 399(3), *414;* 411(22), 412(22), *414*
Rius, G., 353(43), 354(43), *386*
Robinson, B. H., 254(10), 255(10), 265(10), 274(10), 278(10), 279(10), *301;* 305(12), *385;* 413(23), *414*
Roder, R., 66(20), 67(20), 74(20), 89(20), *93*
Rogers, M. T., 305(7), 334(7), 336(7), 365 (7), *385;* 322(31), *386*
Rustgi, S. N., 186(23), 201(23), *252*

Salach, J., 396(9), *414*
Sands, R. H., 404(13), 405(13), 407(13), *414*
Sato, K., 66(25), 74(25), *93*
Scheer, H., 402(12), 403(12), *414*
Scheffler, K., 135(4), *162*
Schmalbein, D., 66(20), 67(20), 74(20), 89(20), *93*
Scholes, C. P., 390(6), 400(6), *414*
Schreurs, L. A. H., 25(15), 30(15), *57*
Schumacher, R. T., 66(13), *93*
Schwartz, R. N., 241(64), *253;* 244(69), 246(69), *253;* 244(70), 246(70), *253;* 244(71), *253;* 249(75), *253*
Schweiger, A., 204(31), *252*

Schwoerer, M., 225(46), *253;* 231(54), 232 (54), *253*

Seidel, H., 66(9), *93;* 144(44), *164;* 166(2), *252;* 171(4), *252*

Singer, T. P., 396(9), *414*

Slichter, C. P., 89(51), *94;* 143(43), *164*

Smigel, M. D., 254(8), 255(8), 270(8), 271(8), 272(8), *301;* 254(9), 255(9), 271(9), *301;* 271(26), *302;* 409(17), *414;* 409(18), 410(18), 413(18), *414*

Sneed, R. C., Jr., 55(35), 56(35), *57;* 76(36b), *94;* 88(42), *94;* 254(3), 255(3), 286(3), 292(3), 300(3), *301;* 305(15), 373(15), *386;* 318(26), *386;* 411(22), 412(22), *414*

Sokolov, E. A., 76(37), 84(37), *94;* 254(7), 255(7), 265(7), 270(7), *301;* 305(16), 380(16), 381(16), *386;* 305(17), 380(17), 382(17), 384(17), *386;* 305(18), 380(18), *386*

Sorokin, P. P., 76(35), *94;* 353(45), *386*

Spaeth, J. M., 186(25), *252*

Srinivasan, R., 179(9), *252;* 232(55), *253;* 388(1), *414*

Starr, M., 369(53), *387*

Steelink, C., 117(25), 120(25), *163*

Stegmann, H. B., 135(4), *162*

Steible, D. J., 322(34), 325(34), 357(34), *386*

Stone, T. J., 270(17), *302*

Strathdee, J., 140(39), 151(39), *163;* 183(14), 201(14), *252*

Stunzas, P. A., 76(37), 84(37), *94;* 254(2), 255(2), 262(2), *301;* 254(7), 255(7), 265(7), 270(7), *301;* 305(16), 380(16), 381(16), *386;* 305(17), 380(17), 382(17), 384(17), *386;* 305(18), 380(18), *386;* 305(19), 380(19), *386*

Sturm, M., 186(25), *252*

Sturner, D., 135(4), *162*

Swanenburg, T. J. B., 25(15), 30(15), *57*

Swann, J. C., 411(20), *414*

Tanaka, S., 76(35), *94*

Terhune, R. W., 23(13), 30(13), *57;* 23(14), 25(14), 30(14), 31(14), *57;* 66(7), *93*

Thomas, D. D., 54(34), *57*

Thuomas, K. A., 184(19), 186(19), *252*

Tinti, D. S., 384(55), 385(55), *387*

Tolles, W. M., 322(32), 347(32), 359(32), *386;* 322(34), 325(34), 357(34), *386*

Toriyama, K., 46(29), *57;* 305(8), *385*

Townes, C. H., 76(35), *94*

Trammell, G. T., 17(9), *56;* 344(41), *386*

Tsibris, J. C. M., 404(13), 405(13), 407(13), *414*

Tuttle, T. R., Jr., 274(31), *302*

Uebersfeld, J., 234(58), *253*

Unruh, W. P., 76(35), *93;* 354(46), *387*

Valenti, J. L., 322(32), 347(32), 359(32), *386*

Vanngard, T., 32(23), *57;* 74(30a),88(30a), *93;* 389 (3), 399(3), *414;* 398(10), *414*

Van Willigen, H., 107(17), 123(17), 132(17), *163;* 135(6), 137(6), *162*

Vedrine, J. C., 135(2), 136(2), 137(2), *162;* 242(65), 243(65), *253;* 244(66), 248(66), 251(66), *253;* 248(74), *253;* 250(76), *253;* 251(77), *253*

Vieth, H. M., 76(39), 84(39), 86(39), *84*

Wagner, B. E., 240(63), 244(63), 247(63), *253;* 254(5), 255(5), 275(5), *301*

Walker, W. H., 396(9), *414*

Wang, P. S., 56(36), *57;* 304(4), 311(4), 339(4), *385;* 305(13), 339(13), 341(13), *385*

Ward, R. L., 274(32), *302*

Watkins, G. D., 66(15), *93*

Weiner, R. F., 322(29), *386*

Weissman, S. I., 274(32), *302*

Wells, J. W., 199(27), 219(27), *252;* 201(30), *252;* 312(23), *386*

Wenckebach, W. Th., 25(15), 30(15), *57*

Wertz, J. E., 59(1), 62(1), *92;* 306(20), 310(20), *386*

Whiffen, D. H., 177(5), *252;* 178(6), *252;* 183(17), 184(17), *252;* 184(18), 186(18), *252;* 186(22), 201(22), *252;* 322(27), *386;* 359(48), *387;* 360(50), *387*

Wilkinson, B. A., Jr., 30(20), *57;* 66(24), 74(24), 75(24), 89(24), *93*

Wilmhurst, T. H., 59(3), *93*

Witte, A., 66(20), 67(20), 74(20), 89(20), *93*

Wolf, H. C., 66(17), *93;* 166(2), *252;* 209(33), *252;* 225(46), *253;* 225(47), 230(47), 231(47), *253;* 231(54), 232(54), *253*

Woodbury, H. H., 66(14), *93*

Woonton, G. A., 89(59), *94*

Yamamoto, T., 66(25), 74(25), *93*
Yoshida, H., 262(12), 263(12), *301;* 305(9), 378(9), 379(9), *385;* 305(10), *385*

Zeldes, H., 17(9), *56;* 344(41), *386*
Zimmermann, V., 225(46), *253;* 231(54), 232(54), *253*
Zoeller, J., 133(33), *163*

Subject Index

Page numbers in **boldface** indicate tables or figures. All compound and radical names have not been included; but see Table 3-4 (pp. 124-130) for liquid phase radicals studied by ENDOR, Table 4-4 (pp. 187-197) for solid phase radicals studied by ENDOR, and Table 4-13 (pp. 226-228) for triplets studied by ENDOR.

Adiabatic rapid passage, 54
Adrenodoxin, **404, 407,** 407
α-Aminoisobutyric acid, 312, **313, 315**
Anisotropic hyperfine interaction, 167
Anthracene triplet in phenazine crystals, 229
Arrhenius equation, 119
Attenuator, 63
Azotobacter vinelandii, 394, 395, 396

Bacteriochlorophyll, 403, 403, **403**
Benzophenone anion, 14
Bloch equations, 145
Bohr magneton, 2
Boltzmann factor, 3, 11
Bruker ENDOR spectrometer, 67

Capillary tube, 62
Cavity sensitivity Q, 61
$\dot{C}Cl_3$, 334, 336
$\cdot CClFCONH_2$, 334, 336, **337**
$CD_2H\dot{C}DR$, 366
$CD_3\dot{C}DR$, 366
$CD_3\dot{C}HR$, 366
$\dot{C}F_2CONH_2$, 321, **321**
$\dot{C}FHCONH_2$, 320, **321**
$\dot{C}H_2COO^-$, 322, **360**
$CH_2D\dot{C}R$, 366
$CH_3\dot{C}HCOOD$, 316
$CH_3\dot{C}HR$, **366**
$CHD_2\dot{C}HR$, 366
Chemical exchange, 19, 47, 274
Chlorine, 31
Coherence effects, 109, 110, 158, 159, 160, 161
Combination lines, 55
Conduction electrons, **27**
Copper picolinate, **237, 238**
Copper Tutton salts, 25
Coppinger's radical, 30, **97,** 110, **111, 159,** 159
 microwave field splitting, 159
 rf field splitting, **111**

Cross-relaxation, 13, 17, 19, 47
Cyclobutyl-1-carboxylic acid radical, 222
Cytidine, 178

ΔT_{1e} Mechanism, 13, 22, 23, 25
Density matrix method, 143, 144
 for ELDOR, 325
Depolarization ENDOR, **23,** 22
Deuteron distant ENDOR, **223**
Differential pulse technique, 97
Dimethylglyoxime radical pairs, **181**
2,5-dimethyl-p-benzosemiquinone radical anion, **113, 114**
Diphenylmethylene triplet, **231**
Dispersion mode ENDOR, 161
Distant ENDOR, 23, 24, 25, 26, 223, 224
 deuterated 1,1-cyclobutane-dicarboxylic acid, 223
 quadrupole coupling tensors, 223
 ruby, **24**
2,6-Di-t-butyl-4-cyclohexylphenoxy, 155, 157, **158**
Double ENDOR, 175, **176,** 178
DPPH, 67, 133, **134, 290, 291, 299,** 274, 275, 376, 377, 378
 powder ELDOR, **376, 377,** 274, 375, 376, 377, 378
Durosemiquinone, **115, 116**

ELDOR, allowed-allowed transition, 36, 44
 applications to oriented radicals, 357-369
 cavity, 77, **78, 79,** 81, **85**
 energy levels, 35
 equivalent electrical circuit, 40
 experimental aspects, 86-92
 forbidden-allowed transition, 37, 46
 forbidden-forbidden transition, 46
 linewidths, 49, 55
 observed transition, 36
 pumped transition, 36
 reduction factor equations, **48**
 resolution, 55
 signal display, **84**

spectral presentation, 82
spectrometer, **77**
ELDOR lineshape, 55, **288**
  effect of field modulation, 55
  effect of large hyperfine splittings, 56
  effect of transverse relaxation time, 55
Electron-nuclear dipolar modulation (END), 43, 150-157, 268, 269
Electronic structure, 122, 123, 132
  conformational study, 132
  galvinoxyls, 122
  ground state orbital degeneracy, 123
  pentaphenylcyclopentadienyl, 123
  phenoxy, 122
  rubrene, 122
  semiquinones, 122
  substituted triphenylmethyl, 122
  tetracene, 122
ENDOR, 12, 26, 31, 168, 171, **173**, 175, 183-185, **200**, **202**, **203**
  Al, 30
  cavity, **69**, 70, **71**, **72**
  copper Tutton salt, 30
  depolarization, 31
  disordered solids, 233
  dispersion signal, 31
  enhancements, 21
  inorganic crystals, 232, 233
  instrumental aspects, 72-90
  Li, 26
  line intensities, 149
  ^{31}P nuclei, 12
  radical pairs, 180
  resolution, 32
  spectrometer, 64, **65**, **66**, **68**
  transitions, 8
ENDOR enhancement, 150
ENDOR-induced ESR, 97, 112, 115, 116, 199, 221
Energy level diagram, 3, 5, 7, 8, 36, 185, 220, 257, 371, 379
  cross-relaxation, 379
  ELDOR, 36
  quadrupole coupling, **185**
  tunneling splitting, **371**
Enhancement of rf field, 28
ESR spectrometer, 64
Excitons in crystals, 381-384

F center, **34**, 53, 171, **173**, 174

Ferredoxins, 405
Field frequency lock, 73
Field swept ELDOR, 50, 185, 199, 256-258, 261, 266-275
  effect of molecular motion, 266-273
  identification of pumped and observed transitions, 257
  lineshapes, 278
  method for obtaining, 257, 258
  microwave power dependence, 262
  reduction factors, 278-285
  saturation transfer by ELDOR, 272
  temperature and concentration variations, 260, 261
  theoretical relationship, 262, 263, 264
Flat cell, 62
Flavoproteins, 390-397, **395**
Fluorine hyperfine splittings, **320**
FMN, **391**
Forbidden-allowed ELDOR lines, **346**
Forbidden ESR transitions, 17
Frequency swept ELDOR spectra, 53, 285-298
  absorption ELDOR, **289**
  dispersion ELDOR signal, 288, **289**
  hyperfine lines and combination lines, 285, 290, 292, 294, 295
  lineshapes, 286-287
  trapped electron, 53

Galvinoxyl radical, 154
Glycine radicals, **350**, **361**, **368**

H_1 dependence of ENDOR response, 145
H_2 dependence of ENDOR response, 146
H-bonded protons, 217
1H, 1H-Heptafluor-1-butanol, **241**
Hall Probe feedback loop, 67
Heisenberg exchange, 19, 47, 271, 273-275
Hemin, **401**, 401
Hemoglobin, **400**
High power ENDOR, 66
  continuous wave, 66
  pulsed, 66
Homogeneous spin packet, 21
α-Hydronaphthyl, 209, 210
17β-Hydroxyl-4′,4′-dimethylspiro[5α-androstane-3,2′-oxazolidin] 3′-oxyl, **273**

SUBJECT INDEX 425

Inhomogeneously broadened, 21
Intramolecular motion, 117, 218
Iris, 63
Iron sulfur proteins, **406**
Isotropic hyperfine modulation, 154

JEOL ENDOR spectrometer, 66, 88

Klystron, 63

L-alanine, 215, **216, 317, 319**
Lattice-induced nuclear spin-flip, 42
L-cysteic acid monohydrate, 213, **214**
Li ENDOR, 27
Line intensity (ENDOR), 106
Line-shift mechanism, 26, 31
Liquid crystal solvents, 137, 138
Longitudinal relaxation time, T_1, 5
Lumiflavins, **391, 392**

McLachlan perturbation, 123
Magnetic field homogeneity, 72
Magnetic susceptability, 50
Magnetogyric ratio of electron, 2
Malonic acid radicals, 46, **324,** 324-326
Matrix ENDOR, 26, 239-249, **245,** 249
  anisotropic interaction, 241
  electron radii, **245**
  isotropic interaction, 241
  lineshape, 242, 243
  linewidths, **245**
  trapped hydrogen atom, 249, **249**
Matrix proton tensors, **203**
Mechanisms of radical formation, 210-218
  cations and anions, 211
  electron transfer reaction, 212, 213
  glycine HCl, 210
  hydrogen abstraction, 212
  proton transfer, 212-214, 218
  proton transfer to a carboxyl anion, 215
4-Methyl-2,6-di-t-butylphenoxy radical, 222
Methyl group tunneling, 218
Methyl-malonic acid crystal, **370**
Metmyoglobin, **401**
Microwave cavity, **60, 61**
Microwave filter, 83
Microwave frequency stability, 73
Microwave helix, 61, 63
Microwave modes, 86
Modulation amplitude, 54

Modulation frequency dependence, 53, 54, 64, 347-349
Molecular motion, ELDOR studies of, 266-271
MTHF radical, 379

N-acetylglycine, 205, 206
NADPH dehydrogenase, **393,** 393, 394
$ND_2H^+CH\dot{C}OO^-$, **368,** 368
Negative ENDOR, 30, **30,** 31
N-galvinoxyl radical, 112
$NH_3^+\dot{C}HCOO^-$, 318
Nicotinamide adenine dinucleotide phosphate (NADPH) dehydrogenase, 390
Nitrogen ENDOR, 135-137, 212
Nitroxide radical, 256, 299
4-N-maleimido-2,2,6,6-tetramethylpiperidine nitroxide radical, 259, 260, **261, 263, 264,** 265, 299
NMR gaussmeter, 73
Nonadiabatic spin exchange, 322
Nuclear frequencies, 9
Nuclear magneton, 6
Nuclear polarization, 24, **25,** 25
  forbidden transitions, 24
  saturation, 24
  of the allowed ESR transitions, 25
Nuclear saturation, 28
Nuclear spin, 24
Nuclear spin transition W_n, 47
Nuclear Zeeman term, 8

Optical detection in polycrystalline matrices, 384
Ordering parameter, 140
Organic single crystal ELDOR, 306-308, **309,** 311, 321-323, 325, 327, 336-347
  chlorine quadrupole interaction, 334-339
  deuterium hyperfine splittings, 339, 340
  ELDOR spin-flip transitions, 343-345
  first order ELDOR transitions, **309**
  hyperfine splitting anisotropy, 319-322
  intermolecular spin diffusion, 349-352
  interpretation, 306, 307
  intramolecular admixture of nuclear spin states-forbidden lines, 326-334
  intramolecular motion-methyl group, 311-316
  modulation frequency dependence, 347-349

overlapped lines, 351
proton spin exchange, 322-326
α-protons in presence of methyl protons, 316-318
resolution of small hyperfine splittings, 341-343
second order corrections, 309-311
temperature dependence for $NH_3^+ \dot{C}HCOO^-$, 319
temperature dependence of R for α protons, 317, 318
torsional oscillation, 321
tunneling methyl groups, 369-373
1-Oxyl-2,2,6,6-tetramethyl-4-hydroxypiperidine (*tanol*), **142**, 142

Packet-shifting ENDOR, 21, 23
Peptostreptococcus elsdenii, 394
Peroxylamine disulfonate dianion radicals (PADS), 274
Phase sensitive detector, 62
1-Phenylnaphthalene anion, **112**
rf field splitting, **112**
Phosphorus-doped silicon, 12, **12**, 13, 19, 20, **15**, **15**, 31
Population diagram, **10**, **13**, **16**, **18**, **20**, **25**, **38**, **44**, **45**
modulation of the hyperfine anisotropy, **44**
nuclear polarization, **25**
spin exchange, **18**
steady state ELDOR, **44**, **45**
transient ELDOR, **38**
T_{x1}, **44**
T_{x2}, **44**
Positive ENDOR, 29
Potassium ENDOR, 31
Potassium hydrogen maleate (KHM), 46, 327, **332**
Powder ELDOR, 373-378
Proton ENDOR, 98-101
line intensities, **104**
line overlap correction, 105
Proton hyperfine tensors, 199-204
α-Proton tensors, **200**
β-Proton tensors, **202**
Pulsed ELDOR, 353-355

Q of cavity, 61
Quadrupole coupling constants, 140, 141, 186

Quadrupole relaxation, 56

Raman scattering, 18
Reduction factor, 41, 276, 277
Relaxation paths, 14, 15, 16, 43, 47, 53
ENDOR, 14-17
isotropic hyperfine modulation, 43
T_{x1}, 15
W_n, W_{x1}, W_{x2}, W_e, 53
Relaxation times, 4
Resolution in solids, 34, 56
RF coherence effects, 109, 110, 158-161
double quantum transition, 161
ESR line splitting, 160
splitting of NMR line, 159
RF enhancement, 28, **28**, 29
RF power, 74, 75
Riboflavin, **391**
Riboflavin radical cation, **397**
Rotational diffusion, 54, 155
Ruby (0.01% Cr^{+3} in Al_2O_3) ENDOR, 25

Sample size, 73, 74
Saturation parameter, 50
Second order effects, 183
Selena-adrenodoxin, **407**
Selenium ENDOR, 407
Separation of overlapping ESR spectra, 298, 299
Sign of isotropic coupling constants, 139
Spectral density, 31, 32
Spectral diffusion, 47, 271
Spectral resolution enhancement, 33
Spin density determination, 181
anisotropic coupling, 182
ring atoms, **182**
Spin diffusion, 52, 350, 378
Spin exchange, 18, 19, 47, 117
Spin Hamiltonian, 6, 167, 184
quadrupole interaction, 184
Spin-lattice relaxation, rate, W_e, 4
time, T_{1e}, 4
Spin packet, 21, **22**, 22, 52, 53
Spin-spin relaxation, time T_{2e}, 4
Steady State ELDOR, 39, **40**
electrical circuit analog, **40**
Steady State ENDOR, **13**, **16**, 39
mechanisms, 39
Stochastic Liouville method, 270, 279

T_{1n}, 4
T_{2n}, 4
Tanol, 289
Tanone, 135
1,3,6,8-Tetra-*t*-butylcarbazyl radical, 235, 236
Tetracyanquinodimethane salt (TCNQ), 381, 383
2,2,6,6-Tetramethyl-4-pyrolidinol-1-oxyl, 272, 283, 284
Thevin's theorem, 41
(*p*-Toly)diphenylmethyl radical, 97
Transient ELDOR, 38, 39, 355, **356**
Transient ENDOR, 10, **10**, 11, 13, 178
Transition probability matrices, 41
Transverse relaxation time, T_2, 5
Trapped electrons, **50, 51, 52,** 380
 ELDOR, **50, 51, 52,** 380
Traveling wave helix, 84
1,2,4-Triazole, 207, **208**
1,3,4-Trimethylpentaphenylcyclopentadienyl radical, **107**
Triphenylmethyl radical, **33, 118,** 233
 intramolecular motion, 119, 120
Triphenylphenoxy radicals, **108**

Stokes-Einstein relation, 267, 271, 274
Succinate dehydrogenase flavin radical cation, **397**
Succinic acid radical, **177,** 183
 double ENDOR, 177
 relative hyperfine constant sign, 177

Triplet fluorene spectrum, 225, **229,** 232
Triplet state ENDOR, 224, **225,** 229-231
 anthracene triplet in phenazine crystals, 229
 diphenylmethylene, 230
 ENDOR transitions, **225**
 fluorenylidene, 230
 matrix proton ENDOR, 231
 nonplanarity, 231
 proton hyperfine tensor measurement, 229
 spin Hamiltonian, 224
Triplet states by ELDOR, 380
Tri-t-butylphenoxy radical, **102, 140**
Tri-tolymethyl radical, **106, 240**
Tunneling rotation of methyl groups, **220,** 221, 369
Tunneling sidebands, 372
Tunneling splitting, 370
Twinned crystals, 199

Ubisemiquinone anion, **121**

Valine, 211
Varian ELDOR spectrometer, 76
Varian ENDOR spectrometer, 67, 69
Vitamin E (α-tocopherol quinone), 408
Vitamin K_1 (phytonodione), 408
Vitamin K_3 (menadione), 408

Xanthine oxidase, **412, 413**

Zeolite, **250,** 251